8/19.95

TEXTBOOK OF

RADIOLOGIC TECHNOLOGY

TEXTBOOK OF
RADIOLOGIC TECHNOLOGY

CHARLES A. JACOBI, B.Sc., F.N.C.R.T. (A.R.C.R.T.), R.T. (A.R.R.T.), M.T. (A.S.C.P.)

Professor and Chairman, Department of Radiologic Technology,
College of Allied Health Professions, University of Nevada, Las Vegas;
Director of Education and Chairman, Education Committee,
American Registry of Clinical Radiography Technologists;
formerly Member, Radiological Safety Board, University of Nevada System;
Member, Health Sciences Preprofessional Committee, University of Nevada,
Las Vegas; Assistant Professor and Chairman, Medical Radiologic Technology;
Member, Radioisotopes Committee, Oregon Institute of Technology,
Klamath Falls, Oregon

DON Q PARIS, B.Sc., R.T. (A.R.R.T.)

Chairman, Department of Radiologic Technology, College of Public and
Environmental Services, Northern Arizona University, Flagstaff, Arizona;
formerly Director, Health Sciences Division, Pima Community College,
Tucson, Arizona

SIXTH EDITION

with 654 *illustrations including* 1 *full-color plate*

THE C. V. MOSBY COMPANY

Saint Louis 1977

SIXTH EDITION

Printed in the United States of America

Distributed in Great Britain by Henry Kimpton, London

The C. V. Mosby Company
11830 Westline Industrial Drive, St. Louis, Missouri 63141

Library of Congress Cataloging in Publication Data

Jacobi, Charles A
Textbook of radiologic technology.

First-3d ed. published under title: X-ray technology.
Bibliography: p.
Includes index.
1. Radiography, Medical. 2. Nuclear medicine.
I. Paris, Don Q, joint author. II. Title. [DNLM:
1. Technology, Radiologic. WN160 J16x]
RC78.J18 1977 616.07′57 76-41715
ISBN 0-8016-2385-5

VH/VH/VH 9 8 7 6 5 4 3 2 1

To students of

RADIOLOGIC TECHNOLOGY

PREFACE

A new edition of a standard textbook must be as up to date as possible. We willingly listen to comments from our colleagues, professional peers, alumni, and current students; and at University of Nevada, Las Vegas, the comments of our "student-teachers" are considered very valuable.

Both additions and deletions are found in Chapters 1, 2, and 3. Chapter 4 has been completely revised. Chapter 5 contains many additions. Many new illustrations are found throughout the entire textbook.

Many of our alumni reward us and themselves with notable contributions to our profession. From among these individuals we have called on Jack D. Stevens, R.T., for a major contribution in Chapter 4. We are most grateful to him and to E. I. DuPont Company for that material and permission to use it.

We wish also to acknowledge our appreciation to many other persons, companies, and hospitals that have aided in this production. Especially we express our thanks to Mr. Danny Dehlinger, Manager, Siemens Medical, Phoenix, Arizona, and Mr. Irven L. Rule, Product Specialist of Siemens Corporation, Torrance, California, for their considerable assistance and advice for the changes in Chapters 2 and 3. We are most appreciative of the assistance and advice given us by Dr. William S. Properzio, Assistant Director for X-ray programs, Division of Training and Medical Applications, Bureau of Radiological Health; Dr. Gregory J. Barone, Chief, X-ray Products Branch, Division of Compliance, Bureau of Radiological Health; and Mr. Thomas C. Sell, Office of Radiation Programs, Las Vegas Facility, Environmental Protection Agency.

We gratefully acknowledge the assistance given to us by and the privilege of using radiographs from Dr. Paul D. Bandt, and Ramon B. Pence, R.T., Southern Nevada Memorial Hospital, Las Vegas, Nevada; Dr. John I. Pretto, Chief of Radiology, Sunrise Hospital, Las Vegas, Nevada; Dr. Frank S. Cavallero, and Richard Fucillo, R.T., Valley Hospital Limited, Las Vegas, Nevada; Department of Radiology, Flagstaff Community Hospital, Flagstaff, Arizona; and Department of Radiology, Scottsdale Memorial Hospital, Scottsdale, Arizona.

Mr. James F. Trantham, Las Vegas, Nevada, made some technical drawings, and we thank him for his efforts. Mr. John Goad, photographer in the Audio-Visual Department of University of Nevada, Las Vegas, and Mr. John Dellinger, student photographer at Northern Arizona University, Flagstaff, Arizona, produced numerous radiograph photographs for us, and we deeply appreciate their efforts. Much of the extensive photographic contribution to the last edition by Daniel P. Giaquinto, R.T., Program of Radiologic Technology, Pima Community College, Tucson, has been retained with appreciation.

Professors Ray E. Goldsworthy, Hiram M. Hunt, and Duane T. Pierce of the Department of Radiologic Technology, University of Nevada, Las Vegas, gave valuable assistance and advice in many ways; for this we are deeply appreciative.

Above all, we give credit to our wives for their continued calming influence and extensive assistance in so many ways not possible to describe; without this steadying influence at home we could not accomplish the task.

Charles A. Jacobi
Don Q Paris

CONTENTS

COLOR PLATE

TEXTBOOK OF
RADIOLOGIC TECHNOLOGY

1 • INTRODUCTION TO RADIOGRAPHY

As a cluster, health-related sciences and corresponding allied health professions represent a rapidly increasing employment field. In conjunction with this growth go advances in sophistication of equipment and techniques of application, all of which require understanding and consequent improved use of technical terminology. Certainly, one allied health profession, radiologic (radiography) technology, qualifies in this category.

Those persons electing to enter a program of study and associated clinical experience leading toward professional competence and growth in radiologic and radiography technology exhibit great need for appreciation and understanding of its scope and interrelations for eventual success in achieving the primary goal of improved patient care.

Radiographic exposure is but one of the several functions of both radiography and radiologic technologists. Radiography is the making of a record or photograph by means of the action of actinic* rays (x rays) on a sensitized surface, and a radiograph, or radiogram, is a film or other record so produced. Stated differently: *a radiograph is a permanent photographic record of the structures through which a beam of ionizing radiation has passed.*

ALLIED HEALTH PROFESSIONS AND MEDICAL SPECIALTIES

Both radiography and radiologic technologists must be expert in the performance of technical procedures requiring the use of x rays. In addition, radiologic technologists possess limited expertise in performance of technical procedures requiring the use of radioisotopes. Growth of the separate, recognized disciplines of nuclear medicine technology and radiation therapy technology permits both radiography and radiologic technologists to concentrate on and develop greater skills in diagnostic radiographic procedures. All these preceding applications of ionizing radiations are ordered by and conducted under supervision of qualified, licensed medical and osteopathic physicians, dentists, and veterinarians. These technologists must perform the medical requests with maximum protection against the possible effects of ionizing radiations both to the patients and to themselves, and may be employed by any of these professional persons or by a hospital or clinic.

Another allied health specialty is medical laboratory technology. A medical laboratory technologist is a person trained to be expert in the performance of technical procedures in the clinical laboratory that require the use of a variety of instruments and that are performed under the supervision of qualified, licensed medical and osteopathic physicians, dentists, and veterinarians. For the most part both radiography and radiologic technologists work directly with radiologists and roentgenologists, and the medical laboratory technologist works directly with pathologists; however, this is not without exception.

Other allied health professional personnel with whom radiography and radiologic technologists perform on the *medical team* include physical therapists, nurses, and pharmacists.

Our discussion of purely professional persons will be restricted to medical (physicians) doctors, since the organizational structure of the allied health profession of radiologic technology is so closely allied to this profession.

Medical doctors are graduates of medical schools. To enter medical school, one must have completed required premedicine course-work, but may or may not have a baccalaureate degree in premedicine. Following graduation from medical school, the medical doctor must spend a period (usually 12 months) of *internship* in an AMA-approved hospital, that is, a hospital approved by the Council on Medical Education of the American Medical Association (AMA) for medical internship. Upon satisfactory completion of the internship, the medical doctor must successfully write examinations required by the State Board of Medical Examiners in states in which he may wish to practice medicine.

If this new medical doctor, or one who has been in medical practice, desires to *specialize* in one field of medical practice, he will enter a *residency* for a specified number of years in a par-

*See Glossary.

ticular AMA-approved hospital. Upon the successful completion of his residency, the doctor will write a prescribed number of *medical specialty board examinations*. Successful performance with the board examinations entitles this doctor to practice his medical specialty in any state in which he holds a license.

Both roentgenologists and radiologists, then—with whom radiologic technologists often work closely—have completed a baccalaureate degree in premedicine (prior to or concurrent with medical studies), a graduate degree (M.D.) in medicine, 1-year internship, and a 3-year residency: approximately 11 or 12 years of intensive study and practice (internship and residency) under strict supervision of skilled and experienced medical doctors.

Medical specialties differ in their requirements as to residency time period; otherwise, their requirements are very similar.

In alphabetical order the medical specialties are as follows:

AM Aerospace Medicine
A Allergy
AN Anesthesiology
BE Broncho-Esophagology
CD Cardiovascular Diseases
D Dermatology
DIA Diabetes
EM Emergency Medicine
END Endocrinology
FP Family Practice
GE Gastroenterology
GP General Practice
GPM General Preventive Medicine
GER Geriatrics
GYN Gynecology
HEM Hematology
HYP Hypnosis
ID Infectious Diseases
IM Internal Medicine
LAR Laryngology
LM Legal Medicine
ND Neoplastic Diseases
NEP Nephrology
N Neurology
CHN Neurology, Child
NA Neuropathology
NM Nuclear Medicine
NTR Nutrition
OBS Obstetrics
OBG Obstetrics and Gynecology
OM Occupational Medicine
OPH Ophthalmology
OT Otology
OTO Otorhinolaryngology
PTH Pathology
CLP Pathology, Clinical
FOP Pathology, Forensic
PD Pediatrics
PDA Pediatrics, Allergy
PDC Pediatrics, Cardiology
PA Pharmacology, Clinical
PM Physical Medicine and Rehabilitation
P Psychiatry
CHP Psychiatry, Child
PYA Psychoanalysis
PYM Psychosomatic Medicine
PH Public Health
PUD Pulmonary Diseases
R Radiology
DR Radiology, Diagnostic
PDR Radiology, Pediatric
TR Radiology, Therapeutic
RHU Rheumatology
RHI Rhinology
ABS Surgery, Abdominal
CDS Surgery, Cardiovascular
CRS Surgery, Colon and Rectal
GS Surgery, General
HS Surgery, Hand
HNS Surgery, Head and Neck
NS Surgery, Neurological
ORS Surgery, Orthopedic
PDS Surgery, Pediatrics
PS Surgery, Plastic
TS Surgery, Thoracic
TRS Surgery, Traumatic
U Surgery, Urological
OS Other Specialty
US Unspecified

A radiologist is a physician with special experience in radiology. Radiology is the science of radiant energy and radiant substances, especially that branch of medical science that deals with the use of radiant energy in the diagnosis and treatment of disease.

Roentgenology is the branch of radiology that deals with the diagnostic and therapeutic use of roentgen rays. A roentgenologist is a physician who devotes himself to diagnosis and treatment by the roentgen rays (x rays).

The other medical specialists and the general practitioners of medicine are the medical doctors for whom the radiologic technologists perform their skills and professional arts.

RADIOLOGIC TECHNOLOGY

History

While experimenting with cathode rays generated in a Crooke's tube, Dr. W. C. Roentgen discovered a "new kind of ray" on November 8, 1895. He called it x ray since it was, at that time, an unknown form of energy. Since Dr. Roentgen's death, consideration has been given to naming these rays roentgen rays in his honor; hence, we find both *x rays* and *roentgen rays* referring to the same energy form.

From this great discovery, given freely to the world by Dr. Roentgen, many medical and industrial applications have grown. Among these is the *science of radiology,* defined as the science of radioactive substances and x rays. However, the discovery of x rays preceded the discovery of radioactivity (see p. 127), and the first radiographic exposures used in medical diagnosis were made with x rays. For the sake of consistency, we must realize that radiography technology preceded radiologic technology (see p. 3).

Near the beginning of the twentieth century many physicians were using x rays in medical practice. As the use of x rays increased, the physicians began to train medical assistants in the techniques of x-ray applications. This resulted in an increasing number of partially trained medical assistants applying ionizing radiations to patients and obtaining varying qualities of radiographs (skiagrams).

When Roentgen's discovery was made public, the application of electric currents in medical practice was receiving considerable attention. Ed C. Jerman, a talented electrician, was engaged with his father, a middle western physician, in this effort. With the release of information pertaining to the production of x rays, Ed Jerman sought to assemble the necessary apparatus to produce x rays. He became experienced in the operation of early x-ray machines and became well known in his own right to the medical profession and to the manufacturers of x-ray equipment; he is credited with starting the allied health profession of x-ray (radiography) technology in 1896.

Because of his knowledge of x-ray machines and the techniques of radiography, Ed Jerman received requests from equipment manufacturers to conduct schools for physicians' assistants; these were in the northern United States and in southern Canada around the Great Lakes. Thus, early in the twentieth century, Ed Jerman became the first professional teacher of *radiography technology* in North America.

Mr. Jerman's driving enthusiasm, skill, and personality stimulated his students to want additional educational opportunities; their common desire caused these persons to gather for educational discussions. These meetings, conducted by Mr. Jerman, led to the formation of the American Association of Radiological Technicians on October 25, 1920. A second meeting was conducted by Mr. Jerman, as President, on June 27, 1921.

During its formative years this Association pressed for the setting of standards, and by joint committee action of the Radiological Society of North America and the American Roentgen Ray Society, a Registry for the purpose of certifying x-ray technicians was established on November 18, 1922. The original Registry Board was composed of both radiologists and technicians, representing their societies.

In 1925 membership in the American Association of Radiological Technicians was restricted to Registered Technicians.

The Second Annual Meeting was conducted in Chicago in April, 1927, after a reorganizational meeting in 1926. During the next several meetings, emphasis was given to improving educational standards and to the establishment of an official journal, *The X-ray Technician.* Annual meetings, now called conventions, have been conducted each year since 1927.

In 1932 it was decided to change the name of the Association to The American Society of X-ray Technicians; this change went into effect in 1934. Also in 1932, the Registry was first called The American Registry of X-ray Technicians.

The American College of Radiology and The American Society of X-ray Technicians became the official co-sponsors of The American Registry of X-ray Technicians on May 6, 1943. In 1945 the Council on Medical Education and Hospitals of the American Medical Association accepted the responsibility of inspecting and approving training schools for x-ray technicians.

Continuous *upgrading* of the profession of radiologic technology through increased and expanded educational requirements is a mark of our progress. The inclusion of academic courses is now an integral part of most training programs.

Continuous progress and expansion is seen in other facets of our allied health profession. During the Annual Convention in 1962 certain name changes were approved and adopted. The American Registry of X-ray Technicians is now The American Registry of Radiologic Technologists (ARRT), with offices in Minneapolis, Minnesota, and The American Society of X-ray Technicians is now The American Society of Radiologic Technologists (ASRT) with offices in Chicago, Illinois. The journal, *The X-ray Technician,* is now called *Radiologic Technology.* These changes in nomenclature indicate the expansion of our knowledge and performance to include the uses of radioactive isotopes.

Upon becoming registered with the ARRT, it is possible to pursue additional studies and training in either of two *specialty fields* and to write the examinations to be certified as either a *Nuclear Medicine Technologist* or a *Radiation Therapy Technologist*.

A combined certifying body and professional society governed solely by the technologist members was formed in 1955. This organization, the American Registry of Clinical Radiography Technologists (ARCRT), concerns itself with the education and certification of diagnostic (radiography) technologists. Until August, 1975, the office was in Enid, Oklahoma. Numerous organizational changes commenced in 1969 and were finalized in August, 1975. The Administrative Office of ARCRT was moved to Oklahoma City, Oklahoma; the Office of Education was moved to Las Vegas, Nevada; the Office of the Examiner was moved to Harrisonville, Missouri. In addition to these two Registries and Societies a few states (at time of writing these were California, New York, and New Jersey) have licensure laws for radiologic technologists and several other states are currently considering licensure of radiologic technologists.

The primary goals of improving patient care and of effecting diagnostic dose reduction through improved and expanded professional growth are common to the personnel of ARRT, ASRT, ARCRT and the licensure states; many of these persons are members of both ASRT and ARCRT, and are registered and/or certified by ARRT, ARCRT, and a licensure state. Many methods of achieving these goals have been introduced, a very recent one being an organization named WICERT (Western Intercollegiate Consortium on Education in Radiologic Technology [in college-based programs]). This was formed in January, 1975, by representatives of seventeen college-based programs in eight western states. It strives to raise teacher qualifications, curriculum standards, and student experiences. The ARCRT certifies instructors in its approved schools, and the ASRT Board of Directors has recommended to the Joint Review Committee (see its composition in a succeeding paragraph) that there be minimum qualifications for instructors and program directors teaching in schools approved by the Council on Medical Education of the American Medical Association. Both ASRT and ARCRT provide continuing education programs for radiologic technologists.

Education

In the beginnings of this profession there was very little education, and essentially no formal education. Most learning was achieved by the students from direct "on-the-job" instruction. Later, semiformal classes were introduced in larger hospitals and were conducted when the patient load permitted.

Formal hospital schools of 12 months appeared in the 1930s and continued into the 1950s. In this time period the requirement for eligibility to write either Registry examination increased to graduation from nothing other than an "approved 24-month school," still hospital based. In September, 1952, the first college-based school of Radiologic Technology was introduced at Oregon Technical Institute (now Oregon Institute of Technology), Klamath Falls, Oregon. This developed into a 30-month program; the first two academic years (18 months) are spent in the classrooms and "live" laboratories, followed by 12 months of continuous clinical experience in an affiliated hospital that meets specific requirements of the Joint Review Committee (JRC) of ACR (American College of Radiology) and ASRT members.

Numerous similar college-based 24- to 36-month programs "sprang up" over the nation in the next two decades. In the 1960s a few colleges and universities developed baccalaureate programs leading to eligibility to write the Registry examinations. In 1967 the first 2+2 program was developed by the Department of Radiologic Technology of University of Nevada, Las Vegas. This program permitted students to matriculate and graduate with an AS degree and write the Registry examination in a period of 28 months. Also, non-college, Registered Radiologic Technologists could, after admission to the University, challenge the "lower division" (radiologic technology) course work and pursue studies leading to a baccalaureate degree in one of six areas of related interest.* These "upper division options" serve the student of radiologic technology much as would a master's degree following a baccalaureate degree in other disciplines. Further experimentation continues in a number of colleges and universities (e.g., Northern Arizona University in Flagstaff, and Weber State College in Ogden, Utah) to find better methods of preparing students of radiography and radiologic technology for better futures and to enable them to deliver better patient care. The course material and clinical experience in each college-based pro-

*For information regarding these offerings, the reader should write to Department of Radiologic Technology, University of Nevada, Las Vagas, Las Vegas, Nevada 89154.

gram is presented somewhat differently; thus each college-based program is properly considered to be experimenting with different approaches to learning for the same purposes.

Graduates of JRC-approved schools (both hospital and college-based) are eligible to apply for and write the examination of the ARRT; successful examinees are authorized to use the initials, R.T. following their names. These initials stand for Registered Technologist and the parenthetical indication of x ray, radiation therapy, or nuclear medicine follows the initials. (Radiation therapy and/or nuclear medicine certification require specific, additional education and experience.) Effective July 1, 1976, ARCRT approved both hospital- and college-based schools, and initiated the policy of differential certification for successful examinees of these programs (schools). The examinations for graduates of college-based programs are appropriately more comprehensive in nature and of greater difficulty than the examinations of hospital programs (schools).*

ETHICS

Ethics relates to the mode of conduct and behavior. A pattern of proper and ethical conduct *at all times* is essential in those who intend to practice any profession. The ethical practices of the profession of radiologic technology are of such broad scope as to make it necessary for those persons engaged in this profession to consider carefully all of their actions and performances both on and off duty.

It is absolutely essential that all allied health personnel and the associated support personnel in the hospitals and clinics appreciate and understand that **patient care has first priority!** If there were no patients, we would be unemployed! In our necessary and very personal associations with each patient, we must always prevent unnecessary discomfort, and treat each one as if he/she is our only concern. Use a kind voice, and always explain carefully what is to be done, being certain the patient understands. Be firm when necessary, but never act rude or sound irritable.

The patient quite naturally exhibits some anxiety during radiographic procedures. Make him/her as comfortable as is possible and consistent with the examination at hand. Although these procedures are quite commonplace to the technologist, they are usually equally strange to the patient. Exhibition of self-confidence and assurance tends to establish a feeling of trust within the patient. During the radiographic exposure(s) be certain that **all radiation protection possible is afforded** to both the patient and the technologist!

A major part of the impression (of the technologist) gained by his/her associates in the department and elsewhere derives from cleanliness, personal habits, neatness, politeness, and punctuality. Each technologist, both new-on-the-job and seasoned veteran, needs to practice these attributes.

The use of fresh linens and proper cleansing of the radiographic table and the cassettes are obvious requirements. When permitted, additional cover for warmth should be applied on both the radiographic table and the stretcher. Constant observation for and preventive measures against shock are required.

In the almost constant associations with other members of different disciplines in allied health we expect respect for our knowledge and experience, and we must show the same respect for the knowledge and experience of our associates. Do not use first names, especially before patients; *always use the professional title* in addressing members of the medical and osteopathic professions and the senior members in your own and other departments.

Discretion with professional information is an absolute must. Information regarding any patient must never be divulged in any manner. Tact and studied statements are an attribute of each successful technologist.

Refusal of radiographic information to both patient and family must be achieved in a manner that precludes antagonism. Divulging any information regarding radiographic interpretation or results is a distinct violation of professional ethics and subjects the violator to severe reprimand.

Knowledge of the economics of the practice of radiology and hospital operation is important to both the employee and the employer. It is of the utmost importance to the employee, since this knowledge will serve to enlighten him about the many facets contributing to the successful operation of the establishment. One cannot evaluate profit by the expedient of comparing film and solution costs with salary. The responsible technologist will investigate new methods that may make the total operation economically more sound. Rea-

*For information regarding Registry examinations and approved schools the reader should write to ARCRT, Suite 400, 2501 N. Stiles, Oklahoma City, Oklahoma 73105 and/or ARRT, 2600 Wayzata Blvd., Minneapolis, Minnesota 55405.

sonable suggestions for improvement are always in order.

Hospitals are, statistically, one of the larger businesses in the United States. A radiologic department is one of the major expenditures in a hospital; properly operated, it is one of the major contributors toward successful operation of the organization.

Courtesy, cooperation, and communication, the three C's of modern medical precept, are the summation of effort in all departments. When each of these items becomes an integral part of the routine of the technologist, he will begin to practice professional ethics.

Ethical activities

The technologist's obligations in his work

The work of the radiologic technologist and of his department is indispensable to the practice of medicine in all its branches. A well-executed radiograph is necessary to the establishment or ruling out of a diagnosis of pathology. In these days of modern lawsuits there are many situations in which a radiograph is not only standard but imperative. For example, any physician who undertakes to treat the "sprained ankle" without benefit of radiologic diagnosis is quite liable for a malpractice suit, since many radiographs of "sprained ankles" demonstrate fractures of the lateral malleolus, or the like.

The importance of good and complete radiographs in the diagnosis of chest pathology and of abdominal pathology cannot be overstated; a negative radiograph (one without demonstration of pathology) is by no means time and effort wasted! A negative radiograph serves to rule out the presence of many suspected conditions of pathology—tuberculosis, cancer, fracture, or the like—and the existence of a properly exposed *negative* radiograph is one step nearer to the diagnosis.

In obtaining radiographs of any part of the body, there is a minimum number of views that must be made, and these views should be supplemented by the technologist (with routine consent of the department head) on his own volition upon recognizing the need. In the past a posterior (A-P) and a lateral view were usually sufficient, but in modern radiologic practice many diagnoses can be missed without further radiographic views. For example, ulnar flexion (radial deviation) of the wrist is, probably, the *single* view that may demonstrate a fracture of the scaphoid. This view is presently a standard (routine) view, and to omit it may be the cause of a missed diagnosis of fractured scaphoid—which may result in a lawsuit. Many orthopedic surgeons, in addition to the routine views of the wrist, will request three lateral views, at different densities (penetrations); it is significant that, more often than not, one of the three lateral views may demonstrate a fracture of the scaphoid. Therefore, do not hesitate to make additional radiographs when they are deemed necessary and when authority is granted. It is better to make one or two additional radiographs than to make the minimum number and have the diagnosis missed.

Another excellent example of potentially missed pathology is in the tangential view of the tibia. In this view the central ray passes parallel with the medial surface of the tibia, and all things projecting from this surface are visualized; if the projection is small, it cannot be seen in either the posterior or lateral view.

An understanding of precisely what the physician seeks is of tremendous help to the technologist; it will enable him to ascertain that the final radiographs present the correct penetration and density at the site of maximum pain. For example, even if the request does not specify it, the technologist should ascertain whether the pain is *on top* of the shoulder (in the acromioclavicular joint) and subsequently make an exposure from the measurement at this area, not at the shoulder proper. If in doubt, make exposures using both penetrations.

Always inspect the finished product before dismissing the patient. Many times an error in technique will be noticed—no one is beyond making such errors. In such instances, retakes are definitely *not* "wasted films." Remember, it is always possible that we will be called to the witness stand at a later date to swear that these are the radiographs we made, and they should be of *good* diagnostic quality demonstrating the correct degree of penetration.

The technologist's obligations to the patient

An injured or ill patient is first of all worried and frequently in pain. The relatives "fluttering" around the door of the radiology laboratory are impatient, irritable, and sometimes unreasonable. In placing the patient in the required position on the table, we may increase pain; perhaps we may even cause the patient to "cry out," again aggravating the relatives and the patient. Go slowly. A comfortable radiographic table remains to be invented. Reassure the patient. Above all, refrain from discussing the results of a radiologic examination with the patient, as this great responsibility belongs to the referring physician! Our slightest word regarding the diagnosis may differ totally from the physician's diagnosis, and this will instill doubt and fear in the mind of the patient.

Questions directed to the technologist by the patient are not rare, and, in fact, many times each day patients ask "How did my 'x ray' look?" The best way to handle such inquiries is to be pleasantly noncommittal, with some gentle statement, such as, "I am not trained to read these radiographs, and I suggest that you ask your doctor." Sometimes the patient on the table will be a personal friend, or a relative or acquaintance, and in these instances we need to be especially careful not to dabble in diagnosis or to make any statement that may reflect discredit upon the doctor, his diagnostic or surgical skill, or the like. Many times we are asked, "How good a doctor is so-and-so?" Here, again, we must be politicians, and a noncommittal reply, such as, "He has a good reputation," or something of like nature will harm no one.

If we encounter excessive pain, or pain that we feel is unjustified by the objective signs, we should so notify the physician and request his advice and assistance in the routine procedures to follow.

Duties of technologists

Depending on individual certification and experience and on departmental requirements, radiologic technologists may perform a variety of duties, all of which are within the scope of the profession.

In small offices a technologist, usually female, may act as receptionist and secretary in addition to her radiologic activities.

In larger establishments such as hospitals, clinics, and nuclear medicine and therapy offices, the technologist may perform routine radiologic duties and certain specialized examinations, or he may function entirely in a specialized field.

Routine functions require complete operational knowledge of all x-ray and processing equipment in the department. A certain amount of recordkeeping is essential in any department, and the chief or supervising technologist is perhaps the best qualified of all personnel in the department to maintain such records; other duties include personnel and patient scheduling.

Specifically, the technologist receives the requests and makes the required exposures on the patients. Next the exposed films are processed, and the technologist either notifies the physician that his radiographs are ready to view, or the radiographs are placed in the reading room for the radiologist.

Specialized duties include those of x-ray and radioisotope teletherapy, and of operational procedures with the specialized instruments in the field of nuclear medicine.

PROFESSIONAL SOCIETIES

These have been discussed in previous paragraphs as to political structure and basic purposes. It is now useful to describe some of the professional aspects. A professional society is the *only ethical medium* through which expression of personal ideals of a professional nature may be communicated. It is through participation in our professional societies—district, state, regional, and national—that continued growth and advancement of professional standards will be achieved. No single individual is sufficiently strong to promulgate particular ideals. Through effort of the group in the society, such ideals, if desirable, are usually achieved.

Current national conditions dictate that our profession have a stronger organization than the purely educational society. Several states have existing licensure laws, and others are pending. There is evidence that a national licensure law will go into effect in the near future in those states possessing no such laws. These will be of the nature of minimum standards to protect patients and equipment operators. Also, hospitals and other employers may be denied federal compensation for radiographic examinations if all technologists are not properly certified. Our efforts toward continuing education must be directed along these lines in addition to the existing demands for greater skills and increased in-depth knowledge of our entire discipline.

X-RAY MACHINES

Regardless of make or model, all x-ray machines have many items in common. An x-ray machine must have a table (Fig. 1-1, *A*) upon which the patient is positioned. For some examinations the patient is positioned against a chest board (Fig. 1-2). (Other examinations are performed in the patient's bed or in surgery.)

An x-ray machine must have a control panel (Fig. 1-3) upon which the determinations of kilovoltage, milliamperage, and time are made. Kilovoltage, milliamperage, and time (in seconds or parts thereof) are the *three prime factors* of x-ray production. This panel may have numerous auxiliary meters and selector switches, such as line amperage, line voltage, etc.

A

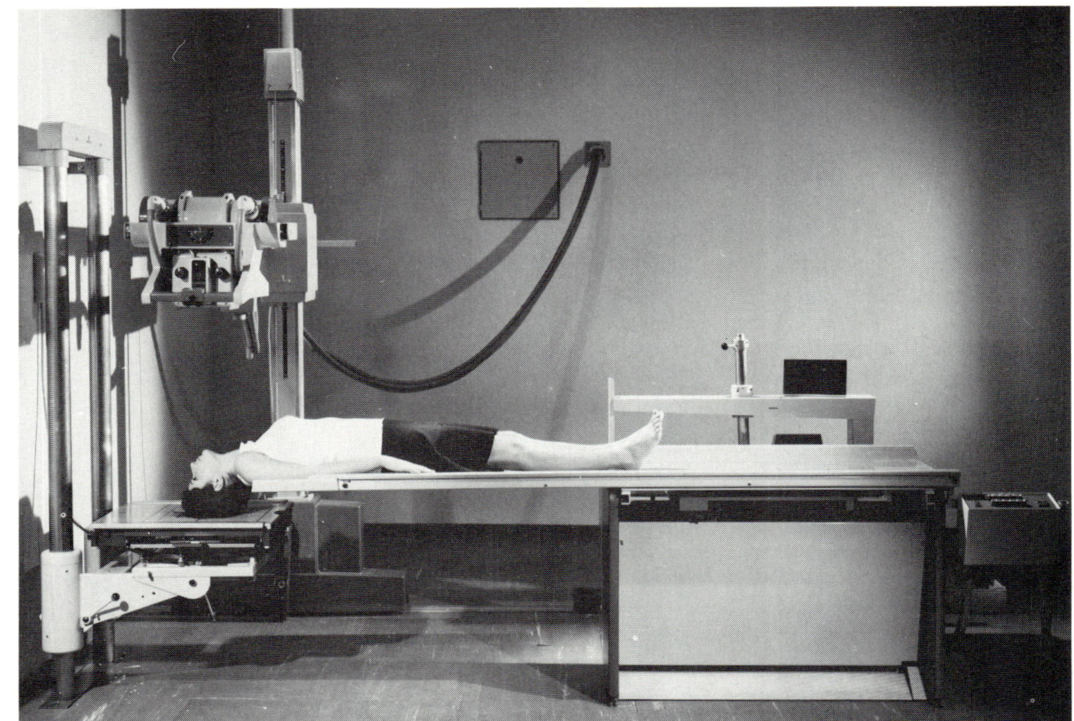

B

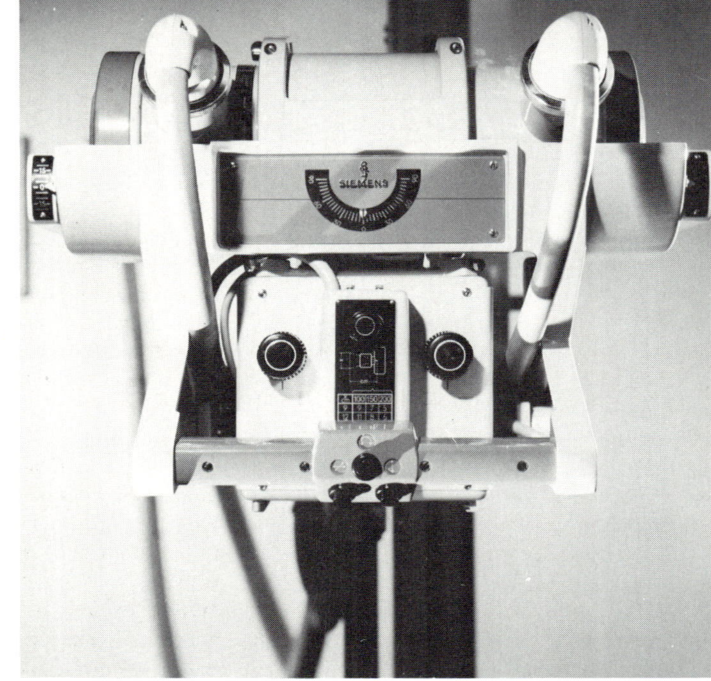

Fig. 1-1. A, Siemens Multi-Planigraph radiographic table. Bucky wall stand is in position for extended skull radiography. X-ray tube, in position over the patient's head, is mounted on a floor-to-ceiling tube stand. Part of the tube stand floor-track is seen on the opposite side of the table. A control panel to select table movements during planigraphy is seen at the foot of the table. **B,** Siemens Multi-Planigraph tube head. **C,** Siemens Multix table and overhead tube crane with planigraphic attachment. **D,** Siemens Tridoros 5S, a six-pulse generator. High-tension generator is on the left; it could be placed in either the control room or the radiographic room. Console control is on the right and would be placed in the control booth. (Courtesy Siemens Corp.)

C

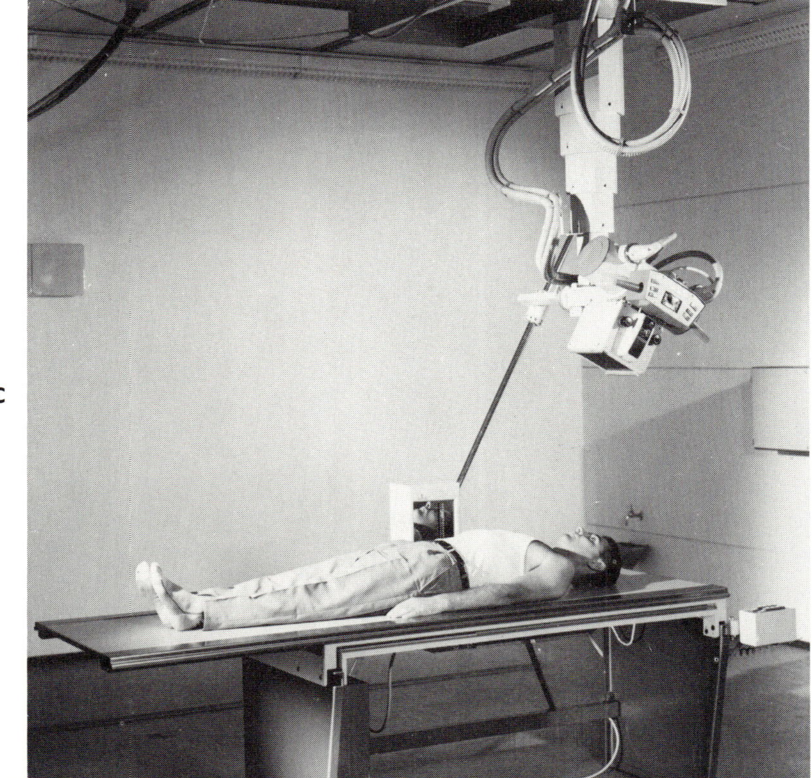

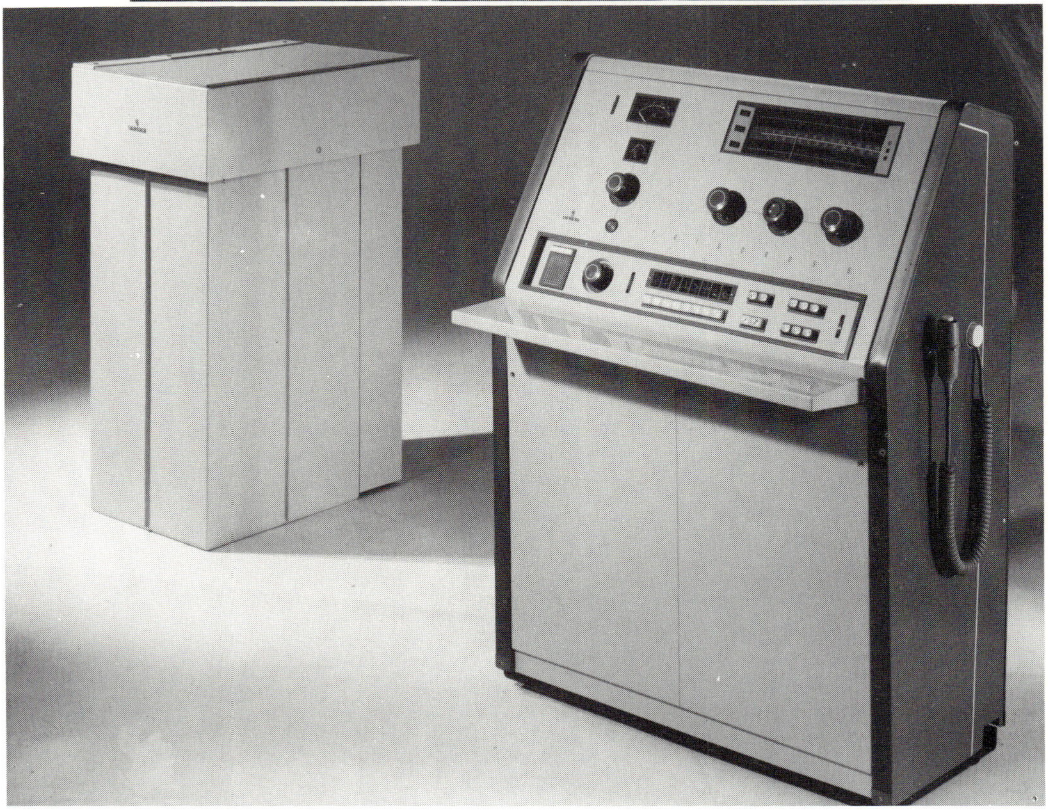

D

Fig. 1-1, cont'd. For legend see opposite page.

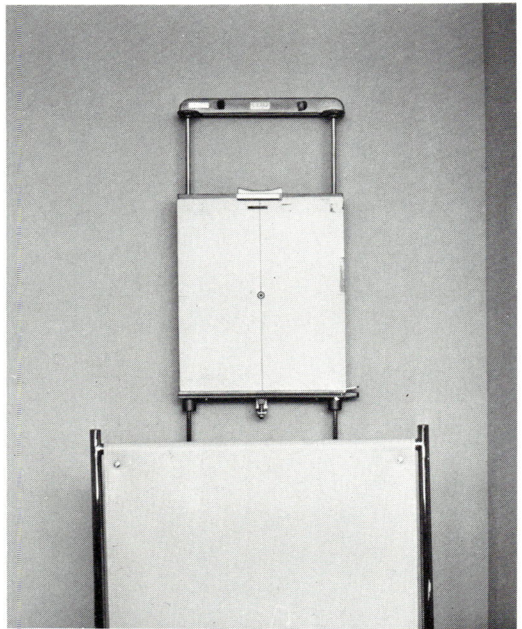

Fig. 1-2. Wall rack for cassette in chest radiography. An aligned grid with a 72-inch focal-film distance is in the cassette slot. Lead curtain is in place on curtain stand.

A

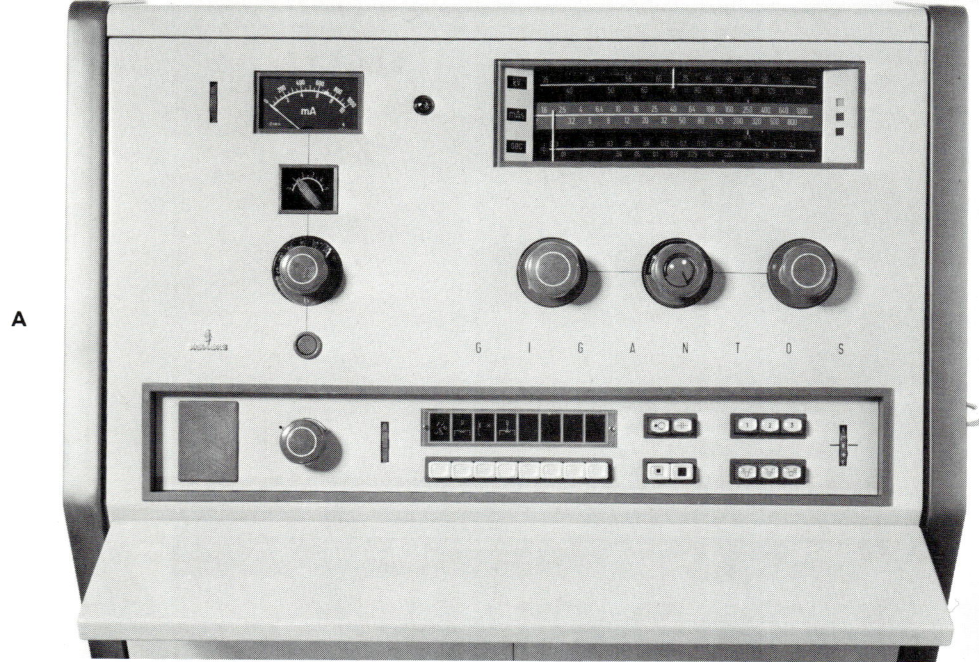

Fig. 1-3. Control panels of five x-ray machines in current use. **A,** Siemens Gigantos (courtesy Siemens Corp.). **B,** General Electric Model DXS 550 (courtesy General Electric Co.). **C,** Picker Model G-500S (courtesy Picker X-ray Corp.). **D,** Keleket 500 MA (courtesy Tracerlab-Keleket). **E,** Standard Model Ultima 600 (courtesy Standard X-Ray Co.).

The control panel will always present (1) an *on-off* (line) switch, which activates most of the circuits of the x-ray machine; (2) a device by which the milliamperage is selected; (3) a device to select the kilovoltage; and (4) a device to select the exposure time. The exposure switch usually extends from the control panel on a short cord (except on mobile units). The kilovoltage (kVp) is the voltage (determining force and penetrating ability) of x rays and is the *tube voltage;* the milliamperage times the exposure time is the milliampere-seconds (mAs) and is the *tube current.* The milliampere-seconds determines the quantity and intensity of x rays produced.

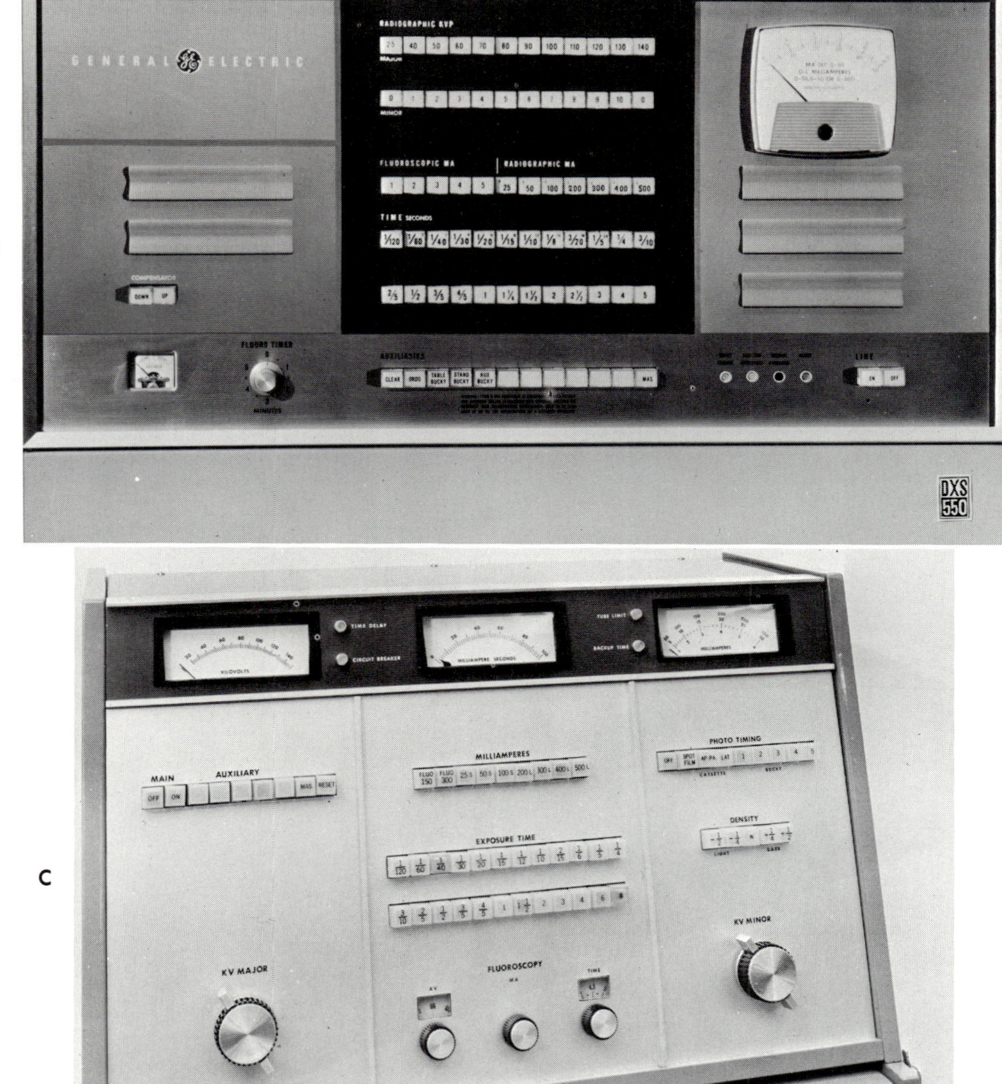

Continued.

Fig. 1-3, cont'd. For legend see opposite page.

D

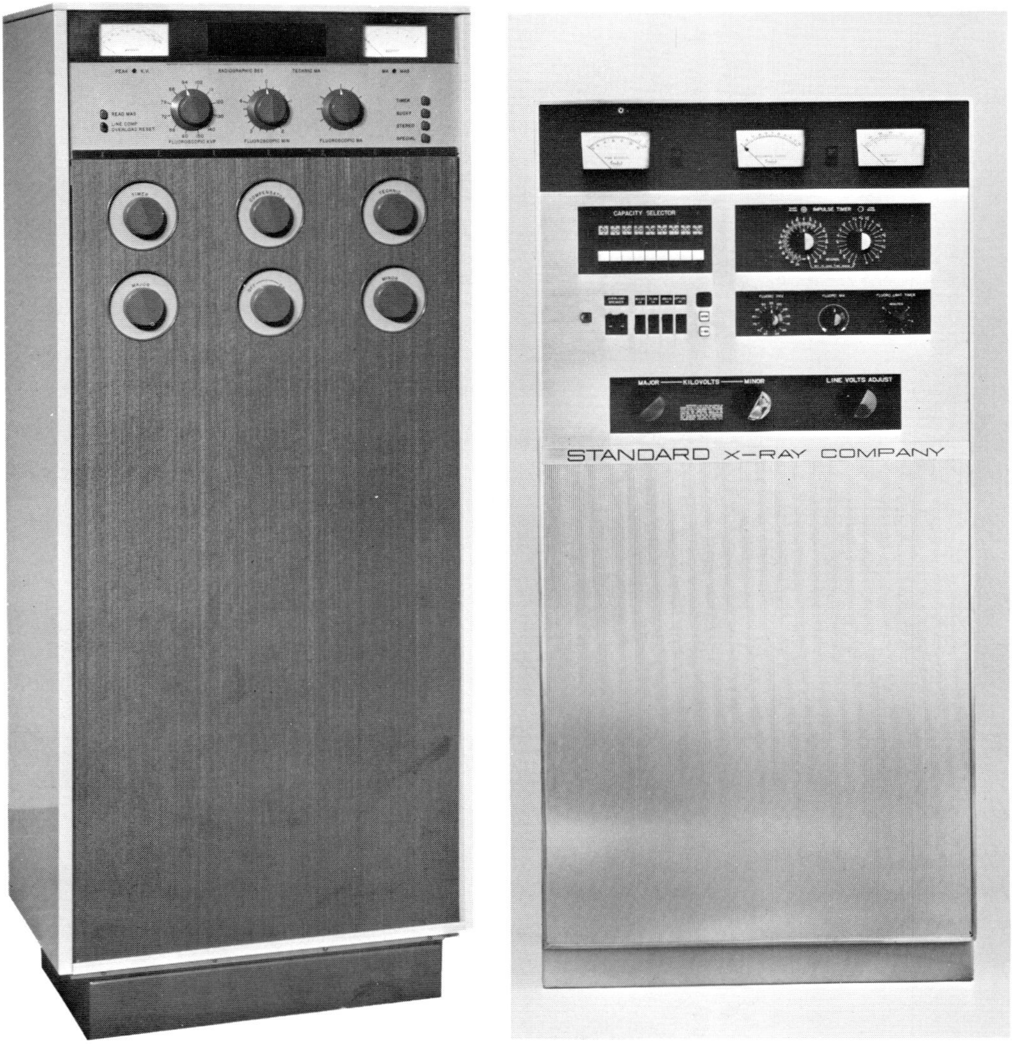

E

Fig. 1-3, cont'd. For legend see p. 10.

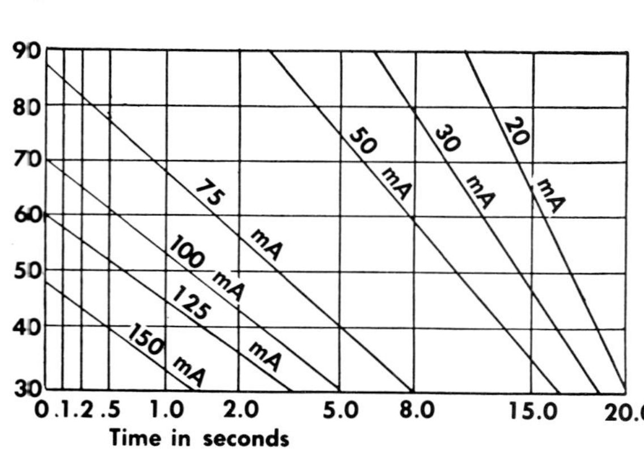

Fig. 1-4. Tube-rating chart. This tube-rating chart has no reference to any specific tube. Any combination of values found to the left of the sloping milliamperage line is acceptable, whereas those on the line and to the right are too high for the tube. Example: 200 mAs at 70 kVp cannot be obtained safely using either 125 or 100 mA, but can safely be obtained when using 50 mA for 4 sec.

A

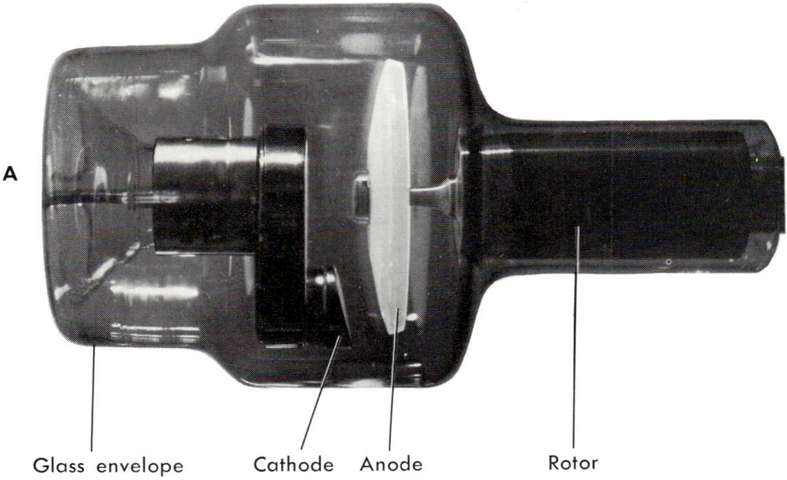

B

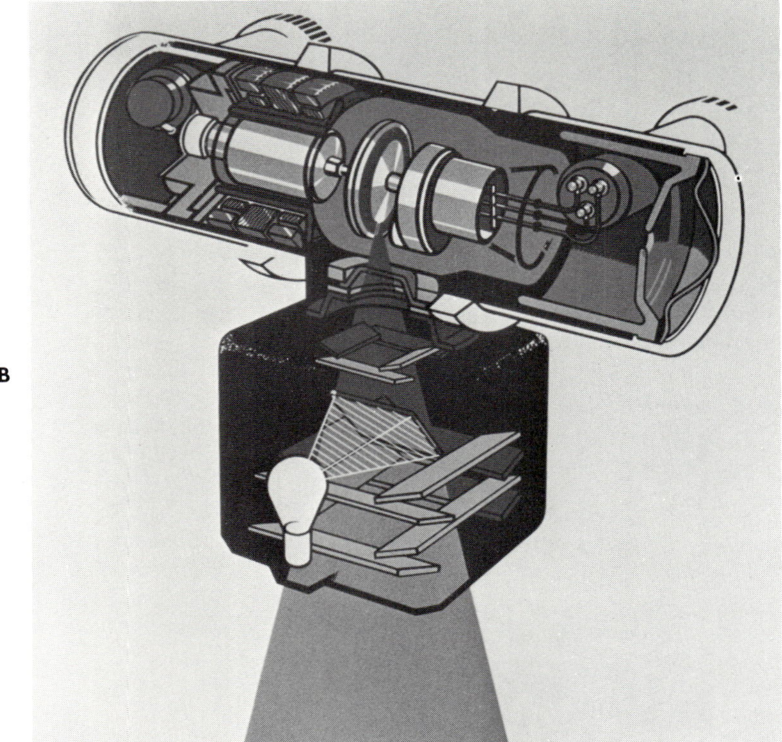

Fig. 1-5. A, Siemens Biangulix rotating anode x-ray tube. Anode disk rotates at 3,000 to 9,000 rpm, depending on specific tube design and use in operation. **B,** Cutaway view of rotating anode tube in shield with collimator attached. (Courtesy Siemens Corp.)

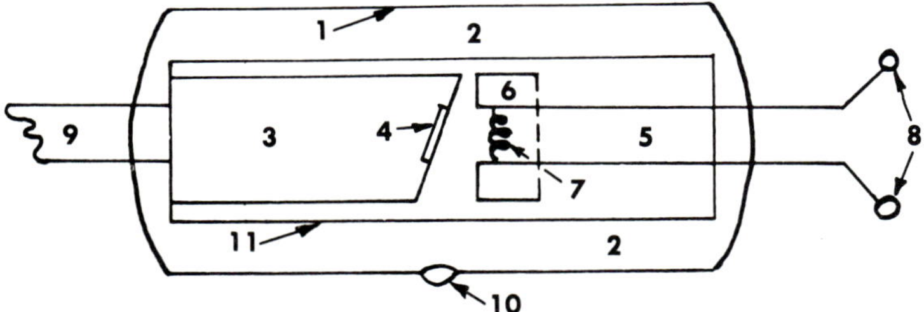

Fig. 1-6. X-ray tube, stationary anode.

1. Metal shielding
2. Insulating oil
3. Anode
4. Tungsten target
5. Cathode
6. Focusing cup
7. Cathode filament
8. Wire connections to secondary side of filament transformer
9. Anode connection to secondary circuit
10. Port (window) in metal shield
11. Evacuated glass envelope

The usual sequence of selection for operation is as follows:

1. Turn line switch to *on* position.
2. Check (and adjust if necessary) the line voltage.
3. Select milliamperage.
4. Select time (and determine that mA × time gives the correct mAs).
5. Select kilovoltage.
6. Check all selections against the tube-rating chart (Fig. 1-4).

An x-ray machine has a number of transformers and other electrical items usually immersed in an oil bath and situated at some distance from both the table and control panel. From the upper surface of the transformer extend the *high-voltage* (high-tension) cables to the various x-ray tubes. A general term applied to the several transformers and other electronic devices is *x-ray generator*.

A most important part of the x-ray machine is the x-ray tube (Figs. 1-5 and 1-6). X rays are generated in the tube and pass from the tube through the *port* (window) in the metal case that surrounds the x-ray tube.

The three principal items necessary in a modern, hot-cathode x-ray tube are the cathode, anode, and an evacuated glass envelope to contain the cathode and anode.

X RAYS

Radiologic technologists must, of course, have knowledge of the nature of x rays and of x-ray production; however, in this introductory chapter no attempt is made to discuss the subject in depth. A few summary paragraphs at this time will suffice; later chapters will treat the subject in greater detail.

X rays are any of the radiations (electromagnetic waves) of the same nature as light radiation but of an extremely short wavelength, about one angstrom (1Å) unit,* emitted primarily as the result of a sudden change in the velocity of a moving electron (electric charge), as when rapidly moving cathode rays strike a solid obstacle, or target, in a vacuum tube, and as the result of changes in the atoms in the target (anode) due to this impact. The unit of measure of x rays is the roentgen (see glossary); it is abbreviated as R.

The most notable properties of these rays are (1) ionization of a gas through which they pass, (2) penetration through various thicknesses of all solids, (3) production of secondary rays, and (4) action on photographic plates, fluorescent screens, etc., like that of light.

X rays are one of the forms of energy existing as electromagnetic waves. Collectively, these several waves constitute the electromagnetic wave spectrum. A spectrum is the series of images formed when a beam of radiant energy is subjected to dispersion and then brought to focus so that the component waves are arranged in the order of their wavelengths.

X rays and the electromagnetic wave spectrum

The longer wavelengths in the electromagnetic wave spectrum are the radio waves; the shorter

*An angstrom unit is a unit of measure of wave length and is equal to one one-hundred millionth of a centimeter. It is written also 1×10^{-8} cm.

Table 1-1. Approximate wavelength range in angstrom units of electromagnetic waves

Radiations	Wavelengths in Å units
Radio waves	10^{14} to 10^{11}
Hertzian waves	10^{10} to 10^{9}
Short electric waves	10^{8}
Infrared rays	10^{7} to 10^{5}
Visible light rays	10^{4}
Ultraviolet light rays	10^{3}
X rays	10^{2} to 10^{-1}
Gamma rays	10^{-2}
Cosmic rays	10^{-4}

wavelengths are the cosmic* waves or rays. *Cosmic rays, consist of high-energy electromagnetic waves, gamma rays, and assorted electrons, protons, neutrons, positrons, etc.*

Table 1-1 lists the electromagnetic waves in their respective positions in the electromagnetic wave spectrum.

X rays are sometimes compared with visible light, and indeed they differ from visible light in but few qualities. Just as light rays strike a film emulsion and cause certain physical reactions within the crystalline structure of the emulsion, in the shape of the source of the reflected light rays (latent image), so do x rays pass through an object or structure and strike the film emulsion to cause a similar sequence of events.

It is the nature of x rays that each travels in a straight line from its source to the object it strikes, including the film. Since the source of x rays in diagnostic x-ray tubes is very small (from as large as 2 square millimeters to as small as 0.3 square millimeters), the x rays diverge from this "point," travel to the structure and through it to the film, and cause an image (shadow) somewhat larger than the actual size of the structure (Fig. 1-7).

The preceding paragraphs present the student with some of the important facts concerning x rays. Basic information on production and use of x rays in relation to exposure of film is presented next. Both kVp and mAs were discussed briefly on preceding pages.

Since the energy of a single x-ray wave (or photon) is a function of the maximum electrical force used to produce the x ray, it is readily understood that increasing the voltage used to produce x rays causes corresponding increases in the resulting x-ray energy. Thus, if it is desired to penetrate an object of either greater density or greater thickness, it will be necessary to use x rays of greater energy (penetrating power) that are produced by use of increased peak (maximum) kilovolts, kVp. Thus kilovoltage controls the penetrability of x rays.

*The electromagnetic portion of cosmic rays is usually referred to as high-energy gamma rays.

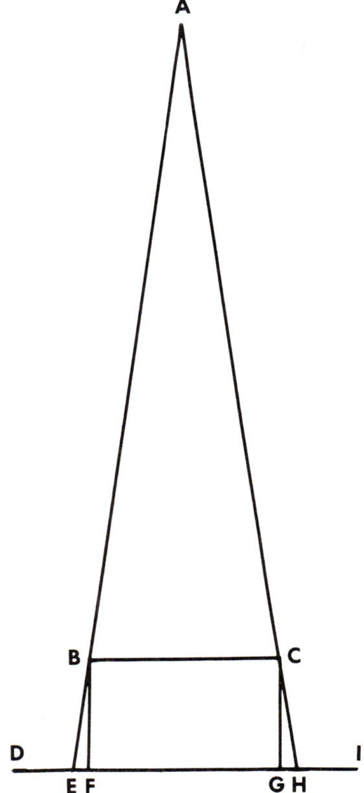

Fig. 1-7. A vertical line from point **A** to the base, **D-I**, is drawn to represent a 40-inch ffd (focal-film distance). Object x-rayed, **BFGC**, is 6 inches thick (vertical) by 10 inches wide. Projected size of **E-H** over **BC** (or **FG**) is an increase of 0.118, or 11.8%.

There is similar relationship between the number (quantity) of x rays produced and the tube-current volume. When greater quantities of line current are used to produce correspondingly greater quantities of tube current (milliamperage), a remarkably greater quantity of x rays is produced. If a structure is properly penetrated and the finished image (on the film) has insufficient density, it is probable that a greater number of x rays should have been employed to produce the desired image density (radiographic effect). Although the *film-reciprocity effect* must be considered, it is proper procedure to vary milliamperage and time (in seconds) inversely with each other to obtain a satisfactory value for milliampere-seconds, mAs. Thus it is seen that milliampere-seconds control the image density just as kilovoltage controls the image contrast.

Thus the image density may be changed (in subsequent radiographs) for improved diagnostic quality by suitable changes in these *prime factors* of kilovolts, milliamperes, and time (in seconds). Along with the factor of focal-film distance (the distance between the tube target [focal spot], and the film, usually stated in inches), kVp and mAs are used in mathematical formulas to determine values of radiographic effect (re) on the exposed film.

Typical *sets* of factors for specific anatomic regions and for specific thicknesses of part are presented as examples of varying requirements for different anatomic structures.

Extremities: Hand, P-A projection, anterior view for 4 cm thickness, use 60 kVp, 75 mAs, and 40-inch ffd on screen (plain) film in cardboard holders; 48 kVp, 10 mAs, and 40-inch ffd may be used on screen film in par-speed screen cassettes.

Skull: P-A projection, anterior view for 18 cm thickness, use 78 kVp, 60 mAs, and 40-inch ffd on screen film in par-speed screen cassettes, and using a 12:1 ratio grid either portable or in the Bucky.

Chest: P-A projection, anterior view for 22 cm thickness, use 64 kVp, 10 mAs, and 72-inch ffd on screen film in par-speed screen cassettes.

Pelvis: A-P projection, posterior view for 20 cm thickness, use 66 kVp, 100 mAs, and 40-inch ffd on screen film in par-speed screen cassettes, and using a 12:1 ratio grid either portable or in the Bucky.

The image so formed is *latent;* that is, the image is not visible and must be rendered *manifest* (visible) by a sequence of chemical events in the processing (dark) room.

Understanding the reference and/or meaning of radiographic positioning terms is of major importance. In general use and particularly in this textbook the following meanings apply. The *central ray* is that portion of the primary beam exiting from the port of the x-ray tube shielding at right angles to its long axis, and *directed* to the center of the film or structure to be *exposed* by the passage of x rays *(radiographed).* The central ray (passes) *projects* through the structure from anterior to posterior (A-P) or from posterior to anterior (P-A), etc. When the patient's (or part's) anterior or ventral surface is closest to the film-holder, the resulting *radiograph (radiographic view)* or *view* is *anterior* or *ventral,* and the patient is in the *anterior* or *ventral* position.

FILM HOLDERS

Since light rays affect film emulsions much as do x rays, it is necessary to contain the x-ray films in lightproof holders. These may be cardboard holders or metal and plastic cassettes.

Cardboard holders are simply constructed and may be either stiff or flexible. These holders (Fig. 1-8, *C*) consist of two pieces of cardboard connected either at one end or at one side by some flexible material. The holders are made in the various film sizes. There is a tube side and a back side in each holder. The back side contains a thin lead foil sheet to absorb the backscatter to prevent fogging of film by secondary rays. (See glossary for definition of backscatter.) Backscatter increases with higher voltages; a piece of leaded rubber should be placed beneath *all* film holders during table top radiography. An envelope to encase the film is glued to the inside of the back. (Note: When loading or closing the envelope, place the larger flap directly over the film.) A clamping device is placed at the end or side opposite the flexible connection between the two cardboards. Since the paper that usually encases the film has no effect on the film in a cardboard holder, this paper may be left around the film as additional light prevention. *The total radiographic effect upon the film exposed in a cardboard holder is from the x-ray energy.*

Cassettes are usually made of aluminum or some other equally radiolucent substance supported within a strong metal framework. A cassette has an aluminum front (tube) side and raised metal sides and ends into which the back fits. The back is hinged to the front on one end (or side). Spring locks are so fitted into the back that when they are locked, the cassette is tightly closed. In order to seal out light, the sides and ends have felt padding on the inner surfaces. A thin lead foil sheet is contained in the back to prevent backscatter. The cassettes contain one pair of *intensifying screens* between which the film is sandwiched. The intensifying screens function to augment the x-ray energy by adding light energy to the total energy quantity striking the film emulsion. Intensifying screens are attached

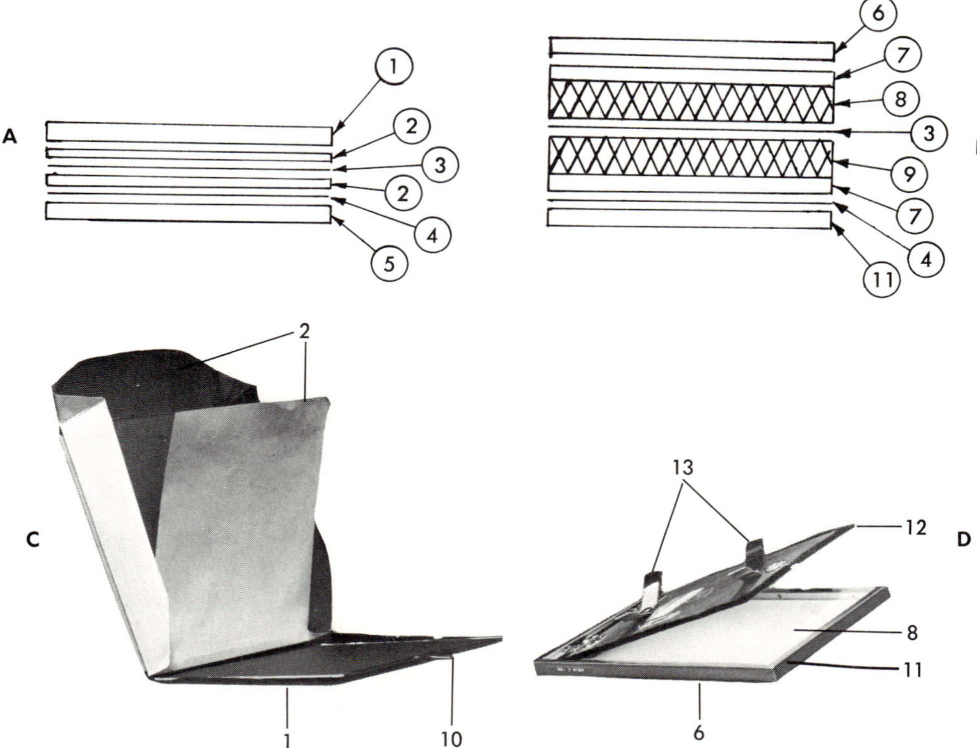

Fig. 1-8. Film holders. **A,** Cross section of a cardboard holder. **B,** Cross section of a cassette. **C,** Cardboard holder. **D,** Intensifying screen cassette.

1. Tube side (front) of cardboard holder
2. Paper envelope to contain x-ray film
3. X-ray film
4. Lead foil (to prevent some backscatter)
5. Cardboard back of cardboard holder
6. Tube side (radiolucent front) of cassette
7. Synthetic base for intensifying screen emulsion
8. Fluorescent emulsion of intensifying screen (of tube side)
9. Fluorescent emulsion of intensifying screen (of back side)
10. Locking clip
11. Metal frame of cassette
12. Cassette back
13. Spring locks on cassette back

to both the front and back sides of the cassette. These screens sandwich the film. Fig. 1-8, *B*, is a cross-section diagram of a cassette.

Like the cardboard holders, the cassettes are made the same sizes as the films. The sizes are 5″ × 7″, 6½″ × 8½″, 8″ × 10″, 9″ × 9″, 10″ × 12″, 11″ × 14″, 7″ × 17″, 14″ × 17″, and 14″ × 36″. Cassettes are either flat or curved. Special cassettes for use with phototimers contain no lead so the remnant rays pass through the cassette to the fluorescent screen in the photo-timing device (pp. 106 and 110).

Cassette screen cleaning

Successful radiograph production depends on a variety of conditions, including the maintenance of clean and lint-free intensifying screens in the cassettes.

Depending on the frequency of use and on other routine conditions, the cassettes should be inspected at periodic intervals. When lint is found on an intensifying screen, it can usually be removed with a special "antistatic" brush.

Other contaminating foreign objects on the screen surface should be removed as soon as possible with one of the following liquid cleaners:

1. Commercial screen cleaner or antistatic solution or both
2. Anesthetic ether
3. Pure grain alcohol
4. Warm water and very mild soap

Screens should be cleaned as often as is necessary and usually on a scheduled rotating basis. Monthly cleaning of all cassettes in small radiologic departments should be considered routine.

To clean screens, moisten a small piece of clean cotton with the liquid cleaner and lightly rub the screen surface in a crosswise motion; then quickly remove any excess cleaner with a dry piece of cotton and place the cassette on its edge like an open book to allow thorough drying before reloading.

A simple card-file index for cassette maintenance should be arranged with corresponding screen-cassette numbers for each series of cassette sizes. Screen installation and cleaning dates should be recorded on a routine basis.

FILM PROCESSING

In this section only the simplest aspects of the rather complicated chemical reactions will be explained in conjunction with the basic mechanical steps of film processing.

In order to make the latent image manifest, it is necessary to change the chemical and physical natures of certain parts of the film emulsion, especially the silver.

Manual processing

Explained simply, the exposed x-ray films are suspended in suitable hangers and immersed for an exact period of time in the developing solution, where the latent image is made manifest. Next the film (in its hanger) is removed from the developing solution, permitting none of the developing solution to drip back into the developing tank. The film is then immersed in the water bath for a few seconds and is next immersed in the acid stop bath for an exact interval of 30 seconds. Following the acid stop bath, the film is immersed in the fixing solution for a period of time long enough to clear and fix the image.* In the fixing bath the film surface is hardened, and the manifest image is fixed. Following the fixing bath, the film is again washed, then rinsed in a Photoflow (detergent) solution, and then dried. The total process may take as much as 45 minutes to an hour in manual processing rooms. Use of automatic processing machines reduces the total time to as little as from 90 seconds to 15 minutes.

To obtain satisfactory results, it is necessary that certain routine procedures be developed and followed. *The proper processing of x-ray film is just as important as the original exposure of the film.* The very best exposure is easily rendered useless or nearly so by careless or improper processing-room technique. In order to develop good habits in any procedure, a strict routine is necessary. The following routine is suggested for a manually operated processing room.

1. Close and lock doors tightly.
2. Be sure that solutions are well stirred and that the amount of solution fully covers the film.
3. Check temperatures of the solutions and water carefully.
4. Set the timer clock accurately.
5. Be sure that all lights except the safelight are out.
6. Hold the cassette with the tube side down and the hinges away from you and place it on the loading bench.
7. Grasp the corners nearest you and remove the film. Be sure to refrain from touching the rest of the film. Avoid dragging the film across the cassette.
8. Place the end of the film that you are holding in the bottom of the hanger, being certain that you have closed the cassette before bringing a hanger across its face.
9. Clamp the corners you hold into the hanger, then turn the hanger over and secure the other two corners. Never allow the film to override on the sides of the hanger or on the ends.
10. Agitate the suspended film as it is immersed into the developer and simultaneously start the timer clock.*
11. Dry your hands and reload the cassette.
12. After the proper time interval has elapsed, remove the suspended film from the developer and rinse it in a running water bath for a minimum of 30 seconds, agitating it *vigorously.* Allow the excess water to drain off the film. No-screen film requires 45 seconds to wash.
13. Immerse the film in an acid stop bath for 30 seconds.
14. Place the suspended film in the fixer and start the timer clock.
15. After the proper time interval has elapsed, remove the suspended film (now the radiograph) and rinse it at least 30 minutes in a running water bath before immersing it in the Photoflow.
16. Place the radiograph in a drier.

*Fixing time is twice as long as "clearing" time; sometimes as little as 3 minutes in fresh fixer.

*Agitation in the developing solution should be continued throughout development (or sufficiently long to prevent the formation of *air bells*).

The solution on the film should never be allowed to drip into the developer tank because the solution that adheres to the film is partially exhausted and will weaken the developing solution earlier than necessary. The fixer is not so weakened. The developer and fixer baths should be maintained at their required levels by frequent additions of specific replenishing solution throughout the day. Following each addition of new replenisher, the solutions should be well stirred. *Remember that there are three equally important solutions in the processing room: developer, water bath, and fixer.*

Equipment

In most processing rooms the developer will be in the left-hand tank as the technologist faces it, the water bath in the center, and the fixer in the right-hand tank. In a strange processing room the developing solution can be identified by its *slippery* feeling. The fixer will have a *vinegary* odor when fresh.

Through-the-wall water baths are highly advantageous in that they enable the physicians to view wet radiographs without disturbing the processing routine.

The processing-room illuminator should be equipped with a light source that has no afterglow.*

The well-designed processing room should be completely light-proof. There should be a clean and dry loading bench away from the solution tanks to eliminate the danger of moisture and chemicals splashing upon the bench. The hangers should be so placed upon the wall over the loading bench that they will not hang over the cassette-loading area, yet will be within easy reach of the technologist.

If the processing room is equipped with an overhead safelight, this light (if indirect) should be located a minimum of 4 feet from the loading bench. The illumination from the safelight should be filtered with a *Wratten 6B* filter and contain a globe no stronger than 25 watts. A direct overhead safelight requires the same filter, a 15-watt globe, and should be a minimum of 6 feet from the loading bench.

The *safeness* of the safelight may be tested in the following manner. With only the safelights on, place an exposed film on the loading bench. Place some opaque object, such as a coin, on the film and expose the film to the safelights for *15 seconds exactly*. Process the film. The visible outline of the coin indicates that the lights are too strong and that some exposure of the film has occurred. Exposed films are seven to eight times more sensitive to safelight fogging than are unexposed films. If unexposed films are used for this purpose, the required time is *2 minutes*.

A film bin should be placed in the loading bench so that films may be obtained from it without disturbing the loading surface. A diagram of such a bin is shown in Fig. 1-9. It is desirable to establish a routine in loading the bin so that the technologist may always be certain of the kind of film located in designated places.

It is advisable to have the film bin wired so that the lights will be turned off when the bin is opened. The safelights need not be in this circuit.

The processing room should have adequate ventilation or an air-exhaust system. Careful installation of an air-exhaust fan will prevent entrance of light and moisture.

Pass boxes between the processing room and adjacent radiographic rooms and halls are a great convenience and help prevent accidental entrance of light.

Entrance into the processing room may be achieved through a variety of methods, each of which precludes the entrance of light. Probably the best method is to use a *light maze* (an arrangement of joined pathways into the processing room). However, there are conditions under which the required space for a maze is unavailable. A second method is that of spacing two

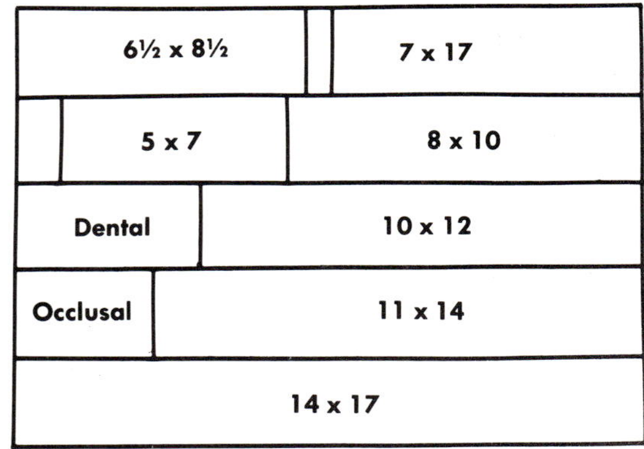

Fig. 1-9. One method of placing films of different sizes in the film bin.

*In this particular use, afterglow refers to a glow of refulgence remaining after a light has disappeared. The radiographic use refers to a condition in an intensifying screen wherein the screen continues to emit light after the x-ray energy has ceased to strike the screen.

doors at either end of a short and darkened cubicle or hall. In this method, one of the doors leads directly into the processing room from the darkened hall and the other door leads from the hall into the outer areas. These doors are then equipped with locks that prevent both doors from being opened at the same time.

Automatic processing

Automatic processing of x-ray film has replaced to a major extent the manual method of x-ray film processing. This came about as a result of the tremendously increased workload in most departments and of the corresponding difficulty in maintaining consistently uniform diagnostic quality in the finished radiographs.

Although the processing principle is basically the same in both manual and automatic processing, the mechanics of operation and the chemistry of both the films and the solutions are changed considerably.

For an automatic processor the film is either marked during exposure or after exposure and prior to processing, just as for manual processing. In a darkened preparation room the exposed film is removed from the film-holder and placed in the receiving slot of the processor. From this time the entire process is mechanically controlled, and the important variables of careful replenishment of solutions, time, temperature, and agitation of the films are eliminated.

All processors include some method of conveying the exposed film (in total darkness, but not necessarily in a darkened room) into the developing solution for an exact time period. The temperature of this and all solutions is maintained automatically within a variation of ±0.5° F. After the proper time period in the developer is completed, the film moves into the fixing bath, again for an exact period of time. After fixation is completed, the film moves into the wash bath for an exact period of time, and then into the hot-air dryer until the radiograph is completely dry and ready for viewing. During this process the recirculation pumps maintain an optimum agitation of all solutions, thus assuring proper agitation of all films. Since all films are driven through each solution at a constant speed and for a predetermined length of time (set on the mechanical control), the diagnostic quality of the radiographs is maintained at a high level of consistency. Radiographic exposure and technique are the remaining variables.

The film-speed, processing chemicals, and exposure factors are all necessarily coordinated with the total time of processing; that is, 90 seconds, 3 minutes, 6 minutes, etc. Fig. 1-10 illustrates the Kodak RP X-OMAT 90-second automatic processor.

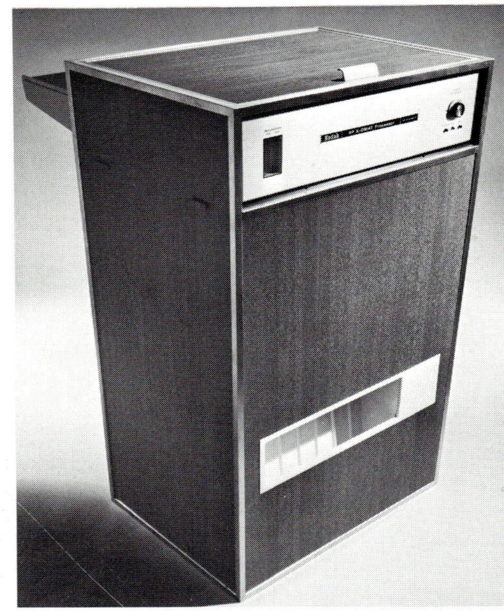

Fig. 1-10. Kodak RP X-OMAT (M6A-N). (Courtesy Eastman Kodak Co.)

QUESTIONS

1. Define radiography.
2. What are actinic rays?
3. What is a radiograph?
4. Describe the general activities of a radiologic technologist.
5. How long does a radiologist or roentgenologist attend college after graduation from high school?
6. Is additional study beyond medical school required of a student of radiology before he can practice his specialty? If so, how much? Explain.
7. What is radiology?
8. How does radiology differ from roentgenology?
9. What led Roentgen to his discovery of x rays?
10. Who was Ed C. Jerman?
11. When was the forerunner of the ASRT first formed?
12. What are the present titles of our registries and our professional societies?
13. Describe the kinds of schools approved by ARCRT and by the JRC.
14. What specialties are available in our profession?
15. What is the address of the ARRT? Of ARCRT?
16. What is meant by professional ethics?

17. What are the three C's of modern medical precept?
18. When is it ethical for a technologist to divulge information regarding the radiologic diagnosis to the patient?
19. What major items are present on all x-ray machine control panels?
20. Why is it necessary to check kilovoltage, time, and milliampere selections against the tube-rating chart?
21. What is the principal effect of kilovoltage during an exposure?
22. What items are absolutely essential in a hot-cathode x-ray tube?
23. To what spectrum do x rays belong? Where in this spectrum are x rays found?
24. What is an angstrom unit? Of what is it a measure? How much (quantity) is an angstrom unit?
25. What is the principal result of milliampere-seconds on the finished radiograph?
26. In a cassette or cardboard film-holder, what is the function of the lead foil backing?
27. What purpose is served by the envelope in a cardboard film-holder?
28. In cassettes, what is the purpose of the intensifying screens?
29. What size cassettes and cardboard film-holders are found in the processing room (or storeroom) of your department?
30. Describe how you would clean a dirt spot from a cassette screen.
31. What are the approximate processing times of manual technique? Automatic technique?
32. What is meant by clearing time?
33. What is meant by fixing time?
34. What type of filter is safe on the safelights in x-ray processing rooms?
35. What temperature variation is permissible with most automatic processors?

2 • BASIC PHYSICAL SCIENCE

The continuing advances in electronic technology as applied to radiologic equipment, specifically diagnostic x-ray machines, require corresponding increases in scientific knowledge and technical capabilities of radiologic technologists. Proliferation of diagnostic radiologic examinations and procedures stems from these same electronic advances. Basic knowledge of chemistry continues to be of high importance; an increasing knowledge of physics, particularly related to electricity, assumes even greater importance than in the past. Fundamentally, mathematics and particularly algebra continue to be the necessary steps leading to an understanding of chemistry, physics, and electricity.

SOLVING ALGEBRAIC EQUATIONS

The following information provides the student of radiologic technology with the basic knowledge necessary to understand and solve problems presented in succeeding chapters. Algebra is the set of all the numbers in a given number field and their combinations in accordance with assigned rules. The essential difference between arithmetic and algebra is that the former deals with concrete quantities (numbers), whereas the latter deals with symbols (letters) whose values may be any out of a given number field.

Examples:

Just as $2 \times 3 = 6$ arithmetically,
so does $a \times b = c$ algebraically.
However, this expression is customarily written as $ab = c$.
Just as $6 \div 3 = 2$ arithmetically,
so does $c \div b = a$ algebraically.
Also $c \div a = b$.

Instead of using a, b, and c we may use common (in the profession of radiologic technology) terms such as milliamperes (mA), time in seconds, and milliampere-seconds (mAs):

10 mA × 0.1 sec = 1 mAs
100 mA × 0.01 sec = 1 mAs
10 mA × 10 sec. = 100 mAs
5 mA × 20 sec = 100 mAs
100 mA × 1 sec = 100 mAs
1,000 mA × 0.1 sec = 100 mAs

Although the total milliampere-seconds value may be obtained by using a variety of combinations, some of these required values may not be available on a particular piece of x-ray equipment. In such instances suitable substitutions are necessitated. However, such items as patient movement, film reciprocity, tube focalspot size, and tube heat-loading and cooling must be considered.

Many time selectors present fractional times such as 1/4 sec, 1/5 sec, 1/8 sec, 1/12 sec, 1/15 sec, etc. Some of these values may be converted to decimal values: 1/5 sec is the same as 2/10 or 0.2. Other values such as 1/12 sec must be used as a fraction in computing mAs:

$$100\text{ mA} \times 1/12\text{ sec} = \frac{(100)(1)}{12} = 8.5\text{ mAs}$$

$$30\text{ mAs} \div 1/15\text{ sec} = \frac{(30)(15)}{1} = 450\text{ mA}$$

FUNDAMENTAL CONCEPTS OF MATTER

With some degree of competence in solving algebraic equations now achieved, the student is next presented with some basic information in physical science. Physical sciences are concerned with the study of the fundamental phenomena of matter. Physical sciences include both chemistry and physics.

Chemistry is the study of matter and of the changes that matter undergoes, whereas physics is the study of the transformation of energy. When one considers the law of conservation of matter and energy, the subject matter of these two sciences appears to be closely related and is often quite similar.

Substance is a form of matter, and *matter is defined as anything having mass or weight and that occupies space.* Matter always exists in one of three states—solid, liquid, or gas. The *mass of a body is the quantity of matter it contains and is determined by its inertia;* that is, the resistance offered to a change in motion. *Weight is the attraction between the Earth and the body of consideration.* Since the attraction between any two bodies is inversely proportional to the square of the distance between the exact centers of the bodies, the masses of the two bodies will be proportional to their respective weights. The preceding statement is true as long as the weights are measured at the same distance from the Earth's center.

Matter represents a given quantity of energy. *Energy is the ability to perform or do work; energy is kinetic when performing a task and potential when available but not operational.* The laws of conservation of mass and energy provide the following information. *The total quantity of mass and energy is constant, although mass and energy may be converted one into the other.*

In one of the three possible states, ninety-two simple forms of matter exist and cannot be further subdivided. These ninety-two simple forms are the ninety-two natural elements. At least twelve additional elements have been produced artificially. Subsequently, all matter consists of one or more of these elements in combination. Any one element in its pure state consists of many atoms, which exist either as single entities or in combination as molecules. A *molecule is an aggregation of atoms, that is, a chemical combination of two or more atoms that form a specific chemical substance. An atom is the smallest quantity of an element that can exist and still retain the chemical properties of that element.*

However, atoms are not the smallest particles found in nature; within the atom are found several much smaller particles including principally the protons, neutrons, and electrons. Protons and neutrons are contained within the nucleus of the atom, and the electrons are considered to orbit about the nucleus. *The proton is a positively charged particle of matter with a mass approximately that of the nucleus of the hydrogen atom. The neutron, which is slightly larger in mass than the proton, is electrically neutral. The electron, which is a negatively charged particle of matter, has a mass approximately 1/1834 of that of the proton.* The radius of the nucleus of an atom has been estimated as approximately 10^{-12} cm,* and the radius of the electron orbits about the nucleus as approximately 10^{-8} cm. The proton mass has been estimated as approximately 1.00758 AMU (atomic mass unit), the neutron mass as approximately 1.00894 AMU, and the electron mass as approximately 0.00055 AMU.

*The expression 10^{-12} cm is a simplified method of writing the number 0.000000000001 cm. The expression 10^{10} is a shortened method of writing the number 10,000,000,000.

The minuteness of each particle (nucleon) in the atomic nucleus is no measure of the energy required to remove a single nucleon from the nucleus of that atom. The energy required to remove a neutron or proton from an atomic nucleus is called the *binding energy* or *force.* If an atomic nucleus were to be assembled from individual neutrons and protons, the energy that would be released would be the total binding force of the nucleus. This binding force is of close range and is enormously greater than the electrostatic repelling force exhibited by two positively charged protons. The binding force of a particular nuclear particle is measured in millions of electron volts. The symbol for one million electron volts is 1 meV.

The binding force varies from one element to another; the greatest variations occur between hydrogen and neon. The following are some of the elements and their corresponding binding forces:

H (hydrogen)	1.0 meV
He (helium)	2.6 meV
^{4}He (helium 4)	7.1 meV
^{6}Li (lithium 6)	5.2 meV
^{20}Ne (neon 20)	8.0 meV
^{70}Ga (gallium 70)	8.7 meV
^{240}U (uranium 240)	7.6 meV

The force increases gradually from elements with atomic weight 20 to those with atomic weight 70, and decreases gradually from elements with atomic weight 70 to those with atomic weight 240. Total understanding of these forces that bind together the nuclear particles remains for the future. It is probable that the protons and neutrons exhibit a constant *milling* motion. If this probability is true, it is equally probable that the binding force derives from continuous and extremely rapid exchange of subnuclear particles such as the pi mesons.*

Under normal conditions, the atom is electrically neutral. There is normally one electron in orbit for each proton in the nucleus. Circumstances often alter the structure and stability of

*Physicists have observed and studied additional subatomic and subnuclear particles including pi mesons, mu mesons, heavy mesons, and hyperons. The rest mass of mesons is compared with that of the electron, and the rest mass of the hyperon is compared with that of the proton. Since these particles do not enter into present considerations of radiologic technology, no discussion of their properties is necessary.

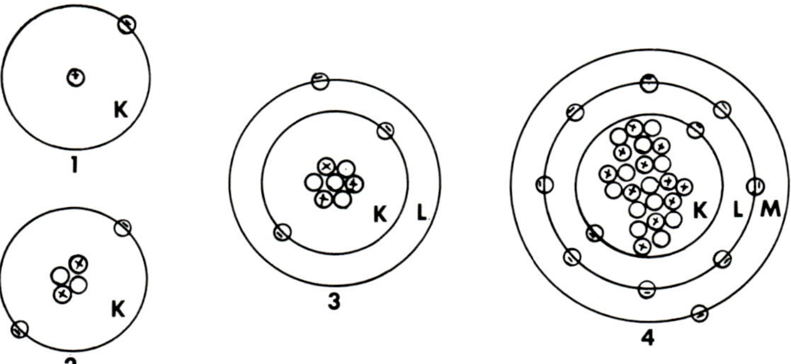

Fig. 2-1. Diagrams of atomic structure. **1**, Hydrogen, with one proton in the nucleus and one electron in the *K* orbit. **2**, Helium, with two protons and two neutrons in the nucleus and two electrons in the *K* orbit. **3**, Lithium, with three protons and four neutrons in the nucleus, two electrons in the *K* orbit, and one electron in the *L* orbit. **4**, Sodium, with eleven protons and twelve neutrons in the nucleus, two electrons in the *K* orbit, eight electrons in the *L* orbit, and one electron in the *M* orbit.

atoms. A deficiency of one or more electrons will render the atom electrically positive, due to the excess of positive charges in the nucleus. A surplus of orbital electrons renders the atom electrically negative because more negative charges exist in the orbits than positive charges in the nucleus. *When an atom either gains or loses one or more electrons, the atom becomes ionized and is either a negative ion or a positive ion.*

The periodic table* is an orderly arrangement of the elements according to increasing number of protons within the nucleus. In this table the elements are in eight vertical *groups* according to family and seven horizontal *periods* according to the increasing atomic number. The *atomic number*† *is the number of protons within the nucleus. The atomic weight is the sum of the number of protons plus the number of neutrons.* In the periodic table, hydrogen is the first element. Hydrogen, a gas, has one proton as its nucleus and one electron in orbit. Since a single proton comprises the entire nucleus of the hydrogen atom, both the atomic number and the atomic weight are 1.

From inside to outside, the labels of the orbits are K, L, M, N, O, P, and Q. Compared to the size of the nucleus, there is an enormous distance between the K orbit and the nucleus and between each two orbits. The orbits are frequently referred to as energy levels because certain measurable quantities of energy are required to move an electron from an orbit near the nucleus to one farther away or to remove an electron entirely from the atom. The electron of the hydrogen atom orbits in the K energy level.

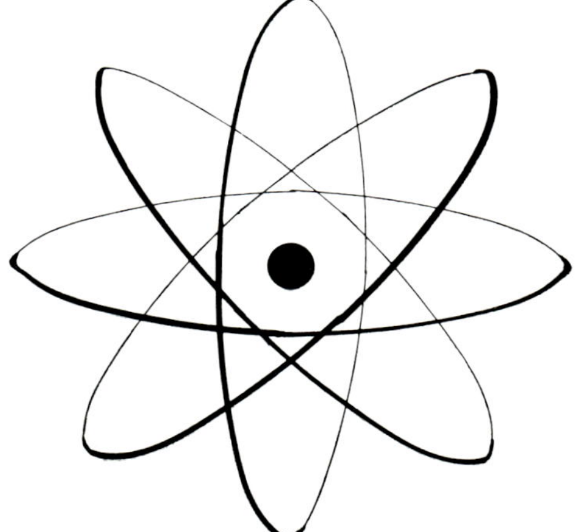

Fig. 2-2. Diagram of one of the modern concepts of atomic structure. Each electron radius is approximately equal in length to all other electron radii in the atom.

Helium, a gas and the second element in the periodic table, has atomic number 2 and atomic weight 4. This indicates the presence of two protons and two neutrons in the helium nucleus. The two electrons of the helium atom orbit in the K energy level. (See Figs. 2-1 and 2-2.)

A major consideration in radiologic technology is the physical nature of tungsten. Tungsten has

*See Appendix for list of elements.

†This is the number that determines the chemical nature of the atom.

atomic number 74 and atomic weight 184. It therefore has 74 protons and 110 neutrons in its nucleus. The orbits require varying numbers of electrons. The arrangement of the 74 electrons in their respective orbits, from inside to outside, is as follows: K-2, L-8, M-18, N-32, 0-12, and P-2.

ELECTRICITY AND MAGNETISM

Electricity

By definition electricity is one of the fundamental quantities in nature, consisting of elementary particles, electrons, and protons. An important characteristic of electricity is that it gives rise to a field of force possessing potential energy. When electricity moves in a particular direction, it constitutes an electric current that gives rise to a magnetic field of force with which kinetic energy is associated. *Electricity classifies as a form of energy because it can perform work.*

Electricity may be of direct current (d.c.) when continuously flowing in a single direction, or of alternating current (a.c.) when alternate pulses flow in opposing directions. Although hydroelectric and steam generators are the principal sources of alternating current,* electricity is produced through *magnetism, chemical reaction,* and *friction.*

Electricity is said to exist wherever electrons are in motion. Since all electrons are alike and bear an electric charge of negative sign and since all protons are alike and bear an electric charge of positive sign and these charges are of equal magnitude (see p. 50), the charge on one electron exactly neutralizes the charge on one proton, regardless of their respective masses.

Since electrons are rather loosely attracted in the outer orbits of atoms, some of these electrons may be removed by friction or other strong, positive attractions. When a silk cloth is rubbed on a glass rod, the silk becomes negatively charged and the glass rod takes on a positive charge. This is the result of electrons being removed from the glass rod by friction and collected in excess on the silk cloth. A deficiency of electrons exists on the glass rod following this procedure. The negative electric charge on the silk cloth can be neutralized by again placing the glass rod in contact with the silk cloth. In fact, the negative charge (excess of electrons) causes the silk to be attracted by the positively charged glass rod, and when it is pulled back to the rod, a neutral condition is produced.

In certain instances the opposite effect occurs. When a flannel cloth is rubbed on an ebony rod, the electrons flow from the flannel to the ebony. As a result the flannel cloth exhibits a positive electric charge (deficiency of electrons), and the ebony rod exhibits a negative electric charge (excess of electrons).

An electrical conductor is a substance capable of readily transmitting electricity, heat, or the like. Some of the better electrical conductors (in order of decreasing conductivity) are silver, copper, gold, aluminum, zinc, platinum, iron, nickel, tin, lead, antimony, mercury, and bismuth. All substances are conductors to varying degrees; that is, there are both good and poor conductors of electricity, and there are no nonconductors of electricity. Contaminated oil and contaminated water are better conductors of electricity than are their pure counterparts.

When electrons are caused or permitted to flow along a conductor, a current of electricity is said to move along that conductor. If a bar of copper and a bar of zinc are placed vertically in a glass or rubber cylinder, the lower halves of each are immersed in sulfuric acid, copper wires are attached to the exposed end of each bar, and a galvanometer, which is an instrument for measuring electric current, is attached to the free ends of the two wires, all the conditions necessary for the production of a flow of electric current and its measurement are present. (See Fig. 2-3.) It will be noted that the galvanometer needle is always deflected in the same direction because the flow of current is always in this same direction. This

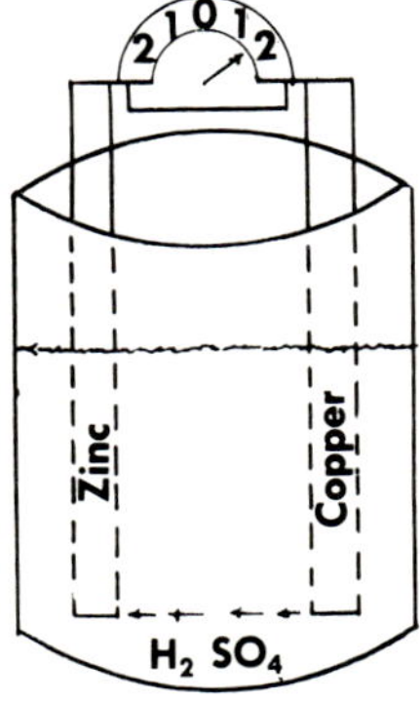

Fig. 2-3. Wet-cell battery. Electron flow is from the negative zinc to the positive copper, making direct current with a positive (right) deflection of the galvanometer needle.

*Generation of electricity through use of nuclear energy is increasingly important.

type of electricity is *direct current.* In this example, a current of electricity flows because the sulfuric acid attacks the zinc and releases negative electrons, zinc sulfate, and hydrogen ions. The electrons move along the zinc to the conductor through the galvanometer and to the copper, where they combine with the hydrogen ions to form hydrogen gas. Note that the number of electrons remains constant in this system but that the chemical reaction releases energy.

An electric current will flow along a conductor whenever a difference in potential (voltage) between two connected points exists. *Electric current may be defined as the rate of flow of electrons along a conductor. The potential difference across or between two points or terminals is known as electromotive force (emf) and is measured in volts.* A difference in potential exists if there is a difference in electron pressure at any two points in the conductor; *emf is also measured in volts and is defined as that which causes a flow of current.*

The emf of a circuit is considered to be the total voltage of the circuit—also, the potential drop across the entire circuit. Electrons will leave a point of low positive charge and travel to a point of high positive charge.

Because the quantity of charge on an electron is very small, it is impossible to detect it by ordinary current-detecting meters. For this reason a larger unit of electric charge is generally used. *This larger unit is called a coulomb and equals the charge on* 63×10^{18} *electrons.* The ampere is the unit used to measure the rate of flow of electricity. *An ampere is a flow of one coulomb per second.* The unit of current is the ampere. Alternatively, *a coulomb is the total quantity of electricity that moves when a current of one ampere flows for exactly one second.* The term ampere-seconds is often used to describe the amount and duration of electric flow.

Just as water flowing through a pipe must overcome the frictional resistance offered by the walls of the pipe, electricity must overcome an electric resistance tending to restrict the passage of electrons along a conductor. *The unit of electric resistance is the ohm. An ohm is the resistance equal to the resistance of a column of mercury having a mass of 14.4521 grams, a uniform cross section of approximately one square millimeter, and a length of 106.3 cm at 0° C.* Ohm's law states: *the current strength in any conductor varies directly as the electromotive force and inversely as the resistance.*

A current of electricity will flow along a conductor because of the emf, but there must be sufficient pressure to overcome the inherent resistance. Greater resistance to the flow of electric current is encountered along a wire of small diameter than is encountered along a wire of large diameter, since the current flows on the outside surface of the wire. A wire of small diameter and short length offers less resistance to the flow of electric current than will a greater length of the same wire.

The previous paragraphs have presented some of the fundamental units of electricity; the volt is the unit of pressure, the ampere is the unit of current, the ohm is the unit of resistance, and the coulomb is the unit of electric charge. A given current will be caused to move along a wire through a given resistance as a result of the pressure of a given voltage. The formula $E = IR$, where E is the electromotive force in volts, I is the current in amperes, and R is the resistance in ohms, expresses this condition. Electric power (rate of doing work) is rated in units called watts. *Watts are the product of volts and amperes.* Electric work is stated in units such as watt-seconds, watt-hours, or kilowatt-hours, which are obtained by multiplying the power in watts by a convenient unit of time. As an example we may state that a given x-ray machine is supplied with 220 volts and 50 amperes. If maximum amperage is used in a given exposure, 11,000 watts will be drawn (used). To find the quantity (ohms) of resistance to the flow of current in this example, divide the 220 volts by the 50 amps; the result is 4.4 ohms.

To obtain certain desired results in using electric currents it is often necessary to *store* electricity for later use at a given instant of time. Instruments designed for this purpose are called condensers or capacitors. The condenser can store a specific charge, whereas a capacitor can store variable charges. A condenser may consist of a unit of two conductive plates separated by a dielectric with appropriate positive and negative connections in the completed circuit. When such an instrument is a capacitor, the plates can be moved to either increase or decrease the space between them.

Alternating current

There are two kinds of current electricity, direct current (d.c.), which we have discussed and alternating current (a.c.). The basic laws and units that relate to direct current also hold for alternating current.

Direct current is a flow of electrons in a single

direction. Alternating current is a flow of electrons in one direction immediately followed by a flow in the opposite direction. Alternating current has proved more efficient than direct current in transmission over great distances, and more easily distributed where used. Most of the electricity used in modern industry and homes is transmitted as alternating current and converted locally to direct current if required. When compared with a d.c. system, the advantages of an a.c. system are numerous and quite evident because of the relative ease with which a.c. potential differences are generated, amplified, and otherwise transformed in magnitude.

If current is plotted against time, alternating current exhibits a characteristic rising and falling curve that, when projected as a graph, approximates a *sine wave. The number of complete cycles that occur each second is the frequency of the current.* A complete cycle includes the half cycle flowing in the positive direction and the half cycle flowing in the negative direction. (See Fig. 2-4.) The usual current supply in American cities is 60 cycles a second. The amplitude of excursion, that is, the distance from the median line to either zenith, is the voltage or driving force of the current in Fig. 2-4.

It is necessary to use high voltage to conduct an alternating current efficiently over long distances. High voltage results when the alternating current passes through a step-up transformer. At distribution points, which supply houses and industrial establishments where voltage requirements are usually much lower, the alternating current passes through a step-down transformer; the result is reduced voltage and increased available amperage.

A single alternating current is termed a *single-phase* current (Fig. 2-4). In a *three-phase* system, three currents flow, differing in phase from each other by 120 degrees (Fig. 2-5). Early in the latter half of this century the use of three-phase generators to obtain increased output from the same values of kilovoltage, milliamperage,

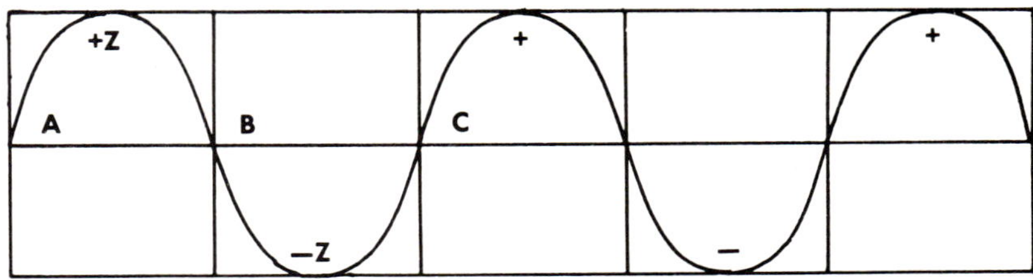

Fig. 2-4. Sine wave diagram. Between *A* and *C* there is one complete cycle. From *A* to *B* the current flows in a positive direction; from *B* to *C* the current flows in a negative direction. In 1 second there are 60 complete cycles, as from *A* to *C*, which contain a total of 60 positive half cycles and 60 negative half cycles. This diagram also represents the flow of an alternating current. The current rises from zero voltage at *A* to its maximum positive peak (the positive zenith) at +Z, falls back to zero at *B*, rises to the negative peak at −Z, and falls back to zero at *C*.

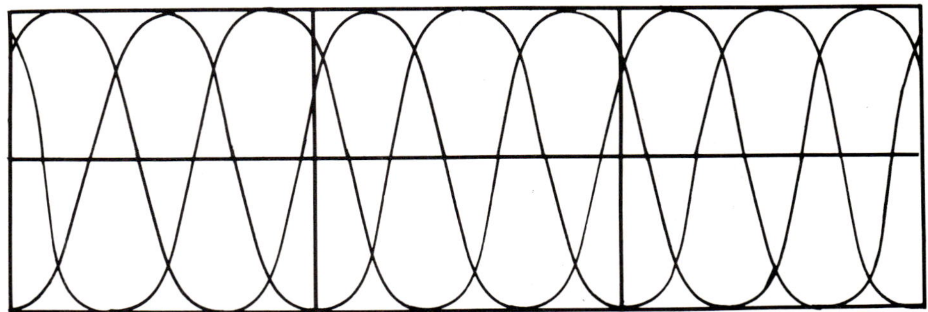

Fig. 2-5. Diagram of three-phase system. Above the center line, or the positive pulse side, there are three peaks; center peak can represent the single peak in a single-phase diagram.

and time increased remarkably. Use of three-phase current results in higher tube loading per exposure and, of great importance, *reduces* the necessary patient skin dose!

X-ray machine circuits require several voltages, which are furnished from the supply line. The supply line voltage is transformed in the x-ray machine according to requirements. To understand the principles involved in transforming alternating current, some knowledge of magnetism is necessary.

Magnets and magnetism

Magnetic ores were first discovered more than 600 years ago, probably in Magnesia, a country in what was formerly named Asia Minor. Presently this name applies to a small region in southwestern Turkey. The word magnet is derived from both Latin and Greek origins and means a stone (or metal) that exhibits the appearance of silver and that attracts other like stones and iron. By definition, *a magnet is a piece of magnetite or magnetic ore that possesses the natural property of attracting iron.*

A piece of soft iron may become a magnet under certain conditions and is always used as the core of an electromagnet. If the iron is in bar form, the magnetic properties will be demonstrated as in Fig. 2-6. If a bar magnet is placed beneath a sheet of paper and iron filings are sprinkled on top of the paper, the iron filings will fall on the paper in the pattern of the "lines of force" exerted by the magnet.

If two magnetized bars are suspended so that each may move freely and the magnets are brought close to each other, it will be noticed that one or both magnets will always swing about so that a particular end of one magnet seeks a particular end of the other. This is because the magnetic lines have direction that gives the magnets north-seeking and south-seeking poles. *Like poles repel and unlike poles attract.* When a magnet is broken into two pieces, each part is a magnet. Each molecule of a magnetizable body, such as iron, is itself a magnet. Therefore magnetiza-

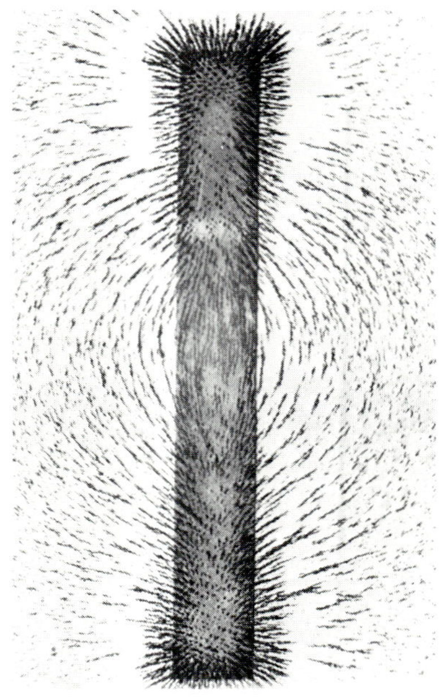

Fig. 2-6. Iron filings sprinkled on a clear surface and falling in the magnetic lines of force surrounding the magnet.

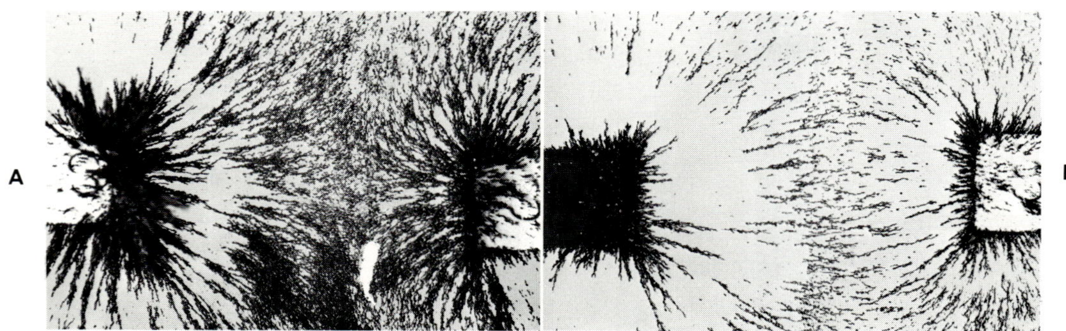

Fig. 2-7. A, Iron filings sprinkled heavily on the south poles of two magnets and between the two poles. Filings fall in the patterns of the two magnetic fields, showing repelling forces of two like poles. **B,** Iron filings sprinkled lightly on the north pole of one magnet and the south pole of a second magnet and between the two poles. Filings fall in the patterns of the two magnetic fields, showing attracting forces of two unlike poles.

tion is essentially the nearly parallel arrangement of the molecular magnets of a given magnetizable body. This experimental evidence demonstrates that there are actually lines of force in a particular pattern about any magnet. (See Fig. 2-7.)

These lines of force are properly called *flux lines.* They also form around a wire when a current of electricity flows along it. The direction of the flux lines and of the flow of the electrical current follow the *left-hand rule;* that is, when the wire is grasped in the left hand with the left thumb extending in the direction of the flow of the electrons, the left fingers point in the direction of the flux lines.

The preceding information is easily demonstrated by passing a bare copper wire through the center of a piece of thin paper or clear plastic and connecting the two ends of the copper wire

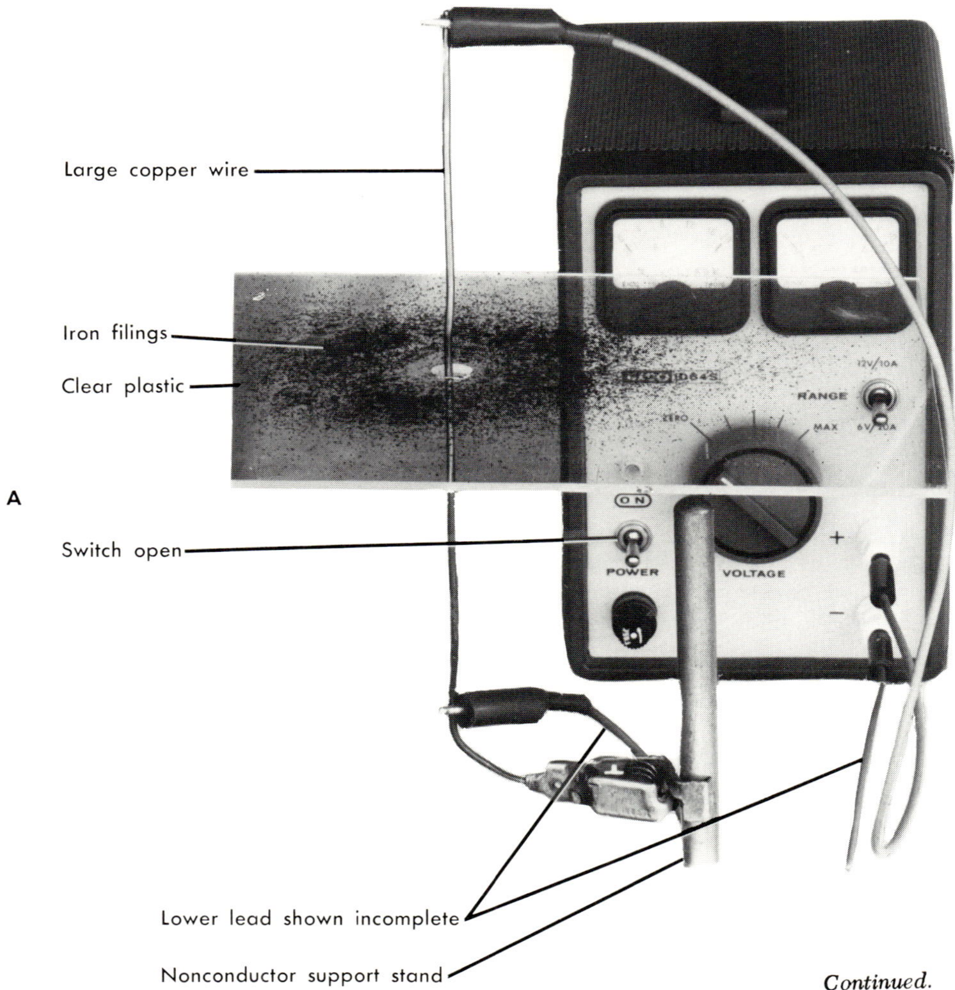

Continued.

Fig. 2-8. A, Iron filings sprinkled on piece of clear plastic surrounding a copper wire. The two ends of the copper wire are connected to a strong d.c. source with the power switched off. Filings have fallen in no particular pattern. **B,** Same apparatus as in **A,** but with the d.c. source switched on. Volts are approximately 1½, and amps are approximately 18. Plastic plate was tapped slightly after the current was switched on, and filings have taken the pattern of the flux lines surrounding the copper wire. **C,** Same apparatus as in **A** and **B,** but with the terminals connecting to the ends of the copper wire reversed. Again the power was switched on, and the plastic plate was tapped slightly; filings have taken a slightly different pattern of the flux lines (in the opposite direction) surrounding the copper wire.

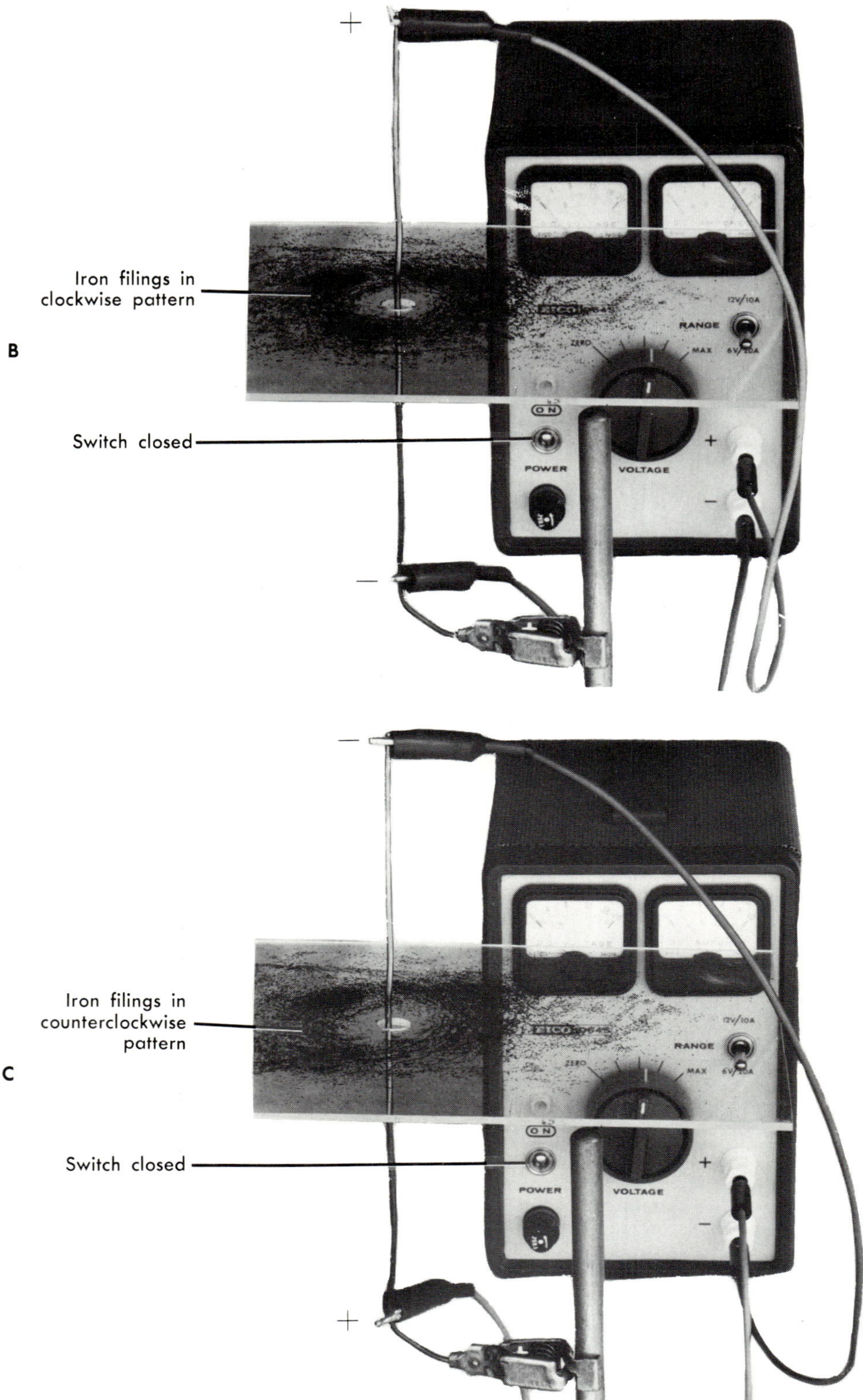

Fig. 2-8, cont'd. For legend see p. 29.

to the terminals of a strong d.c. source (15 to 20 amps). After the connections are made and the current is flowing, sprinkle some iron filings on the paper or plastic near the copper wire; the iron filings will fall in the pattern of the flux lines. If the battery terminals are reversed, new iron filings sprinkled on the paper or plastic will assume a somewhat different pattern. (See Fig. 2-8.)

Transformers

A transformer is an electric device that either steps up (increases) or steps down (decreases) the incoming voltage.

If a copper wire, the free ends of which are attached to a galvanometer, is moved through a magnetic field so that the lines of force are cut by the wire, a deflection of the hand of the galvanometer will occur. If the movement of the wire is in the opposite direction, the deflection of the galvanometer hand will also be in the opposite direction. This process is one of inducing a current of electricity to flow along a conductor—the process of *electromagnetic induction.*

As stated earlier, magnetic lines of force exist around any wire along which an electric current is flowing. If a second wire is placed parallel with and near to a wire conducting an alternating current, an alternating current of electricity will be caused to flow along the second wire; the alternations will be of equal duration but opposite in direction to the inducing current. *This is the principle of mutual induction* and is the process used in most transformers to change or alter the incoming alternating current.

Experimental evidence demonstrates that alternating current flowing in a coil will induce a second alternating current to flow in the opposite direction in a second coil placed within the field of the first coil. This induced current is even stronger when the two coils surround a soft iron core. When such magnetic cores are placed in a magnetic field, they increase the number of magnetic lines and thereby improve transformer efficiency. Fig. 2-9 is a diagram of a twowinding transformer; such transformers operate on the principle of *mutual induction.* Mutual induction is that which is produced on each other by two adjacent circuits. Each of the five turns of the wire on the side N_1 produces its specific number of lines of flux that surround (and cut) the turns (windings) of wire on side N_2 during the time that a current of electricity flows along the wire of side N_1. Since there are twice as many turns on side N_2 as on side N_1, and disregarding inherent losses within the transformer, approximately twice as much voltage will be delivered from side N_2 as was delivered to side N_1. Some of the inherent losses result from the induction on side N_1 from the *induced* current flowing through side N_2.

Transformers and transformer capacities and types may be classified according to ratio. The ratio of a transformer reveals whether the transformer is a step-up or a step-down type and how much it changes the incoming voltage. *The ratio is determined by dividing the number of windings in the incoming (primary) coil by the number of windings in the outgoing (secondary) coil.* Thus if a transformer has one winding in the incoming coil and two windings in the outgoing coil, the transformer ratio is 1:2 and the trans-

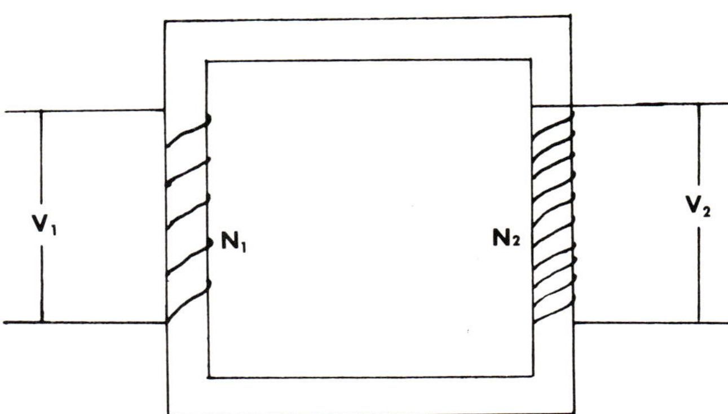

Fig. 2-9. A two-winding transformer. This is a step-up transformer with a 1:2 ratio. (The electrical symbols used throughout the text are copied with kind permission from the American standard graphical symbols for electrical diagrams, approved March 29, 1954, courtesy Institute of Radio Engineers, Inc.)

former is a step-up type. This transformer will deliver *approximately* twice as much voltage as was delivered to it. If the windings were reversed, the transformer would be a step-down type and would deliver *approximately* one half the voltage delivered to it. Voltage is delivered *to* the incoming coil and delivered *from* the outgoing coil of a transformer. If there are more turns on the outgoing side, the transformer is a step-up transformer. Conversely, if there are fewer turns on the outgoing side, the transformer is a step-down transformer.

The outgoing power (watts) cannot exceed the incoming power (watts) and is actually less in quantity due to hysteresis,* eddy current losses,† resistance, and other factors. In ordinary loads the transformer loss usually will not exceed 5%, but in high-voltage transformers, such as those used in x-ray machines, the loss is much greater.

In an x-ray machine, the *autotransformer* is the *kilovoltage selector;* it supplies the primary side of the high-voltage transformer with the predetermined voltage, and operates on the principle of *self-induction.* Self-induction is the inducing of an electromotive force in a circuit by a varying current in the same circuit. The autotransformer consists of a single wire wrapped around a soft iron core. The free ends of the single wire connect to the incoming supply line. A series of taps, for selection of output voltages, is on the side opposite to the primary source. The single wire serves as both the incoming and outgoing coils of the transformer. The output may be determined from the following: *The voltage maintained between the minimum side of the transformer and the outgoing tap selected is in the same ratio to the total incoming voltage as the number of windings between the minimum side and the selected outgoing tap is to the total number of windings.* This statement is expressed in the following proportion: $x{:}V{:}{:}n{:}N$; where x is the voltage delivered from the autotransformer, V is the supply line voltage, n is the number of windings between the minimum side (A) and the selected output tap (B), and N is the total number of windings between the minimum side (A) and the maximum side (C) (Fig. 2-10); that is, $x{:}110 : : 16{:}20$; $20x = 1{,}760$; $x = 88$ volts delivered at B. The maximum kilovoltage (**kVp**) obtained may be determined in the following manner. Multiply the volts delivered at B by the reciprocal of the high-voltage transformer ratio and divide the result by 1,000. For example, when high-voltage transformer ratio is 1:500,

$$(88)\left(\frac{1}{\frac{1}{500}}\right) = 44{,}000, \text{ and } \frac{44{,}000}{1{,}000} = 44 \text{ kVp}.$$

The autotransformer may be designed as a step-down transformer or a step-down-step-up transformer by extending the number of wind-

*Hysteresis is a lagging or retardation of the effect.

†An eddy current is an induced electric current circulating wholly within a mass of metal. Such currents are converted into heat, thus causing serious waste.

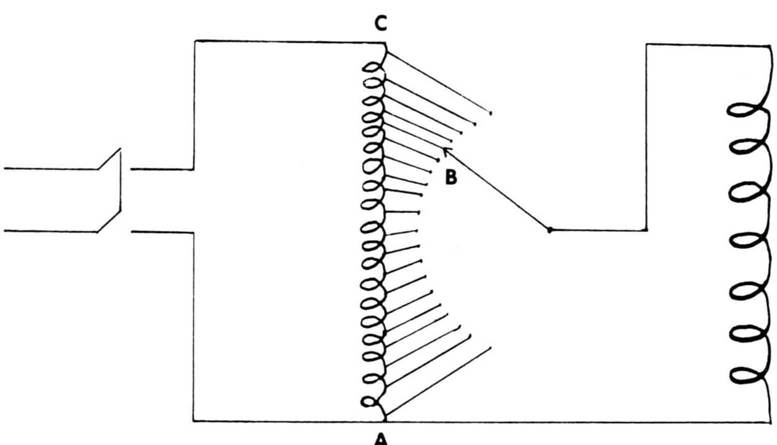

Fig. 2-10. Autotransformer. Supply line furnishes 110 volts. There are 20 windings between *A* and *C* and 16 windings between *A* and *B*. Eighty-eight volts will be delivered to the primary side (incoming side) of the high-voltage transformer from the autotransformer.

ings beyond the maximum side. Fig. 2-10 is a diagram of the step-down type of autotransformer.

BASIC CIRCUITRY OF RADIOGRAPHIC MACHINES

In this era of modern technology the profession of radiology experiences both numerous and rapid changes, among which is the change from single-phase to three-phase x-ray generators. This change makes possible (and necessary) numerous changes in equipment and accessories, all of which enable the production of radiographs of increased diagnostic quality, improved patient care through new radiological procedures, and an increase in patient flow in the department. However the majority of single-phase units over three-phase units in use dictates that this basic textbook continue the simplified explanations of single-phase circuitry, and to add sufficient information regarding the more sophisticated equipment for basic understanding by students and practicing technologists.

A common power supply in most modern buildings has available either single-phase or three-phase current. The single-phase current is usually of 60 cycles per second; three-phase current (from this source) will have 180 cycles per second. The voltage supply (if single-phase) will be either 110-120 or 220-240. Greater power economy is effected by use of three-phase power distribution systems. A common potential between any two of the three principal conductors in a three-phase system is 208 volts.

The **power supply** line consists of either two or three wires; in either case, the voltage may be either 110 or 220. If there are three wires, the middle wire is neutral, and there are 110 volts between it and either of the other two wires, or 220 volts between the two outside wires.

X-ray (machine) generators employ many circuits for operation. Three of these circuits form the basis of all operation: the *primary,* or low-voltage, circuit; the *secondary,* or high-voltage, circuit; and the *filament,* or heating, circuit. However, all of the electricity used in operating the x-ray equipment is obtained from a single source, the supply line.

SINGLE-PHASE CURRENT AND (X-RAY) GENERATORS

Primary circuit

The primary circuit supplies the autotransformer, the primary side of the high-voltage transformer, the timing circuit, and the many other low-voltage circuits necessary for the operation of modern equipment.

A voltage load of 110-120 or 220-240 volts and an amperage load varying from 10 to 100 amperes, according to requirements, flow along the primary circuit. Further requirements of the primary supply are for alternating current, which is usually 60 cycles each second, that is, 60 positive half cycles and 60 negative half cycles. (See Fig. 2-4.)

When the primary switch on the x-ray machine control panel is closed, the following are activated by the primary current: line-voltage regulator and meter, autotransformer, prereading voltmeter (kilovolt meter), ammeter (in older machines), milliampere selector, and filament transformer. Actually, the filament transformers of the valve tubes are also activated at this time.

Since the prereading voltmeter is designed to read in kilovolts and since the technologist must know and select the kilovoltage value prior to exposure, it is obvious that this meter must be connected in the primary circuit with the autotransformer (kilovolt selector) and before the timing circuit.

After the exposure time is selected on the timer and when the timing or exposure switch is closed, the current from the primary circuit passes through this switch, through the magnetic contactor, through the primary side of the high-voltage (x-ray) transformer, and through the circuit breaker. (See Fig. 2-13.)

The supply line voltage is fused at the primary switch. The *primary switch* permits the supply line voltage to enter the primary circuit when the switch is closed. This switch is usually mounted on the control panel and labeled the *line switch.*

The *line voltage regulator* is a part of the primary side of the autotransformer and regulates the incoming voltage. The *line voltage meter* is in parallel with the supply line and shows the voltage delivered to the autotransformer. In some equipment there is a *prereading kilovolt meter* in parallel with the autotransformer between it and the primary side of the high-voltage transformer. The purpose of this meter is to register, prior to exposure, what kilovoltage will be delivered during the exposure. Such a meter requires factory precalibration.

The *circuit breaker* is in series with the exposure switch and magnetic contactor. The timer circuit includes the timer, magnetic contactor, and hand or foot (exposure) switch. The circuit breaker functions to ensure against overload of the delicate equipment of the x-ray machine (pp.

41 and 42), since it may be set to *break* at any desired load; it is quite easily reset.

The *autotransformer* was discussed on pp. 32 and 33.

The *oil-immersed magnetic contactor* acts as a heavy current relay and is actuated by the small current flowing through the hand switch and timer. This condition reduces the danger of shock to the operator and the electrolysis at the contact points, which regulate the heavy current. Closure of the *exposure switch* causes the magnetic contactor to close and complete the circuit to the primary side of the high-voltage transformer.

Timers are incorporated into the x-ray machine to initiate timing and to terminate the exposure. Timers connect, in the primary circuit, to the primary side of the high-voltage transformer. At least three types of timers are commonly used—synchronous, impulse, and electronic. Some manufactures incorporate a synchronous timer and an impulse timer into the same x-ray machine to permit a wider range of accuracy in exposure time. Others combine an electronic timer and an impulse timer for this purpose. A *synchronous timer* is operated by a synchronous motor. The usual range of exposure time for this type is 1/20 second to 20 seconds. An *impulse timer* is operated by impulses of current passing through the timing circuit; there are 60 current impulses each second in half-wave rectified equipment and 120 current impulses each second in full-wave rectified equipment. The usual range of exposure time for this type is 1/120 or 1/60 second to 1/5 second. The impulse timer is quite accurate because the exposure is initiated and terminated at, or very close to, the zero point of the alternating current cycle. The *electronic timer* is operated by means of a series of electronic tubes and relays and is useful over a range of exposures. The minimum exposure time is 1/30 second. Fourteen seconds is a common maximum exposure time. Another method of controlling exposure time uses the *triode valve tube*. This method of timing exposures involves withholding current between the outside (end) plates of the tube until the negative bias* of the middle (third) plate has been overcome by a predetermined voltage stored in a condenser. As a timer, the triode tube is useful in rapid-fire exposures in angiocardiography and other highly specialized radiographic procedures where many exposures are required each minute.

*Bias is the direct voltage in the grid circuit of an electron tube.

There are several conditions under which the timer may either fail completely or function improperly. If the timer accuracy is in question, a spinning top (Fig. 2-11) should be used to check the actual length of exposure with that of the selected time. The factors to use for spinning top radiographs are 60 to 65 kVp, 50 or 100 mA, 0.1 second, and a 30- or 40-inch ffd. No less than five exposures should be averaged for final evaluation. Since there are 120 current impulses in full-wave rectified current, there should be 12 exposure dots on the radiograph in 0.1 second; with 60 impulses in half-wave rectified current, there should be six exposure dots on the radiograph in 0.1 second.

The radiographic density of the dots should be equal in degree. In full-wave rectified units, alternate light and dark dots may indicate either of two conditions: faulty valve tubes or faulty Thyrx timer tubes.

If the filament of valve tube 24A or 24B (Fig. 2-13) emits a quantity of electrons remarkably different from the quantity emitted by valve tube 24C or 24D, correspondingly different valve tube currents will occur in the alternate half-cycles of a given exposure; variations in valve tube current in this instance will cause corresponding variations in the emf of the secondary current.

A Thyrx timer requires a lead power Thyratron tube and a trail power Thyratron tube. If the valve tubes function correctly, it is logical to suspect the efficiency of the Thyratron power tubes. If the lead tube of this timer is faulty, the first, third, and all alternate dots will be light; if the trail tube is faulty, the second, fourth, and all alternate dots will be light. (See item 4, and item 8, p. 42.)

Phototiming, discussed on pp. 106 and 110 is used to obtain the same degree of radiographic density in sequence radiographs as in spot-film fluoroscopy and radiography and other procedures.

The *ammeter* is in series with the primary circuit to register the amperage load of the filament current. In older equipment and in some modern equipment, a certain selection of amperage prior to actual exposure will determine the value of the milliamperage (tube current). Most modern x-ray machines provide an automatic control of the tube current for different kilovoltage values, accomplished through the use of a space-charge compensator (pp. 35 and 52).

The *milliampere selector,* often called the *technique selector,* is in series with a *choke coil,* or rheostat, and the oil-immersed *filament transformer.* This transformer is a step-down trans-

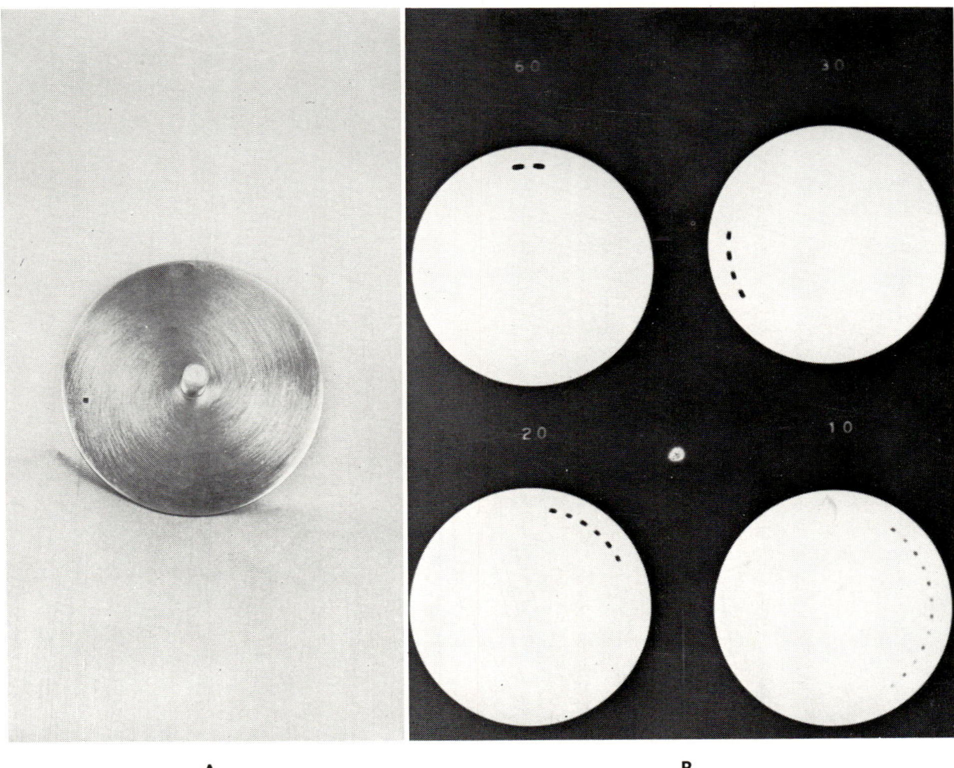

A B

Fig. 2-11. A spinning top is shown in **A.** Photographs of the spinning top in **B** show the following numbers of dots for corresponding times on a full-wave rectified unit: two dots, 1/60 sec; four dots, 1/30 sec; six dots 1/20 sec; and twelve dots, 1/10 sec.

former and supplies the filament of the x-ray tube with sufficient amperage to heat the filament. The filament transformer supplies a current that does not exceed 5 amperes at no more than 15 volts.

The choke coil is an electrical reactor and usually consists of a coil, winding, or conductor of small resistance and large inductance. The core of the coil is so connected to the milliampere selector that increases in milliamperage are obtained when the soft iron core is pulled farther out of the coil; decreases in milliamperage are obtained when the soft iron core is pushed farther into the coil. Such a device offers relatively accurate control over the tube current, especially when used in conjunction with a space-charge compensator.

In comparison with a choke coil, a rheostat is considerably less satisfactory. A rheostat is an electrical device by means of which variable amounts of resistance may be either placed in or removed from the circuit.

Secondary circuit

The secondary circuit begins and ends at the secondary side of the high-voltage transformer and conducts the high voltage used in the production of x rays.

The high voltage is induced in the secondary side of the high-voltage transformer by mutual induction from the primary voltage in the primary side of this same transformer (pp. 31 to 33). Since the primary voltage source is alternating current, it is obvious that the secondary voltage will be produced as an alternating current. Because the secondary voltage is alternating, this power supply must be rectified prior to entering the x-ray tube, since the production of x-rays in the hot cathode tube requires that the high voltage be *unidirectional,* that is, flowing from the cathode to the anode of the x-ray tube (pp. 36 to 38).

The secondary current flows through the following: secondary side of the high-voltage transformer, valve tubes, x-ray tube, and milliammeter. The exposure switch, located in the primary circuit, automatically controls the secondary voltage and current, since they are obtained by mutual induction. (See Fig. 2-13.)

The entire high-voltage transformer is oil-immersed to prevent shock.

The *milliammeter* in modern, shockproof equipment is in series in the high-voltage circuit, mounted in the control panel, and grounded at the midpoint of the secondary side of the high-voltage transformer. The milliammeter measures tube current averages, not the peak values, and registers only during exposure, that is, during the period of time the cathode electrons flow to the anode. *One milliampere is 1/1,000 of an ampere.*

In some modern equipment using tube currents in excess of 300 mA, a *milliampere-second* meter is in series with the *milliammeter.* This meter registers the total milliampere-seconds used in any one exposure. A red signal warning light is usually in series with the milliampere-second meter. The warning light flashes on when the exposure is made, to call attention to the number of milliampere-seconds employed, so that if the selection is great enough to overload the x-ray tube, the operator can terminate the exposure.

The milliampere-second meter also provides a more accurate registration of the true value of the milliamperage during very short exposures.

Filament circuit

The primary circuit supplies current to the filament circuit, which is frequently called the *heating circuit.* The filament transformer induces the heating current, which flows through the cathode of the x-ray tube. The heating current for the valve-tube cathodes arises from the appropriate valve-tube transformer in the generator; the current to the primary side of this transformer originates from a fixed position on the autotransformer. The current functions to produce sufficient heat in the cathode filaments to enable the secondary current through thermionic emission (p. 50 and Fig. 3-5), to flow across the terminals of the valve and x-ray tubes. (See Fig. 2-13.) The cathode filament of the x-ray tube, when heated, is the source of electrons for the tube current (milliamperage) of the secondary current.

Rectification

Rectification is the restriction of the flow of current to a particular direction; that is, the flow of current in each half cycle is in a direction useful in the production of x rays.

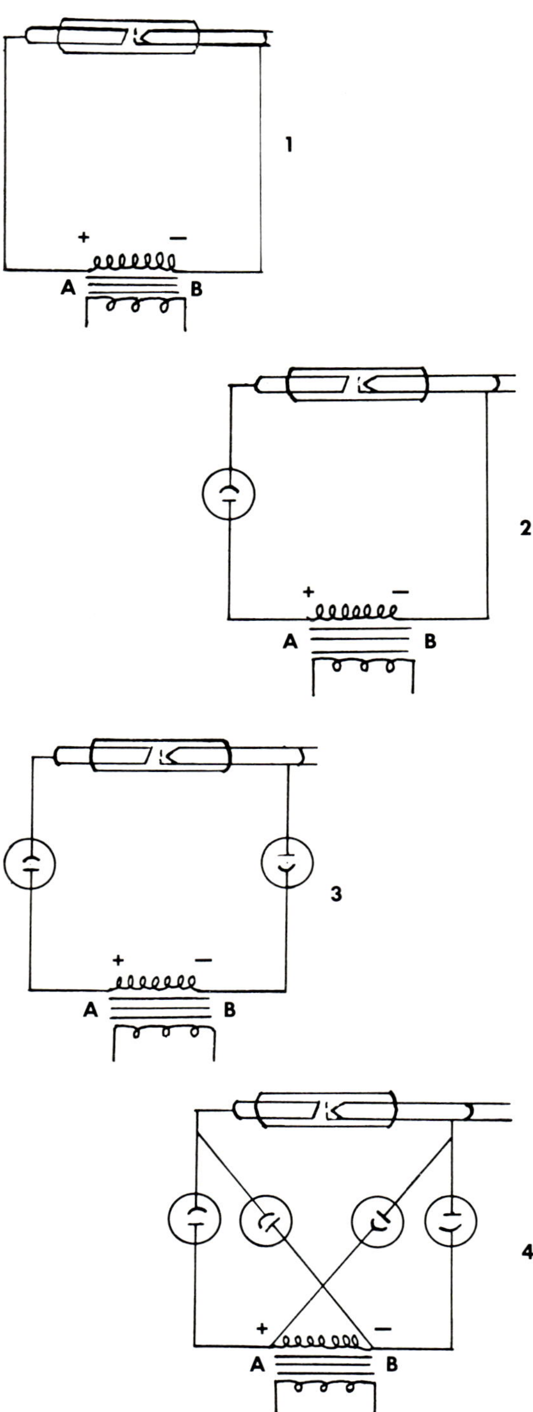

Fig. 2-12. Diagrams of rectification circuitry. **1,** Self-rectification. **2,** Half-wave rectification, one valve tube. **3,** Half-wave rectification, two valve tubes. **4,** Full-wave rectification, four valve tubes.

Rectification may be achieved by use of the x-ray tube alone. In such an instance, the rectification is called *self-rectification.* This type is satisfactory in limited circumstances and is a form of half-wave rectification. In general, rectification is classified as either *half-wave* or *full-wave.* Fig. 2-12 presents diagrams of the current flow in a self-rectified circuit and of the current flow in both half-wave and full-wave rectified circuits.

In the operation of self-rectified or half-wave rectified equipment, *only half the current impulses* produce x rays. Current can flow only from the cathode to the anode. Consequently, current flowing in the opposite direction is blocked.

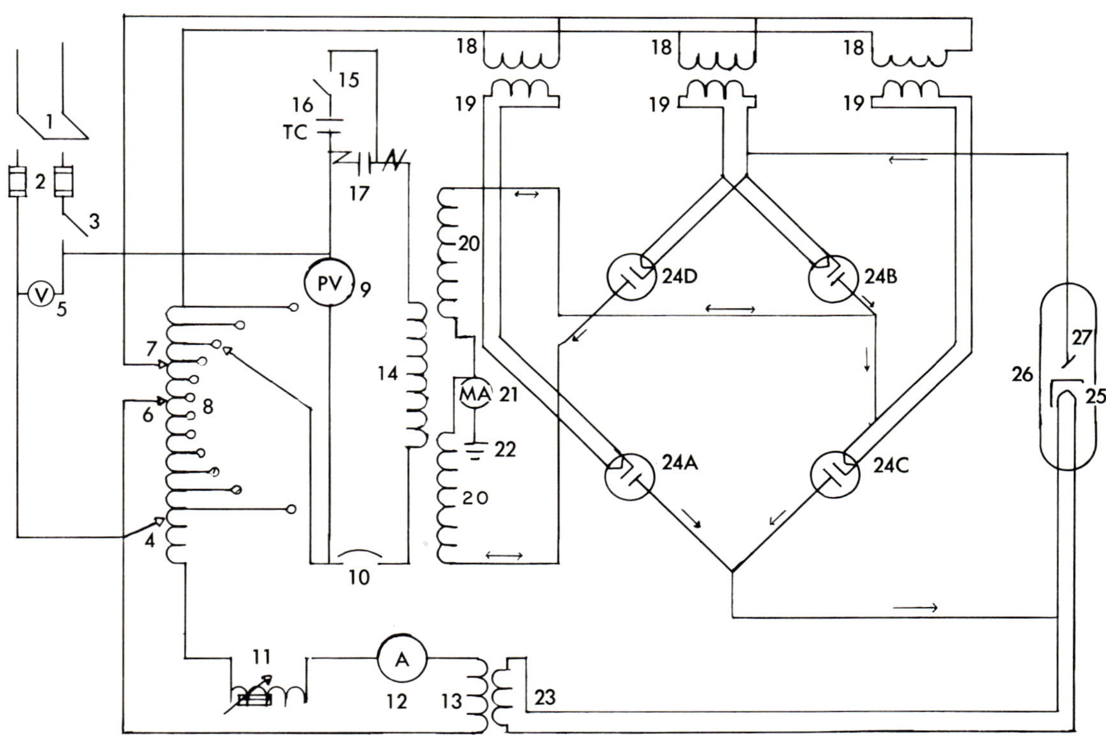

Fig. 2-13. X-ray machine circuitry with full-wave rectification.

1. Power switch
2. Fuses
3. Primary switch
4. Line volt regulator
5. Line volt meter
6. Fixed connection for x-ray tube filament transformer
7. Fixed connection for valve tube filament transformers
8. Autotransformer (kilovolt selector)
9. Prereading volt meter (kilovoltmeter)
10. Circuit breaker
11. Choke coil (milliampere selector)
12. Filament ammeter (present in older machines)
13. Primary side of x-ray tube filament transformer
14. Primary side of high-voltage transformer
15. Exposure switch
16. Timer to close circuit
17. Magnetic contactor
18. Primary sides of valve tube filament transformers
19. Secondary sides of valve tube filament transformers
20. Secondary side of high-voltage transformer
21. Milliammeter
22. Ground
23. Secondary side of x-ray tube filament transformer
24. Valve tubes (rectifier)
    A and **B** in first half-cycle
    C and **D** in second half-cycle
25. Cathode (filament) of x-ray tube
26. X-ray tube
27. Anode of x-ray tube

The cathode in full-wave rectified equipment receives *all the current impulses* from the same direction, thus permitting full current flow.

The valve tubes are in series with the rectifier circuit. There is a slight loss in the kilovoltage during travel from cathode to anode in a valve tube, primarily because the valve tube operates at less than saturation current. (See p. 52.) This loss seldom exceeds 3 kilovolts. Valve tubes are discussed on pp. 50 and 51.

Fig. 2-13 is a diagram of the basic circuits of a full-wave rectified x-ray machine.

THREE PHASE CURRENT AND (X-RAY) GENERATORS

Three-phase (polyphase) currents are generated in the same way as are single-phase currents. In a polyphase system its several single-phase components are displaced equally in time phase from one another. Thus the voltages and the currents of a three-phase system differ by 120 degrees in time sequence.

From pp. 36 to 38 we learn that full-wave rectification enables twice the number of pulses on the positive (upper) side in the diagram and

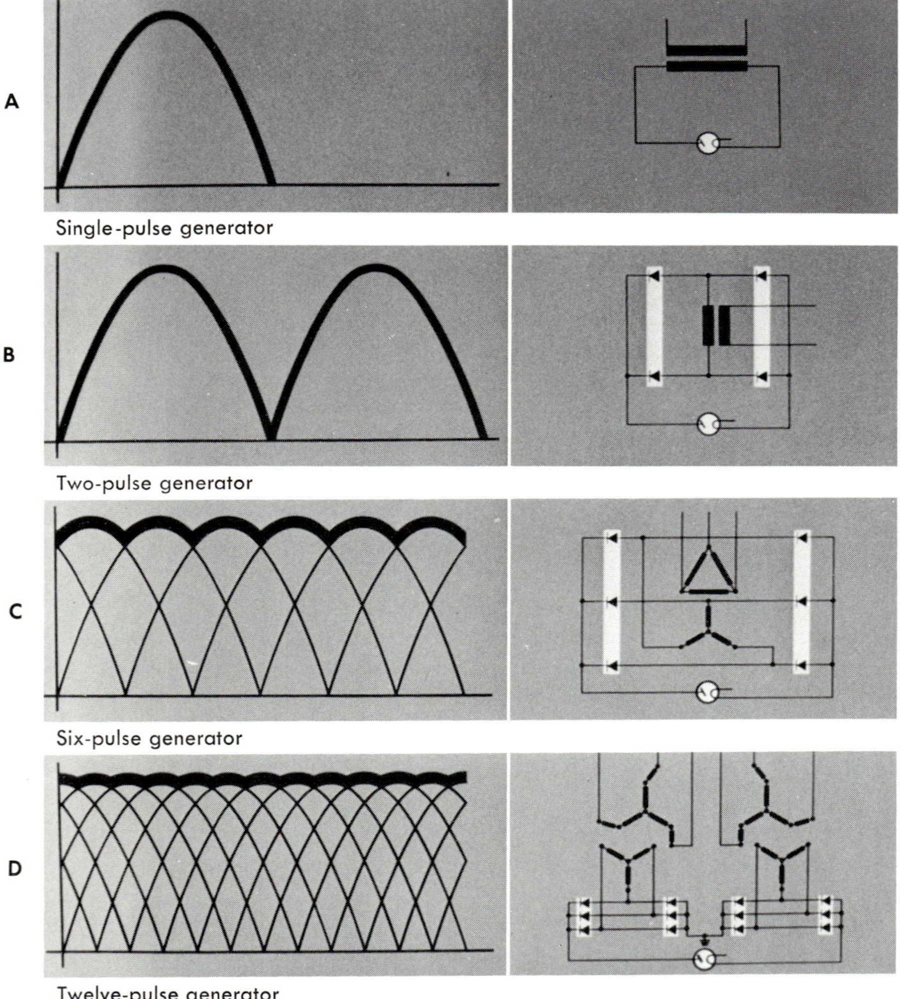

Fig. 2-14. Tube voltage and wiring schemes of diagnostic x-ray generators. **A,** Single-pulse generators; single useful pulse of a half-wave rectified, single-phase current. **B,** Two-pulse generator; two pulses used in a full-wave rectified, single-phase current. **C,** Six-pulse generator; six pulses used in a full-wave rectified, three-phase current. **D,** Twelve-pulse generator; special circuitry permits doubling six pulses as seen in **C.** (Courtesy Siemens Corp.)

actually makes available twice as many pulses of high voltage current for use in x-ray production. Fig. 2-14, *C*, is a diagram of three-phase, full-wave rectified, 60-cycle a.c.; in this diagram there are six positive pulses in each complete cycle. Furthermore, the voltage drop (sloping line) between each pulse (peak) and the subsequent minimum voltage is very slight. In a system of this type the voltage never drops to zero so a high voltage is maintained at all times; thus, harder rays are produced in greater quantity and from less total electrical energy input.

The combined components of the control panel and transformer comprise the x-ray generator. It is the work of this generator to supply the x-ray tube with the range of high voltages necessary to produce the desired quantity and quality of x rays emitted from the tube. A six-pulse generator delivers about 60% more energy to the x-ray tube than a two-pulse generator. It is obvious that radiography performed with three-phase units requires remarkably shorter exposure times than when performed with single-phase units. This results in radiographs having greater definition (sharpness).

In three-phase operation of a six-pulse generator the image-forming radiation is produced continuously. Twelve pulses may be obtained (as diagrammed in Fig. 2-14, *D*) from a six-pulse generator by means of special circuitry. Symmetrical voltage distribution is obtained by grounding the d.c. center point, thus ensuring the most favorable load conditions for the high-voltage cables and tube shield. This generator delivers nearly ideal constant potential (or tube voltage). Such potential has minimal ripple* that permits greater dose yield for a given application of electrical energy to the x-ray tube. (See Fig. 2-15 and Table 2-1.)

The remarkably greater energy delivered to the x-ray tube from polyphase generators requires rectification and timing of even greater precision than the energy from single-phase generators. The rectification must be accomplished in far less time, and the exposures are generally so short as to be possible only with electronic timers.

Rectifiers

Rectification of current for use in x-ray production has progressed from the original mechanical disks through valve tube arrangements into solid state rectifiers. An intermediate development between conventional valve tube rectifiers and solid state rectifiers incorporated a vacuum valve and selenium rectifier. This was followed with a solid state silicon rectifier. Using silicon provided several advantages over vacuum valve and selenium, one of which is that silicon rectifiers withstand far greater voltages than vacuum valve and

*Ripple voltage is the alternating component of unidirectional voltage from a rectifier or generator. The ripple (rise and fall) of voltage from six-pulse and twelve-pulse generators approaches a straight line.

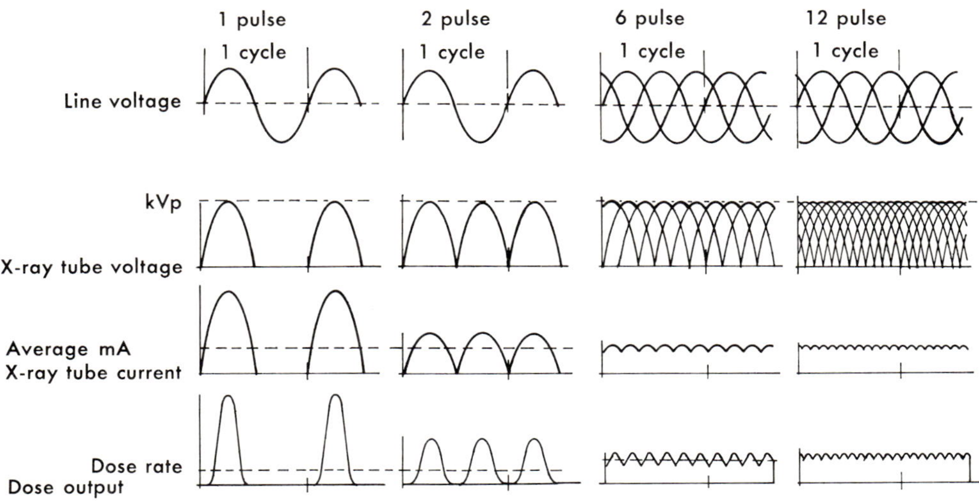

Fig. 2-15. Comparison of diagnostic x-ray generator curves. (Redrawn with permission from Siemens Corp.)

Table 2-1. Diagnostic x-ray generator data* (100 mA average tube current)

	1-pulse				2-pulse				6-pulse				12-pulse			
pkV	**kV eff†**	**mA peak**	**Dose rate rela‡**	**Dose peak**	**kV eff**	**mA peak**	**Dose rate rela**	**Dose peak**	**kV eff**	**mA peak**	**Dose rate rela**	**Dose peak**	**kV eff**	**mA peak**	**Dose rate rela**	**Dose peak**
60	60	314	1	6.8	60	157	1	3.4	57.2	105	1.6	2.3	56	102	2	2.2
80	80	314	4	27.2	80	157	4	13.6	74.5	105	6.4	9.2	72	102	8	8.8
100	100	314	10	68.0	100	157	10	34.0	94.0	105	16.0	23.0	92	102	20	22.0

*Note: Data measured with a 30-mm (thick) aluminum phantom. (Courtesy Siemens Corp.)
†eff = effective.
‡rela = relative.

selenium rectifiers. The silicon rectifier readily handles up to 150 kV and as much as 1,000 mA with an unlimited (almost) life expectancy.

Silicon actually is a semiconductor; i.e., a solid crystal in which the electrons take part in the conduction process only when it has received a certain increment of electrical charge (energy). Silicon can be made into two types of semiconductor, which, when placed together, become a solid state rectifier. One of the semiconductors is an *n-type* in which there is an excess of electrons (negative charges); the other is the *p-type* in which there is a deficiency of electrons (excess of protons, or positive charges). When the two semiconductors are placed together, a *p-n junction* or solid state rectifier is the result.

If a crystal of silicon receives a trace amount of phosphorus impurity, the phosphorus contributes a very loosely bound electron (not necessary in covalent* bonding) that is free to participate in the conduction process (n-type semiconductor). Conversely, if a crystal of silicon receives a trace of aluminum impurity, the crystal will lack one electron required to complete covalent bonding. When electrons migrate to this "hole," it has the same effect as positive charges moving in the opposite direction (p-type semiconductor).

When a p-type semiconductor is joined to an n-type semiconductor a solid-state rectifier is formed; i.e., a p-n junction is established. A p-n junction in a semiconductor permits a large current to flow when the potential direction is from the n-type (side) to the p-type (side), and a very small current to flow when the potential direction is reversed. This arrangement functions to rectify current in a manner that is very similar to that of a valve tube.

The advantages of these small solid-state rectifiers over valve tube rectifiers are numerous. In addition to the much smaller space necessary, the advantages of greater efficiency in conduction of electric current, longer life, decreased cost of insulation, etc., are obvious.

Electronic timers

Electronic timers for x-ray machines are superior to all other types of timer. Electronic timers all operate on the same general principle: *the length of an x-ray exposure is determined by the time required to charge a capacitor to a predetermined quantity.* Two essential items compose an electronic timer; these are a resistor and a capacitor (RC) in circuit. The capacitor is always connected to the grid of a Thyratron type switch.

Fig. 2-16 is a diagram of the basic circuitry of an electronic timer. Since the switch is closed between exposures, the capacitor is short-circuited, and does not collect a charge. The switch is opened at the beginning of an exposure, and concurrently a second switch (not shown) closes the circuit through the x-ray machine and the exposure begins. During the exposure, electrons migrate from the upper capacitor plate to the lower plate. This causes the upper plate, which is connected to the Thyratron grid, to become more positive, thus lowering the negative charge of the grid. Eventually the grid charge is reduced to a point (critical level) that permits current to flow through the Thyratron, thus opening a second switch in the x-ray circuit and terminating the exposure. The rate of electron flow away from the upper plate is controlled by the resistor; the greater the resistance, the slower the flow. The time required for the Thyratron grid charge to be reduced to its critical level is controlled by the

*Covalence refers to the number of pairs of electrons an atom can share with its neighbors. A chemical bond is a mechanism by means of which atoms are held together in a molecule.

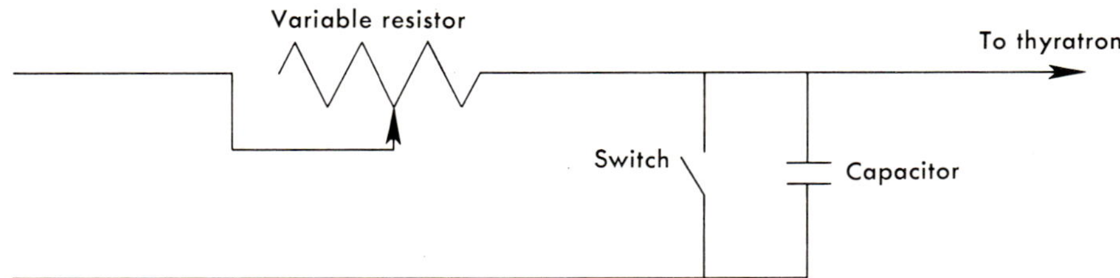

Fig. 2-16. Electronic timer circuit.

capacitor circuit resistance. Selection of an x-ray exposure time changes the resistance in the capacitor circuit and the length of the exposure time varies directly with the resistance.

The RC circuit and Thyratron tube can be used in a variety of connections to control exposure times; this combination always produces an accurately timed electric current. When an electronic timer is employed in conjunction with a silicon controlled electric switch, an x-ray pulse may be as short as 1 millisecond with an activation time* of 1 millisecond. Electronic timers are capable of controlling in excess of 60 exposures per second, and may be connected in either the primary or secondary circuits of the x-ray (high-voltage) transformer.

CARE OF X-RAY MACHINES

Equipment failure

Major repairs on radiographic equipment should be made by specialized personnel in the department or by service personnel from the x-ray machine sales and service company. Recent federal regulations applying to the assembly of collimators require that they be of the positive beam limitation type when assembled into a general purpose diagnostic x-ray system. The only exception is if an uncertified beam limiting device is installed in an x-ray system containing no certified components. After August 1, 1979, all major components added to an x-ray system must be certified. Positive beam limitation may be accomplished automatically or may be a manual system with x-ray lockout until the proper field size is set. Manufacturers of x-ray systems and their major components including collimator are required to provide a certification that they meet all applicable requirements when assembled according to manufacturers' instructions by placing a label or tag permanently affixed or inscribed on the component. The person who assembles major x-ray components into the x-ray system certifies that he has followed the manufacturers' instructions by filing a report to the government and giving a copy to the purchaser.

When an x-ray machine is inoperable, patients are inconvenienced, and income to the department is either delayed or totally lost. Time is a major factor in most departments, and any time saved will be beneficial. Useful information relayed to service personnel *before* they leave their office could save much time lost in obtaining the proper repair parts. For the radiologic technologist, knowledge of preventive maintenance must include the ability to *isolate* the problem through a logical sequence of checks and evaluations, and, whenever possible, to notice the beginning of trouble so that it can be corrected before serious damage occurs.

The checking sequence

1. Prior to calling the x-ray serviceman, evaluation of the problem in the following manner will usually expedite the necessary repair. Make a series of astute observations regarding the problem. Repeat these observations to the serviceman, with the reason for such observations.
2. At the time of exposure:
   a. Observe the various meter readings.
   b. Listen carefully for the normal sounds of the equipment in comparison with the unusual sounds.
   c. Be aware of that "intangible" sense or feeling of normal operation compared with the same type of sense regarding abnormal operation.
3. Verify the exposure problem with all circuit conditions:
   a. Radiography with Potter-Bucky diaphragm in and out.
   b. Fluoroscopy in and out.

*Activation time is the time delay between the "command" to make an exposure and its commencement.

4. Appearance of the radiograph:
   By logical deduction, account for the radiographic deviation according to prime factors, distance, structures penetrated, and film and film holder combination.
5. Sequence of timing sounds:
   a. Was the operation of the equipment normal in regard to the sequence of sounds?
   b. Did the meters read normally? If there were abnormal readings, why and how were they abnormal? How much deviation from normal was observed?
   c. Have the controls been checked? (Move each control and reset to same value. The reason for this is that the stop that mechanically centers the contacts may have been temporarily out of alignment or adjustment, or it may have been broken.)
6. The circuit breaker:
   Circuit breakers may be operated:
   a. By high milliamperage.
   b. By high kilovoltage or high kilovoltage in conjunction with time and milliamperage.
   c. By means of any short circuit to the ground.

   If the circuit breaker "kicks out" during an exposure, there may be a temporary overload resulting from settings too high for safe operation. Repeating the exposure with reduced settings may pinpoint this type of difficulty. The condition of the circuit breaker should be checked if the panel board fails to light up.
7. The x-ray tube:
   Most installations make use of an x-ray tube with a transparent port for observation of the cathode filament. If the filament fails to heat, perform steps a and b.
   a. With the filament circuit closed and while observing the cathode filament through the port, rotate the tube or move the cathode cables. The purpose of such movements is to localize, if possible, a broken wire inside the high-voltage cable or a poor connection in the "plug-in" cable jack.
   b. If the cable is attached with a hand-tightened thread or screw device, attempt to tighten the device.
8. If the machine is full-wave rectified and one of the rectifying valves is burned out, the milliammeter will register somewhat more than one half the selected milliamperage during the exposure.*
9. If one of the high tension cables is punctured:
   a. There will usually be a strong odor of burning rubber.
   b. There will seldom be a "flash" seen or a "hissing" sound heard.
10. Fuses:
    The fuse panel is usually located in an easily accessible area. With the main power supply disconnected, examine each fuse carefully to ascertain which fuse is burned out.
11. A check of all accessible "plug-in" electric connections including the main power cable, if so connected, sometimes will reveal that the trouble is caused by a connection inadvertently loosened by cleaning or by unusual cable movements.
12. Precaution: *Do not* make repeated exposures if the trouble is not readily apparent; further damage may result.

Tube-rating charts

A tube-rating chart is supplied with each installation. In the event of an x-ray tube replacement, be certain to obtain the correct tube-rating chart for the new x-ray tube.

Focal spot size is the principal factor governing the quantity of energy applied to the diagnostic x-ray tube. The (maximum) rate of heat conduction through the target and dissipation from the anode limits the quantity of energy applied as a result of electron bombardment of this small area. It is readily seen that energies producing heat quantities greater than that tolerated by the tungsten target material can melt the tungsten at the focal spot. The rate of conductivity of heat through the target and from the anode of one tube may not necessarily be the same as that for another tube having the same focal spot size.

Proper use of the tube-rating chart tends to prevent overloading the tube; overloading usually necessitates an expensive replacement. The radiographic tube-rating chart is designed to indicate maximum "safe" exposure values for any one exposure. Repeated exposures having these same maximum values can still overload the tube. New combinations of exposure factors should be checked on this chart prior to exposure. From the

---

*See p. 34 for additional discussion of valve-tube failure.

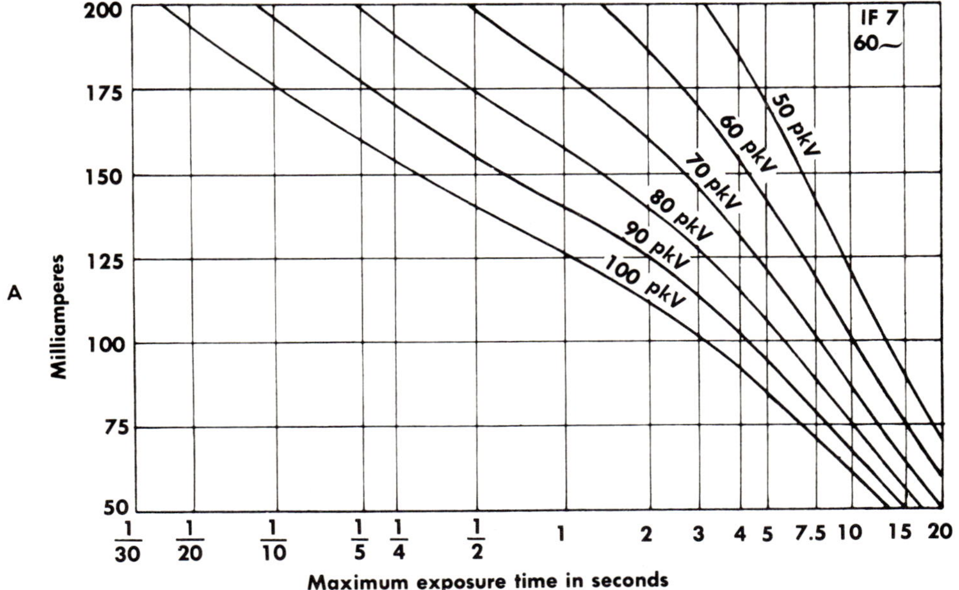

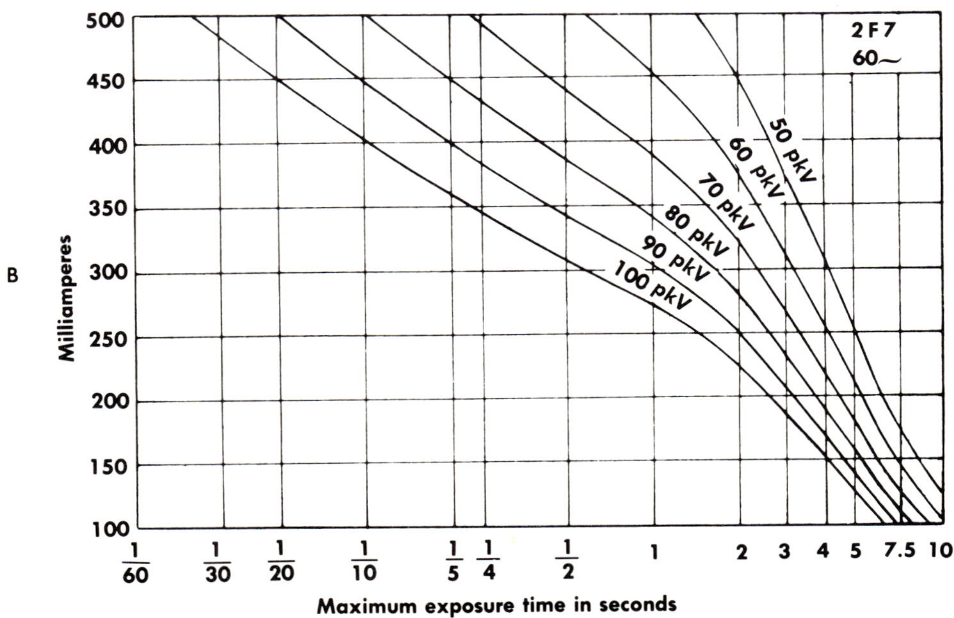

Fig. 2-17. Tube-rating charts. **A,** 1.0 mm focal spot. **B,** 2.0 mm focal spot. (Courtesy The Machlett Laboratories, Inc.)

tube-rating chart it may be found that the required milliampere-second value using relatively high milliamperage is unsafe at the desired kilovoltage. Usually, this same milliampere-second value will be safely obtained if the milliamperage is reduced to one half value and the time is doubled in value, assuming that the load on the large filament is not switched to the small filament. This would make it necessary to check the rating on the small filament-rating chart. (See Fig. 2-17.)

A tube-thermal characteristics chart is developed at the factory from values of maximum anode heat storage capacity and heat dissipation of the anode. The heat units developed in the anode may be calculated from the product of the kilovoltage and the milliampere-seconds.

The rating charts in Fig. 2-17 are for the Dynamax 25 x-ray tube. Two examples of technique factor selections are given.

1. An exposure of 200 mA, for 1/20 second, and at 90 pkV can be used safely on the small focal spot. It is seen on the chart that the maximum allowable energy for 1/20 second is for 200 mA and 97 pkV.

2. An exposure of 100 mA, for 4 seconds, and at 100 pkV cannot be used on the small focal spot. It is seen on the chart that the maximum allowable energy for 4 seconds is for 100 mA and 92 pkV. The technologist may elect either of two options: (a) use the large focal spot*; (b) use the small focal spot but use 50 mA for 8 seconds.

To prevent unnecessary evaporation of the cathode filament, *always open the filament circuit when it is not in use, that is, between patients and between exposures of a single patient,* except during certain special radiographic procedures. (This refers to x-ray tubes and equipment manufactured prior to the 1960s.)

Routine care

An x-ray machine represents a large financial investment to the owner. It is the technologist's responsibility to maintain this equipment in a state of peak efficiency.

Protect the tabletop from scratches and sticky dirt by use of a cotton sheet, except during sinus and skull radiography. The patient is made more comfortable with the use of a smooth sheet. Use a good grade of waxless furniture polish to maintain the tabletop finish. When blood, grease, or other material has inadvertently been spilled on the table, wipe it off with warm water and surgical or green soap. Dry the area thoroughly and then wipe clean with a second disinfectant such as 70% alcohol. Dry again, and apply furniture polish.

The tube shielding, table ends and sides, and parts of the control panel that are black should undergo daily cleaning with a cloth dampened with furniture polish. Monthly attention should be given the counterbalance cables of the fluoroscopic tube and screen and of the Potter-Bucky diaphragm. Any "fraying" or broken strands should be immediately called to the attention of the service personnel. The tube stand and other parts of the equipment that are bright or chrome finished should be cleaned frequently with a special chrome polish to prevent tarnish. Keep the tube stand track clear of dust and lint.

Spilled barium should be removed immediately after the patient is dismissed. If there is crinkled black surface paint on parts of the equipment, use a cloth dampened with warm water to wipe the surface and then rub with a fiber or medium stiff bristle hairbrush and then with a dry cloth.

Some radiographic equipment requires a "warm-up" period prior to use. Allowing this period to elapse ensures greater consistency in radiographs.

The wall power safety switch to stationary equipment should be opened at the end of the work period. When not in use, the power supply cord of mobile equipment should be removed from the outlet and coiled on the hooks provided.

In using either mobile or stationary equipment, avoid unnecessary bending of the high-tension cables.

*However, this increases the penumbra effect.

REFERENCES

Boast, Warren B.: Principles of electric and magnetic circuits New York, 1950, Harper & Brothers.

Delario, A. J.: Roentgen, radium, and radioisotope therapy, Philadelphia, 1953, Lea & Febiger.

Miller, Franklin, Jr.: College physics, ed. 2, New York, 1959, Harcourt, Brace & World, Inc.

Robertson, John Kellock: Radiology physics, ed. 3, Princeton, N.J., 1955, D. Van Nostrand Co., Inc.

Selman, Joseph: The fundamentals of x-ray and radium physics, ed. 5, Springfield, Ill., 1972, Charles C Thomas, Publisher.

Weyl, Charles, and Warren, S. Reid, Jr.: Radiologic physics, ed. 2, Springfield, Ill., 1951, Charles C Thomas, Publisher.

White, Harvey E.: Modern college physics, Princeton, N.J., 1962, D. Van Nostrand Co., Inc.

QUESTIONS

1. When time is 0.1 second and milliamperage is 300 what is the value of milliampere-seconds?

2. How much time is required to produce 10 mAs when 750 mA is selected?
3. In what forms or states may matter exist?
4. What is an atom? What is a molecule?
5. Explain ionization. What transitory and what near permanent effects has this process upon atoms?
6. Which is longer the radius of an atomic nucleus or the radius of average electron orbits about the nucleus?
7. What determines the placement of an element in the periodic table?
8. Name the energy levels of an atom of tungsten (W).
9. What is electricity? Why does electricity classify as a form of energy?
10. Compare the electric charge on a proton with that on an electron. What unit or units did you use in this comparison?
11. Explain your answer and compare saltwater and highly refined oil as conductors of electric current.
12. What causes electric current to flow along conductors?
13. State Ohm's law.
14. Which offers greater resistance to the flow of electric current: a long wire of given diameter or a short wire of the same diameter? (Both pieces of wire are of the same composition.)
15. How may electricity be stored for instantaneous release upon demand?
16. What is a sine wave? What may be learned from such a diagram?
17. What substance is used as core material in electromagnets?
18. What are flux lines? In what direction do these lines exert energy?
19. Explain mutual induction.
20. Explain self-induction and differentiate it from mutual induction.
21. What is transformer ratio?
22. On all x-ray machine control panels is found the external part or parts of an autotransformer. What name is often applied to this device?
23. What basic quantity of electrical information may be determined from application of the formula: x:V :: n:N?
24. Compared with single-phase alternating current, how many peaks (positive impulses) are found in a three-phase alternating current?
25. What are the minimum, basic circuits of x-ray machines?
26. What purpose is served by the circuit-breaker? Why is it located in this particular part of the circuit?
27. In a single-phase alternating current x-ray exposure of $1/12$ second, how many dots should appear on the film if the current is half-wave rectified? (The current is 60-cycle.)
28. Differentiate between the operations of an impulse timer and a synchronous timer.
29. Explain the differences in information obtained from a milliampere meter and a milliampere-second meter.
30. Explain rectification and its use in x-ray machines.
31. How much is the gain in energy supplied to an x-ray machine from a two-pulse generator to a six-pulse generator?
32. Explain why 100 kVp on a single-phase unit requires more mAs for a satisfactory radiograph than 100 kVp on a three-phase unit.

3 • PRODUCTION OF X RAYS

Successful production of x rays for use in both diagnostic and therapeutic radiology results when the large variety of component parts are assembled correctly and function properly. To understand the total production process, it is necessary to study and understand each basic component. After achieving some degree of understanding of electricity and electrical circuitry in the preceding chapter, the next logical consideration is that of electronic tubes, including both x-ray and valve tubes.

X-RAY TUBES

Although x rays are produced when high-speed electrons are suddenly declerated or stopped, successful use of x rays depends on production under certain conditions:

1. There must be a source of electrons, the *cathode filament.*
2. There must be a target, the *anode,* made of suitable material, and so connected as to attract the electrons at the proper time.
3. The electrons must encounter no outside intereference in traveling to the target.
4. There must be a method of accelerating the electrons toward the target.

All these conditions are met in the modern hot-cathode x-ray tube; the *hot-filament cathode* and the *tungsten anode* are contained in an hermetically sealed, *evacuated glass envelope.*

Alternating current flows to and from the cathode in the filament circuit and pulsating direct current flows to the cathode and across to the anode and from it without destroying the vacuum. If the vacuum were not maintained, irregularities in the flow of electrons from cathode to anode would occur. Since the flow of electrons constitutes the *tube current (milliamperage)* it is vital to successful operation of the x-ray tube that the flow of electrons be maintained as near constant as possible during each exposure. If the x-ray tube should become *gassy,* that is, if the tube becomes incompletely evacuated, noticeable fluctuations in milliamperage will occur when the tube is operated.

A metal shielding material containing lead encases the evacuated glass tube (envelope). The metal shield acts as a primary barrier to absorb x rays that are not directed through the port. A port (window) of radiolucent material is placed in the metal shielding directly beneath the anode to permit the passage of the useful x rays through a limited aperture. (See Fig. 1-6.) Highly refined oil completely fills the space between the metal shield and the glass tube to function as an electric insulator, as a heat conductor, and as a filter for soft and useless x rays. The presence of the oil makes the x-ray tube essentially shockproof. During x-ray production enormous quantities of heat result and are conducted from the anode connections outside the glass tube to the metal shield, and then to the air. Between the glass tube (directly below the anode) and the port in the metal shield the oil acts as an *inherent filter* that must be equivalent to a minimum of 0.5 mm of aluminum. Outside the port and built into the metal shield is a slot (or slots) for insertion of additional filters. On older x-ray tube shieldings (housings) a second slot was built in for attachment of various sizes of cones. On the more modern x-ray tube shieldings the collimator is attached to the metal shielding in this location. (See Figs. 1,5, *B,* 3-1, and 3-2.)

Anodes

The anode of the x-ray tube is positively charged during the time of x-ray exposure; that is, during the time that the exposure (secondary) switch is closed. The positive charge on the anode attracts the electrons as they are released from the cathode, thus completing the high-voltage (secondary) circuit.

The anode is usually comprised of a copper bar or cylinder, with one end extending out of the glass tube and connected to the high-voltage transformer. The other end faces the cathode and has a small tungsten button embedded in its center. The face of the anode is beveled; that is, angled away from the cathode at a 10- to 20-degree angle, depending on the make and style of the x-ray tube. The angle of the anode controls to a considerable degree the strength of the rays (or quantity of total-beam energy) emitted toward the cathode end and toward the anode end of the x-ray tube. (For additional discussion of this phenomenon, *heel effect,* see Fig. 4-11 and

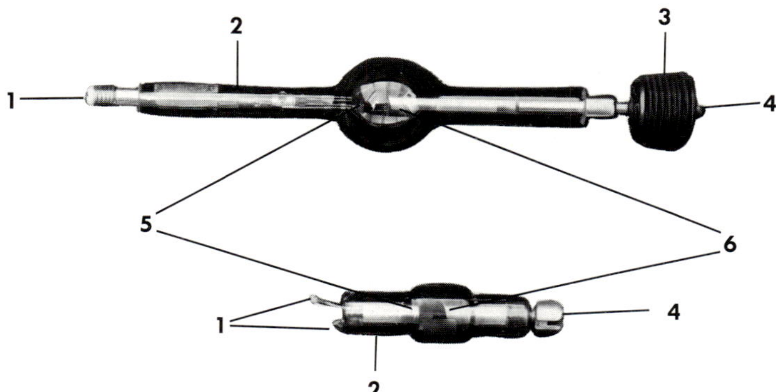

Fig. 3-1. Stationary anode x-ray tubes. Upper photograph is of an early Coolidge, nonshock-proof tube; lower one is of a tube encased in metal and surrounded with oil.

1. Cathode connections
2. Evacuated glass envelope
3. Metal fins for air cooling
4. Anode connection
5. Cathode
6. Anode

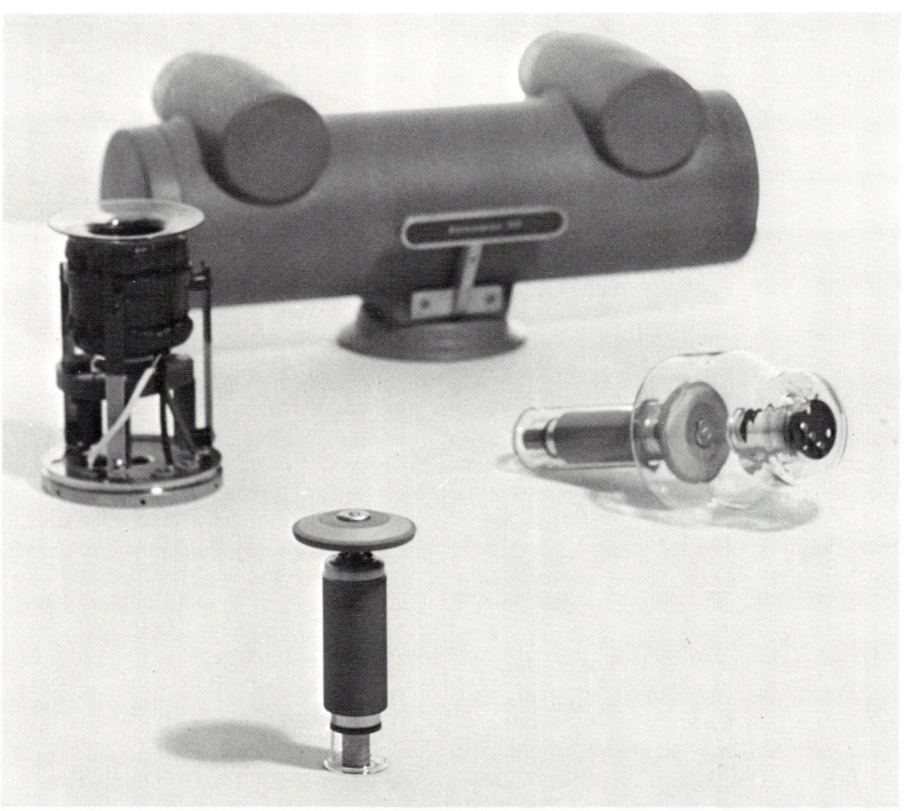

Fig. 3-2. Dynamax "50" x-ray tube components. Clockwise from top; metal casing for tube, anode and cathode in evacuated glass envelope, rotor and target, and stator windings. (Courtesy The Machlett Laboratories, Inc.)

pp. 89 and 90.) The tungsten block is about 2 mm thick and serves as the target for the cathode electrons. The kinetic energy of the cathode electrons impinging on the tungsten button is transformed into two forms of energy: x ray and heat. The heat dissipates quite rapidly from the tungsten via the copper anode through the oil to the tube shielding.

There are several methods of dissipating the generated heat from the anode to the tube shielding. One method of anode cooling uses oil to transfer the heat to the shielding which, in turn, radiates the heat to the air. Other methods of anode cooling use fins or radiators to dissipate the heat. The fins are at right angles to the long axis of the anode. Most high-capacity radiographic tubes have a motor-driven fan attached to the shielding to aid in cooling the shielding material.

The anodes of diagnostic x-ray tubes may be either stationary or rotating. In many rotating anode tubes, the beveled (angled) edge of the *disk* circumference forms a 15-degree angle with the transverse plane of the x-ray tube. The beveled edge slopes away from the cathode so that the useful x-rays may project through the port. A focusing cup directs the electrons to the lower edge of this bevel. (See Figs. 1-5, *A*, and 3-2.)

A molybdenum focusing cup surrounds the cathode filament. The focusing cup concentrates the electrons emitted from the filament onto a small area of the anode target. Since the filament is linear in shape, the electrons impinge upon the target in a line. The anode angles slightly away from the cathode so that the x rays emitted at right angles to the electron beam appear to be coming from a point instead of a line (Figs. 3-3 and 3-4). The stream of electrons is called both the electron stream and the cathode rays.

Tubes designed for use in x-ray therapy are similar to radiographic tubes; the chief differences are that the anodes and targets of therapy tubes are larger and usually stationary, and the electrons do not impinge on as small a spot.

The cathode electrons are caused to strike the anode in an area (electronic focal spot) determined by the molybdenum focusing cup, the shape of the cathode filament, and the angle of the anode. Early radiographic tubes had the anode angle of 45 degrees. Modern stationary anode tubes have the angle at approximately 18 degrees, to decrease the *optical* focal spot size. (See Fig. 3-3.) Early focal spots also included elliptical and rectangular shapes.

The present *linear focus* in stationary anode tubes evolved from numerous attempts to reduce the optical focal spot size. The terms *electronic (actual) focal spot* and *optical (effective) focal spot* are often confused and frequently misunderstood. *The electronic focal spot is the actual area of bombardment by the cathode electrons.* The size of the area struck by electrons is controlled for the most part by the shape and size of the focusing cup and filament of the cathode; the angle of the anode obviously influences the size of this area, but is not its principal control. *The optical focal spot is the projected area of the electronic focal spot; this projected area is at right angles to the cathode electron stream.* The electronic focal spot is, of course, considerably larger than the optical focal spot. The optical focal spot is the term used to describe the focal spot of a given x-ray tube. (See Fig. 3-4.) The size of the optical focal spot is finally a result of the angle of the anode and the actual area of bombardment of the target (area of electron beam bombardment). Obviously, use of a smaller optical focal spot produces radiographs evidencing greater definition.

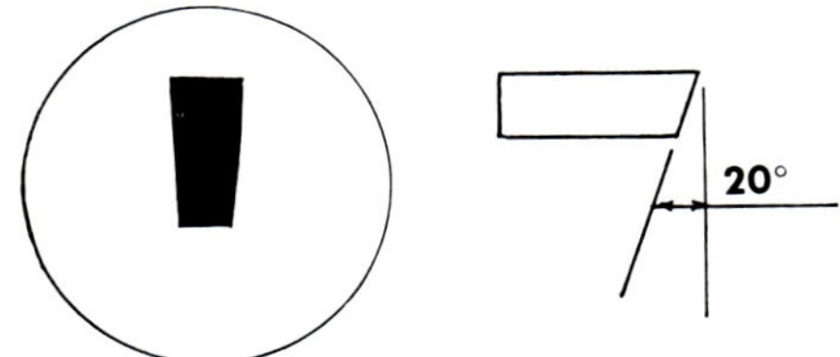

Fig. 3-3. Stationary anode. Left diagram is an end-on view of the anode (shaded) in the copper core. Right diagram demonstrates a 20-degree angle of the bevel.

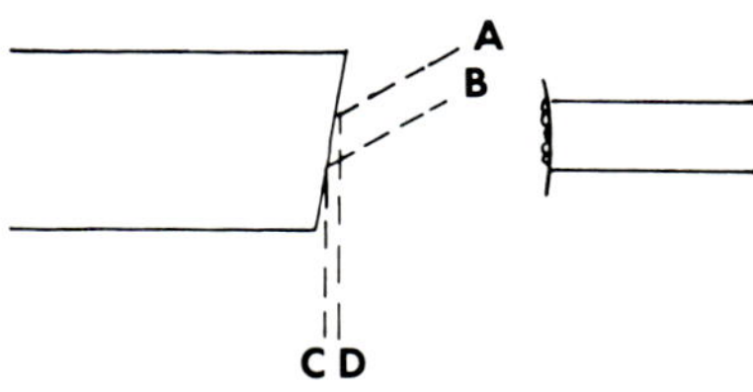

Fig. 3-4. Optical focal spot. Electronic focal spot is the length (in this figure) of the line **A-B.** Projected length of the line **A-B** is imaginary line **C-D,** which is the length of the optical focus. **A-B** is 3.5 mm and **C-D** is 1 mm.

The rotating anode is a disk approximately 3 inches in diameter (Fig. 1-5). An external rotor induces this anode to spin upon its axis at approximately 3,000 or 9,000 rpm. Because of the spin, there is a constantly changing target area on

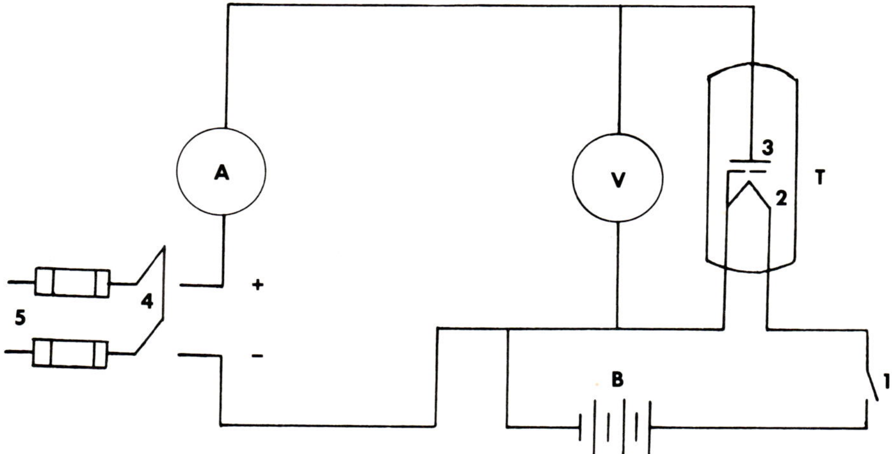

Fig. 3-5. Thermionic emission; secondary current conduction.

1. Single pole switch in battery circuit
2. Cathode filament in vacuum tube
3. Anode of vacuum tube
4. Double pole switch of alternating current
5. Fuses of alternating current line

B Battery
A Ammeter
V Voltmeter
T Vacuum tube

which the cathode electrons impinge. This condition permits the use of greater kilovoltages and milliampere-seconds within the safe limits of tube operation—determined on the specific tube-rating chart (pp. 12 and 43). The circumference of the disk is the actual area of bombardment. As in the stationary anode tube, the cathode filament is the source of electrons. The electrons bombard a small portion of this circumference at any specific instant. Introduction of the rotating anode tube permitted great advances in the development of high-speed radiography, which utilizes high tube current and short exposure time.

A double focal spot is used in many modern x-ray tubes (both rotating and stationary anodes). This tube usually has two cathode filaments, independent of each other. Some x-ray tube manufacturers use a single filament with two sets of connections to the filament circuit. Each connects to the continuous filament, which has a smaller portion (small filament) usually in the center of the larger. When there are two independent filaments in the cathode, they are usually side by side. Some *double-focus* tubes have a separate switch to select focal spot size. Usually the milliamperage (technique) selector incorporates this selection.

Cathodes

The cathode has a negative charge in relation to the anode. The filament circuit of the x-ray machine supplies the cathode filament with the necessary heat. The x-ray tube filament current requires approximately 12 to 15 volts for normal operation. Also, one side of the cathode filament connnects to the secondary side of the high-voltage transformer to conduct the secondary current across the x-ray tube.

The construction of the focusing cup, the relation of the focusing cup to the cathode filament, and the application of high voltage to the x-ray tube cause the electrons, which are emitted from the filament, to strike the anode target in a very small area.

The filament is small, approximately 0.0085 inch in diameter, and offers considerable resistance to the flow of the heating current. The filament usually consists of either pure tungsten or silver-tungsten alloy. This heating (filament) current raises the filament temperature to a sufficiently high value to cause the electrons of the filament to *boil off* and surround the cathode in a cloud (the electron cloud). Increases in the filament current cause corresponding increases in the kinetic energy of the filament electrons, thus causing proportionately more electrons to be emitted from the coil of wire. This process of releasing electrons by heat is called thermionic emission and is further explained in the following paragraphs and Fig. 3-5.

THERMIONIC EMISSION

The conduction of current across the terminals of valve and x-ray tubes is made possible by thermionic emission. *Thermionic emission is the release of electrons by application of heat.*

Experiment has revealed that current flows between the cathode and anode (in a hot-filament vacuum tube) *only* when the cathode filament releases electrons. Fig. 3-5 and its text explain the necessity of electron release for current flow.

The number of electrons released (thermionic emission) depends on the filament heat. When saturation current exists (p. 52), the relation between tube current and filament temperature is expressed in Richardson's equation as modified by Dushman:

$$I = AT^2e - \frac{b}{T}$$

Using tungsten as the filament material, the elements of this equation are as follows:

A and b are constants of the tungsten filament; A = 60.2 amp/cm²degrees²; T = the absolute temperature in degrees Kelvin of the filament (for x-ray and valve tube filaments operating between 10 and 500 mA the absolute temperatures are from 2200°K to 2700°K); e = 2.71828 the approximate value of the base of natural logarithms; $-\frac{b}{T}$ (the exponent on e) is a unitless quantity since $\frac{b}{T} = \frac{e\phi}{kT}$, where $e\phi$ is work (e is the electron charge, ϕ is the work function of the metal), k is the Baltzmann constant (work per degree K), and T is in degrees; I = current density in amperes per square centimeter of the thermionically emitting surface.

The electrons flowing from cathode to anode each second constitute the tube current (milliamperage); the magnitude of the tube current is a function of the total number of the electrons flowing between the cathode and the anode. Tube current can be calculated as follows:

Where the charge on one electron is 4.8002×10^{-10} esu,* and one ampere-second = 3×10^9 esu, and an electronic charge = 4.8002×10^{-10} esu, or 1.6019×10^{-19} coulombs:

$$1 \text{ mAs} = \frac{3 \times 10^9 \text{ esu}}{10^3} \times \frac{1}{4.8002 \times 10^{-10}}$$

$$= (3 \times 10^6)\left(\frac{1}{4.8002}\right)(10^{10})$$

$$= \frac{3 \times 10^{16}}{4.8002}$$

$$= 6.24 \times 10^{15} \text{ electrons}$$

To produce x rays, it is necessary that the liberated electrons strike the target with high velocity; that is, the kinetic energy of the electrons (cathode rays) is converted into x-ray energy, heat energy, and other nonuseful rays. This occurs when the anode is positively charged in the high-voltage circuit. Following closure of the exposure switch, the secondary voltage is quite high at the cathode in relation to the anode. Therefore, the voltage drop between the cathode and anode accelerates the liberated cathode electrons across to the positively charged anode with a force that is approximately proportional to the impressed secondary voltage. The midpoint of the high-voltage transformer is grounded to make practical insulation possible. Since the rectifier circuit is supplied from both legs of a transformer grounded at its midpoint, the result at any one moment is a high positive potential in one leg and a high negative potential in the other. This condition, with rectification of the current, provides a high potential drop between the cathode and the anode.

In a self-rectified unit the generation of heat in the anode is usually insufficient to permit release of electrons; therefore, current cannot flow from anode to cathode in the inverse half cycle. However, if the anode becomes excessively heated from continuous or prolonged usage, it will emit electrons. Insertion of a valve tube in series between the x-ray tube anode and the high-voltage transformer prevents the rectification of current by the x-ray tube. The valve tube anode cannot reach a degree of heat that would permit release of electrons, due to a lack of appreciable potential drop.

VALVE TUBES

Valve tubes differ somewhat in construction from x-ray tubes. The valve tube anode face is at right angles to the cathode stream. The electron stream strikes the entire anode face. There is no tungsten block in the valve tube anode. (See Figs. 3-6 and 3-7.)

It has been stated (pp. 35 to 38) that the valve

---

*esu = electrostatic unit.

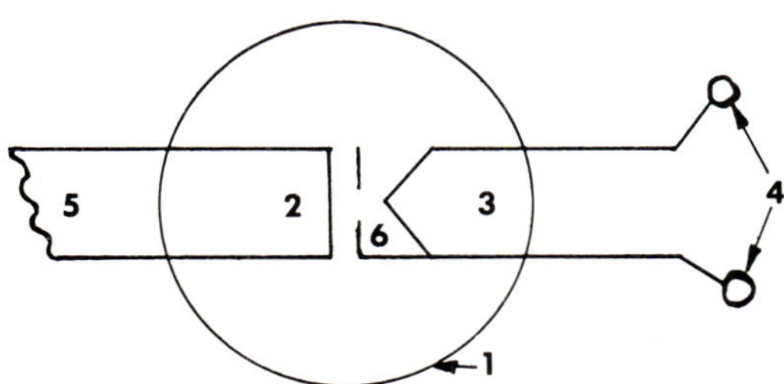

Fig. 3-6. Valve tube diagram. (See also Fig. 3-7.)

1. Evacuated glass envelope
2. Anode
3. Cathode
4. Cathode connections to secondary side of valve-tube transformer
5. Anode connection to high-voltage circuit
6. Cathode filament

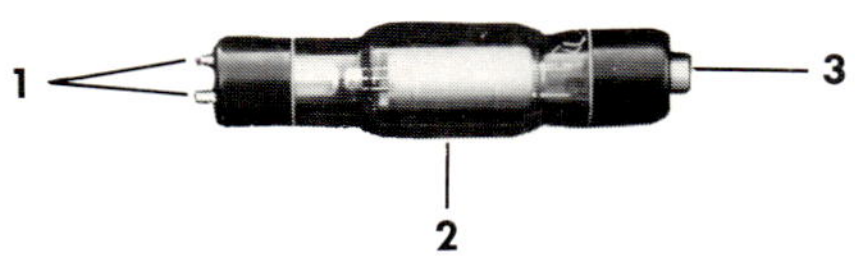

Fig. 3-7. Valve tube photograph. Cathode and anode are hidden from view by the metal sleeve surrounding them.

1. Cathode connections
2. Evacuated glass envelope
3. Anode connection

tube's function is to conduct the secondary current along a predetermined circuit.

A good valve tube will *not* produce x rays because the electrons cannot cross the valve at high speed. The design of a good valve tube is such that the tube current is maintained well below saturation. Consequently, the voltage drop is very small (p. 50).

Two types of valve tube filaments are available, and each type performs satisfactorily. The principal difference between the two types permits considerable difference in operation. The *tungsten filament* valve tube requires approximately 12 volts to operate the filament current. The *thoriated tungsten filament* valve tube requires approximately 6 volts to operate the filament current; the thorium coating becomes the source of electrons and permits the lower operating voltage, thereby prolonging tube life. Considerably less heat of the cathode filament is required to remove electrons from the thorium dioxide (ThO_2) coating on the filament wire than from the tungsten filament. To prevent tube current fluctuations and other abnormal conditions, all valve tubes in a given rectifying circuit must have uniform filaments; that is, all filaments must be either tungsten or thoriated tungsten. When all filaments are uniform in construction, it is possible to achieve balance in high-voltage flow between sequential components of the high-voltage transformer, the valve tubes, and the x-ray tube.

X RAYS

Characteristics of x rays

X rays* are a form of radiant energy having both a wave nature and a quantum nature. Since these rays possess a wave nature and travel with the speed of light, they are properly classified as electromagnetic waves. *An electromagnetic wave is produced by the oscillation of an electric charge.* All electromagnetic waves travel with the speed of light, which is approximately 3×10^{10} cm per second in a vacuum (186,000 miles per second is a frequently used value and is less than 1% in error).

X rays are electrically neutral, are capable of penetrating all matter to varying degrees, and are reflected and diffracted by certain crystals. The angle of incidence equals the angle of reflection, and the dispersion by diffraction is a function of the atomic arrangement and the wavelength of the particular x ray.

X rays can cause numerous biologic, physical, and chemical effects. Among the biologic effects are bactericidal and lethal ones, chromosome aberration, tissue ionization, depilation, tissue desquamation, erythema production, and sterilization. Among the physical effects are the photographic effect on x-ray and other films, the ionization of nonliving substance, and the ability to penetrate matter. Among the chemical effects are the liberation of iodine from solutions of iodoform in chloroform and the discoloration of certain alkaline salts.

Since x rays are a definite form of energy, it is necessary to expend energy to produce x rays. Application of the heating current to the cathode

*The roentgen (R) is the unit of measurement of quantity of roentgen radiation (x rays): when the secondary electrons are fully utilized and the wall effect of the chamber is avoided, a roentgen produces in 1 ml of atmospheric air at 0° C. and 760 mm of mercury pressure such a degree of conductivity that one electrostatic unit is measured at saturation point. (Actually, it amounts to the degree of ionization produced in 1 ml of air by exposing the chamber to x rays.)

filament raises the resistance of the filament to the flow of current. This resistance causes the filament to acquire a certain degree of heat in relation to the quantity of current amperage used. An increase in current causes an increase in the heat of the filament. The heat energizes the electrons of the filament atoms; some of these electrons then move away (are liberated) from the filament as a result of increased kinetic energy. Increases in the cathode filament temperature cause correspondingly greater numbers of electrons to be liberated from the filament. Application of the tube voltage (kilovoltage) drives the liberated electrons to the anode target to produce x rays. In this manner, electric energy is expended in the production of x rays.

In addition to the electromagnetic wave nature of x rays, these rays have also a quantum nature and arise as discrete packets (photons) of energy. (Planck's quantum theory). *A photon is a particle (quantum) of x-radiation or gamma radiation. A quantum is a definite amount of energy ($h\nu$: Planck's constant $\times$ frequency).* The x ray arising as a result of a single electron bombardment of the target is considered as a single photon of energy approximately equal to the electron energy.

Space charge and saturation current

At a given operating temperature of the filament the total number of electrons liberated from the filament is constant regardless of the voltage. The liberated electrons surround the filament in a cloud. Each electron carries a negative electric charge; therefore, each electron repels every other electron in the cloud. Each atom that has lost an electron is then positively charged; therefore, there is an electrostatic charge between the electron cloud and the filament. The continuing heat of the filament liberates additional electrons. The effect of the filament heat is sufficient to overcome the electrostatic attraction between the liberated electrons and the filament ions. *The total effect of these combined forces is the space charge.* It follows that the tube voltage necessary to drive the liberated electrons to the anode must be great enough to overcome the space charge.

When the tube voltage is low, the anode attracts only those electrons that are nearest the anode; therefore, the tube current (milliamperage) is low. When the filament temperature is constant, an increase in kilovoltage attracts greater numbers of electrons to the anode; as a result there is a corresponding decrease in the number of liberated electrons repelled to the filament.

If the kilovoltage is increased, eventually a kilovoltage value is reached at which all of the electrons are driven to the anode as fast as they are liberated and none are repelled to the cathode filament. *This kilovoltage value is the saturation voltage, and its corresponding current value is the saturation current.*

Experimental evidence reveals that *corresponding to each filament current is a maximum value of the tube current that is independent of the applied voltage.* Operation of x-ray equipment at saturation voltage and current permits independent variation of kilovoltage and milliamperage. However, when tube current values exceed 50 mA, it becomes necessary to apply sufficient tube voltage to overcome the effects of the space charge.

High values of filament current cause correspondingly greater values of the space charge. To prevent destruction or damage to the x-ray tube during application of high filament current values, a *space charge compensator* is incorporated into the circuit. The effect of this compensator if tube voltage increases is an automatic decrease in the filament current; thus the compensator maintains the correct tube current value.

Since the number of liberated electrons depends on the heat of the filament, this number is then indirectly dependent on the magnitude of the filament current. Thus, there can be no more electrons driven across the tube each second than there are electrons available each second from the filament. Construction of hot-filament x-ray tubes permits control of tube current either by utilization of the space charge or by total emission of the electrons from the hot filament. When saturation current is achieved, the milliamperage will depend entirely upon the total electron emission. In such an instance, increasing or decreasing the filament current regulates the milliamperage. Therefore, very slight changes in the filament current will produce quite large changes in the milliamperage. Experimental evidence reveals that in a given tube an increase in the filament current from 4 to 4½ amperes will cause the milliamperage to increase from 40 to 100.

The importance of maintaining a constant filament amperage becomes evident. Consequently, voltage stabilizers of various designs are incorporated into the primary circuit. *A voltage stabilizer tends to maintain voltage fluctuations at a minimum; therefore, the amperage fluctuations are maintained at a corresponding minimum.*

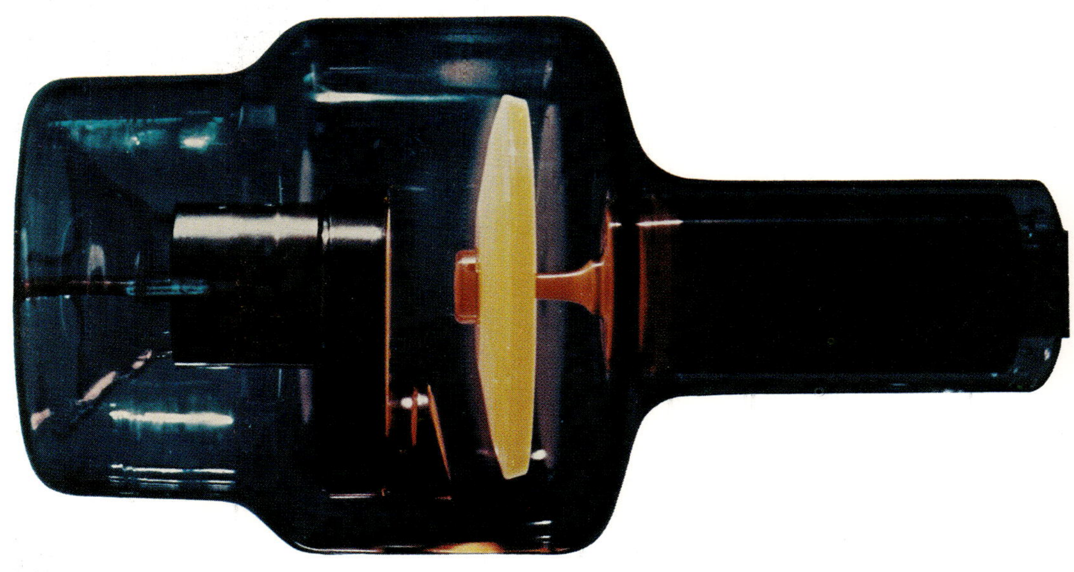

Plate 1. X-ray tube showing heat resulting from electron bombardment of anode. Rotating anode disk and spindle show the enormous quantity of heat energy, approximately 99% of total kinetic energy, generated in an exposure. Approximately 1% of the kinetic energy (of the moving cathode electrons) is converted to useful x-ray energy. (Courtesy Siemens Corp.)

X-ray production

The actual target of the anode upon which the cathode electrons impinge is composed of pure tungsten. We have learned that tungsten has quite high density (74 is the Z number), and that density is the ratio of a mass of homogeneous matter to its volume. Consideration of the preceding information leads to the conclusion that the very small piece of tungsten in the anode-face contains literally millions of atoms.

To produce x rays, it is necessary to decelerate suddenly or stop the high-speed electrons from the cathode. When a high-speed cathode electron strikes a tungsten atom, the electron will penetrate the atom in proportion to the energy of the electron. In modern diagnostic x-ray tubes, the speed of many of the bombarding electrons, when energized by very high kilovoltages, reaches approximately 0.9 the speed of light. The impressed voltage accelerates the electrons between the cathode and anode. Thus, since the electron moves in a strong electric field, the speed of the electron becomes increasingly greater as it approaches the target. The kinetic energy can be calculated approximately if the kilovoltage is known because energy in electron volts (eV) is equal to the kilovoltage: $E = eV$, where E is the energy, e is the electron charge, and V is the kilovoltage.

A simple statement of the energy released within an x-ray tube when it is operated is expressed in the following equation:

$$\text{Kilovolts} \times \text{Milliamperes} \times \text{Seconds} = \text{Joules}$$

A joule is a unit of work or energy equal to 10^7 ergs and is practically equivalent to the energy expended in 1 second by an electric current of 1 ampere in a resistance of 1 ohm. One joule is approximately equal to 0.7376 foot-pound.

Problem: How much energy is expended inside an x-ray tube when the technique selection requires 80 kVp at 30 mAs (15 mA × 2 sec)?

80 kVp × 30 mAs = 2,400 joules. The work performed in such an exposure is 2,400 joules × 0.7376 foot-pound, or 1,770 foot-pounds. A man weighing 170 pounds and climbing a single flight of stairs in a two-story house will expend approximately 1,770 foot-pounds of work.

According to the law of conservation of energy, when a fast-moving cathode electron is decelerated or stopped by an atom, it must give its energy to that atom. An electron expends energy to penetrate an orbital shell. This causes deceleration of the penetrating electron.

In some ways the action and reaction of a single electron striking the target, specifically one tungsten atom, can be likened to a pebble tossed into the surface of a placid pool of water. In the latter instance waves are seen to radiate outwardly in a circular pattern from the point of entry of the pebble into the water. Since vision is limited, essentially, to the two-dimensional surface of the water, we consider wave radiation only in two dimensions. Actually, waves form and radiate downward as well as laterally. So it is when the cathode electron strikes the tungsten atom. Waves radiate outwardly in all directions of a sphere from a given point. These waves (or rays) include not only x rays, but also heat rays and other nonuseful forms of energy. Thus it is readily understood that much of the kinetic energy of the bombarding electron is lost as far as being useful in radiography is concerned. (See Plate 1.)

This stated analogy between x rays and water waves is correct only as explained above, and in the fact that some of the electron energy is converted into x rays and some of the stone's energy is converted into water waves. However, it must be realized that x rays travel as separate packets (photons) and that water waves are continuous.

In penetrating the three outer (P, O, or N) orbits of the tungsten atom, the electron gives up energy to the atom, which emits this energy in the wavelength range of infrared (heat). It is in this manner that most of the applied energy (approximately 99%) is expended. (See plate 1.) With sufficient voltage, many of the electrons are driven to the anode with enough energy to penetrate the M and L orbits and to the K orbit. *This very high energy given to the atom by the electrons and emitted from the atom as excess energy is in the wavelength range of the continuous x-ray spectrum.* The emitted energy is approximately 1% of the applied energy.* *The continuous x-ray spectrum is called the general or white radiation; it is also called the continuous spectrum, Bremsstrahlung or "braking" radiations, and is formed as a result of the deceleration of highspeed electrons penetrating an atom.*

*The efficiency of the anode may be determined from the relation of the x-ray photon energy to the cathode electron energy. This is expressed in an empirical (experimental) formula: Efficiency = $(1.4)(10^{-9})(ZV)$; where Z is the atomic number of the target element, V is the tube voltage, and 1.4 and 10^{-9} are constants. At 100 pkV (peak kilovoltage) the efficiency of tungsten is 1.036%.

When liberated from the filament, the accelerated electron may strike and dislodge an orbital electron of the target atom. When this occurs, another electron must fill the vacated space. Remember, when the cathode electron is stopped or decelerated, its energy is given to the atom. In Chapter 2 it was stated that the orbits of any atom are frequently referred to as energy levels. This statement refers to the requirement of a certain quantity of energy to remove an electron from its orbit. More energy is required to remove an electron from the K orbit than from the L orbit, from the L orbit than from the M orbit, and so on. The orbital energies are considered as *negative* energy, whereas the cathode electron energy is considered as *positive* energy. It follows that the orbits farther from the nucleus have greater *positive* energy.

Removal of an electron from its orbit usually includes removal of the electron energy also. When a bombarding electron strikes and dislodges a K electron from a tungsten atom, another electron must fill the vacated space. This atom emits energy in the form of a *characteristic x ray* during the transition. The energy quantity is the difference between the negative energy of the K electron and the lesser negative energy of the transitional electron. *Characteristic x rays are of definite wavelengths, are characteristic of a pure substance, and are emitted by this substance when properly excited.* Since a K orbit electron of tungsten represents approximately 70 keV (1 keV = 1,000 electron volts) of energy, it would require a cathode electron with approximately 70 keV of energy to dislodge a K electron. An L orbit electron of tungsten represents approximately 11 keV of energy. If an L orbit electron fills the vacated K space, the atom radiates 59 keV (the difference between 70 keV and 11 keV) of energy as characteristic x rays; it also radiates the remaining energy as infrared rays. *The structure of the atom determines the energy of the characteristic radiation (this does not apply to the continuous spectrum, Bremsstrahlung).*

The M orbit electron of tungsten represents approximately 2.5 keV of energy. If an M orbit electron fills the vacated K space, the energy emitted during this transition is 70 minus 2.5, or 67.5 keV, which is a much greater amount of energy than that given off during an L to K transition. All this emitted energy is in the form of electromagnetic waves. When an M orbit electron fills a vacated L space, the difference in energy levels is 11 minus 2.5, or 8.5 keV of energy given up in the form of an electromagnetic wave.

Removal of a K electron causes the atom to emit a characteristic ray. *Characteristic rays of tungsten radiate from tungsten only when the tube voltage equals or exceeds approximately 70 kVp (kilovolts peak).* Elements having atomic (Z) numbers greater than 74 require greater voltages to dislodge K electrons, and the wavelengths emitted following such a transition in energy are characteristic of these more dense elements.

Corresponding rays are those rays arising from the same transition in energy level. Corresponding rays may arise from transitions between the same named orbits of any two atoms. When corresponding rays arise from transitions into the K orbits, these rays are also characteristic.

The impressed voltage controls the force of the bombarding electrons and so controls their energy. Therefore, the voltage controls the energy of the emitted electromagnetic wave, or x ray.* Since the voltage controls the energy of the x-ray photon, the voltage peak determines the orbit from which the most energetic x-ray photon radiates and thereby determines the shortest wavelength emitted. It follows, then, that wavelength depends on the voltage. Experimental evidence reveals that the shorter wavelengths are harder (more energetic), so hardness depends on wavelength. If a wave is harder, the wave is capable of increased penetration; therefore, penetrability depends on wavelength. *These three properties of x rays—wavelength, hardness, and penetrability—are called the qualities of x rays and are all controlled by the kilovoltage.*

Quantum nature of x rays

Since the current of the secondary circuit is alternating, the impressed voltage must rise from zero to the predetermined peak, then return to zero, then rise to the peak, and so on in single-phase units. The voltage neither falls nor returns to zero in three-phase units. The constantly varying amounts of voltage propel the cathode electrons to the target; therefore the resulting energy of the x-ray photons will vary in propor-

*The energy of an x-ray photon may be determined from the formula:

$$\text{Photon energy} = \frac{12.4 \times 10^3}{\lambda\ \text{Å}} \text{ electron volts}$$

tion. As a result, the x-ray beam is a heterogeneous bundle of many wavelengths (the continuous spectrum).

It was previously mentioned that x rays have both a wave nature and a quantum nature, also that x rays originate as a heterogeneous bundle of many wavelengths. These wavelengths originate in the target from bombardment of cathode electrons possessing particular quantities of kinetic energy; therefore, the wavelengths possess a certain energy. Electrons at low energy produce longer wavelengths that are less energetic. Greater electron energy produces shorter wavelengths possessing greater amounts of energy. Thus, each individual wavelength of x ray represents a specific quantity (quantum) of energy. Regardless of the source of a given wavelength, it invariably possesses the same quantum of of energy.

The atom emits one burst of energy for each single addition of energy. *An atom cannot give off energy unless energy has been added to the atom.* If the cathode electron penetrates to the K orbit and dislodges a K electron, the atom emits a quantum of x-ray energy proportional to the K orbit energy. Since the emitted x-ray quantum originates from the K orbit, it follows that this quantum possesses a shorter wavelength than a quantum from the L orbit would possess.

Experiment proves that the shortest wavelength is solely dependent on the maximum voltage impressed upon the x-ray tube. For the sake of convenience, x-ray wavelengths are expressed in angstrom units (Å). An angstrom unit is expressed as 1×10^{-8} cm and is 1/100,000,000 of a centimeter in length. Following is a formula to determine the wavelength of any x ray:

$$\text{Shortest wavelength in Å} = \frac{12396.44^{*}}{\text{Maximum voltage}}$$

The Duane-Hunt relation. The energy of an x ray, or light photon of frequency ν is found by experiment to be $E = h\nu$, where h is Planck's constant, equal to 6.62×10^{-27} erg-sec. In terms of wavelength:

$$E = \frac{c}{\lambda} \text{ (ergs)}$$

*Although 12.4×10^3 is a less accurate value for this constant, practical consideration permits use of this more easily remembered number. (The resulting error is less than 1%.)

If metric units are used, the energy is expressed in ergs. However, a more convenient experimental energy unit is the electron volt. Since the electron charge e is equal to 4.80×10^{-10} esu (electrostatic units) and one volt = 1/300 esu of potential, 1 eV $= 4.80 \times 10^{-10} \times 1/300 = 1.60 \times 10^{-12}$ ergs. Converting (1) to electron volts:

$$E = \frac{hc/\lambda}{1.6 \times 10^{-12}} (eV)$$

But $h = 6.62 \times 10^{-27}$ and $c = 3 \times 10^{10}$. Substituting these values:

$$E = \frac{(1)}{(\lambda)} \frac{(6.62 \times 10^{-27})(3 \times 10^{10})}{1.6 \times 10^{-12}} = \frac{1.24 \times 10^{-4}}{\lambda(\text{cm})}$$

Finally, if λ is to be in angstrom units:

$$E = \frac{1.24 \times 10^{-4}}{\lambda(10^{-8})} = \frac{1.24 \times 10^{4}}{\lambda} \text{ or } E = \frac{12396.44}{\lambda}$$

If the energy involved is that emitted during an electronic transition ($\triangle$W):

$$\triangle W = \frac{12396.44}{\lambda}$$

Or, if the energy is known and the wavelength is desired, $\triangle$W and λ can be interchanged (λ is in Å units; $\triangle$W is in electron volts):

$$\lambda = \frac{12396.44}{\triangle W}$$

By the use of the formula for determining wavelength, it is possible to calculate the wavelength range most commonly used in diagnostic radiography. With a maximum voltage of 30 kVp, the minimum wavelength (λ) in angstrom units is as follows:

$$\lambda = \frac{12.4 \times 10^3}{30{,}000}, \text{ or } \lambda = 0.413 \text{ Å}$$

With a maximum voltage of 150 kVp, the minimum wavelength in angstrom units is as follows:

$$\lambda = \frac{12.4 \times 10^3}{150{,}000}, \text{ or } \lambda = 0.08 \text{ Å}$$

The above information establishes the approximate wavelength range in diagnostic radiography to be from a minimum of 0.08 Å to a maximum of 0.413 Å. The maximum wavelength in the x-ray spectrum is approximately 4.96Å. Since 2,500 volts (2.5 kV) is the minimum voltage that will produce x rays from tungsten, the wavelength is obtained as follows:

$$\lambda = \frac{12.4 \times 10^3}{2.5 \times 10^3}$$

$$\lambda = 12.4 \div 2.5 = 4.96 \text{ Å}$$

A mathematical relationship exists among the factors of wavelength (λ), velocity (υ), and frequency (ν). The following formula expresses this relationship: $\upsilon = \lambda\nu$ (upsilon = lambda nu). Substituting values of wavelength from above in this formula demonstrates that shorter wavelengths possess proportionally higher frequencies:

$$3 \times 10^{10} = (0.413)(1 \times 10^{-8})(\nu)$$
$$\nu = 7.26 \times 10^{18} \text{ vibrations/sec (approximately)}$$
$$3 \times 10^{10} = (0.08)(1 \times 10^{-8})(\nu)$$
$$\nu = 36 \times 10^{18} \text{ vibrations/sec (approximately)}$$

MEASUREMENT OF X-RAY PENETRABILITY

Penetrability is one of the important qualities of x rays, equally with hardness and wavelength; all three qualities are interdependent and all are dependent upon kilovoltage. Increasing kilovoltage either increases the depth of penetration of the cathode electrons into the target atoms or increases the number of cathode electrons having sufficient energy to penetrate into the K shell of the target atoms. In either event, an increased penetrability of the primary beam is the result; that is, either x-ray photons of greater penetrability or more numerous x-ray photons of high penetrability are produced.

The factors for a highly satisfactory technique on one machine will not necessarily be the same as those for another machine, even though the two machines are of the same make and capacity. The differences in x-ray energy output are due to the unpredictable variations in transformers and x-ray tube targets.

Because it is almost impossible to ascertain or develop a technique by purely mathematical processes, it becomes necessary to determine the penetrability of specific x-ray photons by some standard method. The device usually employed in this determination is the *penetrometer*. A penetrometer (Fig. 3-8, *A*) may be of any suitable metal but should be in the form of a *step wedge* with increasing thicknesses in each step. Aluminum is the usual metal of choice. In a step wedge, each successive step is ⅛ inch greater in thickness. The steps may have lead numbers on them to indicate the greatest step that a varied kilovoltage will penetrate. The milliampere-seconds used in this type of

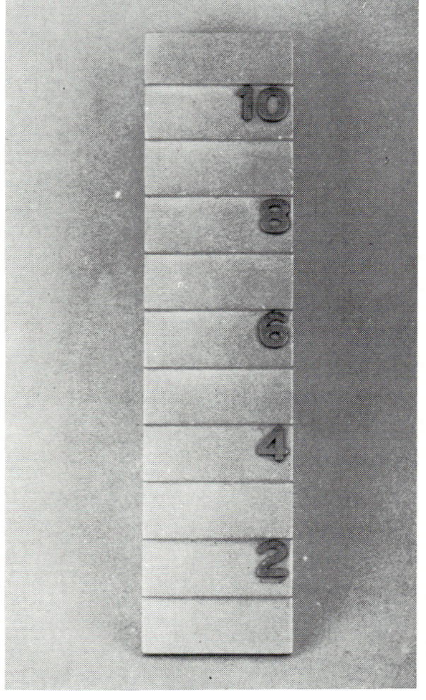

A

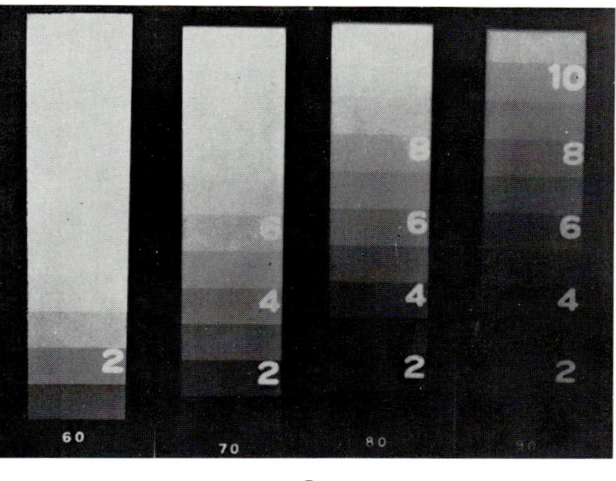

B

Fig. 3-8. A, Penetrometer. **B,** Penetrometer exposure series. Penetrometer exposure factors are 60 kVp, 70 kVp, 80 kVp, and 90 kVp; all exposures were made at a 40-inch ffd and at 50 mAs.

calibration must be constant in each series of exposures; it is equally important to maintain a constant distance (ffd) in each series. Fig. 3-8, *B*, represents such a series of exposures. The information gained from such a series is useful in developing techniques on new equipment or in making technique adjustments on equipment in use.

It is usually possible to visualize density or penetration differences of 1 kilovolt in penetrometer radiographs made with 50 kVp or less. Those radiographs made at voltages between 60 kVp and 70 kVp usually require 2 kilovolts for an appreciable visualization of change in penetration; above 70 kVp, this requirement increases to 3 kilovolts. This applies to high contrast technique. When high kilovoltage is employed the grayness (latitude) precludes *seeing* these differences.

THE X-RAY BEAM

As was mentioned earlier, the energy emerging from the x-ray tube consists of a heterogeneous bundle of many wavelengths. Since the x-ray photons arise as waves, these waves diverge from the face of the anode in all directions. Actually, x rays radiate in all degrees of a sphere from the point of bombardment on the anode face. The protective devices that surround the x-ray tube prevent escape of most of the useless rays. Many of these rays are also so soft that they are incapable of traveling any great distance from the target.

The angle of the anode also provides for the emission of the primary (useful) x rays through the side of the x-ray tube. X rays emitted from small focal areas produce radiographs exhibiting the greatest definition, since there is very little overlap of the emitted rays.

In radiography, the chief concern is with the *primary beam*. The primary beam consists of all the rays escaping from the tube shielding through the port and arising from the original bombardment of the target by the cathode electrons. Prior to penetration of the object of radiography, it is necessary to remove many of the softer rays from the heterogeneous beam to reduce unnecessary exposure.

The primary rays diverge in all forward directions with the *central ray*. The central ray is that portion of the primary rays that leaves the port at right angles to the long axis of the x-ray tube and is *the portion of the primary beam directed to the center of the film or structure to be radiographed.* It is necessary to control the divergent portions of the primary rays. Collimators and diaphragms, when properly attached over the port, effectively control most of the diverging x rays.

SECONDARY RAYS

When a beam of x rays passes through any substance, the substance tends to absorb or remove part of the energy. Many experiments on the reduction in intensity of an x-ray beam by passage through an absorbing layer have been performed. The effect of air as an absorbing material is most important. Although air consists, for the most part, of relatively loose molecules of lighter elements, the primary rays must interact with these atoms and molecules in one or more of the three ways discussed on pp. 58 to 60. Exact data for air absorption may be obtained from the National Bureau of Standards. To obtain the exact intensity of an x-ray beam at a given distance from its target, the value obtained by calculation from the inverse-square law must be multiplied by the correction factor for this distance in air. (See pp. 87 to 89.)

When the primary rays pass through the tissues of the body or other organic material, several phenomena occur. Among these phenomena is that of secondary ray production. *Secondary rays are the rays generated in the patient and surrounding objects by the passage of the primary x rays.* The student must realize that only the primary rays are x rays. Secondary rays are not x rays, since they are not generated as a result of sudden deceleration or stoppage of high-speed electrons. However, many of these secondary rays may possess characteristics and capabilities of x rays.

Experiment reveals that these secondary rays are usually of at least two kinds: scattered or secondary scatter rays (some possess wavelengths identical with the primary rays and others possess longer wavelengths) and characteristic fluorescent rays (these are characteristic—possess the same wavelength—of the radiator material). *Secondary scatter rays* diverge in all directions from the point of generation in the object (radiator). The greater intensity of these rays is in the forward direction. In therapy, because of the effect of these rays on human tissues, the secondary scatter rays are of extreme importance when the primary wavelength is short. *Characteristic fluorescent rays* are identical with characteristic rays, but the method of generation of each is different. *Characteristic rays result from cathode electron bombardment of the x-ray tube target; characteristic fluorescent rays result from the impact of an exciting primary x-ray photon on the radiator.* The voltage required to produce characteristic rays is proportional to the square of the atomic number of the target material. Additional information on secondary rays in relation to image formation may be found on pp. 69 and 70.

REMNANT RAYS

During the exposure of an object (patient, part, or phantom) many of the primary (x) rays are either absorbed (stopped) in the object or are modified (lose energy); thus the rays that actually expose the film are a combination of primary (x) rays and secondary rays generated within the object radiographed. These emerging rays are called *remnant rays,* and compose that ionizing radiation that produces the radiographic (latent) image. Of the remnant rays, primary rays cause the radiographic density and secondary rays cause the latent image. The quantity of secondary rays in the remnant radiation depends on the secondary ray wavelengths and the methods employed to control secondary ray production.

X RAYS AND MATTER

We have learned (p. 51) that x rays have the ability to cause numerous biologic, physical, and chemical effects. In one way or another, most of these effects are important in radiology, some being of great importance. It is the latter with which we will concern ourselves.

Physical phenomena, such as fluorescence and the photographic effect of x rays, are of major importance in diagnostic radiology. All biologic effects are of major importance in therapeutic radiology, and some are equally important in diagnostic radiology. Of particular importance in diagnostic radiology are the methods and results of interaction between ionizing radiations and living matter and between those radiations and nonliving matter. If such interactions did not occur, there would be neither biologic nor photographic effects. Such effects result in lasting changes, and these changes occur only if radiant energy is absorbed in the irradiated medium. When radiations pass through a medium without losing energy in the process, no effects can occur.

X rays are of quite short wavelengths, especially when compared with the radii of atomic nuclei and of the electron orbits about the nuclei. Because of this relatively large space in atoms, many of the shorter x rays are capable of passing between a nucleus and its orbital electrons and striking neither the nucleus nor an orbital electron. In the following discussion of ionizing ray interaction with matter it is convenient to consider these rays as photons of energy rather than as electromagnetic waves.

X rays are capable of penetrating all matter; however, the material through which these photons pass absorbs much of the x-ray photon energy. This energy loss is in the form of secondary ray production. Photons of energy may interact with and penetrate matter in any one of three different manners. These are explained in the following paragraphs (see Fig. 3-9).

1. *Photoelectric emission and true absorption.* When sufficiently high-energy photons of

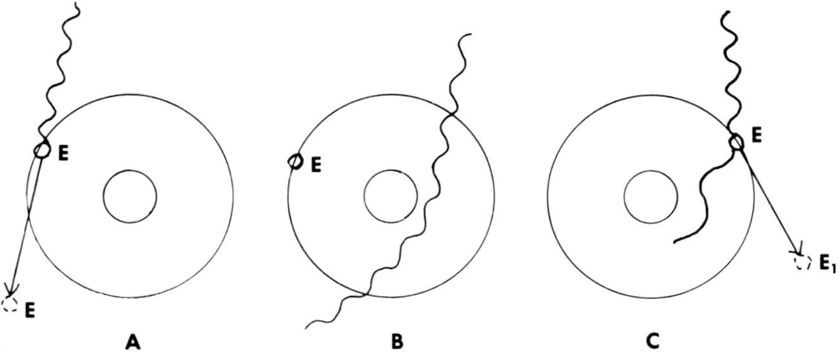

Fig. 3-9. Interactions of energy photons and matter. **A,** True absorption with photoelectron emission. **B,** Unmodified or true (Thompson) scattering. **C,** Compton effect: the Compton photon, less some of its energy, travels onward in a different direction; the recoil electron (E_1) continues in a different direction from the Compton photon; the recoil electron possesses less energy than the Compton photon.

the primary beam collide with and remove an electron from the K orbit of an atom of the material penetrated, the atom emits a characteristic ray and another electron fills the vacated space. The removed electron receives all the energy of the photon remaining (left over) after electron removal; then the electron immediately travels away from the atom, perhaps striking and ionizing other atoms. This type of interaction is photoelectric emission with true absorption; the electron is a *photoelectron** and travels with the transferred kinetic energy of the photon. The photon has given up all of its energy.

2. *Unmodified scattering (Thompson scattering).* A high-energy photon from the primary beam may strike an atom and deflect in another path without entering the atom. The photon retains all its original energy, so it is *unmodified* (modification refers to a reduction in energy with an increase in wavelength). A photon may also pass between the nucleus and the K orbit and touch neither, but since the nucleus attracts the photon, it deflects slightly in exit direction.

3. *Compton effect.* The Compton effect is an interaction between the photon and a free (unbound) electron or between the photon and an orbital electron. A high-energy photon of the primary beam may strike an orbital electron at an angle; the photon imparts a small part of its energy to the electron to eject this electron from its orbit; the photon deflects from its original path and continues through the atom. The ejected electron is a *recoil electron* and may strike other electrons before leaving the atom and thereby cause additional ionization of this atom or other atoms in its path. *Ion pair*† formation may result from such action. The photon retains the major portion of its original energy and may cause additional ionization. *This modified photon is a Compton photon.*

Another condition of pair formation results when photon energy is at least 1.02 meV. In such an instance the photon energy may interact with the magnetic and electric nuclear fields to produce the following situation. The photon is stopped and all or part of its energy is converted into mass as two particles, an electron and a positron, each possessing 0.511 meV of energy. When the photon energy exceeds 1.02 meV, the excess energy is kinetic and is that which produced the two high-speed particles. This is true pair production.*

According to the degree of penetration by x rays, animal tissues are classified as follows: *radiopaque*—bones and other tissues containing calcium salts; *intermediate*—muscle, the epidermis, blood, cartilage and other connective tissues, and stones containing either cholesterol or uric acid; or *radiolucent*—adipose tissues, gas, and air.

The degree to which x rays penetrate tissues depends on the atomic and molecular structures of the tissues and the energy of the primary photons; the physical condition of the patient also affects the penetration. This characteristic of x rays to penetrate matter to varying degrees makes x rays useful as a diagnostic tool in medicine and in industry. The fact that x rays do not penetrate all animal tissues equally permits the use of x rays in the demonstration of the varying densities of these tissues.

X RAYS AND FILTERS

It has been explained that passage of x-ray photons through matter results in a decrease in the emerging photon energy because of absorption.

In radiography, it is necessary to reduce unwanted wavelengths in the primary beam by inserting an aluminum filter† in the tube-shielding port (p. 95). *Present requirements are that*

*The emission of negative charges by the action of light on a surface is the *photoelectric effect,* and the emitted charges are *photoelectrons.* For any given material there is a minimum light frequency (maximum wavelength) below which electrons will not be emitted; this maximum wavelength is called the *photoelectric threshold.* For a given surface, the number of photoelectrons emitted each second (the photoelectric current) is directly proportional to the intensity of the light; also, the kinetic energy of the emitted photoelectrons depends only on the light frequency and is independent of light intensity.

†When an atom loses an electron that attaches to another atom, each becomes an ion and the two are called an ion pair. Some authorities consider ion pair formation as an additional method of interaction of photon energy and matter.

*Additional information relating to triplet production and annihilation radiation is dealt with on page 124.

†The use of the words *filter* and *filtration* in relation to the absorption of the photon energy must not be confused with the same terms as used in chemistry. Chemical filtration refers to the actual holding back of some of the material in suspension. Physical filtration refers to absorption of some of the energy by the filter (absorbing layer).

at least 2 mm of aluminum be used in addition to the inherent filter. Additional thicknesses of aluminum require a slight upward adjustment in the kilovoltage, as discussed on p. 95. Aluminum filters are used because the characteristic fluorescent rays of this element are so soft that the energy of these rays is expended in a few centimeters of air. As a result, there is no visible effect on the radiograph.

Federal performance standards for measurement of HVL using aluminum require that Type 1100 aluminum be used. Type 1100 alloy is 99% minimum aluminum with no more than 0.12% copper. The density of aluminum can be a factor if there is to be a choice between rolled and cast aluminum. However, provided the density and purity are that of Type 1100 the use of 2 mm of aluminum *added* filtration in the primary beam meets present minimum requirements.

Other pure-substance materials have been employed experimentally as filters, and in certain instances such materials present potential advantages. The use of iron as a filter in diagnostic radiography was explored by Bösche and Frik in 1962, and results of experimentation with it are reported in an article by Schanze. The experimental evidence reported in this article in-

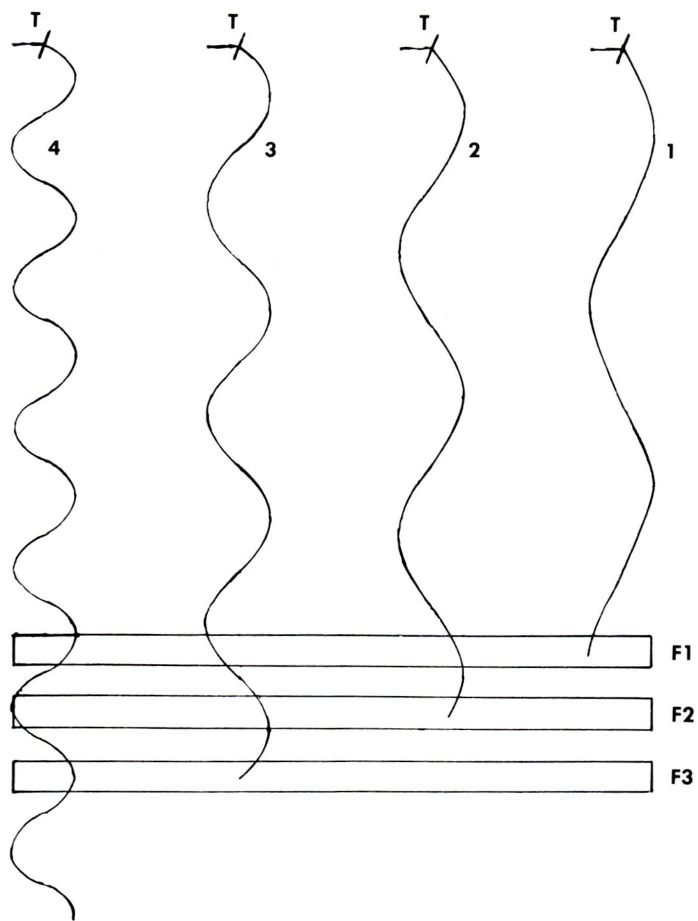

Fig. 3-10. Absorption of wavelengths by filters.

T. Target of x-ray tube
F1. Filter no. 1
F2. Filter no. 2
F3. Filter no. 3

1. Wavelength whose energy is absorbed by filter no. 1
2. Wavelength whose energy is absorbed by filter no. 2
3. Wavelength whose energy is absorbed by filter no. 3
4. Wavelength whose energy is great enough to penetrate all three filters

dicates that between 60 and 120 kVp iron absorbs equal quantities of soft (primary) rays as the same thickness of pure aluminum and increases the total energy striking the film by from 6% to 20%. The increase is obtained through the production of hard secondary rays that cannot be absorbed by the patient.

Fig. 3-10 is a schematic representation of the manner in which filters absorb certain of the weaker x-ray photons and permit other photons to penetrate the filter. If sufficient filters were added in the primary beam, the resulting x-ray beam would contain waves of all the same length. Such an x-ray beam is *monochromatic* or *homogeneous:* all of the waves are of the same length and contain identical energy quanta.

X-RAY INTENSITY

Radiographic processes depend on the quantity of radiographic intensity that strikes the x-ray film; however, x-ray therapy processes depend on the total quantity of intensity absorbed by the tissues. Intensity of radiation is that energy carried by the radiation in a unit of time through a small surface perpendicular to the direction of the radiation, divided by the area of the surface. The quantity of radiation is the product of *intensity times time.* The nature (intensity) of an x-ray beam depends on both the current and voltage between the cathode and anode.

The number of cathode electrons generating x rays during anode bombardment has a direct relation to the intensity of this beam of x rays. If this number increases, there will be corresponding increases in the number of x rays generated. Increases in number of available electrons are achieved either by increasing time or by raising current.

It follows that intensity is associated with milliamperage. Then quantity of radiation (exposure) is the product of milliamperage times time. Milliampere-seconds is an expression of radiographic (intensity) exposure. Milliamperage times time in seconds equals milliampere-seconds. Stated algebraically this becomes $\text{mA} \times \text{s} = \text{mAs}$.

If mA and mAs are known:

$$\text{s} = \frac{\text{mAs}}{\text{mA}}$$

If both s and mAs are known:

$$\text{mA} = \frac{\text{mAs}}{\text{s}}$$

Although specific values of mAs may be obtained in a variety of combinations of different values of mA and s, it is essential that certain precautions be observed in making different selections of these factors. A short exposure time is essential to stop motion as in visceral studies. However, it must be remembered that changing the mA selector from 50 or 100 to 200 and above almost always switches (automatically) the heating current from the small to the large focal spot. This is not necessarily objectionable in most visceral studies.

Reciprocity* of x-ray film is discussed on pp. 70 and 71. It is important here to introduce the following information. In reciprocity failure where E = mAs, 1/60 sec vs 1 sec and appropriate mA do not always produce the same degree of radiographic and object density.†

Experimental evidence reveals that there are two types of radiation: continuous and characteristic (pp. 53 to 55). Continuous radiation consists of the several wavelengths and does not require excessively high voltage. Characteristic radiations occur *only* when the voltage is sufficiently high. The continuous (general) radiation intensity (1) is directly proportional to the milliamperage; (2) varies approximately with the square of the voltage; and (3) varies with the Z number of the target material.

Each type of radiation, continuous and characteristic, affects tissues similarly. No biologic change can occur from energy acting upon living tissues *unless energy is absorbed by these tissues.* The degree of ionization is a measure of the quantity of interaction of energy and matter. Many methods of x-ray intensity measurement have been developed. Probably the most satisfactory of these is the one that depends upon the measurement of the degree of ionization of air at a given distance from the x-ray tube target; measurements of this type must be made in air to avoid backscatter (the radiation scattered back from the underlying materials).

---

*In 1876 Bunsen and Roscoe formulated what is known as the reciprocity law which states: "The effective action of light is constant when the product of the intensity times the time of action is constant." This law has been found invalid, and deviations from it are considered reciprocity law failure.

†It is possible that the total number of pulses in each of the two exposures exerts a strong influence, if not partial control, on the final density.

Common radiation measurement and detection instruments*

The **condenser R-meter** (R is the unit of measure of quantity of roentgen radiation) is commonly used to measure the radiation intensity of x-ray therapy machines (Fig. 3-11). A brief explanation follows. The R-meter consists of a box containing an electroscope that is insulated from the box, a device for charging the electroscope and its attached electrode, and a battery-operated lamp to illuminate the scale, which reads directly in roentgens. A movable scale marker is attached to the electroscope and a small microscope permitting visualization of the illuminated scale. The ionization chamber tube fits into a receptacle in one end of the box. When the tube is placed in contact with the electroscope electrode, a connection is made between this electrode and a second electrode in the ionization chamber in the opposite end of this tube. When operated, the electrometer is charged so the scale marker points to zero. Insertion and contact of the tube, whose chamber has been ionized by the passage of x rays, causes a loss in potential of the electrometer according to the degree of ionization in the cham-

*For more on detection instruments see p. 132.

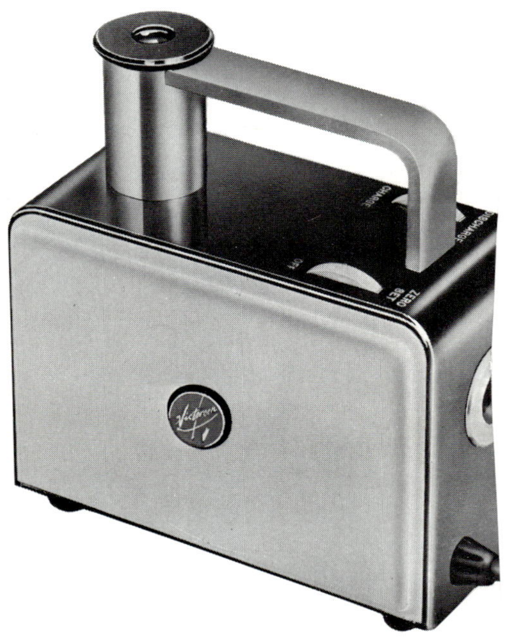

Fig. 3-11. Condenser R-meter, Model 570. (Court
The Victoreen Instrument Co.)

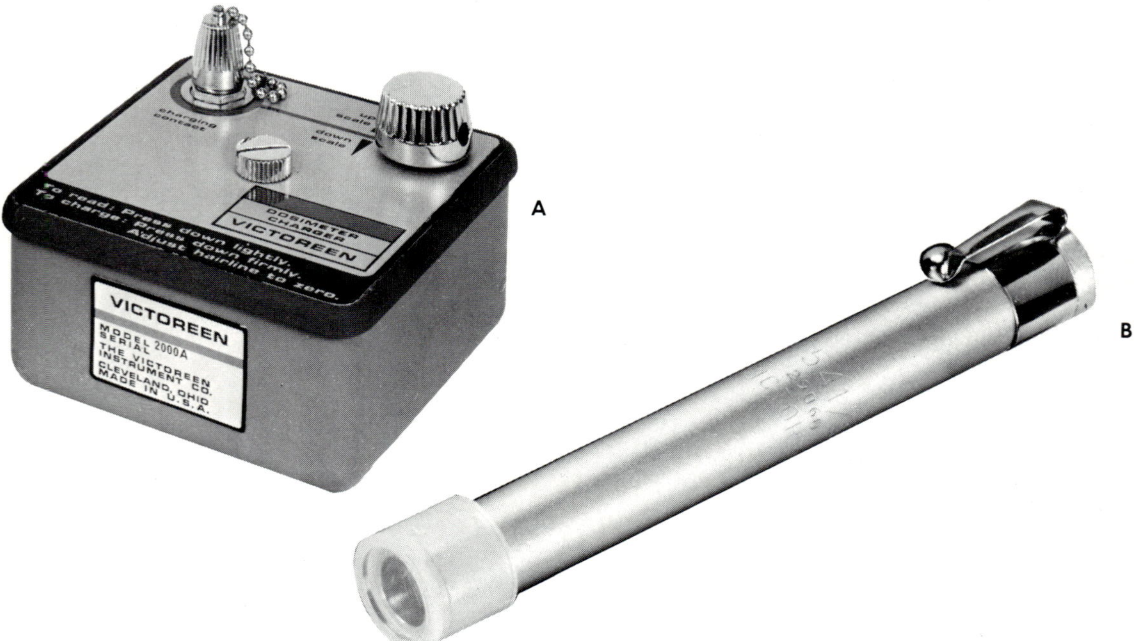

Fig. 3-12. A, Victoreen dosimeter charger. **B,** Victoreen direct reading pocket dosimeter. (Courtesy The Victoreen Instrument Co.)

ber. The scale marker then moves from zero to indicate a certain number of roentgens. After operation, the air in the ionization chamber returns to its normal state and the electroscope is again charged. Measurements are made by exposing the chamber to a certain quantity of radiation at a specific distance from the x-ray tube target for a *specific* (usually 1 minute) *period of time.*

The **dosimeter pencil** (pocket dosimeter) is another device used to measure ionization by radiation (Fig. 3-12). This device, carried in the pocket of the personnel when they are around sources of radiation, operates somewhat differently from the R-meter. The particular advantage of this device is that the wearer can read it at any time, simply by placing one end to his eye and the opposite end to a light. The device nearly always has a *drift,* so that any measurement accruing over a 1-day period is somewhat in error.

A dosimeter pencil is essentially a small Lauritzen electroscope to be worn on the person for recording the quantity of ionizing radiation encountered. This electroscope consists of a fine fiber loop attached to an insulated electrode that is encased in a tube containing lenses and a graduated reticle for viewing and calibrating the motion of the fiber. A refinement of this instrument in the dosimeter pencil is the provision of a reticle scale for determining the rate of radiation received. The rate is determined by the movement of the fiber for a set period of time.

Another device used similarly to the dosimeter pencil is the **minometer** (Fig. 3-13). This instrument can be read only when it is applied (connected) to the charger.

R-meters and dosimeter pencils are operated *after* they are given a static charge. The quantity of charge given to the instrument varies, and there is usually some means of *bleeding off* any

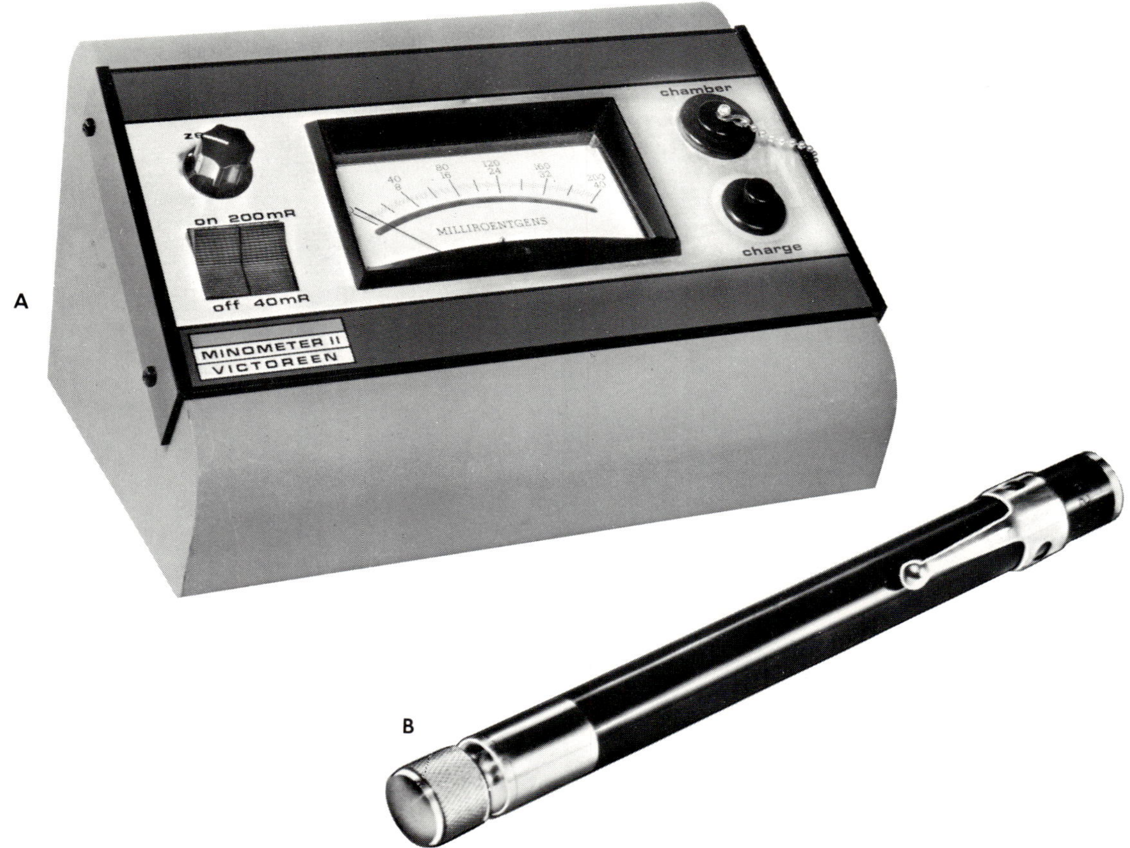

Fig. 3-13. A, Victoreen Minometer II. **B,** Victoreen indirect reading pocket dosimeter. (Courtesy The Victoreen Instrument Co.)

excess charge prior to use of the instrument. Dosimeter pencils are charged by use of a battery-powered electronic circuit. The R-meter charger produces a static charge by friction, and any excess charge placed on the instrument is bled off through high resistance.

The foregoing instruments are employed principally in conjunction with relatively constant x-ray intensities. Ionization-type radiation detectors used to detect high or varying radiations are the ionization chamber, proportional counter, and the Geiger-Müller counter.

The **ionization chamber** consists of a gas-filled envelope and two electrodes of different electrical potentials. The envelope may be one of the electrodes, and the gas may be any number of materials, including air. An ionizing radiation particle or photon entering the gas-filled envelope produces ions, which, because of the applied potential, drift toward the electrodes. The ions drift to the oppositely charged electrode. The applied potential causes an electric current to flow until the potential balance is restored. The current from the chamber is very small, requiring electronic amplification of the signal before it can be recorded on a meter. Ionization chambers do not record individual radiation particles or photons but integrate (add up) the signals produced as an electric current.

The **Geiger-Müller counter** (commonly called the Geiger counter or GM counter) is similar in design to the proportional counter. The chief differences are in the mode of operation and the gas in the detector tube. The potential across the electrodes of a Geiger counter detector tube produces enough gas multiplication* from a single radiation particle to discharge the tube below its operating threshold. The detector tube is then recharged by the high-voltage supply and is again ready to record another particle. Since the Geiger tube discharges below its operating threshold each time it functions, the tube does not discriminate between types of radiation. Furthermore, the Geiger tube operates over a range of several hundred volts without gross changes in its counting rate. The *Geiger plateau* is the voltage range over which only small changes in the counting rate occur.

The **proportional counter** consists of a gas-filled envelope with two electrodes, one of which is a cylinder concentric with very fine wire that

*The formation of new ions by driving the original ions through the gas is called *gas multiplication.*

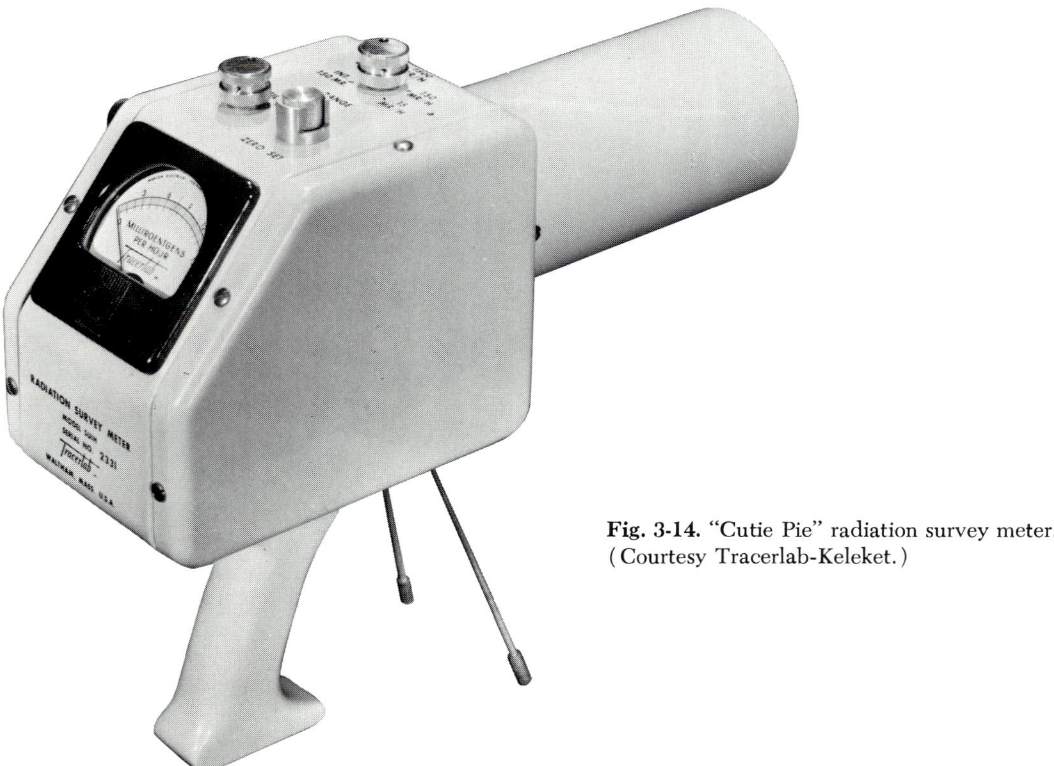

Fig. 3-14. "Cutie Pie" radiation survey meter. (Courtesy Tracerlab-Keleket.)

acts as the other electrode. A potential difference drives radiation-formed ions through the gas with sufficient energy to produce new ions. The pulse produced in a proportional counter is proportional to the number of ions produced, whereas all pulses from a Geiger counter tube are essentially the same size. The advantage of the proportional counter is that through the use of an electronic discriminator pulses below a selected size can be excluded.

Other instruments employed for varying radiation intensity measurements include the Cutie Pie and scalers (Figs. 3-14 and 3-15).

The **Cutie Pie,** an ionization chamber type of survey meter, is an actual rate meter device. The device records instantly both x- and gamma-radiation levels. Equipping the device with a suitable "window" material makes possible its use for beta-ray monitoring. The usual range of sensitivity in the Cutie Pie is from 2 mR per hour to approximately 5R per hour. The extreme sensitivity of this dose-rate meter makes it a most valuable instrument for radiation surveys of x-ray installations, radium and radioisotope storage facilities, and patients undergoing therapy or diagnosis by means of radionuclides. The instruments are calibrated usually against known radium standards; however, instrument response to diagnostic x rays seldom deviates more than 20% from the correct amount. There are both advantages and disadvantages to use of these instruments not pertinent to discussion in this text.

The **scaler,** or scaling circuit, is an electric counting apparatus. This device uses a supply of constant voltage in the order of 1 to 2 kV. Detection or "seeing" radiations by this counter causes very small pulses that must be amplified for counting. Amplification of other electrical "noises" originating in the circuit occurs concurrently with amplification of the desired pulses. The artificial noises are blocked from the counting of pulses by another electronic device incorporated after the amplifier. Finally, the clean, amplified pulses are counted with the time necessary for the counting being determined with great accuracy. Division of the observed counts by the time of observation results in a "counts-per-second" or "counts-per-minute" figure.

Film badges

Film badges are very satisfactory devices to be worn by all persons engaged in work with radiation to record the quantity of radiation received. It is to be remembered that the film will record only that radiation striking it and received at the place where the film is worn. If the technologist (or other operator) or supervisor feels that a second or even third film badge should be worn for specific examinations, these must be worn concurrently with the first, and the locations of the extra film badges be logged in the department record book. Film badges in the form of *finger rings* and *wrist bracelets* are available for specific procedures.

There has been controversy as to whether the film badge should be worn outside the lead apron or beneath this apron during fluoroscopy. The principal, and often only, film badge should be worn in the same place each day. If additional information regarding the amount of radiation striking the apron is desired, a second film badge should be worn on the outside of the apron.

Film badges are not protective devices! They are worn to record radiation received. The radiation may be x rays, gamma rays, or beta particles. Special film badges are available to record radia-

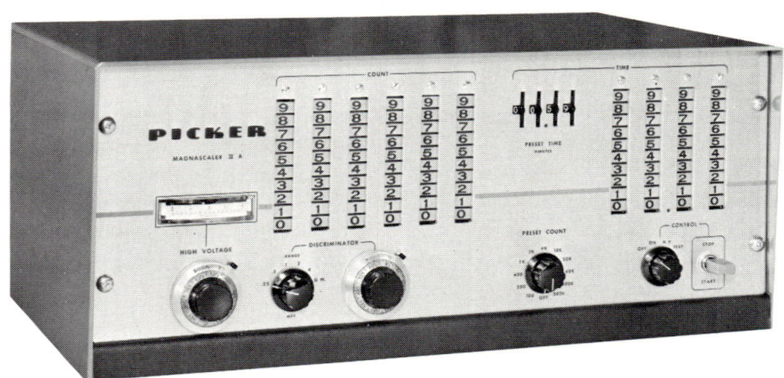

Fig. 3-15. Picker Magnascaler II A. (Courtesy Picker Nuclear.)

tion received from neutrons. All film badges are constructed with some form, usually plastic, of radiolucent material sandwiching a small film, much like a dental film, between laminated, wedged, or spaced filters. The filters may be of different materials. Cadmium and copper are commonly used materials. The degree of darkening on specific parts of the film is read on densitometers by skilled technologists. The degree of darkening is compared with known standards and indicates a quantity of specific radiation (x, gamma, or beta) between certain maximum and minimum levels. The service is available on a time-period basis best suited to the particular departmental work load.

A report of darkened film is an indication that the wearer received a certain quantity of radiation in a specific period of time. If the quantity is in excess of what is considered safe and within set standards, steps will be taken by the supervisor and operator to prevent reoccurrence. However, there are other causes of darkened films, and reported results of some of these can become a source of confusion in the department, especially since lifetime radiation records are kept on file by most agencies supplying film badge service. Careless handling and use of the film badge may permit excessive or unusual exposure to the badge when it is not worn. (See pp. 110 to 112 for maximum limits of radiation received.)

Periodic blood counts

Periodic blood counts on all personnel employed in radiation areas are made so that changes in the hemogram that may be the result of excessive radiation may be determined. However, periodic blood counts are *not* a measure of quantity of radiation received.

A blood count usually includes the following as a minimum: erythrocyte count, leukocyte count, hemoglobin estimation in grams per 100 ml of whole blood, and differential leukocyte count in percentages. Many other indices are often requested and may constitute a part of the routine. It is to be noted that ionizing radiations have an almost immediate effect on the leukocyte count, particularly the lymphocytes, since lymphoid tissue is very susceptible to these radiations. The lowered lymphocyte percentage may result from other factors, however.

REFERENCES

Clark, George L.: Applied x-rays, ed. 4, New York, 1955, McGraw-Hill Book Co.

Glasser, Otto: Medical physics, vol. 2, Chicago, 1950, Year Book Publishers.

Goodwin, Paul N., Quimby, Edith H., and Morgan, Russell H.: Physical foundations of radiology, ed. 4, New York, 1970, Harper and Row.

Reimann, Arnold L.: Thermionic emission, New York, 1934, John Wiley & Sons, Inc.

Robertson, John Kellock: Radiology physics, ed. 3, Princeton, N.J., 1955, D. Van Nostrand Co., Inc.

Schanze, Ulrich O.: Iron filters in diagnostic radiology, Radiologic Technology 37(3):137, 1965.

QUESTIONS

1. How are x rays produced?
2. What kinds of electric current flow to the cathode of an x-ray tube?
3. What functions are served by the oil in the x-ray tube shielding?
4. Differentiate between the electronic and optical focal spots.
5. Explain why tube current is named milliamperage.
6. What causes the liberated electrons to strike the anode with high velocity? How can this velocity be regulated?
7. Why are x rays not produced (normally) in a valve tube?
8. In a hot cathode x-ray tube, what is the source of energy that results in increased kinetic energy of the liberated electrons?
9. What makes possible the photographic effect of x rays on film emulsions?
10. Explain saturation current and its effect on the intensity of x rays.
11. What is meant by the space charge?
12. What are the rays of Bremsstrahlung?
13. Do continuous x rays arise concurrently with characteristic x rays? If so, why? If not, why not?
14. What is the percentage of cathode electrons that ultimately strike the patient? Explain your answer.
15. What is the energy in electron volts of an x-ray wave of 0.2 Å in length?
16. What is the minimum wavelength in angstroms of an x ray produced from 70 kVp?
17. What is the frequency of the wavelength in question 16?
18. Why are secondary rays not x rays?
19. Is ionization an essential occurrence in the process of latent image formation?
20. In the process of exposing a patient to x rays to produce a radiograph, does ionization occur (a) in the patient, (b) in the film emulsion, or (c) in both patient and film emulsion?
21. In which of the four possible types of interaction between energy and matter are positive ions formed? Negative ions?

22. How much total filtration is required in the primary beam? How much added filtration?
23. Why is aluminum required as the external filter?
24. What is the function of filters as used in x-ray therapy?
25. How is the quantity of radiation in a given exposure determined?
26. On what single occurrence does biologic change depend?
27. Why are short exposure times preferred in visceral studies?
28. What is the reciprocity law?
29. What is meant by reciprocity law failure?
30. What detecting instruments are usually employed where high or varying radiations may be encountered?
31. What purpose is served by the wearing of a film badge?
32. What tissue is highly susceptible to ionizing radiations?

4. RADIOGRAPH PRODUCTION

Producing a radiograph of the greatest possible diagnostic quality, with the least possible discomfort and greatest possible protection for the patient, should be uppermost in the mind of the technologist as he performs each examination. Production of high-quality radiographs involves a multitude of operations—many are controlled or performed automatically and others are performed manually by the technologist. It is to be remembered that most automatic operations are "programmed" by the technologist; therefore the end result is invariably attributable either to human skill or to human error. Whether it is radiography or photography that is underway, the same truism holds, *good radiographs (and pictures) do not just happen;* they result from the use of a combination of factors that is just right for the occasion. Perhaps the technologist (or photographer) calculated these factors from his knowledge of all pertinent information, or perhaps he "lucked-out." Regardless of his method, he applied the correct factors.

Since the ultimate objective is a radiograph of the best possible diagnostic quality, it is essential that the student have knowledge of all the factors of diagnostic quality and that he understands how each both affects and effects the end result. Understanding the interrelationship of the factors of diagnostic quality dictates that the student develop prior appreciation and understanding in two related areas of knowledge: (1) film construction, that is, the film base and the emulsion applied to each side of it, and (2) latent image formation.

RADIOGRAPHIC IMAGE

Chemical aspects

Many radiographic phenomena are quite similar to, and many are the same as, comparable photographic phenomena. A considerable degree of useful and practical information concerning radiography may be attained by making proper comparison with photography. In each art the first image on the film is achieved through a physical principle, the result of which is the latent image. *The latent image is the invisible image produced by a physical effect of electromagnetic wave energy upon certain members of a family of chemicals called the halogens.** This image can be rendered visible by the subsequent chemical developing process. A property of the halogen family, that of *photosensitiviity,* sets these elements apart from all others.

Chief interest in the halogens is restricted to bromine, which combines readily with silver to form silver bromide (AgBr). This particular silver halide is probably the principal silver salt used in the film emulsion, although the silver salts of iodine and chlorine are often used in conjunction with silver bromide.

Initially in our profession the end result of x-ray exposure of a patient on a sensitized emulsion was called a *skiagraph* or *skiagram.* A skiagraph is a shadowlike image or picture made on a sensitive surface, especially by x rays. The "light-sensitive" surface was an emulsion of one or more halogens in combination with silver and other chemicals evenly dispersed over glass. Glass presented many problems, especially in handling and storing, and was soon replaced with a thin sheet of cellulose nitrate. This latter material presented the serious hazard of being highly flammable and was the cause of many fires in the radiograph storage area in hospitals. Cellulose nitrate was replaced with essentially nonflammable cellulose acetate. This material was the base of "safe" x-ray film for many years, but has been replaced with the modern synthetic materials, which are approximately 0.0073 inch thick and somewhat thinner than cellulose acetate. Less storage space is required and, of far greater advantage, the synthetic bases do not absorb water!

The finished film consists of the base coated on both sides with a dehydrated suspension of silver bromide in gelatin. The structure of the silver bromide crystals may be explained simply as a combination of positive silver ions and negative bromine ions. Both coats are of constant thickness, approximately 0.001 inch, and the dispersion of the photosensitive crystals is homogeneous. A blue tint is usually added to the base material to increase the diagnostic quality of the

*The halogen family of elements includes fluorine, chlorine, bromine, iodine, and astatine.

radiograph. Most manufacturers apply a scratch-deterring coating to both surfaces.

Different proportions of silver salts are used in the production of different types of x-ray films. With most no-screen film, the photosensitive coating is slightly greater in thickness than the same coating on plain film. The no-screen film coating is more sensitive to x-ray energy than to light energy, and it contains about 40% more silver crystals than the plain film coating. The plain film coating is highly sensitive to light energy.

Fig. 4-1 reveals the dispersion of the reduced (developed) silver grains in a radiograph of a child's hip. In Fig. 4-1, *A*, the circled part on the photograph of the radiograph indicates the area of photomicrography in Fig. 4-1, *B* and *C*. The indicated points, *I*, *E*, and *S* within the circle, are respectively points on the ilium, epiphysis, and joint space on which densitometer readings were made. The readings are as follows: *I*—2.92, *E*—3.1, and *S*—3.21. Fig. 4-1, *B*, is a photomicrograph with low power (25×) of the reduced silver grains in the area between *I* and *E*. Fig. 4-1, *C*, is a photomicrograph with oil immersion (400×) of the same area as in 4-1, *B*. The sharp, black objects in Fig. 4-1, *C*, are the silver grains on the upper side (nearest the microscope objective) of the x-ray film, and the blurred, black objects are those silver grains on the underside of the x-ray film.

Formation of the latent image in the photosensitive coating of the film results from the action of the energy passed through and from the object radiographed when this energy (remnant radi-

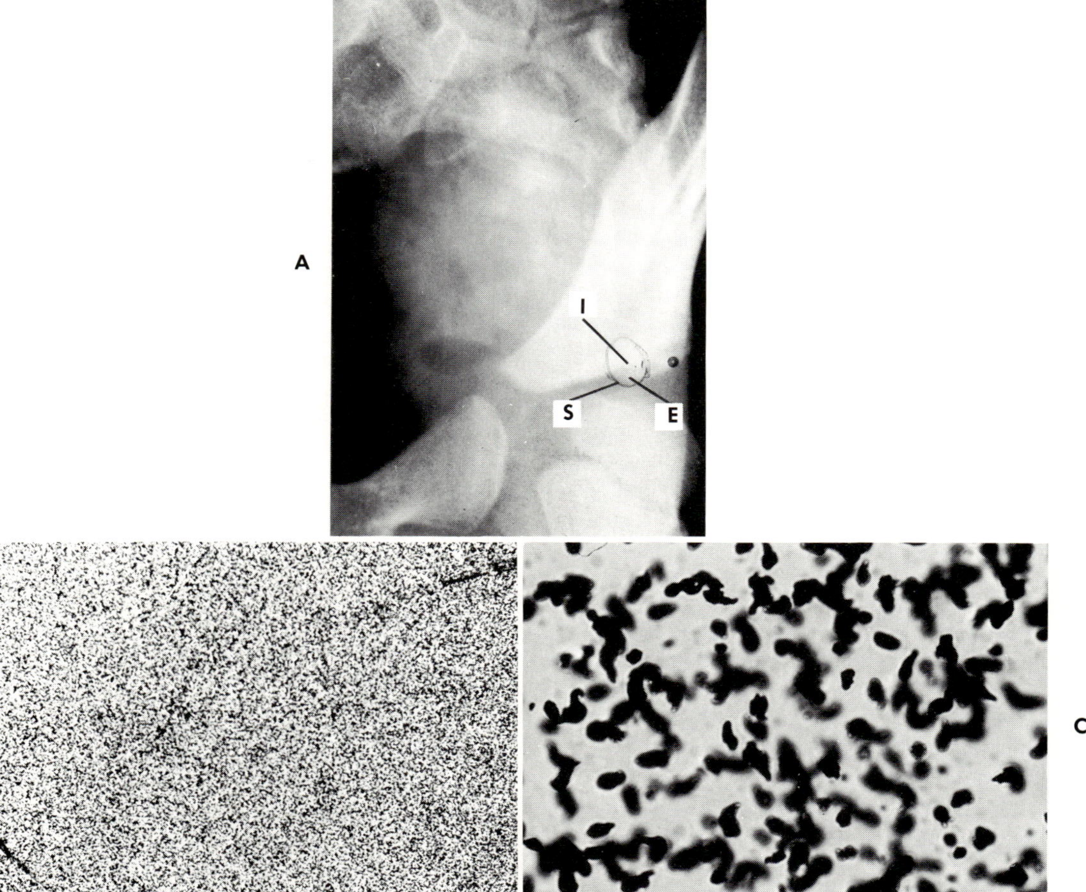

Fig. 4-1. A, Photograph of radiograph of child's hip. *I*, *E*, and *S* are points on which densitometer readings were made. **B,** Photomicrograph with low power of silver grains (after reduction) in area of circle in **A. C,** Photomicrograph with oil immersion of center of same area as in **B.**

Table 4-1. Lattice structure of silver bromide crystals

Ag^+	Br^-	Ag^+	Br^-	Ag^+	Br^-	Ag^+	Br^-	Ag^+
Br^-	Ag^+	Br^-	Ag^+	Br^-	Ag^+	Br^-	Ag^+	Br^-
Ag^+	Br^-	Ag^+	Br^-	Ag^+	Br^-	Ag^+	Br^-	Ag^+
Br^-	Ag^+	Br^-	Ag^+ *Ag*+	Br^-	Ag^+	Br^-	Ag^+	Br^-
Ag^+	Br^-	Ag^+	Br^-	□	Br^-	Ag^+	Br^-	Ag^+

ation) strikes the silver bromide grains. Actually, the x-ray (primary ray) part of the remnant rays serves in the final radiograph to produce only film (background) density. Only the secondary rays (generated in the object struck and traversed by the primary beam) are responsible for the eventual object image. It is to be considered that the film density is a part of the total manifest (when processed) image. When the latent image is developed, it is called the actual image *(manifest image).* Upon striking the silver bromide grains, the x-ray energy (and/or light energy when cassettes are used) causes the grains to separate into positive silver ions ($Ag+$) and negative bromine ions ($Br-$). This reaction may be written simply as follows:

$$\text{Light}^* + \text{AgBr} \rightarrow \text{Ag} + \text{Br(gas)}\uparrow$$

The complete *lattice structure* of silver bromide provides a situation in which the silver is free to move. This is probably the principal reason for the selection of this particular silver halide in these photosensitive emulsions. The lattice structure of silver bromide consists of alternate silver and bromide ions as shown in Table 4-1. This is a uniform structure except for the misplaced $Ag+$ ion (in italics). This condition is known as *Frenkel's disorder;* the misplaced silver ion is known as an *interstitial ion.*

Physical aspects

The degree of density in the radiograph probably depends on the total number of silver ions present in each specific area of the radiograph; that is, where greater energy absorption occurred, greater tissue density existed; therefore fewer silver ions were available for eventual development.

The theory of latent image production is very involved; therefore only a portion of the theory is presented.

Experimental evidence suggests the existence of minute specks of both metallic silver and silver sulfide on the unexposed silver grains in the film emulsion. It is further considered that the metallic silver specks are on the surface, and the silver sulfide specks are beneath or inside the surface. When x-ray (or light) energy strikes the silver halide grains, electrons are released and their kinetic energy causes them to move. In their ambient motion most of the electrons collect at *sensitization specks** on or near the surface of the emulsion grains; thus these specks exhibit a rather strong negative electric charge. The silver ions, being electrically positive, migrate to the specks and collect in the form of atomic silver. (When atomic silver is reduced, or developed, it becomes metallic silver and is black.) The number of electrons collecting at the sites of sensitization determines the number of silver ions attracted to these sites. Silver ions will not collect if electrons are absent; hence, there would be no potential development sites.

In general it is correct to assume that milliampere-seconds control *radiographic density,* since the number of cathode electrons made available to bombard the target controls the number of x-ray photons in any exposure. Radiographic density *is the amount of film blackening—the degree of gradation of blackness in the radiograph.*

It is also correct to assume that kilovoltage controls *contrast,* since the voltage impressed on the tube controls the energy of the bombarding cathode electrons, thereby controlling the resulting photon energy. Contrast may be explained as the comparative difference in transmitted light between the lighter and darker areas in the radiograph.

In a footnote on p. 61 it is stated that the reciprocity law has been found to be invalid. Additional information regarding this law, its facts and its failures, will aid the student in better understanding of latent and manifest image formation. Such understanding is enhanced through comparison of pertinent facts of radiography with similar facts of photography. X-ray energy and light energy are similar in that both x rays and light rays are members of the electromagnetic wave spectrum, and that both travel at the constant speed of 3×10^{10} cm per second. Additional comparisons are presented in Table 4-2.

*X-ray energy is substituted for light energy when cardboard holders are used and is augmented by light energy when intensifying screens are used.

*Sensitization specks is an expression used in the explanation of the latent image formation. In theory, more of these specks form when greater energy strikes the silver halide crystal.

Table 4-2. Comparison of x-ray and light exposures on film emulsions

Description	X rays	Light rays
Brightness	mA	I (intensity)
Time	s	t
Exposure	mAs	I•t

From Table 4-2 and p. 61 one can see that, in theory, the effective exposure (E) is equal to the mAs in radiography and to I • t (intensity of the light times the time of exposure) in photography. In some of the early research on reciprocity (I • t) failure, it was determined that exposure depends on the specific values of I and t (mA and s), not solely on their product. Stated differently, exposure depends on the level of illumination (photographically). In radiography the foregoing applies when mA is substituted for I, and s for t. Finally, it has been determined that the exposure effect depends on the rate of energy striking the emulsion.

The numerous effects of reciprocity failure result from the fact that latent image formation depends on several energy photons striking each single grain of silver halide. With both extremely high and low milliamperage values the silver halide response* falls off, this results in decreases in contrast at high mA values and in increases in contrast at low mA values. According to the Gurney-Mott theory, high intensity (mA) with short exposure time either causes or permits such slow migration of the silver ions that the electronic part of latent image formation is lost. As a result some migrating electrons are repelled away from the sensitization specks. With exposure made at low mA and long exposure time, the sensitization specks form slowly, thus resulting in electron losses and in silver ion diffusion.

Contrast, which must be considered with density, *is the visible difference between adjacent densities resulting from subject and film characteristics.* Tissues of different structural characteristics and different compositions are never penetrated to the same degree in any one exposure.

The greater the number of high-energy photons contained in the primary beam, the greater will be the degree of penetration of the object being radiographed; therefore the numbers of silver and bromine ions liberated in the film will be greater.

*Silver halide response, or film response, is usually expressed as film speed.

ENERGY PACKAGE

Understanding the results of the energy causing the exposure requires consideration of the *total energy* as a *package;* e.g., 25 mA × 2 sec at 60 kV is a different energy package than is 100 mA × 0.5 sec at 60 kV. Both energy packages are different from that of 100 mA × 1.0 sec at 50 kV. Each of these three energy packages has a different exposure effect* on the film emulsion. (See Fig. 4-2 *A* through *C*). However, the *visual* density and contrast and the visibility of detail in each of the three views is so nearly the same *in this kilovoltage range* as to make all three techniques highly acceptable. This fact simply proves the "rule of thumb" stated on p. 114, item 4 under technique changes. The density readings obtained using a Photovolt Densitometer and the *calculated*† delivered R dose are listed in the legend for Fig. 4-2, *A* through *C*.

The response (speed) of x-ray films must be considered along with the energy package.

Film speeds (types)

There are at least four speeds of x-ray film. In order of increasing response to applied energy, the first three are no-screen, regular (screen), and fast films. The fourth speed approximates fast film in rate of response and was developed for processing in rapid automatic processors; it is generally called RP film. The regular, fast, and RP films are very sensitive to light energy and are to be used with intensifying screens. The density obtained in these films is superior (greater) to that obtained in no-screen film. No-screen film is quite sensitive to x-ray energy and usually exhibits increased latitude with excellent soft tissue and bone detail. No-screen film is not popular in most departments because of the probabilities of improper film and film-holder combinations. In most departments no-screen film is replaced with regular film in cardboard holders for extremity radiography, *although this increases radiation dose to the part examined. Use of regular film in cardboard holders demands that the technologist use greater than usual gonadal protection!*

*Continuing investigation of the effects of the energy package on image density will include use of three-phase equipment and up to 1,000 mA with appropriately shortened exposure times.

†The calculations are made from information contained in Table 4-11.

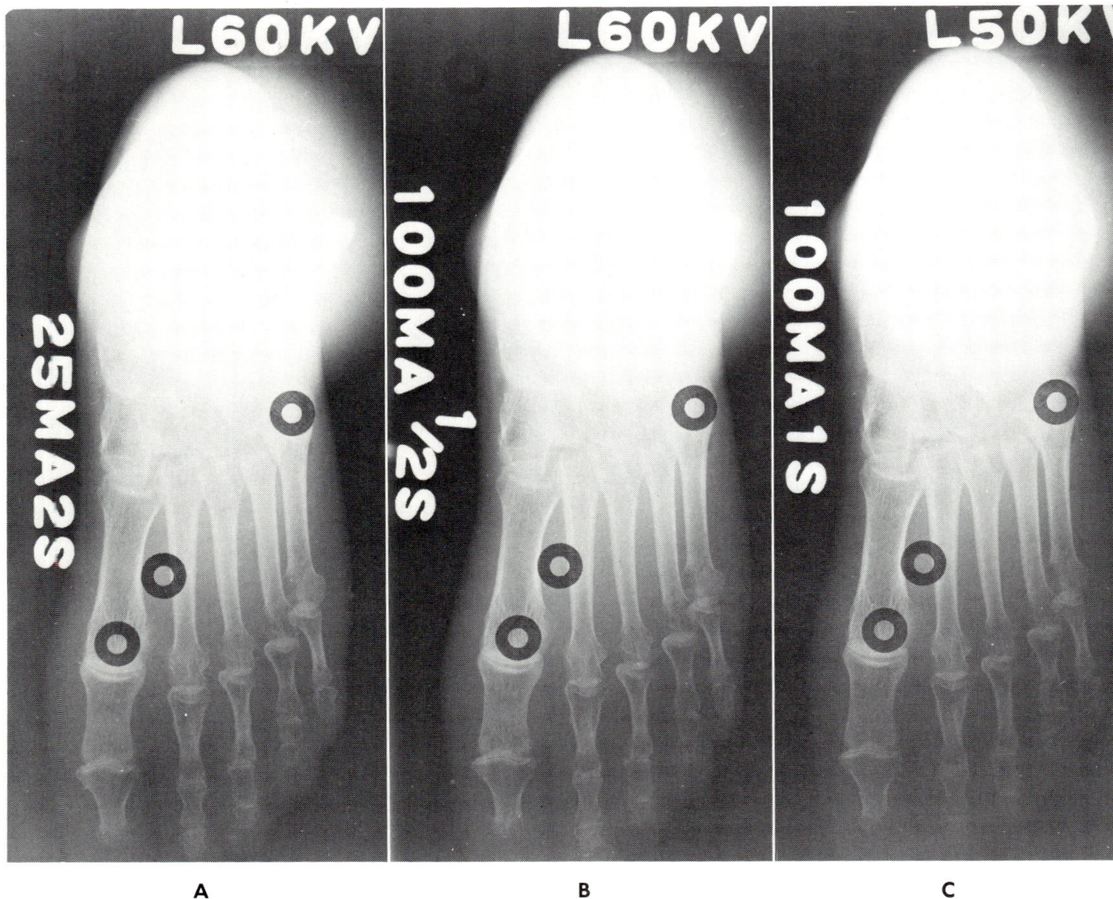

Fig. 4-2. Energy package exposures. The density readings are averages of three each. The R dose is calculated from Table 4-11. **A,** 25 mA, 2 sec., 60 kV, 3.956 density of background, 110 mR, 2.5 density end M-5, 2.88 density end M-1, 2.823 density space between M-1 and M-2; **B,** 100 mA, ½ sec., 60 kV, 4.0 density of background, 110 mR, 2.556 density end M-5, 2.896 density end M-1, 2.846 density space between M-1 and M-2; **C,** 100 mA, 1 sec., 50 kV, 4.2 density of background, 150 mR, 2.623 density end M-5, 2.943 density end M-1, 2.936 density space between M-1 and M-2.

RADIOGRAPHIC QUALITY

A radiograph is a permanent photographic record of the structures through which a beam of ionizing radiation has passed. However, it may be rendered useless by lack of visibility of detail. This condition may be caused by either overexposure or underexposure. Consequently, definition (radiographic sharpness) may be present but obscured.

Radiographic (diagnostic) quality is apparent (manifest) as the image in the remaining parts of the original film emulsion. Since the image is visible, the quantity of visibility of the image present in any radiograph is of major importance. This condition is called **visibility of detail;** it is a photographic property, and is therefore *subjective. Visibility of detail is the clearness with which we perceive the image on the radiograph.*

The other major condition present in a radiograph and affecting radiographic quality is called **definition;** it is a geometric property, and is therefore *objective. Definition* (sharpness) *is the distinctness with which images of anatomic structures are recorded.*

A "perfect" radiograph will have both maximum definition and maximum visibility of detail. Although it is not likely that a perfect radiograph is produced each time an exposure is made, we must always strive for maximum definition and maximum visibility of detail; anything less must be considered a poor radiograph.

The five major factors contributing to the understanding and appreciation of radiographic quality are: definition, visibility of detail, density, contrast, and sensitometry. Many variable conditions and/or accessories either control or influence these major factors. We use *control* to mean the ideal primary method of producing a major change in a subsequent radiograph. We use *influence* to mean methods other than the primary one that may intentionally or unintentionally produce change in a subsequent radiograph. Discussion of the controlling and influencing conditions and accessories for each of the five major factors comprises the next several pages.

Definition

Definition is the distinctness or clarity of detail or outline, as in a picture; it is the sharp demarcation of outlines or limits. It is controlled by focal spot size, motion, magnification, distortion, intensifying screens, and film-screen contact. Definition is influenced by density, contrast, fog, and film processing.

When definition is considered, it is always necessary to be aware of what the eye "sees" as being sharp, that is, without blur. As long as the structural detail (of the object radiographed) is optically without blur, it is considered to be an image of good definition. When a radiographic (or photographic) image is without blur, its points and/or lines do not exceed the maximum size of the circle of confusion.*

Detail is the quantity of visibility of fine structures and overall sharpness that is radiographically demonstrated. Definition results from many factors that either influence or control it. (Note that definition and visibility of detail are *not* the same. If visibility of detail is lacking, it may prevent the "seeing" of definition.)

Circle of confusion

Definition (sharpness) in a radiograph (and in a photograph) is said to be present when no point in the reproduced subject has a circle of confusion of diameter greater than 1/1,000 its distance from the eye. Experiment has shown that distinct vision is achieved when the object viewed is at least 10 inches from the eye.

The eye views a radiograph (or scene) as a collection of points, and if the points are of no greater diameter than 1/100 inch and the viewing distance is 10 inches, all points appear sharp. When it is recalled that the image viewed in the film emulsion is a two-plane image of a three-dimensional object and that the image so formed is the result of thousands of tiny grains of metallic silver remaining in the emulsion, it is readily understood that the eye sees this collection of tiny points as a solid image.

Radiographs appear perfectly sharp if the circles of confusion corresponding to all single points in the object shadow converge at the eye with angles not exceeding three minutes of an arc of a circle, or a maximum diameter of 1/100 inch.

Conditions controlling definition

Focal spot size. The x-ray tube focal spot (target) is the most important mechanical factor controlling definition. The smaller the focal spot size, the sharper the image. In order to maintain maximum definition when focal spot size is increased because of a different machine or x-ray tube, it becomes necessary to compensate for this difference by an increase in the focal-film distance.

The necessity of using the smallest possible focal spot cannot be overemphasized. Any source, other than a point source, of x rays causes a degree of image unsharpness. Good radiographic practice requires that the technologist use *all* possible methods to improve and/or enhance diagnostic quality. Use of very small optical (effective) focal spots ultimately improves visibility of detail, since such practice improves definition. The effects of large and small focal spots are visualized in Fig. 4-3, a diagram of umbra and penumbra effects.

In terms of light and shadow, umbra is a complete shadow within which no light is received from a given source. Penumbra is the space of partial illumination on all sides between the umbra and the full light. In radiography the x-ray energy can be compared to light energy, but it must be remembered that although light energy does not pass through an opaque object, x-ray energy will. The light umbra may be compared with the sharp radiographic image and the light penumbra with the degree of radio-

*The circle of confusion is the disk, of measurable diameter, by which a point in the object is represented in the image formed by a lens. (X-ray beams follow light beam laws to the extent that these photographic principles apply.)

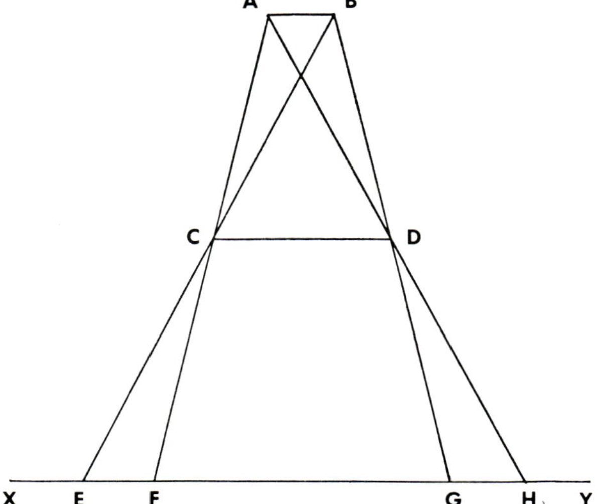

Fig. 4-3. Penumbra. Penumbra effect is demonstrated by the lines *E-F* and *G-H*. *F-G* is the true shadow, *A-B* is the light source, and *C-D* is the object. *X-Y* is the film.

graphic unsharpness caused by object-film distance, focal-film distance, and focal spot size. Study of Fig. 4-3 will reveal certain of these principles.

In Fig. 4-3, the line *A-B* (or a point source in the center of this line) represents the light source; line *C-D* represents the object; *F-G* represents the umbra or true shadow on the film *X-Y;* and *E-F* and *G-H* represent the areas of pneumbra, or radiographic unsharpness. (Because the objects of radiography possess three dimensions, completely sharp reproduction of them is not possible. *This lack of perfect sharpness in radiography is called unsharpness.*) It is evident that smaller light sources will produce proportionally less penumbra. Also, smaller focal spot sizes will produce less areas of unsharpness when both object-film distance and focal-film distance are optimum. Use of smaller optical focal spots results in radiographs of increased definition.

Impingement of the cathode electrons on very small focal spots causes less blurring and improves proportionally the definition in the resulting image in the radiograph. In most stationary anode tubes the small spot range is from 1.8 to 2.6 mm and the large spot from 2.8 to 4.6 mm. In a rotating anode tube the small spot is usually 0.8 to 1.0 mm and the large spot usually 1.5 to 2.0 mm. However, fractional focus tubes may have small focal spots of 0.3 mm or less. These tubes are designed to permit the use of rather long object-film distances, not only to obtain maximum radiographic enlargement but also to retain definition.

Motion. During exposure, motion of the part blurs the image and results in a loss of definition. There are four methods by which motion may be minimized: (1) by the use of immobilization devices such as sandbags, compression bands, etc.; (2) by the use of the shortest possible exposure time, which usually necessitates the use of intensifying screens (the slight decrease in definition caused by intensifying screens is not objectionable in the attempt to minimize motion); (3) by requiring the patient to suspend respiration during the exposure, except during extremity radiography; and (4) by the elimination of possible motion of the tube support arm and stand.

Magnification. Magnification inevitably causes losses in varying degrees of definition. However, magnification may be reduced to a minimum by two factors: object-film distance and focal-film distance. These are usually considered the major factors affecting magnification. In some instances magnification is desirable when visibility of a part is more important than maximum definition. Magnification usually is accompanied by a degree of blurring. *Magnification is the symmetric enlargement of the image on the radiograph.*

The radiographic image size may be enlarged or reduced within certain limits by using either of two methods. The enlargement is achieved when object-film distance is increased or when focal-film distance is decreased The reduction is achieved when object-film distance is decreased or when focal-film distance is increased. An increase of object-film distance will blur the radiographic image, producing *unsharpness*. The same effect results from a decrease of focal-film distance. The formula for determining the quantity of magnification is written:

$$\frac{\text{ofd}}{\text{ffd} - \text{ofd}} = \%\ \text{magnification}$$

Magnification is desirable in certain instances, for example, to emphasize certain bone sections, hairline fractures, or other suspected diseased areas. A good procedure is to strive for the same percentage of magnification in each successive radiograph of a sequence of a fracture. To use the magnification formula, ofd and ffd must be converted to the same unit of measure. Either multiply inches by 2.5 or divide centimeters by 2.5. (One inch = 2.54 cm; however, 2.5 is a satisfactory conversion factor.)

Example: ffd is 36 inches, ofd is 15 cm. What is the percentage of magnification?

$$\frac{15}{2.5} = 6; \frac{6}{36 - 6} = \%\ \text{magnification};$$

$$\frac{6}{30} = 0.20 \text{ or } 20\%$$

A certain degree of unsharpness is inevitably present in radiographs. In special cases some sharpness is sacrified in favor of magnification. In some of the standard techniques a low degree of unsharpness is expected. When using the unsharpness formula, all numerical values may be used as found and need not be converted to a common unit.

A formula to determine the quantity of unsharpness has application only when marginal

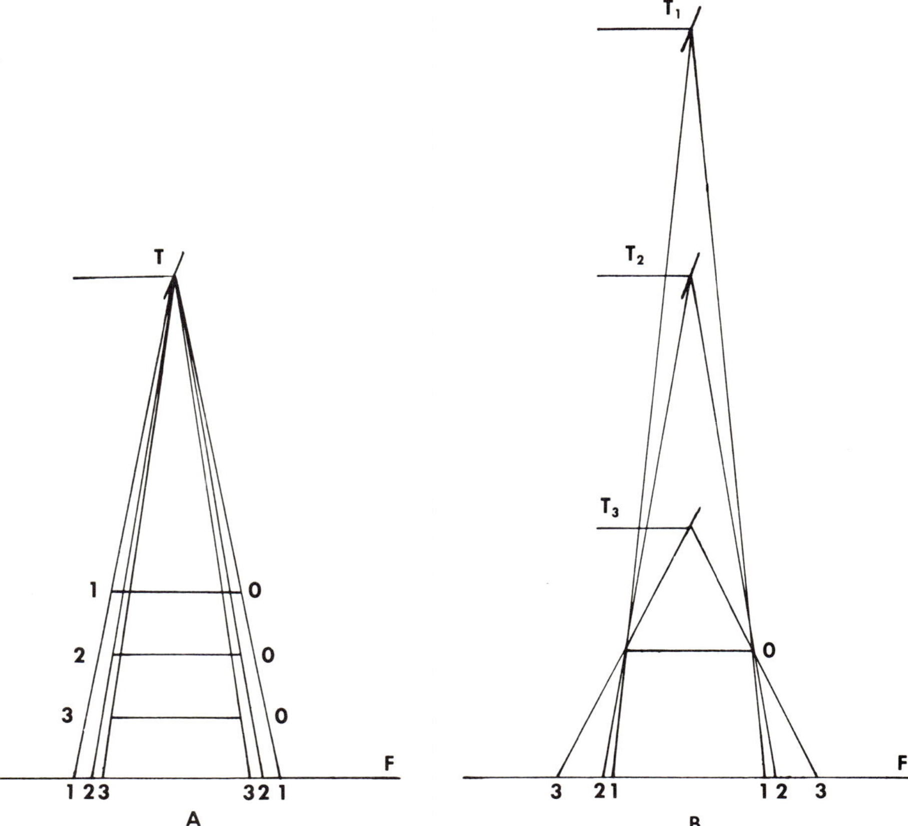

Fig. 4-4. Effects of object-film distance, focal-film distance, and focal spot size on the radiographic image. In **A**, *T* is the focal spot at a constant distance from the film *F*. *O* (the object) is of constant length in the three positions, but as ofd is decreased from position *1* to *3*, the size of the image of *O* is decreased. In **B**, *O* is the object at a constant distance from the film *F*. As *T* (the focal spot) is brought closer to the film from position *1* to *3*, the size of the image of *O* is increased.

sharpness and detail are too blurred for diagnostic purposes. The optimum value of unsharpness is 1.0; however, any value for unsharpness of 2.0 or less is satisfactory.

$U = \dfrac{dF + DM}{D - d} + S$; where U is the quantity of unsharpness, d is the ofd, F is the focal spot size in millimeters, D is the ffd, M is motion of part in millimeters, and S is the factor for screen blurring. The blurring factor for most modern screens is 0.15.

Example: In a standard lateral (frog-leg) hip technique, the following applicable factors are found: d = 10 cm (½ the thickness of part), F = 1.0 mm, D = 40 inches; the factor of 0.15 for screen blurring applies.

$$U = \frac{(10)\ (1) + 40}{40 - 10} + 0.15$$

$$U = \frac{50}{30} + 0.15$$

$$U = 1.81$$

If a focal spot of 2.0 mm had been used:

$$U = \frac{60}{30} + 0.15$$

$$U = 2.15$$

This is concrete evidence of the necessity of always using the small focal spot when possible.

Focal-film distance. *The focal-film distance is the distance (usually in inches) between the focal spot of the x-ray tube and the film.* Most radiographic techniques presently require a 40-inch focal-film distance. Fig. 4-4, *B*, demonstrates the varying effects of increased and decreased focal-film distances, using the same length line for the object as used in Fig. 4-4, *A*. Study of Fig. 4-4, *B*, will reveal that longer focal-film distances (when practical) are highly desirable (as in teleroentgenography), since longer focal-film distances tend to produce an image size approximating the size of the object.

Although equipment capacity, room size, and common sense restrict focal-film distances to reasonable limits, it has been found that the greater is the focal-film distance, the greater the radiograph definition. In many departments where room size permits, chest radiography and some erect (sitting) skull radiography are performed at a focal-film distance of 10 feet.

This distance also controls magnification to a large extent. Examination of Fig. 4-4 reveals the importance of focal-film distance to the size of the ultimate image. Magnification is maintained at a minimum when long focal-film distances are employed; the opposite of this is also true.

Another consideration with use of short focal-film distances is that of the effect of parallel rays on image size and definition.

PARALLEL RAYS: As x rays radiate outward from the point of origin in the x-ray tube target, the weaker x rays radiate at wider angles from the central ray than the stronger x rays. As a result fewer of the weaker primary rays strike the object and film at increased focal-film distances. The stronger primary rays strike the object and film at increased focal-film distances and travel in paths more nearly parallel with each other. (See Fig. 4-11.) These are called parallel rays.

Parallel rays are employed in *teleroentgenography* to present image shadows of the various viscera in nearly correct relative size. Since the various viscera of the thoracic cavity are situated at remarkably different distances from the film in routine chest radiography, the parallel rays avoid, to a great extent, the enlargement obtained when the more angular rays are employed in producing the radiographic image.

Object-film distance. *The object-film distance is the distance between the object being radiographed and the film.* Since the art of radiography involves the use of three-dimensional subjects, it is impossible to radiograph a part of the human anatomy that possesses no thickness. Study of Fig. 4-4, *A*, will reveal that as the object-film distance is increased, the size of the resulting image is proportionally increased. It is obvious that magnification may, and usually does, cause increases in marginal unsharpness (areas of penumbra in light and shadow). When marginal definition (sharpness) losses are visible, internal definition and detail losses are also present. (See Fig. 4-5.) The necessity of keeping the film as close as possible to the structure under radiographic consideration cannot be overemphasized.

The radiographs of the phantom right arm (Fig. 4-5) were exposed with 60 kVp, 80 mA, for 1 second at a 40-inch ffd. Readings on the densitometer were made on both radiographs at the sites of the arrows. At tabletop the bone tissue density is 3.33; the soft tissue density is 3.51. At 5.5-inch ofd the bone tissue density is 2.99; the soft tissue density is 3.115.

Comparison of the visible silver grains in Fig. 4-5, *B*, with those in *G* shows greater density (more silver grains reduced to metallic silver) in *B*. Comparison of *C* with *H* shows this condition more clearly.

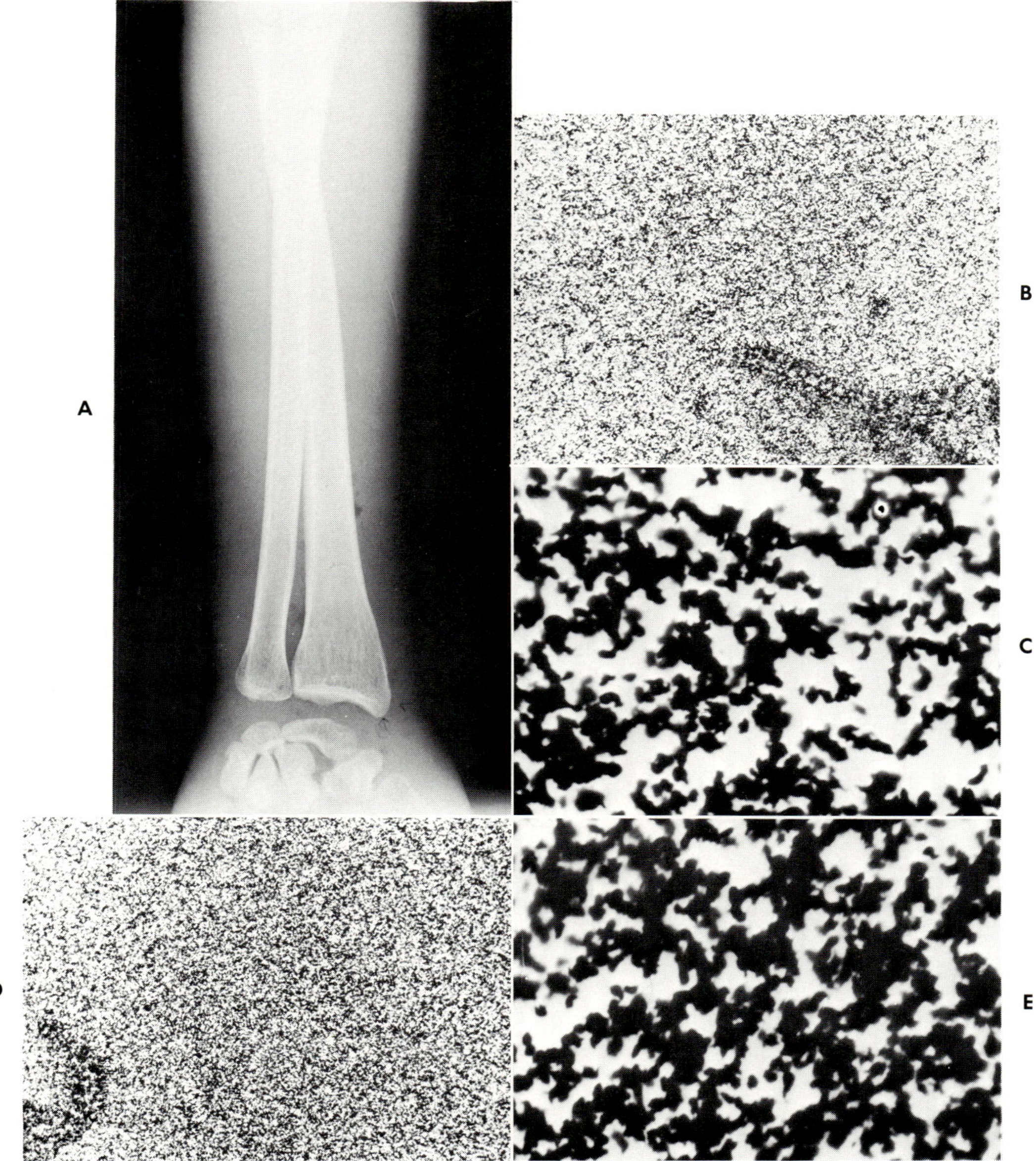

Fig. 4-5. A, Radiograph of phantom right arm with no (increased) ofd (tabletop). **B,** Photomicrograph (25×) of radiograph of bone tissue with no increased ofd. Note tiny arrow pointing proximally to the bone tissue in the laterodistal point of the radial head in **A**; dark shadows in the lower margin are the end of the arrow. **C,** Photomicrograph (400×) of radiograph of bone tissue with no increased ofd (site is same as in **B**). **D,** Photomicrograph (25×) of radiograph of soft tissue with no increased ofd. Note tiny arrow pointing medially to the soft tissue adjacent to the laterodistal point of the radial head in **A**; dark shadow in the lateral margin is the end of arrow. **E,** Photomicrograph (400×) of radiograph of soft tissue with no increased ofd (site is same as in **D**).

Continued.

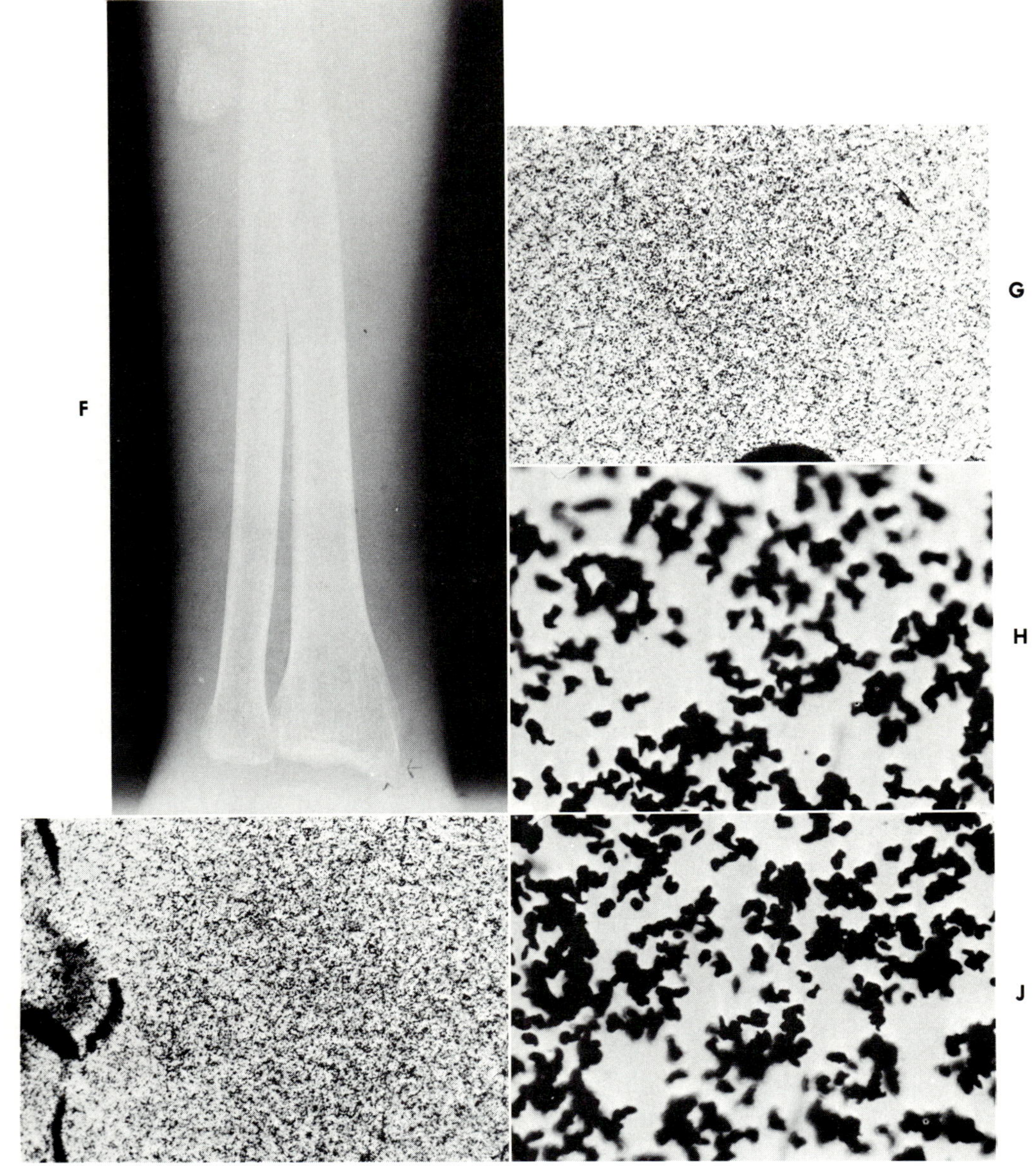

Fig. 4-5, cont'd. F, Radiograph of phantom right arm with 5.5-inch ofd; that is, arm was raised 5.5 inches above tabletop. **G,** Photomicrograph (25×) of radiograph of bone tissue with 5.5-inch ofd. Note tiny arrow pointing proximally to the bone tissue in the laterodistal point of the radial head in **F**; rounded dark shadow in the lower margin is the end of the arrow. **H,** Photomicrograph (400×) of radiograph of bone tissue with 5.5-inch ofd (site is same as in **G**). **I,** Photomicrograph (25×) of radiograph of soft tissue with 5.5-inch ofd. Note tiny arrow pointing medially to the soft tissue adjacent to the laterodistal point of the radial head in **F**; dark shadows in the lateral margin are the end of the arrow. **J,** Photomicrograph (400×) of radiograph of soft tissue with 5.5-inch ofd (site is same as in **I**).

Similar comparisons between *D* and *I* and *E* and *J* of Fig. 4-5 show similar results. Although greater density appears toward the center of the photomicrographs in both *D* and *I*, the silver grains appear to be more evenly dispersed in *D* than in *I*. This condition can be explained as "losses in internal definition and visibility of detail."

True distortion

Distortion is the perversion of shape in a radiographic image. Foreshortening or elongation or both are the manifestations of distortion resulting from the change in radii of the two sides of an object. Distortion may result when the central ray is angled or when the object is not centered to the vertical central ray. (See Fig. 4-6.)

Control. Distortion, like magnification, causes losses in varying degrees of definition (detail sharpness). (See Fig. 4-6.) Distortion is controlled by proper alignment of target-object-film. In radiography of certain parts, such as a lateral mandible, it is necessary, and permissible, to distort slightly the object image in a desired radiograph. In this particular instance the target angulation distorts (elongates) the image of the mandible.

TARGET-OBJECT-FILM ALIGNMENT. In general the central ray is directed at an angle of 90 degrees to the surface of the film; positioning instructions often state that the central ray (CR) is to be directed at 90 degrees to a plane of the object that is parallel with the surface of the film or film-holder. If for any reason (intent or mistake) other than a 90-degree angle is obtained on one side of the center of the object radiographed, the other angle will be 90 degrees plus the difference from the first side.

Alignment of target-object-film other than 90 degrees (Fig. 4-6) of necessity causes increased unsharpness (penumbra effect) on the elongated side of the image.

Intensifying screens. Intensifying screens are one of the greatest aids to the production of high-quality radiographs. Use of these screens reduces exposure time, reduces exposure quantity, and minimizes motion of part, since the screen crystals respond to the applied x-ray energy with a correspondingly produced quantity of light rays that is added to the quantity of primary rays striking the film surfaces.

Intensifying screens are composed of a dehydrated suspension of x-ray excitable phosphors* coated on one side of a sheet of radiolucent material. The modern synthetic materials cannot absorb water and are classed as *stainless,* since any solutions splashed on them are easily removed when allowed to dry. The phosphors are finely divided and of uniform size (0.015 mm or less) in the suspension, which is of constant thickness. The screens are mounted within the cassette to increase the effect of the applied x-ray energy. This increased effect is achieved because x-ray energy causes the phosphors of the screen to glow with a blue-white light.

The radiographic effect upon the film in a cassette is achieved by a combination of the

*A phosphor is a phosphorescent substance or body, that is, it shines in the dark.

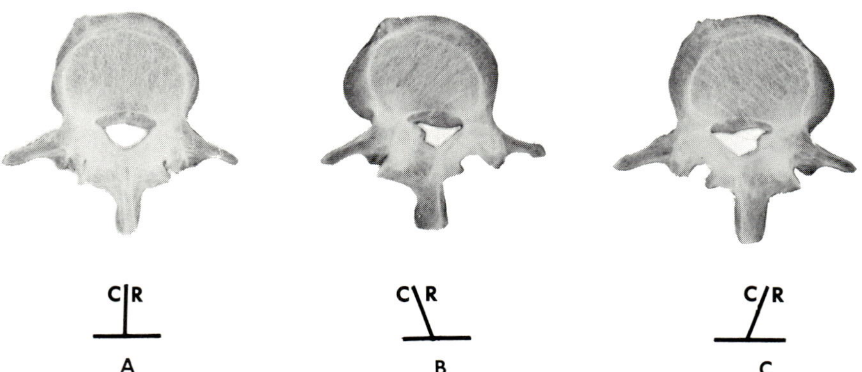

Fig. 4-6. Distortion. In **A, B,** and **C** the kVp was 45; the mAs, 1.25; and the ffd, 40 inches. All used a cardboard filmholder with plain film. In exposure **A** the central ray is directed to a 90-degree angle with the filmholder surface. In exposure **B** the central ray is directed 20 degrees to the right and to the center of the vertebra. In exposure **C** the central ray is directed 20 degrees to the left and to the center of the vertebra.

x-ray energy plus the fluorescent light energy of the phosphors. In general the screens may increase from ten to sixty times the applied energy of the x rays as they pass through the screens. The quantity of intensification depends on the chemical composition and size of the phosphors in the screen emulsion. The x-ray energy accounts for approximately 2% of the total exposure in intensifying screen cassettes through actinic action.*

Quantity of intensification means the same as speed of intensification and is called *screen speed,* and as with film, actually means response to x-ray energy. Phosphor size affects speed and definition in the radiograph.

In the latter part of the 1960s and in the current decade, research on screen speed and resolution has brought about many changes in screen emulsion composition, and in the *decreased* requirements for extremely high energy "output" from x-ray generators.

Earlier screen emulsions used calcium tungstate and other phosphors along with certain dyes to achieve specific screen speeds. Since many of these kinds of screens continue in use, particularly in small departments and in rural areas, limited information regarding speed of such screens is furnished in Tables 4-3 and 4-4.

*The results of one series of experiments indicated that 98.3% of the total exposure was the result of screen intensification.

Table 4-3. Intensifying screen types

Screen speed	Purpose
Detail Slow or High definition	Requires greater exposure but produces excellent detail, contrast, and definition
Average Medium or Par	Requires moderate exposure and produces good definition and detail
Fast or High	Requires very short exposure and produces slightly less definition and detail

Table 4-4. Speeds of intensifying screens

Screen	Relative speed	Average unsharpness
Average speed	2	0.3
High speed (resolution)	4	0.25
Detail speed	8	0.15

Calcium tungstate is much less efficient in converting x-ray energy into light ray energy than are the newly developed phosphors. These are barium fluorochloride, gadolinium, and lanthanum. Each of these phosphors responds to shorter wavelengths than does calcium tungstate. As a result, the newer intensifying screens permit shorter exposure times and obtain increased subject contrast in the radiographs with increases in definition (decreases in unsharpness). One manufacturer lists available relative speeds as 4, 3, 2, and 1. Comparison of these with the stated relative speeds in Table 4-4 reveals significant increases in available speed of intensification.

It is generally true that changes in exposure technique are usually required when kilovoltages are less than 75.

Intensifying screens perform several distinct functions in radiography. Since the screens increase the effect of the applied energy to the film, it is possible to use less electric energy, which results in lower roentgen output (smaller roentgen doses) to the patient—a safety factor. The same increased effect on the film permits the use of relatively low-voltage equipment to obtain good radiographs. Use of intensifying screens decreases exposure time considerably and, as a consequence, minimizes motion of part.

The use of intensifying screens contributes to loss in definition; however, this loss is minimal. The loss of definition depends on the size and chemical nature of the crystals used in the emulsion. Since all screens are manufactured to specific standards, there is little noticeable difference in definition between any two speeds of the same brand (manufacture) of screen. Most screens are manufactured with the emulsion crystal size comparable to earlier standards for medium speed. This size crystal is small enough to permit excellent detail and large enough to respond quickly to a relatively intense exposure. Consideration and understanding of how screen emulsions, particularly phosphor crystal size, can cause a decrease in definition necessitate that the student have some understanding of the *circle of confusion.* (See p. 73.)

Film holders are discussed on pp. 16 and 17. Screens are always contained within a cassette that may have either a rigid or a flexible structure. The screens function primarily to reduce the amount of exposure required (dose delivered to the patient), thus shortening exposure time and improving definition. However, since the screen emulsion glows with blue-violet light as a result of the applied x-ray energy, there is a distinct increase in image contrast; that is, the black and dark gray areas will be darker, and the light gray to white areas tend to remain essentially the same if correct exposure factors are employed.

A change in technique from cardboard holders to intensifying screen cassettes increases contrast. Use of cardboard holders in routine procedures obtains a radiograph of less contrast and density and with improved visibility of both soft tissue and bone detail.

Good radiographic definition is achieved through the resolving power of the screen expressed in lines per millimeter. The resolving power of a film or plate is the ability of this film or plate to reproduce the fine detail of the optical image. Resolution is the act or property of rendering visible the separate parts of an object. The resolving powers of the commonly used intensifying screens are as follows: detail, 9 to 10; par, 7 to 8; high speed, 6 to 7; and extra fast, 5 to 6.

Film-screen contact. When film is placed in cassettes, extreme care must be taken to achieve good *film-screen contact.* This term means that the two screen surfaces that sandwich the film must be in total contact with the film and must exert equal pressure over the entire surfaces of the film. The condition of poor film-screen contact is seldom consistent throughout the cassette; the film is in good contact with the screens in some areas and in poor contact in others. A film exposed in such a cassette will have sharp shadows with good detail in one area and blurred indistinct image shadows in another. (See Fig. 4-7.)

Poor film-screen contact affects definition considerably, since the area of poor contact produces a blurring effect in the radiograph. There are several conditions that cause poor contact. Among these are a warped cassette, improperly installed intensifying screens, and improper tension of the cassette clamps. Some of these conditions can be corrected; in other instances, new cassettes or screens must be purchased.

Several methods of film-screen contact determination have been developed. Among them is one that is quite simple. New paper clips are placed in any pattern desired over the surface of the cassette to be tested, being certain that all paper clips are *lying flat* and singly on the tube-side surface. The cassette contains an unexposed film. A routine exposure for average (par) speed intensifying screens, as used in Fig. 4-7, is as follows: 55 kVp, 5 mAs, and 40-inch ffd. The film is processed in the usual manner. If the screens are in good contact with the film *on both*

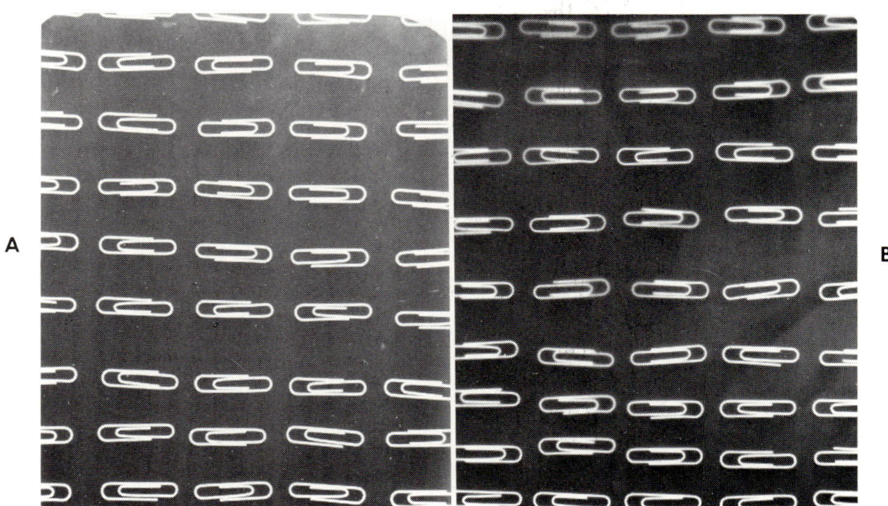

Fig. 4-7. Film-screen contact. **A,** Sharp margins of paper clips demonstrate that the two intensifying screens are in good contact with the film throughout the entire surfaces. **B,** Unsharp paperclip shadows in the upper and left upper parts of the radiograph demonstrate that at least one screen is in very poor contact, if it is in contact at all, with the film in this area of the cassette.

sides, the shadows of the paper clips will be quite sharp; if not, noticeably blurred shadows of some paper clips will be seen in certain areas of the radiograph.

Since the intensifying screens are quite expensive and easily damaged, they must be handled with care. If dirt is attracted to the screen surface, the dirt should be removed with a camel's hair brush. If this is not successful, a lint-free cloth should be dampened with pure grain alcohol and gently wiped over the affected area. Screens should be kept free of splashed water, developer, or fixer, since any of these agents may cause spots, which are removable only from stainless screens. Light spots in the radiograph occur from decreased activity of spotted areas in the screens.

There are certain phosphors that will continue to glow after the source of energy has ceased; phosphors containing impurities will do this. This *afterglow* is called *screen lag* and would be present only if intensifying screens contained such phosphors. Screen lag is not encountered if the screens are obtained from reputable suppliers and manufacturers.

Conditions influencing definition

Density. Losses in definition are inevitable as a result of excess density. When more silver grains are reduced to metallic silver than is necessary for good definition, fine details may be inadvertently obscured. Definition consists of both objective and subjective components. *Objective definition is the breadth of image blur; subjective definition is the rate of change from one density to another.*

When the radiologist must *spotlight* an area of a radiograph to enable interpretation, he is denied a certain amount of definition in this region. Thus the patient may receive an incomplete or erroneous diagnosis as a result of technologic error or carelessness!

Film speed. Film speed, that is, the rate of response of the sensitized emulsion on the film base to the energy striking the emulsion, is regulated by the manufacturer and results to a large extent from the chemical composition of the additives in the silver halide, the percentage of silver in the silver halide, the thickness of the emulsion, and the size of the silver halide grains (or crystals). If speed is gained through the use of larger crystals, definition is lost or, at least, is decreased.

Experimental evidence indicates that, in general, definition is inversely related to film speed.

Contrast. In-depth discussion of contrast starts on p. 97; in these paragraphs we are concerned principally with the influence that contrast exerts on definition. Very high contrast can result in adjacent shadows having extreme density and extreme opacity (lack of radiographic density). As discussed in the preceding paragraphs, definition may be reduced. (See Fig. 4-8.)

The relationship of contrast to photographic properties of radiographic quality is discussed on p. 97. The present consideration is how contrast may exert influence on definition.

We have seen in the preceding paragraphs that density influences definition rather strongly, especially excess density. As a general rule, high contrast is obtained with a small range of x-ray intensities. Stated differently, the greater the range of x-ray intensities, the less is the contrast obtained in the radiographic image. Provided that the object is penetrated correctly, it follows that decreases in contrast (increased latitude) tend to increase definition. Finally, it is correct to state that definition may be decreased (and even lost) when contrast is excessively great. Moving in the other direction (see Fig. 4-15), small decreases in contrast may show slight improvement (increase) in definition.

Kilovoltage. Kilovoltage (penetrability) influences density and controls contrast. If the peak kilovoltage is increased, the density is increased and the contrast is decreased. Conversely, if the peak kilovoltage is decreased, the density is decreased and the contrast is increased. (See Fig. 4-15.)

Recognizing that kilovoltage has a definite effect on *both* contrast and density, a *standard* technique maintains a constant milliampere-second value (relative to the structure) and varies the peak kilovoltage according to the thickness of the part. With the current emphasis on decrease of radiation to the patient and greater latitude in the radiograph, a different concept in radiographic practice uses a constant, *optimum peak kilovoltage** (usually 120) with the milliampere-

*Experimental evidence indicates that there may be a maximum kilovoltage optimum for a given anatomic part or structure. Further research may establish kilovoltage levels as optimum to employ for specific structures, with milliampere-selections between established minimums and maximums. On this theory it can be assumed that high kV technique does not necessarily imply 90, 100, 120, or even 150 kV.

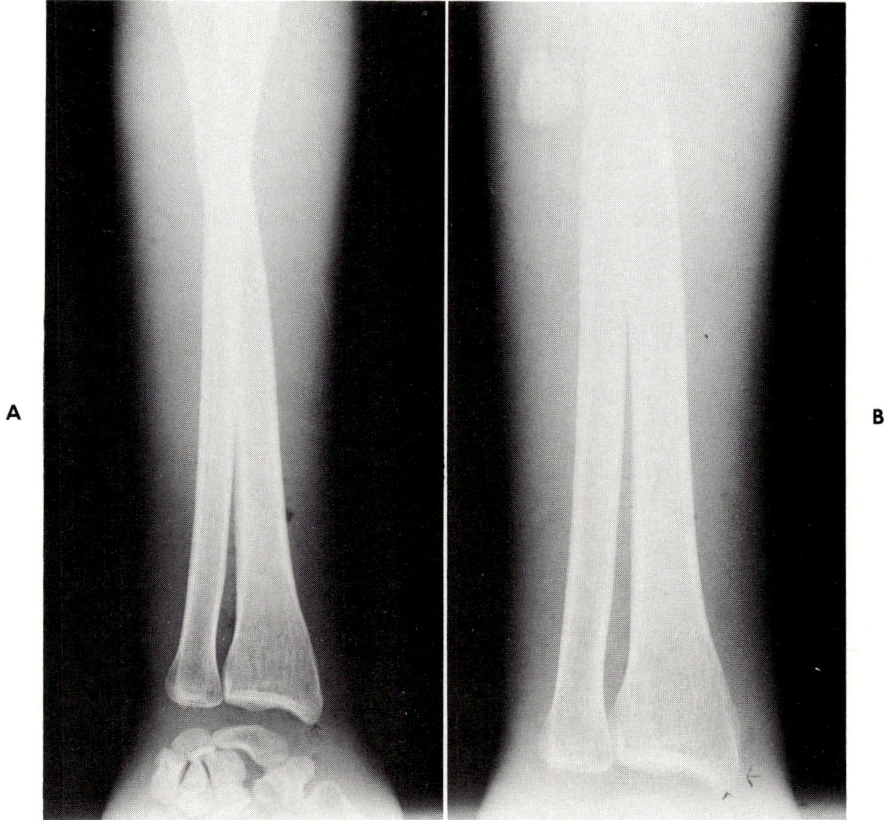

Fig. 4-8. A, Normal density with no increased object-film distance. Phantom arm was exposed at tabletop with 60 kVp and 80 mAs at 40-inch ffd. Density reading of the bone tissue is 3.33; density of the soft tissue is 3.51. (Note: Both density readings were made at sites indicated by arrows.) **B,** Decreased density with 5.5-inch object-film distance. Phantom arm was exposed with the lower surface of the arm elevated 5.5 inches above the tabletop. Factors were the same as those used in **A.** Density reading of the bone tissue is 2.99; density reading of the soft tissue is 3.115.

seconds as the variable. It is generally preferable to vary the time and maintain a constant milliamperage.

Fog. Detailed discussion of fog, and the several kinds of fog, as well as the conditions causing it begins on p. 91. Fog exerts strong influence on definition by preventing the correct amount of silver grain reduction (to black, metallic silver) in any and all areas where fog exists.

Just as density, when increased, can cause definition loss, so can fog (in any amount) cause definition loss. The greater the amount of fog, regardless of cause, the greater is the amount of definition loss. When silver grains reduce and cause black points in an image, other than those desired, it is obvious that less definition in the image is the result.

Film processing

It is now necessary to explore the chemical processes occurring in the formation of the manifest image. The exposed film emulsion contains the latent image. It is necessary to make this latent image manifest by reducing the exposed silver salts to (black) metallic silver in the shape of the image. Following reduction (development) in the developing solution, it is necessary both to fix the manifest image and to clear the emulsion of the silver bromide.

Automatic processing. As partially explained

on p. 20 x-ray films are processed by either an automatic or manual method, depending on the needs of the department. The manual method will be discussed on subsequent pages. In the automatic method the exposed x-ray films are manually fed into an automatic processor, and development, fixation, washing, and drying are performed automatically in the processor. In both methods the same *basic* principles are involved.

Considerable information regarding the composition of the film emulsion and of the processing solutions in manual processing is available. The formulas for both the film emulsions and solutions for processing these films in automatic processing are proprietary information and are closely guarded by the manufacturers.

There are two types of automatic roller transport processing. One is designed to process conventional medical x-ray films in cycles varying from 3 to 10 or 15 minutes, depending on the model and make of processor employed. The other is the rapid processor (RP) that requires the newer RP series of medical x-ray films and processes them in approximately 90 seconds. For both types of automatic processing special chemical solutions had to be formulated to permit processing in shorter cycles than in manual processing. Additionally, these solutions are required to function in (and withstand) much higher temperatures than those used in manual processing. Finally, new film emulsions were necessary for these same reasons and had to be transported successfully by the roller transport system without sticking to the rollers.

Manual processing. A modern manual processing room usually contains the following solutions: developer, water bath, acid stop bath, fixer, water bath, and Photoflow solution. (Note: If the fixer tank is positioned in the wall between the processing and drying rooms, the last water bath and the Photoflow will then be in the drying room.)

Processing. With automatic processing of x-ray films special care must be given to correct maintenance of the processor. Regular attention to cleaning, solution temperatures and volumes, recirculation pumps, and all processor systems is of cardinal importance. The technologist who neglects these daily "duties" must expect frequent trouble and processor failure.

Regardless of whether the films are processed automatically or manually, incorrect processing will inevitably decrease the quantity of contrast in the radiograph.

The *optimum* developing temperature for manual processing of x-ray films is 68° F. Most films require a minimum of 2½ minutes for development. Plain and high-speed film may be developed in 5 minutes at 68° F. (or 4 minutes at 70° F.). No-screen film may require different developing times. All films should be fixed for a minimum of 3 to 6 minutes; *fixing time is considered to be twice the "clearing time."**

When removed from the developer, a single 14″ × 17″ film will have absorbed approximately 3 ounces of solution in its emulsion; hence, it is necessary to replenish the solution frequently.

In certain areas, especially in high altitude, algae may grow in the water bath; thus correct fixation is prevented. This condition may be improved by suspending a small sheet of pure copper in the water bath. Both sides of the copper sheet must be scoured each day for greatest effectiveness.

Correct processing of exposed films results in the maximum definition possible as a result of the exposure technique, accessories employed, and general condition of the patient. Prolonged processing or processing at temperatures higher than those recommended will most certainly increase radiographic density. Such density increases result in losses in definition. The opposite of this is true within lesser limits.

Changing the latent image into the manifest image is a complicated series of chemical reactions, collectively termed an *oxidation-reduction reaction.* A brief explanation follows.

Chemical changes are classified either as those involving no change in valence or those in which a change in valence occurs. The latter is an oxidation-reduction reaction, and the atoms of the involved elements undergo new combinations and replacements. These changes involve rearrangements of the electrons of the atoms. Results of electron interchange dictate that certain elements gain in valence whereas other elements lose in valence. Oxidation is that process in which an atom gains in positive valence (gives up electrons). Reduction is that process in which an atom loses in positive valence (receives additional electrons).

Oxidation and reduction are processes mutually dependent upon each other; that is, neither event can occur without the other, and the events must occur simultaneously. The reducing agent is that which is oxidized; conversely, the oxidizing agent

*Clearing time is the minimum time required in a given fixing solution for removal of all the unexposed silver halides and is usually not less than 1½ minutes.

Table 4-5. Composition of the developer

Chemicals	Function
Elon-hydroquinone Elon—$(CH_3NHC_6H_4OH)_2 \cdot H_2SO_4$ Hydroquinone—$[C_6H_4(OH)_2]$	Brings out latent image in film emulsion by action of Elon (an activator) and hydroquinone (a developer) (Elon is another trade name for Metol); developer removes bromine ions from energy-struck silver bromide and leaves black metallic silver in emulsion; Metol is strong and stable and brings out *softer* tones; hydroquinone is weak and unstable and brings out *brilliant* blacks; both Metol and hydroquinone are reducing agents, and react concurrently in this oxidation-reduction reaction (phenadone replaces Metol in automatic processing developer)
Sodium carbonate Na_2CO_3	Produces developer pH of approximately 11.0; also accelerates reducing action and softens emulsion
Potassium bromide KBr	Acts as restrainer; regulates and slows reducing (developing) action of Elon-hydroquinone, thereby preventing smudging (running together) of blacks and whites
Sodium sulfite Na_2SO_3	Acts as preservative; slows down oxidation; is reducing agent

Table 4-6. Composition of the fixer

Chemicals	Function
Sodium thiosulfate $Na_2S_2O_3 \cdot 5H_2O$	Dissolves excess silver bromide salts in inverse proportion to amount of exposure in given area; in area where part of the object radiographed did not cover film, no silver salts will be dissolved; this part of film will be totally black
Potassium alum $KAl(SO_4)_2 \cdot 12H_2O$ (potassium aluminum sulfate)	Hardens film emulsion by shrinking and *tanning* action on gelatin
Acetic acid CH_3COOH	Acts as acidifier of this fixing solution and as neutralizer of alkalinity of wet film when acid stop bath is not used; removes animal fats from gelatin
Sodium sulfite Na_2SO_3	Acts as preservative

is that which is reduced. (Further explanation of this process is not pertinent in this text.)

COMPOSITION OF THE DEVELOPER. See Table 4-5 for a listing of the necessary chemicals and their function.

Developing agents are used to produce a visible image corresponding to the latent image. Development is accomplished through either of two methods: *physical,* wherein the developing solution supplies the silver to form the developed image, or *chemical,* wherein the silver is in the film emulsion and the developing solution reduces the ionic silver to metallic silver, which is black. Our interest is in chemical development, in which each silver halide grain is either developable as a unit or is not developable. The formula for the oxidation of silver bromide grains is as follows:

Silver bromide + Hydroquinone ⟶ Free bromine and silver ions + Quinone + Hydrogen ions

$$2AgBr + C_6H_4(OH)_2 \longrightarrow 2Ag^+ + 2Br^- + C_6H_4O_2 + 2H^+$$

The total density of a radiograph depends for the most part on the number of silver halide grains struck by the exposure energy. Each grain in the emulsion is protected by a chemical layer that breaks down in one or more sites depending on the total energy striking the grain. The number of these sites determines the speed with which the developing agent reduces the grain. As a result, some grains may not develop simply because of insufficient time. However, all silver halide grains will develop (reduce) when left in contact with the developing agent for a long enough period of time. Density resulting from reduction of unexposed grains is a form of fog.

WATER BATH. The water bath is just as important as the developer and fixer. After the film has been removed from the developer, the water bath washes out the alkaline developer in the film emulsion.

ACID STOP BATH. Improved radiographic quality results when the films are immersed for 30 seconds in an acid stop bath consisting of a 28% solution of acetic acid. The pH of the stop bath effects an almost instantaneous neutralization of the alkalinity of the "wetted" film emulsion. This, of course, stops the developing process.

COMPOSITION OF THE FIXER. See Table 4-6 for a listing of the necessary chemicals and their functions.

WATER BATH. After the fixer, the water bath removes the excess fixer and helps prevent streaking of the films.

Under normal conditions, it requires approximately 1 hour to process a radiograph in proper manner if a hot-air dryer is available in the processing room.

In both automatic and manual processing of x-ray films, exactness in all steps and correctness of both time and temperature are absolutely essential! Any deviations will result in changes in density with corresponding losses in definition.

Visibility of detail

As defined on p. 72 visibility of detail is the clearness with which we perceive the image on the radiograph. It is also mentioned on this page that visibility of detail is subjective; i.e., the quantity of visibility of detail is governed by the individual's bias and visual limitations, and is judgmental and cannot be measured with a common unit.

The production of radiographs of high diagnostic quality depends on many elements. Radiographic quality is the characteristic summation of the various elements that combine to produce a radiograph and is determined by the degree of tissue differentiation. Tissue differentiation in the radiograph occurs because x-ray energy quantity is absorbed in proportion to the tissue density. *Maximum tissue differentiation* is present only when the radiograph demonstrates *maximum definition and maximum visibility of detail.*

The end result of a given series of a radiologic technologist's professional endeavors is one or more radiographs of the maximum tissue differentiation consistent with circumstances. Radiographic (diagnostic) quality depends directly on the quantity of tissue differentiation.

For maximum *visibility of detail* to exist, it is necessary that all parts of the image possess some density; that is, each part of the image is made visible by the presence of reduced silver. Visibility of detail exists when all structures necessary for interpretation can be seen when no additional optical aids are required. Increased visibility of detail is often called latitude.

Comparing radiography with photography, it is well known that photographs with very poor (low) contrast are obtained when the exposures are made between the hours of 10:00 A.M. and 2:30 to 3:00 P.M. This is because the sunlight is at its maximum quantity.

Just as sunlight is (controls) the energy in the energy package (light, F-stop, and shutter speed) in photography, so does kilovoltage *control* the energy in the energy package (kVp, mA, and time) in radiography.

It follows that increasing kilovoltage (in a subsequent exposure, and beyond certain limits) *flattens* (decreases contrast) the image, and latitude* is so gross that visibility of detail diminishes inversely.

As a result it is obviously appreciated that *too much* energy negates contrast and visibility of detail (diagnostic quality).

Density

Elsewhere in this chapter it is stated that *density is the amount of radiograph blackening.* We emphasize that the quantity of energy (striking the unexposed film) exposes the emulsion in proportion to that energy (primary and secondary rays), and that the degree of blackness in all parts of the radiograph results from the quantity of silver grains that are present and reduced to metallic silver.

It should be remembered also that the number (quantity) of energy photons striking the film is governed (controlled) by the milliampere-seconds of exposure; i.e., milliampere-seconds controls density.

The degree of blackening in a radiograph is the

*In this respect latitude refers to a condition within the radiographic image, that is, the range between and limited by the maximum and minimum densities throughout which visibility of *fine* detail is possible. This is radiographic latitude and must not be confused with either exposure latitude or film latitude.

radiographic (photographic) *density.* It is defined by the equation

$$D = \frac{I_o}{I_t}$$

where I_0 is the intensity of the light falling on the area being measured (with a densitometer) and I_t is the intensity of the light transmitted by (passing through) this area.

In addition to the fact that milliampere-seconds controls density, consideration must be given to those laws and conditions that influence it. These are the *inverse square law* and the several conditions causing fog.

Milliampere-seconds

In general, milliampere-seconds are considered to affect only the density; however, in radiography of some of the more dense structures, a change in milliampere-seconds will affect both density and contrast. Kilovoltage determines the penetrability, and milliamperage determines the intensity of the x-ray beams.

Since each cathode electron that strikes a target atom and has sufficient kinetic energy causes x-ray production, it is obvious that larger numbers of cathode electrons striking the anode will cause the production of correspondingly increased numbers of x rays. Thus total milliampere-seconds (considered as the tube current) controls the number of x rays produced, or the intensity of the x-ray beam, and the ultimate density of the radiograph.

Primary influence

Two sets of conditions influence (affect) density. The factors of primary influence are the following: processing, kVp, film type, focal-film distance, heel effect, and pathology of structure. In addition to pathology of structure it is necessary to consider tissue opacity, since tissue of greater density (to x rays) absorbs greater quantities of the primary rays. This fact results in fewer remnant rays reaching the film. The factors of secondary influence include the following: fog, screen composition, grids, filters, and the type of beam restrictor employed, such as cones, collimator, or diaphragm.

Focal-film distance

Varying the focal-film distance may be useful in affecting only density. The shorter the focal-film distance, the greater the amount of radiographic intensity reaching the film; therefore the greater the film density. (However, when the focal-film distance is decreased, definition is sacrificed.)

The following factors (distance and radiographic intensity, inverse square law, heel effect, and pathology of structure), which influence both contrast and density, are discussed in order of importance.

Distance and radiographic intensity. X-ray intensity diminishes at a rapid and predictable rate as the distance from the source (focal spot) increases. This reduction in intensity is in accordance with the *inverse square law,** which states that the *intensity is inversely proportional to the square of the distance.*

If any degree of accuracy in the description of a beam of x rays is to be achieved, both the *quality* and *intensity* of the beam must be considered. The qualities of x rays are discussed on p. 54. The intensity of x rays is discussed on p. 61. Intensity measurements are necessarily made at a specific distance from the source. As has been pointed out, x rays diverge in all directions from the point of origin, but their escape, except through the port provided, is prevented by the tube shielding. At this time proper consideration should be given to the primary beam and its intensity at a given point. Proper measurements of the beam intensity must include consideration of the fact that x rays travel in straight lines and that passage through any substance (including air) causes a reduction in intensity as a result of scattering or absorption or both. In other words, true measurements of intensity must be made in air at specific distances from the origin and in the central portion of the direct primary beam.

---

*The *radiographic effect formula,* an empirical formula, has been derived from the inverse square law and is written as follows:

$$re = \frac{(\text{mA})\ (\text{s})\ (\text{kVp}^2)}{d^2}$$

In the radiographic effect formula, *re* stands for radiographic effect and refers to the total actinic energy resulting from kilovoltage and milliampere-seconds at a given focal-film distance; *mA* stands for milliamperage; *s* stands for time in seconds (or parts thereof), *kVp* stands for kilovolts peak, and *d* stands for focal-film distance.

Use of this formula will obtain approximate results when applied to plain film in cardboard holders. (See Fig. 4-2.) The values for *re* may be of any numerical quantity and have no specific relation to radiographic intensity.

Fig. 4-9, *A*, represents a geometrically perfect four-sided pyramid 4 feet in height and 4 feet square at the base. This figure illustrates all of the intensity energy entering at point *P* and passing through planes *ABCD* and *A′B′C′D′*. If 100 units of intensity fall upon plane *ABCD*, which is an area of 4 square feet, each square foot will receive one fourth of 100, or 25 units, of intensity per square foot. The same quantity will pass through plane *ABCD* and fall upon plane *A′B′C′D′*, which is an area of 16 square feet. Thus each square foot here receives 6.25 units of intensity. In summary, doubling the distance reduces the intensity to one fourth of the original per unit area for unit time. The methods for measuring intensity are discussed on pp. 61 to 65.

Inverse square law. The inverse square law is written algebraically as:

$$I : : \frac{1}{d^2}$$

where *I* is the intensity of the radiation, and *d* is the focal-film distance (ffd).

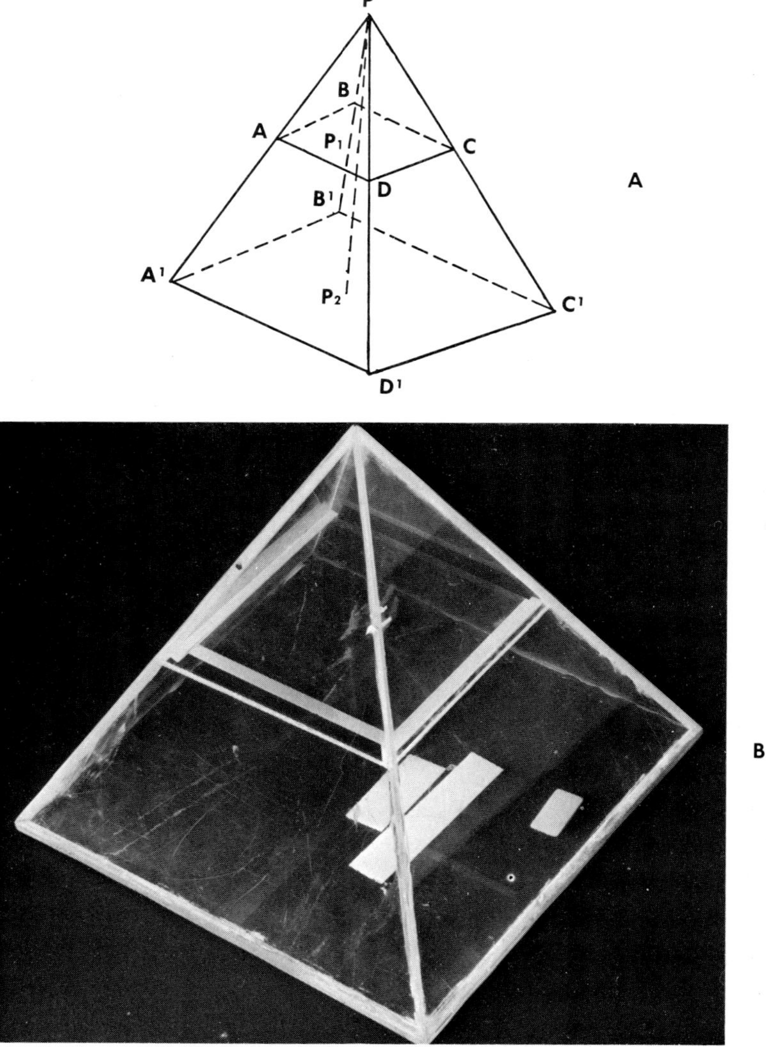

Fig. 4-9. Four-sided pyramids. In **A**, the distance from *P* to P_1 is 2 feet. It is 2 feet from P_1 to P_2. *ABCD* is a square, side *AB* being 2 feet long. *A′B′C′D′* is a square, with side *A′B′* being 4 feet long. **B** is a clear plastic construction. Its dimensions are as follows: base sides, 1 foot; vertical height, 1 foot. The small base (at the 6-inch vertical point) is removable.

In a given examination the mAs employed is 8, and the ffd used is 40 inches. What will be the new mAs value at an ffd of 30 inches when the radiographic density is to be approximately the same in both radiographs?

1. Determine the mAs per unit of square area in the original exposure.
   a. Each side of the plane at 40-inch ffd is 40 inches long.
   b. 40 inches squared = 1,600 square inches.
2. $8 \div 1{,}600 = 0.005$ mAs/sq. in.
3. a. Each side of the plane at 30-inch ffd is 30 inches long.
   b. 30 inches squared = 900 square inches.
4. $900 \times 0.005 = 4.5$ mAs at 30-inch ffd.

This is slightly more than one half the mAs required to produce the same radiographic intensity at the film surface when the ffd is reduced 25% (to 30 inches).

Since intensity and milliampere-seconds are used as being equal, the following formula can be used.

$$\frac{\text{Old mAs}}{\text{New mAs}} = \frac{\text{Old ffd}^2}{\text{New ffd}^2}$$

The formula may be applied as in the following example:

In a given examination the mAs employed is 10, and the ffd used is 6 feet. What will be the new mAs value at an ffd of 8 feet? (Of course, the intent is to achieve a radiograph whose density is approximately that of the original.)

Substituting in the second formula, we obtain:

$$\frac{10}{x} = \frac{(6)^2}{(8)^2} = \frac{(3)^2}{(4)^2}$$

$$9x = 160$$

$x = 17.77$; that is, the new mAs at an 8-foot ffd is 17.77

Consideration of both distance and intensity normally involves only focal-film distance. However, it is necessary to consider the effects of increased object-film distance on radiographic intensity (within the true image shadow in the film emulsion). Secondary rays generated within the patient include both soft and moderately hard rays. As the object-film distance is increased, these softer secondary rays, which normally form part of the image, may be absorbed* in air. As a result the image density is decreased with increased ofd.

Heel effect. Fig. 4-10 illustrates the cathode heel effect on radiograph density. In modern equipment the heel effect is of no great significance; however, it may be employed to maintain, in the same radiograph, comparable density of both thick and thin anatomic parts. *The heel effect obtains a slightly more penetrated image on the cathode side of the radiograph than on the anode side;* this increased density is just visible. This is the result of the emission of the more intense rays from the part of the anode nearest the cathode. (See Fig. 4-11.) When the long axis of the x-ray tube is parallel with the long axis of the table, the heel effect is seldom visible. It is greater when shorter focal-film distances are used.

In a posterior (A-P) view of the thoracic spine, it is possible to employ the heel effect to advantage. The patient should be so positioned that the anode end of the x-ray tube is nearest the patient's head. This permits the stronger rays to penetrate the thicker parts of the spine.

X rays generated with modern three-phase, high-voltage equipment and from modern x-ray tubes have different penetrating characteristics than do x rays generated with older equipment

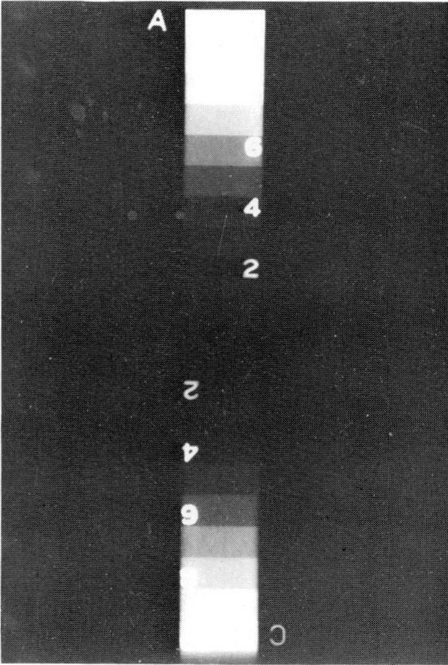

Fig. 4-10. Cathode heel effect on radiographic density. KVp here was 65; mAs, 10; and ffd, 40 inches. Par-speed screens and plain film were used. Density value at anode end on step 6 = 3.08. Density value at cathode end on step 6 = 3.14.

*Experimental evidence indicates that there is a measurable loss in image density (Fig. 4-8).

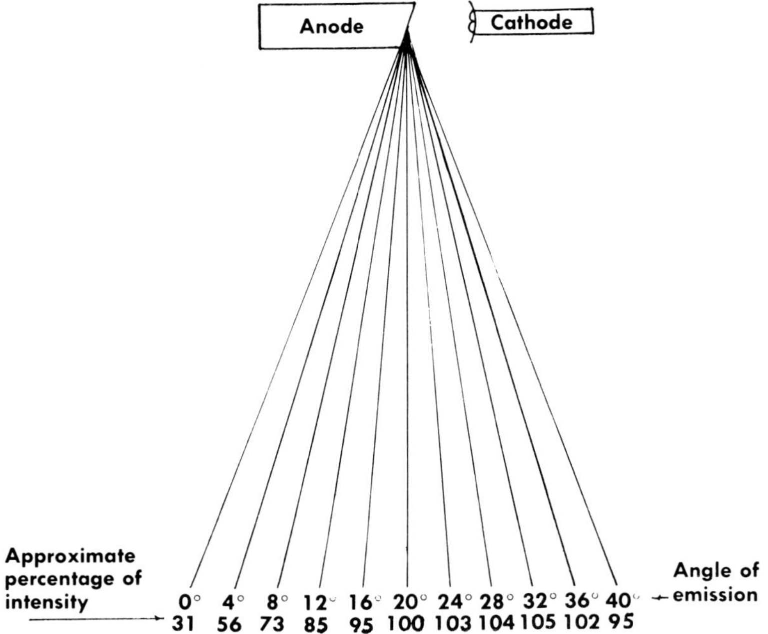

Fig. 4-11. Heel effect. With a tube target angle of 20 degrees, the heel effect is demonstrated in this diagram by comparing the angles of emission (upper numbers) with the percentages of intensity (lower figures). The greatest percentage of intensity occurs with the 32-degree angle of emission and is 105%.

(much of which is currently in use). As a result, heel effect is of little significance today.

Pathology of structure

CARDBOARD HOLDERS. To reduce radiograph density it is a common practice to use cardboard holders in the radiography of relatively thin parts; the maximum thickness of the part usually recommended is 13 cm. (For parts thicker than 13 cm, it is more practical to use cassettes with intensifying screens.) Regular (plain or screen) film is most commonly used in cardboard holders; although no-screen film is specially made for this purpose. The coating on this type of film is much more sensitive to x-radiation than the coating on screen film.

No-screen film in cardboard holders gives excellent detail of both soft tissue and bone when a somewhat longer exposure time than cassette exposure is used.

CONTRAST MEDIA. Because most of the internal viscera possess essentially the same radiographic densities as the surrounding structures, it becomes necessary to add contrast media to the viscera for purposes of radiographic demonstration. In some instances, a contrast medium that is opaque to x rays is used; in other instances, a contrast medium that is radiolucent is employed. Some of the vicera studied by use of contrast media include the gallbladder, kidneys, ureters, urinary bladder, esophagus, stomach, small and large intestines, arteries, veins, ventricles of the brain, spinal canal, heart, etc. The use of contrast media increases contrast because of the differences in relative absorption of x-ray energy between the tissues and the medium employed. The radiopaque media absorb the x rays, whereas the radiolucent media are more easily penetrated than the surrounding tissues.

The contrast media are prepared in several forms, each according to requirements of visualization of a specific viscus or structure. The various forms include solutions, suspensions, emulsions, pastes, powders, tablets, and gases. The viscera or structures visualized, the examination name, and the media employed are listed in Table 13-1.

GENERAL BODY CONSIDERATIONS. Consistent production of high-quality radiographs requires development of an easily followed technique that is satisfactory in most instances. It is useful to develop a technique chart that shows the maxi-

Table 4-7. Grid (Bucky) and nongrid conversion table

		Nongrid to grid		
5:1	6:1	8:1	12:1	16:1
add 10-12 kVp	10-15 kVp	12-18 kVp	15-21 kVp	18-24 kVp
		or mAs multiplied by		
2	3	4	5	6
		Grid to nongrid		
5-1	6:1	8:1	12:1	16:1
subtract 10-12 kVp	10-15 kVp	12-18 kVp	15-21 kVp	18-24 kVp
		or mAs divided by		
2	3	4	5	6

mum permissible deviations from the norm. *The best total results can be obtained only when the time-temperature method of film processing is employed in manual processing.* This method is inherent in automatic processors.

All possible anatomic and physiologic variations in patients cannot be explicated here. Listed below are some of the variations requiring consideration. The exposure changes are approximate and are to be varied within set limitations according to the requirements of the patient. All exposure increases should be made with increased aluminum filtration in the primary beam. See Table 4-7.

Physical condition	*Exposure change*
Extremely obese	Increase
Muscular	Increase (kilovoltage)
Very thin	Reduce
Child	Reduce
Elderly person	Reduce
In wet cast	Increase 3 to 4 times
In dry cast	Increase 2 times

Pathologic condition	*Exposure change*
Sclerosis	Increase (kilovoltage)
Osteomyelitis	Increase slightly
Osteoporosis	Reduce
Paget's disease	Increase
Bone atrophy	Decrease

Secondary influence. The following items (fog, intensifying screens, grids and Potter-Bucky diaphragms, filters, and beam restrictors) are those exerting a secondary influence on radiographic density. In many instances it is to be noted that these same items exert comparable influence on radiographic contrast.

FOG. Radiograph fog, which may be caused by a physical force or a chemical reaction, is a condition of cloudiness or partial opacity of a processed film (radiograph) that should be clear. By definition, *fog is undesirable cloudiness of a radiographic image.* Exposing the film to stray light or other radiant energy or using incorrect development procedures causes fog on the final radiograph.

The condition of fog on a radiograph may be localized in one area or it may be general. Radiograph fog tends to obscure some of the minute details of the demonstrated structures and thereby interferes with the ultimate diagnostic quality of the radiograph.

Oxidation may weaken or partially exhaust the developer, and the use of such a developer may result in chemical fog because prolonged developing time is required. Overdevelopment and normal development at excessively high temperatures* may cause chemical fog. Also, it is likely that development at lower than proper temperatures will cause chemical fog, and will cause losses in contrast.

Prolonged inspection of films during development in manual processing is a frequent cause of fog, due to a combination of light and accelerated oxidation of the developer.

Fog frequently occurs on films that are outdated when exposed.

Fog is controlled by the following: radiation, chemicals, and light; fog is influenced by these conditions: temperature, film storage, and film age.

Physical forces capable of causing radiograph

*Special mixing formulas or solution concentrates or both in which the restrainer is partially or wholly absent are available from the film manufacturers. Such solutions are used for rapid development and fixation in conjunction with surgical procedures. These techniques are designed for rapid processing at high temperatures for 1 minute in each solution in manual processing and should not be confused with automatic processing.

fog include heat, daylight, artificial light, x rays, and gamma rays.

HEAT. Prolonged storage of x-ray film in rooms where temperature is much above 80° F. may cause fog.

LIGHT. White light that leaks around doors or through cracks in the walls will cause fog. The wrong type of safelight filter will permit passage of rays that cause fog. Wattage beyond specifications in the safelight globes will cause fog. Overlong exposure of films to the "safe" rays of the safelight will cause fog.

X RAYS AND GAMMA RAYS. When x-ray film is stored in the processing room or other areas that are not adequately protected from x rays in adjacent therapy or diagnostic rooms, it is possible that x radiation or gamma radiation and even beta particles from isotopes may cause fog. X rays may penetrate improperly protected pass boxes and fog the films either before or after exposure.

GRIDS AND POTTER-BUCKY DIAPHRAGMS. A grid is a stationary arrangement of thin lead strips interspaced with a radiolucent material. The purpose of the grid is to remove (absorb) a considerable quantity of the secondary (scattered) rays and some primary rays, which cause unnecessary density in the radiograph. (See pp. 57 and 58, secondary rays and remnant rays.) Since the lead strips of the grid absorb the rays that strike them, inevitable shadows (*grid lines*—absence of radiation effect on the film) will appear in the radiograph.

Experiment proved that proper arrangement of the lead strips (parallel with the long axis of the grid and table) in a grid that moved in the direction of the short axis of the x-ray table prevented these grid lines in radiographs. This work of Dr. Potter and Dr. Bucky resulted in the Potter-Bucky diaphragm, which is commonly called the Bucky. Grids are used where the use of the Bucky is either impractical or impossible. The grid is light and portable and may be used in conjunction with mobile radiographic equipment. Lysholm and wafer are common names of grids. (See Fig. 4-12, *A*.)

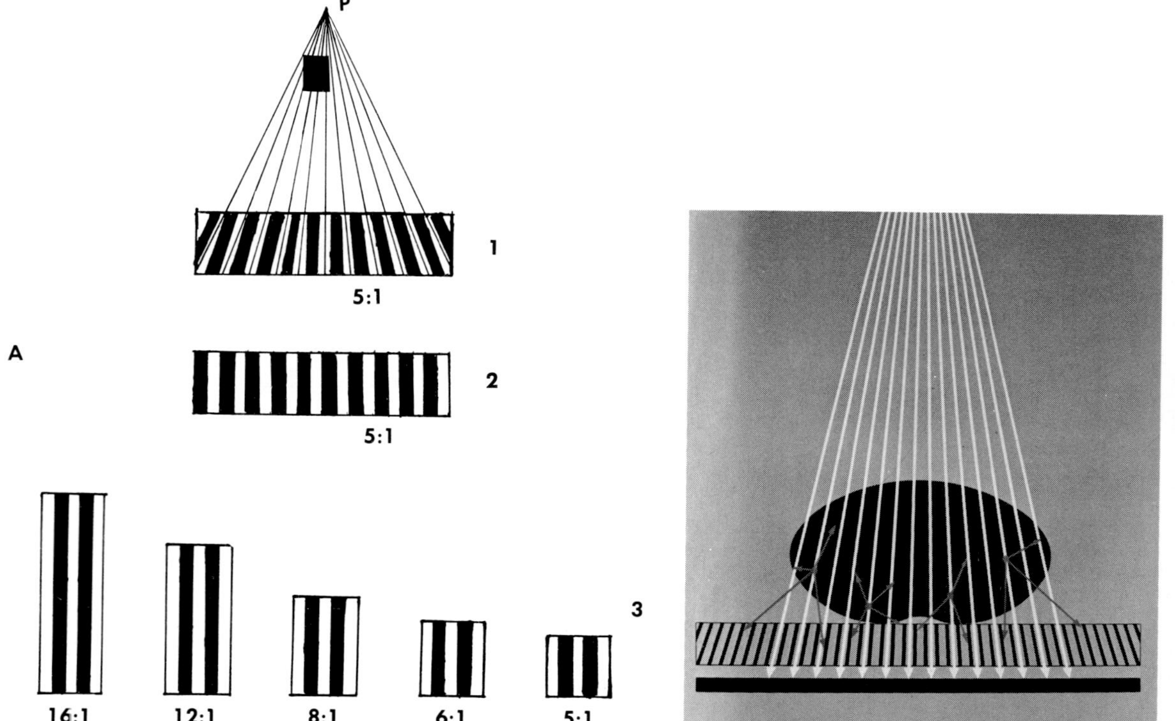

Fig. 4-12. A, Grid ratios. Arbitrarily the relation between the width of the lead strip (black) and the intervening radiolucent material has been drawn as being equal. This is done for purposes of easy comprehension. Actually, the lead strips are exceptionally thin. **B,** Grid action. (Courtesy Siemens Corp.)

The Bucky is beneath the x-ray tabletop and moves a flat grid in the direction of the short axis of the table. A cassette tray is below the grid, and the entire device is placed on a pair of tracks so that the entire Potter-Bucky diaphragm can be moved the length of the x-ray table. The purpose of the Bucky is to facilitate radiographic exposure of thick or dense anatomic parts and to decrease the scattered or secondary rays that strike the film. As a result, a Bucky improves detail visibility and contrast. Because the grid moves, grid lines are not produced in the radiograph. The lead strips in a grid are exceedingly thin. A distinct relationship, expressed as the *grid ratio,* exists between the height of the lead strips and the width of the intervening spaces.

*"The grid ratio is the relation of the height of the lead strips to the distance between them."** Thus a grid in which the thickness or vertical height is 8.0 mm and in which the space between each two lead strips is 1.0 mm would have a ratio of 8:1. The other ratios are 16:1, 12:1, 6:1, 5:1, and 4:1.

In Fig. 4-12, *A, 3,* the comparative heights of five grids are diagramed and greatly enlarged (1 mm = 0.1 inch). To reach the film, the x rays must travel between the lead strips in the grid. The required distance that x rays must travel in a 16:1 grid is twice that in an 8:1 grid. A 16:1 grid absorbs twice as many scatter rays as an 8:1 grid. Everything else being constant, radiographs made with a 16:1 grid will be considerably less dense than those made with an 8:1 grid. Increased scatter-ray absorption improves radiographic contrast. However, if scatter-ray absorption (clean-up) is maximum in a particular examination and a grid of higher ratio is substituted in subsequent examination of the same part, it is highly probable that contrast in the radiograph will be decreased. Under average conditions the use of a grid when one has not been used previously, or the use of a grid of higher ratio (as above), removes secondary rays that have been responsible for (excessive) density; thus visibility of detail is improved. With normal or average use of a grid the following conditions exist: *film contrast varies directly with grid ratio; scatter-ray absorption varies directly with grid ratio; radiograph density varies inversely with grid ratio.* Remember that the use of a Bucky or grid will increase contrast because of the reduced amount of secondary (scattered) radiation reaching the film. If a grid or Bucky is not used, the radiograph will have greater density because of the scattered radiation. It is, then, correct to assume that if a grid or Bucky increases contrast, density is decreased.

The distance between the tube target and the grid surface becomes more critical with the use of higher ratio grids because fewer primary rays are capable of passing between the lead strips of the grid.* For example: a 36-inch focal film distance is quite satisfactory with an 8:1 grid in the Bucky, whereas a 40-inch focal-film distance is equally satisfactory with a 12:1 or 16:1 grid in the Bucky. This principle is explained in terms of the *grid radius. The flat grid radius is the vertical distance from the center of the tube side of the grid to the target of the tube.*

Fig. 4-12 *A, 1,* is a diagram of a *focused (aligned) grid* in which the x-ray beams pass between the lead strips. Fig. 4-12, *A, 2,* is a diagram of a *parallel grid.* A focused grid absorbs more scattered rays than a parallel grid; also, the focused grid is more critical than the parallel grid. Parallel grids inevitably absorb more of the useful rays than focused grids.

Although there is a definite optimum distance (radius) for a specified grid, usually sufficient latitude exists with each 40-inch grid to permit minimum distances of 26 to 28 inches and maximum distances of 44 to 48 inches before the problem of *off-distance cutoff* becomes serious. If an aligned grid is employed at a distance other than that specified by the radius, certain areas of the film may not be exposed because the x rays have been absorbed or "cut off" by the lead strips.

Off-center and off-level cutoff may occur when aligned grids are used and the tube or table is angled or not centered. (See Fig. 4-13, *A.*)

The grid radius determines the optimum distance between the x-ray tube and the grid. The use of these grids at this distance permits a maximum penetration by the useful rays because of the arrangement of the thin lead strips.

Although the *crossed grids* are not shown in Fig. 4-13, *B,* some discussion of them is pertinent. Crossed grids are usually constructed as two linear (parallel) grids; one grid is placed directly above the other with its lead strips at right angles to those of the lower grid. Crossed

*From Characteristics and applications of x-ray grids, Cincinnati, 1968, The Liebel-Flarsheim Co.

*Reference is made to a situation where interchangeable grids are available.

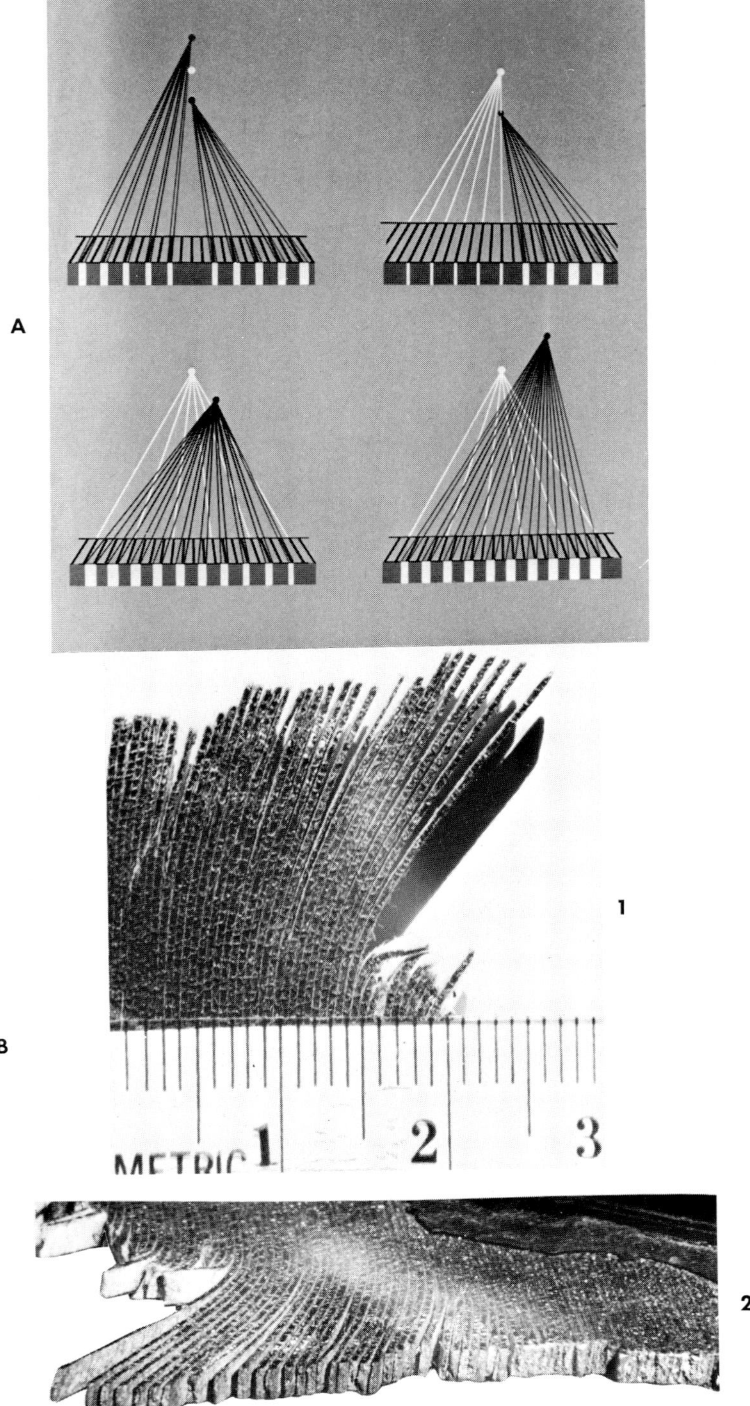

Fig. 4-13. A, Grid: centering and focus. **B, 1,** Photograph of the lead strips and intervening radiolucent substance of an 8:1 focused grid. **2,** View of the lead strips. (**A** courtesy Siemens Corp.)

grids have both advantages and disadvantages when compared with linear grids.

In general, the crossed grid will remove more secondary radiation than a linear grid of ratio equal to the combined ratios of its two equal parts; for example, a crossed grid each of whose parts has 5:1 ratio will remove more secondary radiation than a linear grid of 10:1 ratio. This advantage is most striking at voltages under 100 kVp.

The advantage of the linear grid over the crossed grid is that it may be used in tilted tube techniques without undue "cutoff" in the radiograph.*

A Bucky is operated by any of three methods: mechanical cocking followed by mechanical release; mechanical cocking followed by electronic release; and complete electronic control of reciprocation.†

The following is an explanation of the grid travel in a manually cocked Bucky. Cocking the Bucky moves the grid in position at one edge of the table. Closing the exposure switch electronically releases the grid, which then begins to travel to the opposite side of the table. A spring regulates the rate of travel. The Bucky timer determines the total travel time. The actual radiographic exposure occurs only during the grid travel.

The recipromatic Bucky differs from the manually cocked Bucky in that the grid travels in both directions across the table during the exposure. The manually cocked Bucky requires two selections: one of exposure time on the control panel and a corresponding one on the Bucky. The recipromatic Bucky requires selecting only the exposure time; the length of the exposure determines the number of times the grid travels.

Since there is a considerable amount of useful as well as scatter-ray absorption when a grid is used, more penetrating x rays must be made available; this is accomplished by increasing the peak kilovoltage. (Increasing the milliampere-seconds frequently accomplishes a comparable result; however, it is more practical to add to the peak kilovoltage because increasing the milliampere-seconds markedly increases the exposure intensity.)‡ (See Fig. 4-2.) The conversion factors for nongrid to grid (Bucky) technique and for grid (Bucky) to nongrid, along with conversions for lower to higher and higher to lower grid ratios, are listed in Table 4-7.

In converting technique from higher grid ratio to lower, it is advisable to reduce the milliampere-seconds, which also reduces the quantity of radiographic exposure to the patient.*

Higher kilovoltage requires still higher ratio grids, and probably a change from moving grids to stationary grids with increased numbers of lines per inch. The modification of existing technique factors to compensate for changes in grid ratio should allow for changes in the number of lead strips per inch.

FILTERS. Filters are inserted into the filter slot in the tube shielding to remove the softer rays, which cause increased and undesirable densities in the radiograph. These softer rays cause needless radiation to the patient and are therefore objectionable. *Filters are used in radiography, to protect the patient and to improve radiographic quality.*

Aluminum filters of 1 to 3 mm total thickness are used in addition to the inherent filter. Too much reliance on the inherent filter is hazardous. Prior to all exposures, an inspection is essential to determine the presence of 2 mm of aluminum in the filter slot. (See pp. 59 to 61.) The use of 3 mm of aluminum requires a slight increase in kilovoltage; 2 to 4 kVp are added to the technique for every 1 mm of aluminum in excess of 2 mm, since additional filtration decreases the radiograph density.

Filters absorb the softer x-ray photons (pp. 59 and 60). If the filter material is aluminum, any secondary rays will be so weak that they expend their energy in a very few centimeters of air. (See Fig. 3-10.)

Filters should be used with all diagnostic x-ray equipment. The minimum recommended filtration is 2 mm of aluminum in addition to the inherent filter. In high-kilovoltage techniques the use of additional filtration improves radiographic contrast.

BEAM RESTRICTORS. Any device placed in the

---

*From Characteristics and applications of x-ray grids, Cincinnati, 1968, The Liebel-Flarsheim Co.

†Oscillating grids are incorporated as a part of certain specialized equipment.

‡When the standard, high-contrast technique is routine, the thickness of the part penetrated determines the kV to employ. In such instances it is better to compensate for changes in grid ratio with corresponding changes in mAs.

*An empirical formula based on the grid index is as follows:

$$\text{Known mAs}\ \frac{(\text{index of grid desired})}{(\text{index of grid used})} = \text{New mAs}$$

The grid index is the numerical value by which the nongrid mAs is multiplied to obtain the desired mAs for a specific grid.

path of the primary beam that will contain the beam within predetermined limits is a beam restrictor, that is, it will permit only a certain sized field of exposure. Such devices function to reduce the quantity of secondary rays produced in the patient, thus reducing radiographic density. Secondary benefits derived from use of these devices include, in addition to patient protection (dose reduction), increased visibility of detail and oftentimes improved (increased) definition (p. 100). Beam restrictors include cones, collimators, and diaphragms.

Radiographic cones. Cones are used to limit *the field of exposure, to decrease the amount of secondary scatter, and generally to improve detail visibility in the radiograph.* Although cones differ in size, length, and shape, all are used for the same three purposes.

Cones are made of a light metal with a radiopaque liner material. They may have a round, flared end that permits a round field of exposure, or they may be designed to provide a rectangular field of exposure. There are also modifications that vary the field of exposure by manipulation of single or double diaphragms built into the device. There is a choice of field shape in these single- and double-diaphragm devices; the shapes may be round, square, or rectangular and of variable size within the shape of the diaphragm.

Collimation must be employed in all radiographic exposures! Recent federal regulations require that all new equipment be fitted with an *automatic collimator,* one that will automatically close to the exact size of the film during the exposure. This essentially precludes "the having of" an unexposed margin of approximately ⅛ inch on each edge of each radiograph. (That would present *certain* evidence that the patient received no excessive radiation in that single exposure. Of course, improper centering can cause reexposing the patient; thus, the R dose would be doubled.)

In instances that require numerous exposures over a specific area, *coning down* is highly desirable. Coning down refers to the use of an extension, dental, or mastoid cone or finely collimated beam to emphasize certain structures by eliminating secondary scatter. This procedure on a specific structure is recommended for certain areas of the body, for example, for a lateral or posterior (A-P) view of the lumbosacral joint (even when a single view for emphasis is requested following a routine exposure).

Use of a collimated beam (or properly sized cone) reduces the secondary (ray) dose to the gonads to as much as ⅙ or ⅛ of the noncollimated dose.* In both skull and chest radiography, the gonadal dose is from secondary radiation. In these examinations proper collimation of primary beam and correct direction of the central ray reduce the gonadal dose considerably.

Use of very small collimated beams (cones) necessitates an increase in the exposure quantity. This may be accomplished by an increase in peak kilovoltage or in milliampereseconds; however, it is preferable to increase the peak kilovoltage. Table 4-8 lists the required increases for the various-sized cones.

Various types of collimating devices are replacing the standard "set of cones." The use of cones requires accuracy in alignment and direction of the central ray to prevent the condition called *cone cutoff.* The use of collimators requires even greater accuracy for the same reason. When a circular cone or collimator is employed, the *cone coverage formula* may be used to predetermine the diameter of the field of exposure at different distances:

$$\frac{(L)(d)}{l+z} = D$$

where L is the focal-film distance, l is the length of the cone, z is the distance between the cone slot and the focal spot, d is the large diameter of

*These figures are from *Patient care and special procedures in radiologic technology* by John C. Watson.

Table 4-8. Cone-technique conversion

Size of cone, inches	Increase kVp by	or	Increase mAs by
3 × 10	6 to 8		60%
5 × 10	2 to 4		20%
8 × 10	None		None
Fully extended	6 to 8		60%
Nonextended	4 to 6		40%

the cone, and D is the diameter of the field of exposure.

Example: $L = 40$ inches, $l = 10$ inches, $z = 3$ inches, $d = 8$ inches.

$$\frac{(40)(8)}{10+3} = D$$

$$\frac{320}{13} = D$$

$$D = 24.61 \text{ inches}$$

When no cone is employed, remove the l from the formula. When a square or rectangular collimator is employed, d becomes one of the aperture sides and D becomes the corresponding side in the field of exposure.

The use of cones and other devices to limit the area of exposure increases contrast and decreases density. If a small cone such as an extension cone is used, the primary radiation can enter the patient in an area proportional to the size of the cone and the distance between the patient and the cone. Therefore the use of a small cone limits the amount of secondary radiation generated in the patient. When the amount of secondary radiation is so limited, there is less remnant radiation. As a result, density is decreased and contrast is increased. In order to maintain density while using small cones, peak kilovoltage or millampere-seconds must be increased. (See Fig. 4-14.)

The information in the preceding paragraphs is not necessarily restricted to radiographic cones. Some of the same principles apply to use of both collimators and diaphragms.

Collimators. Most modern radiographic units are installed equipped with a collimator. The collimator is usually a double-diaphragm device installed in the pathway of the primary beam and attached to the x-ray tube shielding at the port. Manual controls for each diaphragm permit the operator to regulate the size and shape of the aperture through which the x rays pass; thus the collimator functions as a beam restrictor. The modified cone coverage formula (see under cones) can be applied to determine the area of exposure.

Diaphragms. Another beam-restricting device usually made of iron, steel, or lead is a diaphragm. It has a certain size and shape of aperture in the center through which the x rays pass (as with the collimator). It may be permanently mounted, or it may be designed to be attached at the port of the x-ray tube shielding. It differs from a collimator both in design and in the fact that the aperture size and shape is fixed; otherwise it functions similarly to the collimator.

It is stated on p. 82 that kilovoltage controls contrast. This is discussed (elsewhere in this chapter) also on p. 70. On p. 80 influencing factors of contrast include the effects of screens on contrast. The following section treats contrast directly.

Contrast

As defined on p. 71 *contrast is the visible difference between adjacent densities resulting from subject and film characteristics.*

Photographically defined, contrast is the property of a photographic material that determines the magnitude of the density difference resulting from a given exposure difference. It is explained as the ratio of the maximum to the minimum transmission of a negative or of the maximum to the minimum reflecting power of a print, or positive. The student should appreciate the fact that there is contrast both within the image shadow (between its dark and light areas) and between the black parts of the radiograph and the image part of the radiograph. The black parts and the image part together constitute the total radiograph.

Control

There is no doubt that kilovoltage controls contrast, although millampere-seconds exert a strong influence on contrast, along with focal-film distance and other factors.

Kilovoltage. It is mentioned on p. 82 in the discussion of kilovoltage as related to density that the standard technique in early practice was to vary kilovoltage with thickness of part and to maintain a constant milliampere-second value. This technique generally produces radiographs exhibiting a high degree of contrast.

A radiograph of extreme densities and opacities (blacks and whites) has high (short-scale) contrast. The contrast in such a radiograph may be so great as to obscure small but significant shadows. Reduction in contrast is a move toward several shades of gray instead of extreme blacks and whites; such a change is toward *latitude* (long-scale contrast). (See Fig. 4-15.) Latitude in a radiograph is the extreme range of demonstrated tissue densities over which diagnostic potential is present; it represents the maximum and minimum deviations from optimum tissue differentiation in a single radiograph. When high kilovoltage technique is employed in contrast studies, both radiopaque and radiolucent pathology is often visualized.

Demonstration of how kilovoltage controls

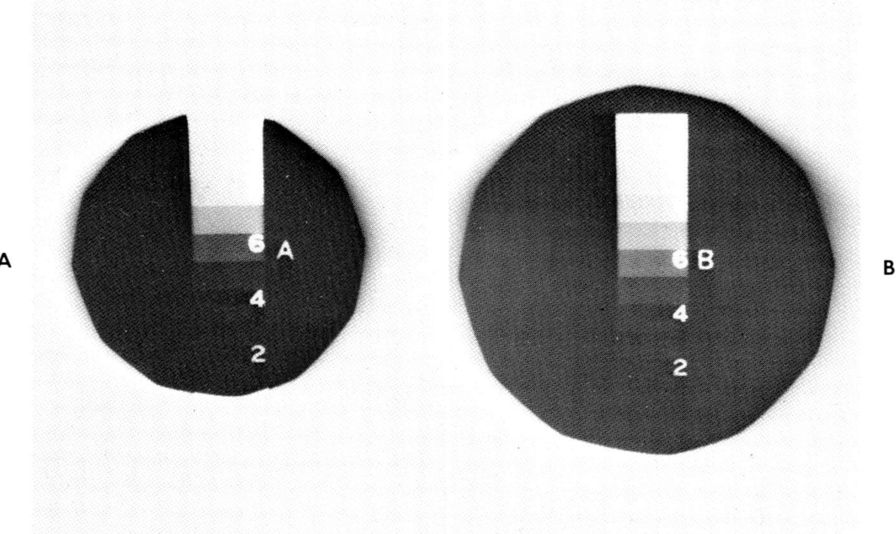

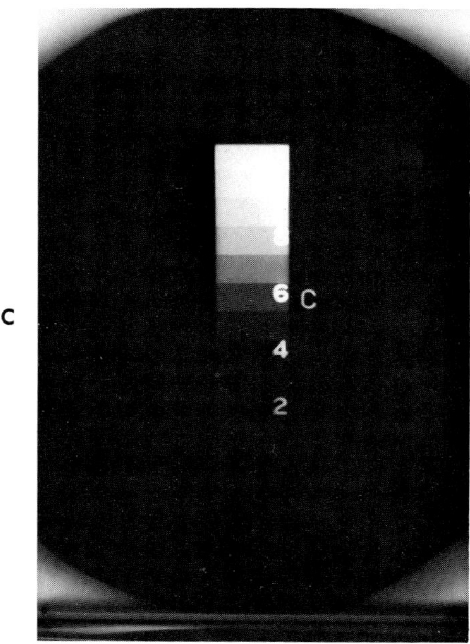

Fig. 4-14. Effects of collimator opening size on film density. In **A**, **B**, and **C**, kVp was 45; mAs was 5; and ffd was 40 inches. Par-speed screens, cassettes, and plain film were used. (Note: Density readings were made between the **A**, **B**, or **C** and the number 6 on the step-wedge.)

Film	*Field size*	*Density*	*Background density*
A	$7\frac{3}{16}$ inches	3.15	1.95
B	$10\frac{1}{4}$ inches	3.18	1.95
C	$16\frac{1}{8}$ inches	3.20	1.95

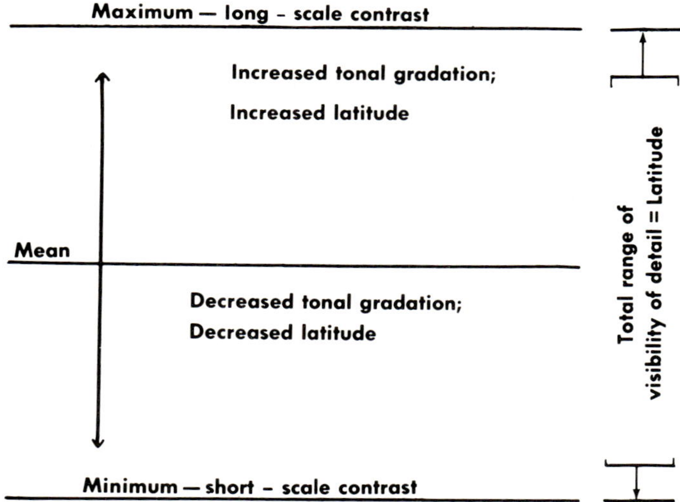

Fig. 4-15. Latitude chart. As x-ray energy increases and exposure quantity decreases, the radiograph demonstrates many shades of gray. Conversely, as x-ray energy decreases and exposure quantity increases, the radiograph demonstrates sharply distinct blacks and whites.

contrast may be achieved in a series of radiographs made of a phantom with several tissue densities in the following manner. Starting with a radiograph of average or acceptable tissue differentiation, greater tonal gradation (long-scale contrast) is achieved when kilovoltage is increased and milliampere-seconds are decreased correspondingly (a 10 kV increase has essentially the same effect as doubling the mAs; therefore the mAs must be halved). Conversely, lesser tonal gradation (short-scale contrast) is achieved when kilovoltage is decreased, and milliampere-seconds are increased correspondingly. It is possible to increase tonal gradation to an extreme limit wherein tissue differentiation ceases. It is also possible to decrease tonal gradation (increase contrast) to an extreme limit wherein tissue differentiation ceases.

Milliampere-seconds. On previous pages it has been stated that mAs and kVp exert considerable effect upon both density and contrast. A discussion of how kilovoltage controls contrast is found on pp. 97 to 99; however, it is to be emphasized that mAs certainly has secondary influence upon contrast, since mAs has control of density. If there were a decrease in mAs used in exposing a particular part, there would be a corresponding decrease in radiograph density. With this decreased density there is an obvious decrease in contrast, since contrast is the magnitude of difference in adjacent densities. The opposite of this is true also.

Primary influence. On p. 91 is a discussion of how fog exerts a secondary influence on density. Of equal importance and exerting a somewhat greater effect is the primary influence of fog on radiographic contrast. It is to be emphasized that contrast is determined quantitatively by the magnitude of density differences within the image shadow and between the image shadow and the black parts of the radiograph. Since fog consists of extraneous densities existing (oftentimes) on all parts of the image shadow, it is readily understood that these densities will reduce contrast.

FOG. Fog reduces contrast by increasing density both in light areas where the density is always visible and in the adjacent darker areas where the density increase may be less visible. Stated differently, fog reduces contrast by reducing the magnitude of density differences.

Secondary influence. The several effects of secondary influence are, for the most part, less obvious than the effect of primary influence of fog on contrast. Many of these secondary factors have been discussed previously in relation to a particular effect on density, and others embrace entirely new considerations.

PATIENT. Since there is no possibility of selecting our patients or of altering their sizes for more or less contrast, it is necessary to understand how different body shapes, sizes, physical conditions, and ages may influence contrast. This knowledge will assist the technologist in selection of appropriate kVp and mAs values to regulate contrast to near that which is desired.

Contrast of internal structures such as the stomach, intestines, gallbladder, arteries, veins, lymph vessels, heart, lungs, brain, and spinal cord to adjacent tissues is made possible through the use of contrast media. Most of these preparations are radiopaque; however, some are radiolucent. See pp. 90 and 91 and Table 13-1.

FILM SPEED. The four kinds of film and associated film speed are discussed on p. 71. Use of "faster" film emulsions is usually a process of gain in one element of diagnostic quality and a corresponding loss in another such element. Use of faster film may gain definition because of reduced exposure time, but will almost always cause losses in contrast. (It is to be noted that increases in definition are not assured with use of fast film.)

As stated on p. 69, plain film emulsion is highly sensitive to light energy. Use of different combinations of silver halides to increase film emulsion response to light energy often causes a radiograph of greater latitude and decreased contrast.

GRIDS. Grids are discussed on pp. 92 to 95. A primary use of grids, either stationary or moving, is to remove (clean-up) the undesirable secondary rays generated in the patient by passage of the primary rays. However, grids remove both secondary and some primary rays.

When correct exposure factors are employed, a grid will increase (improve) contrast by removing nonuseful rays that increase overall density.

FILTERS. Since it is shown on pp. 59 to 61 and 95 that filters remove softer rays from the primary beam, it is obvious that filters will decrease radiographic density to a certain degree. When these densities are of such a nature that the entire radiograph is overly dark, then the use of filters will increase (improve) contrast. However, if filters are used beyond a certain amount of thickness, it follows that contrast will decrease and latitude will increase.

COMPRESSION. Compression may be applied to a particular part of the patient as in pyelography; the compression is applied over the ureters to "hold back" the contrast medium in the kidneys, thus improving contrast. Compression may be applied also in such a manner as to "push aside" tissues or structures that will add unwanted density, thus increasing contrast and diagnostic quality.

The preceding pages of this chapter convey information regarding radiographic quality. With the knowledge and understanding that result from this study, the student is prepared to consider sensitometry as it applies to radiograph production.

SENSITOMETRY

Jack D. Stevens, B.S., R.T.

Sensitometry is the study and measurement of relationships among exposure, processing conditions, and film response. Knowledge of sensitometry and its application assists both students and practitioners of radiography to control the variables that occur in radiographic systems. The most common method of showing the response of a film to exposure is with an H & D* (characteristic) curve.

Fig. 4-16 is an approximation of a *characteristic curve;* on its vertical axis are numbers representing density readings and on its horizontal axis are exposure values. For better understanding of sensitometry and its application a review of terms associated with sensitometry is provided.

*H & D refers to Hurter and Driffield, who developed the curve in 1890.

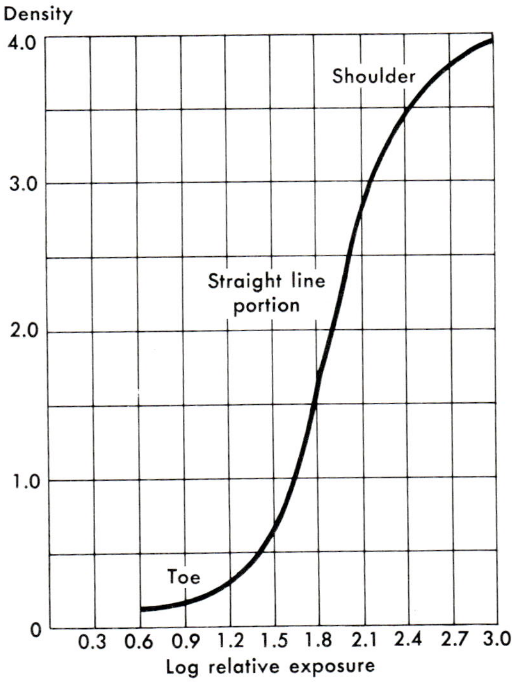

Fig. 4-16. Characteristic curve (approximation). (Courtesy Du Pont Company.)

Density

Radiographic density has been defined as the "amount of film blackening" that results from a deposit of metallic silver remaining in the radiograph after exposure and processing. A useful method of measuring the amount of film blackening is to determine the manner and degree to which it interferes with a beam of light passing through a radiograph. The amount of light absorbed by the radiograph is measured by a densitometer in terms of density.

Sensitometrically, density is the logarithm of the ratio of the amount of light striking one side of the radiograph compared with the amount of light that passes from the other side (passes through the radiograph). When the metallic silver in the emulsion allows 1/10 of the light to pass through, this ratio is 10:1. The logarithm of 10 is 1 and the silver deposit is said to have a density of 1.

$$D = \log \text{ of } \frac{I_o}{I_t}$$

D = density
I_o = light incident to the radiograph
I_t = light transmitted through the radiograph

Exposure

Exposure is the intensity multiplied by the time and can be expressed either in absolute exposure units (ergs per square centimeter of x-radiation) or in relative units. Relative exposure is much more convenient and equally useful. In radiography we think of exposure in terms of milliampere seconds (mAs). When the mAs is doubled the exposure is doubled, kVp remaining constant.

In plotting a characteristic curve we plot density against *log relative exposure*. If the kilovoltage remains constant, the ratios of the exposure reaching the film through two different regions of the subject are always the same, no matter what the values of milliamperage, time, or focal-film distance may be. On a logarithmic scale any two exposures whose ratio is constant will always be separated by the same distance on the exposure scale, regardless of the absolute values. For example, two exposures, one of which is twice the other, will always be separated by 0.3 on the logarithmic exposure scale. The logarithm of 2 is 0.3. So, on the horizontal axis representing exposure is seen the log relative exposure scale.

The position of the curve designated as the *toe* demonstrates the response of the emulsion to relatively small amounts of radiant energy. With increases in exposure, the density builds up slowly until the *straight-line* portion of the curve is reached. Along this straight-line portion the density increases uniformly with the logarithm of the exposure until the *shoulder* of the curve is reached. In this region additional exposure results in smaller increases in density to a point where additional exposure does not produce greater density. In fact, if sufficient exposure is applied the density actually decreases.

Contrast

The dictionary definition of contrast is "to stand out, to exhibit noticeable difference when compared side by side." Radiographically, contrast is the difference in two or more densities. As a radiograph is viewed on an illuminator the difference in brightness of the various parts of the image is called radiographic contrast. This is the product of two distinct factors: (1) film contrast—inherent in the film and influenced by the developing process; and (2) subject contrast—result of differential absorption of radiation by the object.

Sensitometrically, contrast refers to the slope or steepness of the characteristic curve of the radiograph between two points. In radiography we

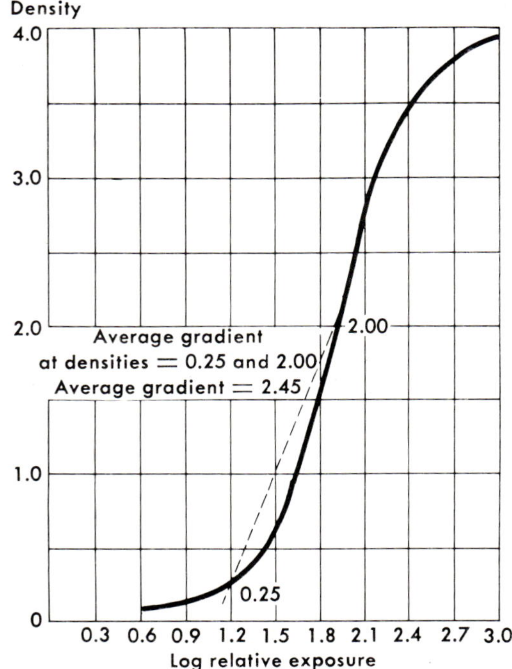

Fig. 4-17. Density, average gradient. (Courtesy Du Pont Company.)

usually use the *average gradient* between densities (Fig. 4-17) 0.25 and 2.0. Usually the *net* densities 0.25 and 2.0 are used. This means that base + fog is subtracted from the total; i.e., if there is a base + fog of 0.18 we would measure the average gradient between 0.43 and 2.18.

Gamma

Gamma is the slope of the straight-line portion of the characteristic curve. This term is seldom used in radiography since the curves of radiographic films have relatively short straight-line portions. Also, this portion of the curve may not coincide with the density range that is most useful in radiography.

Speed

It has been determined that the contrast of a film is indicated by the shape of the characteristic curve. Speed is indicated by the location of the curve along the exposure axis. The faster film will lie toward the left of the graph. In Fig. 4-18, film A is a faster film than is film B. Notice the steepness of the straight-line portion; film A also has higher contrast.

Latitude

The dictionary defines latitude as "freedom from narrow limits." Radiographically we think of latitude in terms of the freedom of exposure ranges and processing times and temperature.

Of the variable factors used we consider that film exposure is controlled by varying the time of exposure, mA, or kV. Exposure latitude is simply a measure of the magnitude of error that is permitted in each of these factors while still yielding a useable radiograph. When a film is said to have *wide latitude* it has the ability to accept large changes in exposure without producing excessive density changes. In Fig. 4-19, film D has wider latitude than film C since an equal change in exposure to both films produced a less abrupt change of density on film D—a graphic demonstration of the rule, *as contrast increases latitude decreases.*

With this basic knowledge of sensitometry and the proper equipment it is possible to evaluate the radiographic quality (produced) in a given department by analysis in four informational areas: (1) fog, (2) speed, (3) contrast, and (4) maximum density.

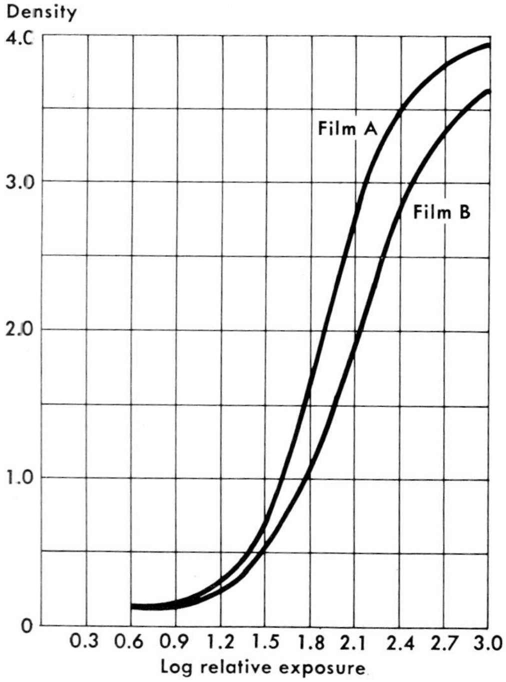

Fig. 4-18. Curves showing comparison of film speeds. (Courtesy Du Pont Company.)

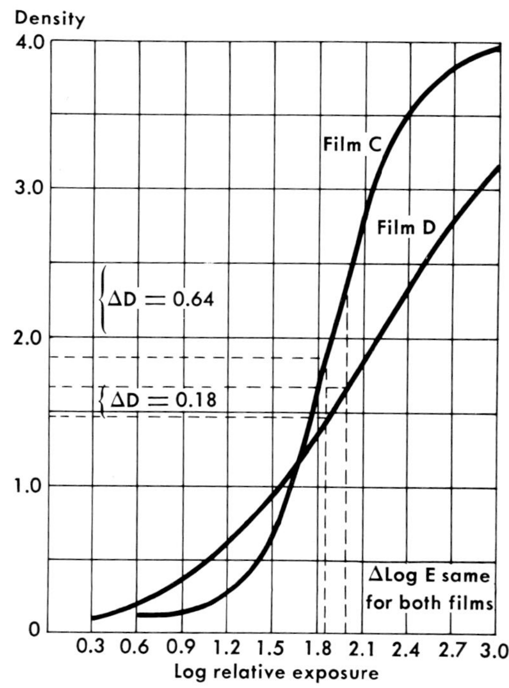

Fig. 4-19. Comparison of latitude of two films. (Courtesy Du Pont Company.)

Four basic steps must be taken to apply sensitometry to radiograph production.

Exposure—effect on the radiograph can be measured with an electroluminescent sensitometer (a laboratory instrument) or a common aluminum step-wedge.

Processing (development)—The film is processed by whatever method is in use (in the particular department).

Measurement (of density)—can be made with either a densitometer or by visual comparison.

Interpretation—achieved from a full-curve plot, a single-density plot, or visual reference with a standard.

A very important part of the learning process in this discipline is the recognition of processing problems and of methods useful in recognition and prevention.

MAJOR PROCESSING PROBLEMS

In addition to fog, which is discussed on pp. 91, 92, and 99, the technologist may face other serious processing conditions that detract from, and may even destroy, radiographic quality. Among these problems are the following: static, exhaustion, stains, and artifacts.

Static

Static marks on radiographs are the result of electric discharge on the film surface. Static electricity may collect on the person or clothing of the technologist who processes the film. This is especially true in high altitude. Static marks may occur as *tree* or *branching* static: the static marks resemble the branching of tree limbs. Other forms of static include *smudge* marks and small black pinpoint areas on the finished radiograph (Fig. 4-20). Films need to be stored in an upright position to prevent static marks that would result from pressure.

Exhaustion

Exhaustion of the developer and fixer occurs progressively despite proper replenishment of solutions. Exhaustion of these solutions refers to a gradual decline in strength as a result of several conditions.

The process of reducing atomic silver to metallic silver liberates bromine ions from the sil-

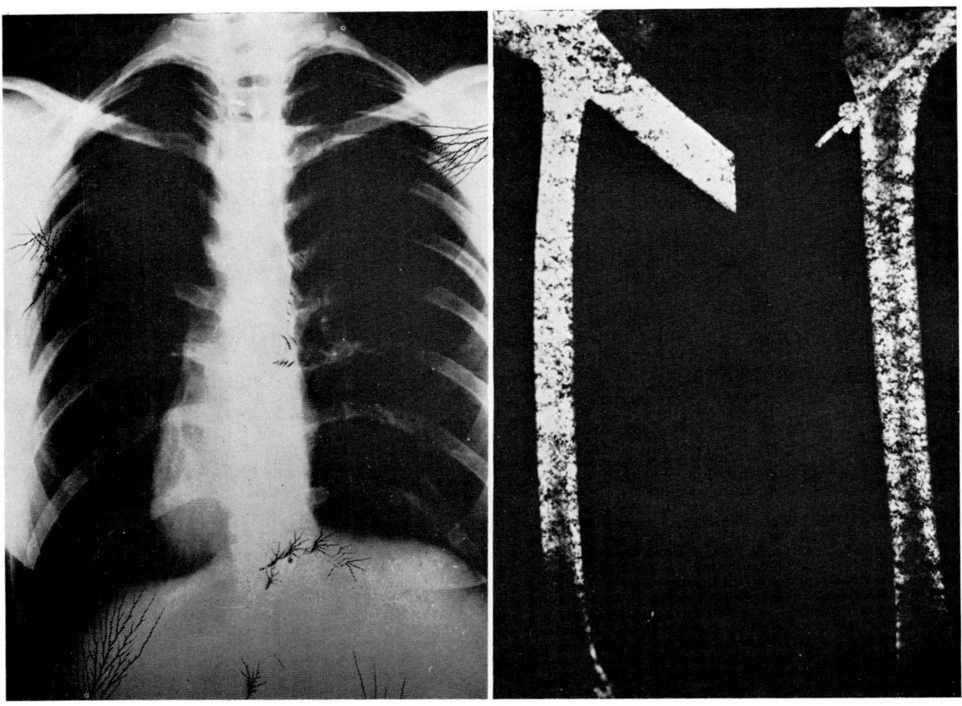

A B

Fig. 4-20. A, Tree or branching static. **B,** Smudge static.

ver bromide crystals. These bromine ions combine with sodium in the developer to form sodium bromide. The presence of sodium bromide tends to impede or decrease the rate of activity of the remaining developing solution. Another deleterious result of the reducing action is the release of hydrogen ions in the developer, which also occurs as a result of time. The release of hydrogen ions tends to lower the pH of the developer, and therefore a longer time is required for development. Age contributes considerably less to the exhaustion of the fixer than to the exhaustion of the developer.

To maintain maximum efficiency in the manual processing room, the technologist should incorporate the following into his routine. He should stir the solutions each morning before use to prevent uneven development and fixation. He should always cover the developer tank, since light and air tend to decrease the effectiveness of this solution rapidly. He should adhere strictly to the *time-temperature* method of processing. This method uses a constant-temperature control device (such as a thermostat) in the incoming water supply to maintain a definite optimum time of processing.

Since exhausted solutions may be the cause of colored stains on the radiograph, the technologist should make frequent checks for exhaustion. He should check periodically the pH of both the developer and the fixer. A milky appearance of the developing solution denotes gross exhaustion. The fixer pH ranges between 4.5 and 4.8. To check the fixer for exhaustion, add one drop of the fixer to 1 or 2 ml of a 10% solution of potassium iodide. If the solution turns milky or cloudy, the fixer is exhausted and should be discarded.

Stains

Automatic processing has, to a great extent, eliminated the problems of stains and some artifacts.

In manual processing routine inspection for accumulation of fixer in the corners and tops of the hangers should be made. The accumulation should be scrubbed off with a stiff brush and a nonabrasive scrubbing compound. Such an accumulation may cause colored streaks and stains on an otherwise good radiograph. Stains can also be caused by incomplete fixation and incomplete washing after fixation and by improperly cleaned tanks.

Artifacts

In manual processing as the films are placed in the developer, they should be agitated for at least 1 minute to loosen any air bubbles that may be on the film surface. If these bubbles were left on the film, there would be undeveloped areas at the site of each air bubble (airbells).

Rough handling of the films prior to exposure, especially bending, will cause black crescent marks on the finished film surface. These crescents will be surrounded by definite white or lighter

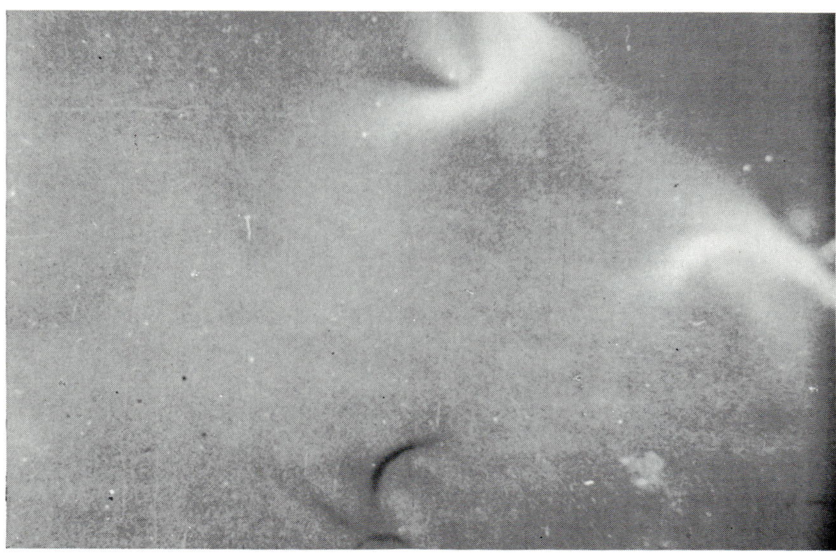

Fig. 4-21. Pressure crescents.

areas. Similar handling after exposure produces distinct black crescents in the emulsion of the processed and finished radiograph; however, the latter crescents are often only slightly more dense than the surrounding parts. (See Fig. 4-21.) The manufacture of certain films tends to prevent the formation of these crescents.

Improperly stirred solutions cause layers of increased or decreased radiograph density as a result of increased or decreased activity of the developing or fixing solutions.

A rather serious but infrequent artifact of improperly processed radiograph emulsions is that of reticulation. *Reticulation is defined as a network of corrugations produced accidentally or intentionally by a treatment producing rapid expansion and shrinkage of the swollen gelatin in processing.* Reticulation occurs as a result of a too great difference in temperature between any two of the several processing room solutions.

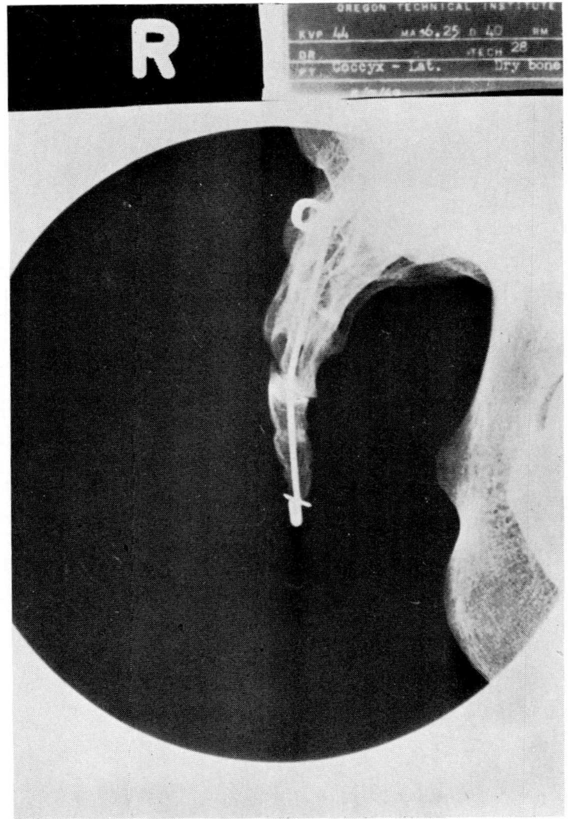

Fig. 4-22. Streaked silver deposit. Black line extending vertically downward from the tip of the coccyx is a heavy deposit of metallic silver.

The emulsion on a film suspended in the developing solution becomes quite loose as a result of the quantity of solution absorbed. The parts of the emulsion containing large quantities of metallic silver are heavier than surrounding areas of emulsion containing less metallic silver; the heavier emulsion may slide downward in the less heavy emulsion and cause typical streaking. (See Fig. 4-22.) This artifact may occur in areas of density greater than the surrounding area and so contribute to a loss in visibility of detail, and even to a loss in definition.

Graininess is a mottling of the radiographic image and is controlled by screen and film emulsion composition. Graininess is influenced by processing.

SPECIAL RADIOGRAPHIC ACCESSORIES

The numerous and highly technical procedures and processes of radiograph production employ a variety of accessory devices. Many of these devices are quite common and are found in all departments of radiology. Others are less common and are found, for the most part, in large departments of radiology. Some technical procedures require no special accessory devices, but employ special usage of existing parts of the x-ray machine. Among these items are four that are discussed in subsequent paragraphs.

Stereoradiography

Stereoradiography is the process of making stereoscopic radiographs. A three-dimensional effect of these radiographs is obtained by the proper mounting and viewing of two very slightly dissimilar exposures of the same structure. A special device called a *stereoviewer* is employed for this purpose.

The two radiographs required for this projection are made at angles of the same degree but on opposite sides of a vertical plane through the center of the structure radiographed. Consequently, the tube is shifted from approximately 1¼ inches from one side of center to the same distance on the opposite side of center, a total shift of 2½ inches. In each shift, the tube is angled to the same point in the structure being radiographed.* For a shift of 2½ inches, the optimum distance between the radiographs

*Completely satisfactory results are obtained when the central ray is angled at 90 degrees to the film surface, especially if the tube shift does not exceed 2½ inches.

and the reflecting mirrors of the viewer is 25 inches. Also, a 2½-inch tube shift is best employed with a 25-inch focal-film distance. Approximately 2½ inches represents the distance between the pupils of the eyes (interpupillary distance*).

Most tabletop and Bucky radiography is performed at a 40-inch focal-film distance, and most chest radiography at a 72-inch focal-film distance. When the focal-film distance is greater than 25 inches, an adjustment in the distance of the tube shift will improve three-dimensional visualization of the structures. A proportion that explains the interrelationship of tube shift, focal-film distance, interpupillary distance, and viewing distance is:

Tube shift:ffd :: Interpupillary distance: Viewing distance†

Practical application of this proportion will develop an appreciation of the relationship. When the viewing distance is 25 inches, the tube shift is one tenth the focal-film distance. An increase of the focal-film distance to 40 inches requires a tube shift of 4 inches, although a tube shift of 2½ to 3 inches will obtain useful results.

Stereoradiographs may be viewed in any one of several devices. Probably the most commonly used device is the Wheatstone Reflectoscope or a modification. This device has two adjustable mirrors and two connected illuminators (viewing boxes) mounted on a sliding carrier so that each illuminator is always the same distance from its corresponding mirror.

Stereoradiography is employed chiefly for medical interpretation of structures within the body. Stereographic visualization makes apparent the separation of overlapping structures or the depth and shape of a single structure or both.

In stereoradiography, varying conditions govern the direction of the tube shift. Among these conditions are structures under consideration, heel effect (if a grid is used), and mechanical devices available on the equipment. The tube shift is usually at right angles to the dominant anatomic lines. If the tube shift is at right angles to the Bucky or grid lines, there will be no change in density in comparable anatomic parts. However, if the tube shift is parallel with the grid lines, density variations may exist in the resulting radiographs unless the heel effect is properly employed. Strict adherence to correct collimation and gonadal protection are of extreme importance in stereoradiography. There will be noticeable differences in density in the radiographs if the optical focal spot size is different in the two exposures.

*The interpupillary distance (IPD) is 2$\frac{9}{16}$ inches or 6 cm.

†From Selman, Joseph: The fundamentals of x-ray and radium physics, Springfield, Ill., ed. 5, 1972, Charles C Thomas, Publisher.

Tomography

Other methods of producing radiographs to demonstrate internal structures have been developed. Although the principle is essentially the same in most of these methods, numerous names are applied to the patented apparatus: planigraph, laminagraph, stratigraph, tomograph, etc. The basic principle employed is that of maintaining an exact focus at one depth of structure while the tissues above and below this structure are blurred. The relationship between the ffd and the ofd remains constant, although both distances change during the exposure (and during tube travel in the planigraph). Fig. 4-23, *B*, is a diagram of the basic geometry in this type of radiography. In this procedure the patient must remain motionless while both the tube and cassette are moved in opposite directions throughout the specific time interval. The exposure time in this procedure will vary, in accordance with the equipment and requirements, from a few tenths of a second to several seconds.

Fig. 4-23, *A*, illustrates the x-ray tube at the start of its travel (with the length of the x-ray table) for the exposure of the depth cylinder as shown in Fig. 4-24, *D*. This is a single-plane device.

Fig. 4-25, *A*, the Multi-Planigraph 2,* enables planigraphy with both linear and elliptic blurring to be carried out on recumbent patients. This unit also makes possible zonographic work with linear and circular blurring.

Zonography is planigraphy with a small planigraphic angle. Zonography provides improved diagnostic capabilities in visualization of extensive objects or processes separated from their surroundings, such as the kidney, sternum, hip joint, and gallbladder.

Phototimers

A phototimer is a device beneath the Potter-Bucky diaphragm and cassette tray used to du-

*Manufactured by Siemens Corp., Erlangen, Germany.

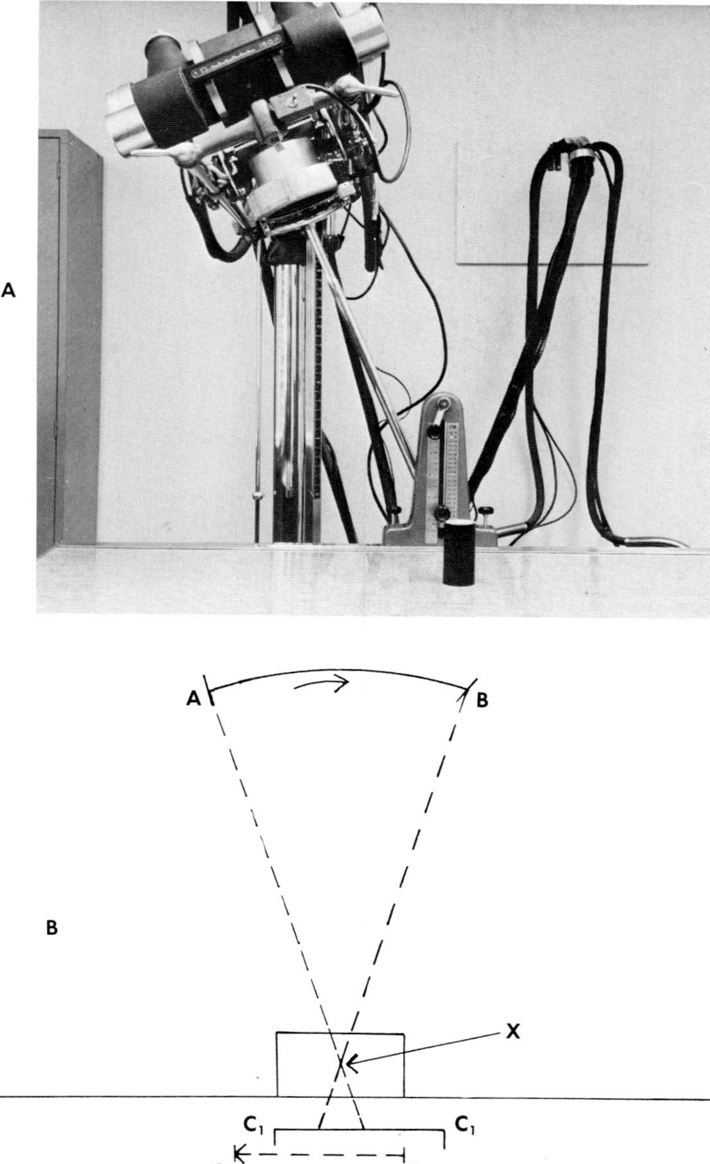

Fig. 4-23. A, Planigraph attached to x-ray machine. Planigraph rod is seen angled and between tube arm and Bucky tray. Planigraph rod is attached at fulcrum to the depth selection. Depth cylinder is positioned in center of x-ray table in front of fulcrum. **B,** Body section radiographic principle. A fulcrum is attached on the level of structure *X*. As the x-ray tube is moved from *A* to *B* during the exposure, the cassette is moved in the opposite direction from a position as in C_1 to a position as in C_2; the cassette is moved in the same horizontal plane. Structure at *X* is in constant focus; all other structures are blurred.

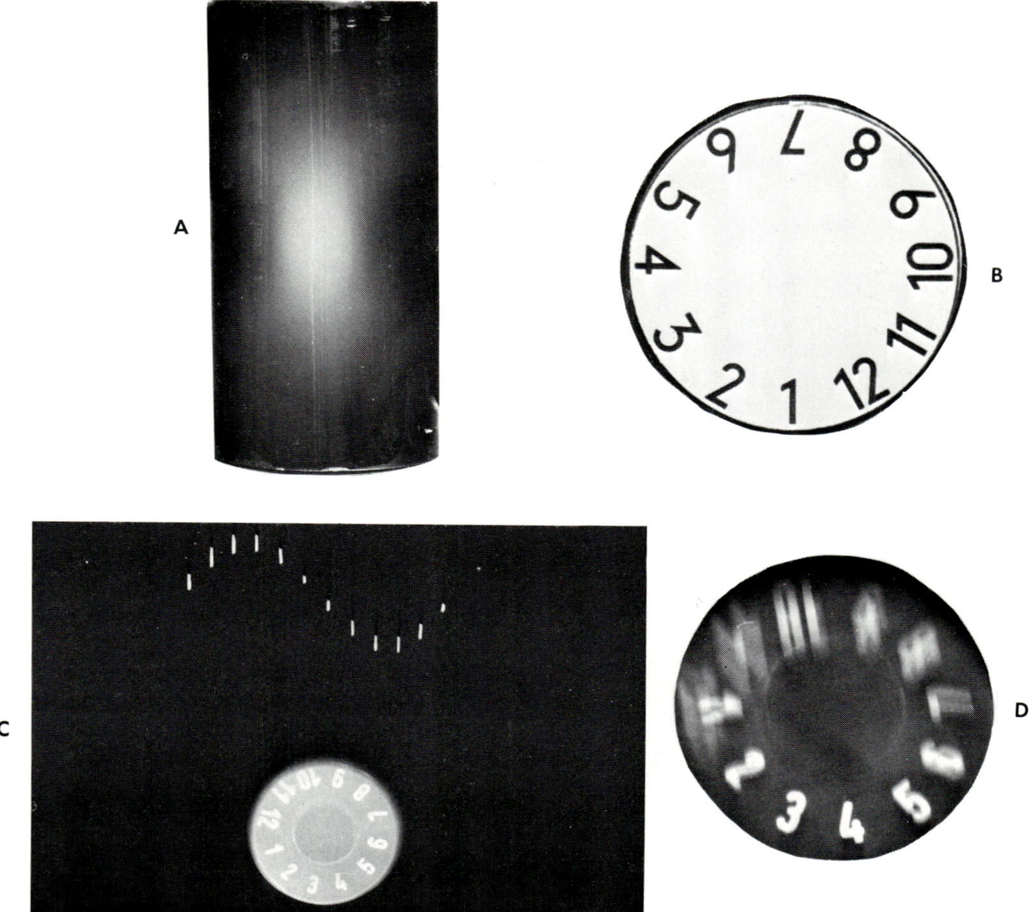

Fig. 4-24. A, Depth cylinder used for **D** here. **B,** Top of depth cylinder used for **D. C,** Depth cylinder radiographs. **D,** Depth cylinder radiograph with fulcrum at 4 cm above tabletop.

Fig. 4-26. Schematic diagram of a phototimer circuit.

1. X-ray power supply
2. X-ray tube
3. Object x-rayed
4. Tabletop
5. Cassette (with no lead backing)
6. Fluorescent screen
7. Phototube
8. Capacitor (condenser)
9. Relay
10. Exposure switch
11. Power line
12. Thyratron

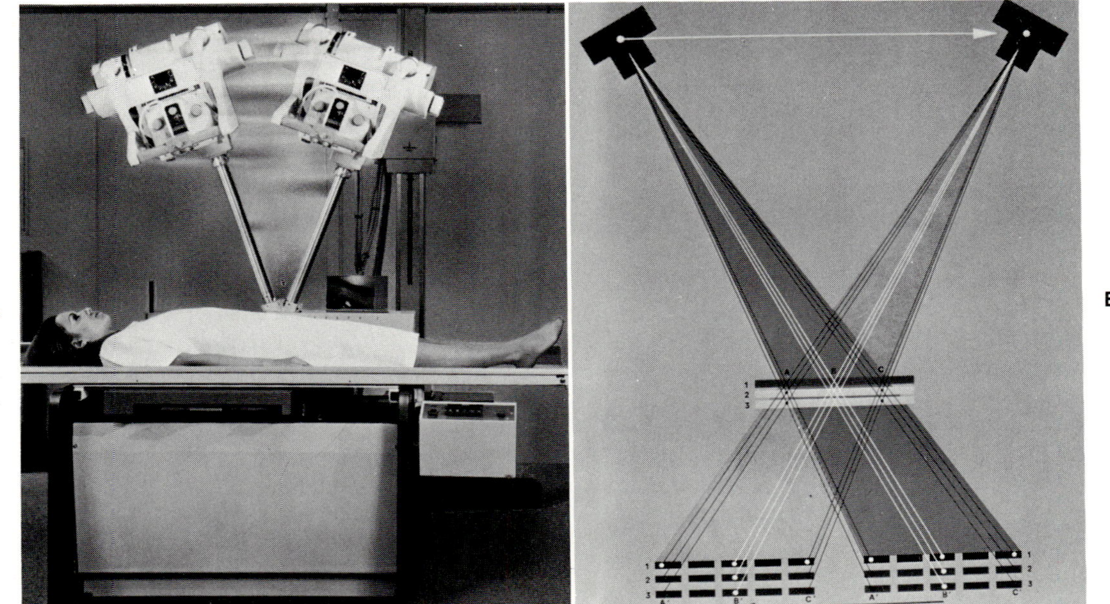

Fig. 4-25. A, Multi-Planigraph 2. X-ray tube is shown in two positions indicating the path of tube motion. **B,** Schematic for simultaneous multisection radiography. (Courtesy Siemens Corp.)

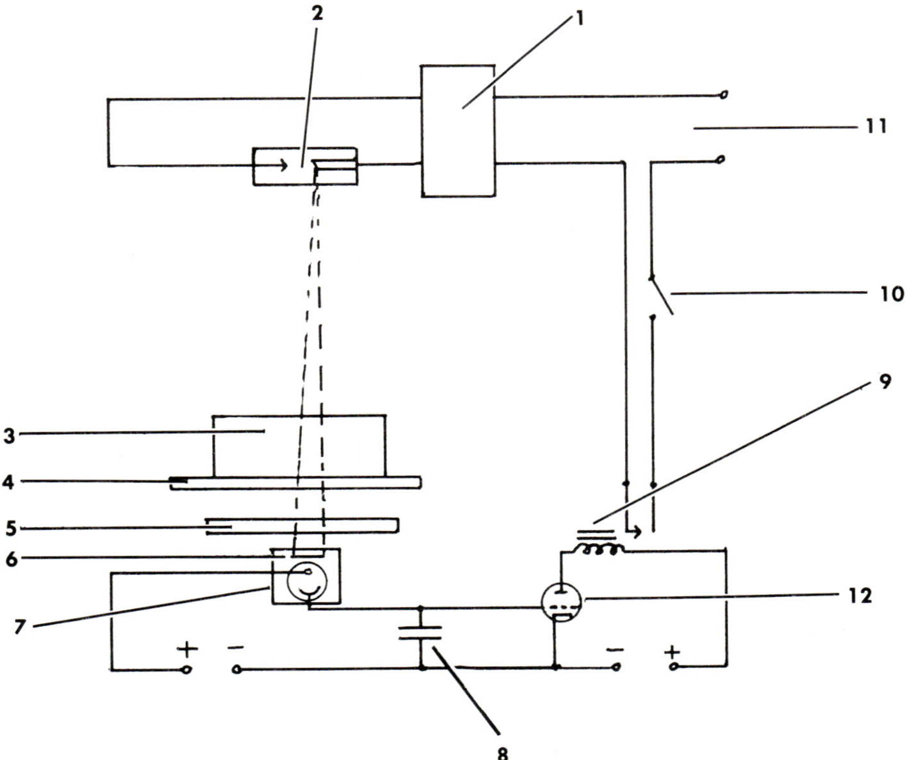

Fig. 4-26. For legend see opposite page.

plicate radiographic density in successive exposures. A phototiming device has its separate controls on the control panel; however, the milliamperage and kilovoltage selectors are the same ones used in routine radiography.

The following statements explain the principle of the phototimer. A special cassette with no radiopaque material in the back permits x-ray energy to penetrate the cassette. A fluorescent screen mounted directly below the cassette tray receives the remnant rays from the cassette. The energy of these rays causes fluorescence in the screen. The fluorescent light energy falls on a photoelectric cell. The electricity generated in the cell flows to a condenser until it has sufficient current to permit discharge. Upon discharge of the condenser, a Thyratron tube ionizes, causing a relay to open and terminate the x-ray exposure. It is in this manner that a phototimer controls radiographic density. (See Fig. 4-26.)

Fluoroscopy

Fluoroscopy is a radiologic examination by means of a fluoroscope. The patient is placed on or against the radiographic table, depending on a recumbent or erect position. A fluoroscopic screen is positioned in front of the patient; that is, between the patient and the radiologist. The radiologist is then in position to observe the viscera in motion, thus adding to the clinical information necessary in diagnosis.

Fluoroscopic screens

Intensifying screens are used to aid in the production of a permanent image in the radiograph. *Fluoroscopic screens are used by the radiologist to observe actions of the various viscera with or without the presence of contrast media.*

A fluoroscopic screen is generally made of a layer of a phosphor (zinc sulfide) coated on a piece of durable plastic. This screen, to seal out dirt, is sandwiched between a protective cover on the tube side and a sheet of leaded glass, which is the viewing side. The protective cover on the tube side permits x-ray penetration; the lead in the glass *partially* protects the operator from direct radiation.

Zinc sulfide is used in a modified state so that the generated light rays are between 5,200 Å and 5,400 Å; maximum sensitivity of the eye to light rays is from 5,000 Å to 6,000 Å. The color of the light from a fluoroscopic screen is usually modified to a greenish yellow and is of such low intensity as to permit, for the most part, only light perception with the rods of the retina; that is, mostly *rod vision* is obtained unless milliamperage is increased, a practice that is not condoned.

Image intensification

Fluoroscopic examinations are conducted increasingly by means of image amplification; this method requires less exposure both to the patient and the radiologist and makes possible vastly improved visual acuity, since both rod and cone perception obtains.

Accessory devices marketed variously as image amplifiers or intensifiers operate in one of two ways. One system receives the low light from the fluoroscopic screen on a photoemission surface. The light rays are electronically amplified and converted to a much greater (higher) light level. In a second system of image intensification, the (remnant) radiation passing through the patient directly bombards a photoconductor to produce a direct electric signal. As in the first system, this signal is electronically amplified and directed onto a viewing screen (such as a television screen). In the second system the fluoroscopic screen is eliminated. (See Fig. 4-27.)

Spot-film radiography

Spot-film devices are incorporated into the construction of the fluoroscopic screen support, along with a low-ratio grid. These devices include a carrier for an 8″ × 10″ or 10″ × 12″ cassette and either mechanical releases or electronic relays for moving the cassette under the screen during fluoroscopic examinations. Other relays automatically switch the tube voltage and tube current to produce radiographic images of the particular area of examination.

When the x-ray machine includes such a device, a second x-ray tube is mounted beneath the tabletop as a part of the fluoroscopic device. This tube has its own relays and factor selections separate from the main radiographic tube.

PROTECTION IN RADIOGRAPHY

It is extremely important to use filters in radiography to control radiographic quality and to furnish adequate protection to the patient. *The ability to avoid retakes is the best protective device the technologist can employ to benefit the patient.*

The increasing use of radioactive materials and x rays affects *all persons.* The present maximum permissible dose for radiologic technolo-

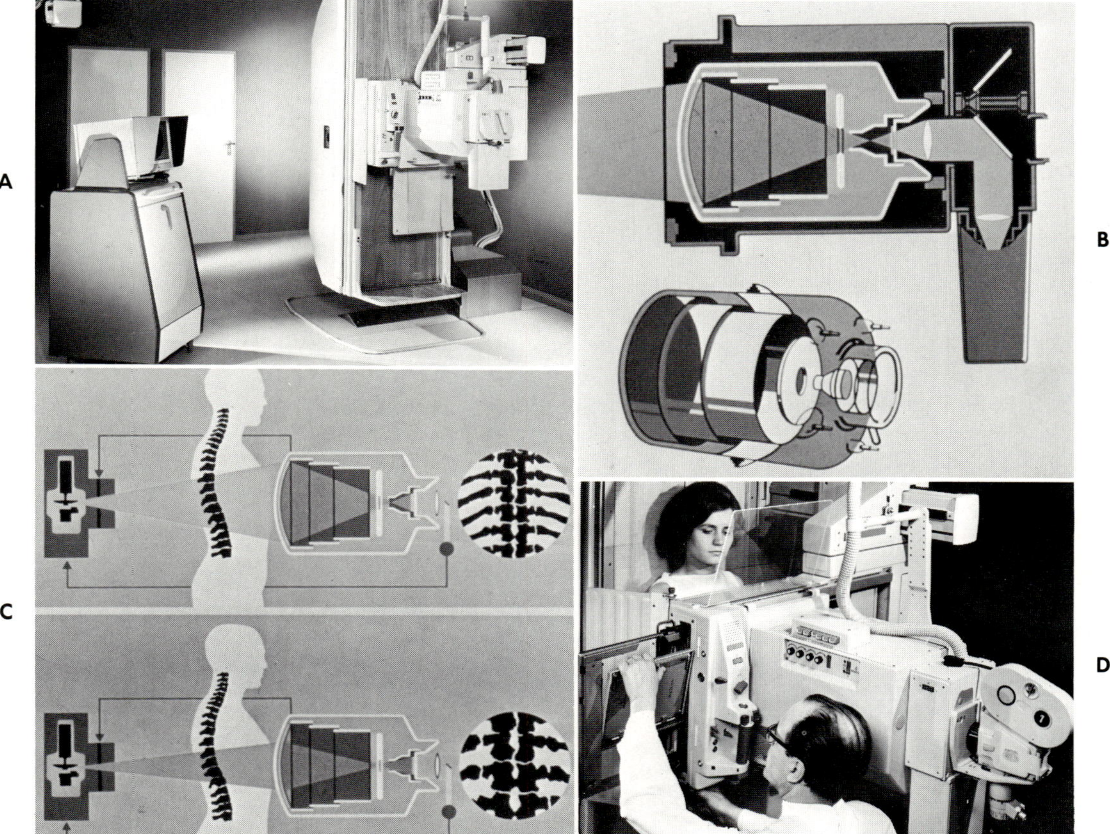

Fig. 4-27. A, Sireskop table with Sirecon image intensifier and television system. Sirecon duplex image-intensifier unit incorporates electron-optical magnification. **B,** Sirecon image-intensifier television unit. **C,** Sirecon duplex image intensifier with image magnification switch. **D,** Sireskop table with Explorator P (spot-film device), Sirecon image intensifier, and a 35 mm Cine camera. (Courtesy Siemens Corp.)

gists is 0.1 R* (100 mR) per week. The MPD (maximum permissible dose) in any 13-week period must be no greater than 25 Rems (roentgen-equivalent-man) to the hands, forearms, feet, head, neck, and ankles, and in any 13-week period no greater than 3 Rems to the skin of the whole body, the gonads, blood-forming organs, and lens of the eye.†

All animal tissues are sensitive to radiation; that is, absorption of radiation doses above certain minimum roentgen values will change or alter the tissue. The following tissues (the sequence in which they are listed is not significant) are most readily affected by the ionizing energy of x rays and gamma rays: dermis, lymphatics, hemopoietic and leukopoietic (blood-forming) tissues, bone (especially the epiphyses in growing children), and the specialized germinal epithelium (gonads). These tissues are also equally sensitive to alpha and beta particles and other high-energy particles.

Aluminum has a marked effect on filtration of the softer x rays. Insertion of an additional 1 mm of aluminum into the path of the primary beam increases the permissible milliampere-seconds from two and one half to three times. This does not indicate a required increase in milliampere-seconds. It does effect a reduction in radiographic intensity to the patient, thus permitting

*The numerical value of the dose equivalent in Rems is assumed to be equal to the numerical value of the dose in roentgens.

†From NCRP Report no. 33.

an increase in milliampere-seconds without an increase in the roentgen dose to the patient. Increased aluminum filtration also generally improves latitude and visibility of detail concurrently with dose reduction to the patient.

It is impractical to measure radiation intensity during radiographic procedures. Such practice would also unduly alarm the patient. However, it is practical to have a working knowledge of radiation dose in terms of milliroentgens per milliampere-second. Some of this information is presented as Table 4-9. Since the patient receives the direct x-ray beams, it is necessary that the technologist be aware of the milliroentgens per milliampere-second delivered to the patient. Should the radiographic request require large amounts of milliroentgens or roentgens, the technologist should consult his radiologist or other supervising physician.

Both the quality and quantity of radiation increase in proportion to a corresponding increase in kilovoltage. Doubling the kilovoltage increases the roentgen output approximately four times.* X-ray quality is discussed on p. 54. The maximum voltage applied to the x-ray tube controls the minimum wavelength emitted from the tube. Thus if voltages in the range of therapy are applied (250 kVp and upward), the wavelengths will be much shorter than those emitted when voltages in the normal radiographic range (30 to 150 kVp) are applied. The student must realize that tubes designed for use in radiography are structurally different from tubes designed for therapy.

Therapy is to be administered only by, or under the direct supervision of, a radiologist. It is recommended that a period of 4 weeks (minimum) should elapse after specific areas of the body have received certain maximum roentgen values in radiography or therapy before there is additional exposure to the same areas. This period of time is considered sufficient in most instances to allow the injured tissues to recuperate and form new cells. X rays and other high-energy forms are used in therapy to effect a destruction of malignant cells and tissues.

X rays are cumulative in effect; however, the x rays do not continue to exist. The ionization that results from exposure to x rays and other high-energy rays constitutes the cumulative effect. They can destroy all living tissue. Scattered radiation is less harmful than primary radiation but still very harmful. A cone that is small enough to expose only the required area effectively controls scattered radiation. The use of such cones is extremely important to adequately protect the patient's gonads. The male infant's gonads are especially susceptible to x rays because of their location. *When possible, cover the gonads in both sexes with pliable leaded rubber* during radiographic exposures, especially in those cases in which the primary rays can strike the gonads.

Good protection practices

1. Always use a collimator when possible, and always use the smallest aperture possible.
2. Limit the collimator or diaphragm opening when using a round cone so that a small and identical amount of cutoff is visible in each corner of the radiograph. Limit the aperture size when using a collimator* so the field of exposure is slightly less than the film size.
3. Avoid *retakes:*
   a. By being absolutely certain of proper positioning.
   b. By being absolutely certain of proper exposure factors.
   c. By being absolutely certain of correct patient, film, and part identification.
   d. By observing proper immobilization procedures. Use sandbags or other such devices to achieve patient comfort and proper immobilization and positioning.
4. Be sure to use the protective lead screen (or cubicle) to protect yourself. If this is impossible, stand a minimum of 6 feet from the widest primary beam. (All mobile equipment should have a timer cord at least 6 feet long or other arrangement to achieve a distance of 6 feet between x-ray table or bed and the operator.)
5. Never stand in the direct x-ray beam or hold the part to be radiographed.
6. Be certain, when using personnel from other departments to help in holding the patients, that they are not called upon too

*A standard electrical formula states that $E = IR$, electromotive force equals current intensity multiplied by conductor resistance. The power formula states that $P = EI$, power equals electromotive force multiplied by current intensity. Substituting IR for E, the power formula becomes $P = IRI$ or $P = I^2R$.

*Automatic collimators preclude this possibility.

Table 4-9. Milliroentgens per milliampere-second*

Added filter (mm al)	kVp 50	60	70	85	100	130	
Radiation intensity using a high-voltage rotating anode tube							
None	7.6	10.2	13.3	18.4	22.5	29.6	mR/mAs at 40″ fsd
0.5	4.8	6.8	9.2	13.2	15.8	20.4	
1.0	3.2	4.6	6.3	9.6	12.0	15.9	
2.0	1.5	2.2	3.2	5.3	8.0	11.3	
3.0				3.1	5.8	9.2	
Radiation intensity using a stationary anode tube							
None	8.2	11.6	14.9	19.8	25.0		mR/mAs, 40″ fsd
0.5	5.0	7.4	9.8	14.0	17.0		
1.0	3.3	4.8	6.7	10.0	12.8		
2.0	1.5	2.3	3.4	5.6	8.4		
3.0				3.2	5.8		

Multiplying factors to determine radiation intensity at distances other than 40 inches

FSD, inches	35	34	33	32	31	30	29	28	27	26	25
Multiplying factor	1.30	1.38	1.47	1.56	1.72	1.79	1.9	2.04	2.19	2.37	2.56
FSD, inches	24	23	22	21	20	19	18	17	16	15	
Multiplying factor	2.78	3.02	3.31	3.63	4.0	4.44	4.94	5.87	6.25	7.1	

*From Trout, E. D., Kelly, J. P., and Cathey, G. A.: Amer. J. Roentgen. **67**:946, 1952.

frequently. These persons must also wear leaded aprons and gloves.

7. Always wear a leaded apron when assisting in fluoroscopy; always wear leaded gloves if your hands are in the direct beam.
8. Be sure to supply the doctors with red goggles at least 20 minutes prior to fluoroscopy so that they are enabled to *accommodate* (dilate the pupils of) their eyes. Supply the doctors with leaded aprons and gloves for the fluoroscopic examination.

X rays generated at voltages up to 100 kVp require 1.5 mm of lead as protection in the walls of the control booth (or in a portable protective screen); for x rays generated at voltages between 100 kVp and 150 kVp, the lead thickness requirement is 2.5 mm. Certain therapy installations require various combinations of poured concrete, concrete blocks, and lead. Other materials used to absorb radiations include barium plaster and pure sand. For certain cobalt 60 installations, especially in industrial establishments, walls 3 feet thick and containing sand of a certain minimum weight per cubic yard are most satisfactory. Such low-density materials as Formica and polyethylene are useless as protective items.

Ionized particles are capable of producing both deleterious and desirable results. Since x rays ionize the air as they pass through it, it is necessary that therapy, radiographic, and fluoroscopic rooms be well ventilated.

The technologist should lock the doors into the fluoroscopic room to prevent entrance of unnecessary light. Entrance of light will prolong the fluoroscopic examination and increase the radiation exposure to the patient and the department personnel.

The minimum precautions to observe with ionizing radiations are stated in the NCRP Report no. 33, *Medical X ray and Gamma ray Protection for Energies up to 10 meV.*

The following statements are of particular interest regarding fluoroscopy. The minimum distance between the fluoroscopic tube target and the tabletop must be at least 12 inches. The total filtration placed permanently in the useful beam must be equal to that in a radiographic tube primary beam, 2.5 mm of aluminum or its equivalent. The source-skin distance of image intensifier equipment *should not* be less than 15 inches. The exposure rate of fluoroscopes operated at 80 kVp *shall not* exceed 3.2 R/mA-min and *should not* exceed 2.1 R/mA-min with the exposure measurement made in air at the position where the beam enters the patient. The exposure rate employed in fluoroscopy *shall not* normally exceed 10R/min measured as above. The maximum permissible milliamperage to be used during fluoroscopy is 5; the recommended range of fluoroscopic milliamperage is from 3 to 5, or less.

In addition to being aware of the effects of x rays, one must also remember that radiographic procedures require extremely high voltages. Therapy voltages are, of course, much greater. Be careful to prevent accumulation of dirt, dust, and moisture around high-voltage equipment, as these can cause short circuits.

Practical technique changes

Working knowledge of radiographic principles enables the technologist to perform efficiently, that is, to produce radiographs of consistently high diagnostic quality at top speed and under all conditions. No two radiologists will desire necessarily the same degree of contrast and latitude, so each technologist must finally produce radiographs to satisfy the particular requirements. Keeping these qualifying statements in mind, the following items may be employed to enable quick and practical technique changes.

1. Practical use is made of the inverse square law in changing technique factors: a normal chest radiographed at 6 feet requires 10 mAs with a given kVp. The same kVp at a 3-foot distance requires 2.5 mAs (one fourth the mAs at one half the distance).

2. In the normal diagnostic range of kilovoltage, each increase or decrease in thickness of 1 cm of anatomic part requires the addition or subtraction of 2 kVp for plain film and 3 kVp for no-screen film.

3. Each inch of distance change, for a maximum of 10 inches, requires the addition or subtraction of 1 kVp.

4. If the mAs is halved, 10 kVp must be added; if the mAs is doubled, 10 kVp must be subtracted. (In either instance, the quantity of kVp added or subtracted depends on the kilovoltage range.)

5. To penetrate a grid whose ratio is 8:1, increase exposure four times; for 12:1, increase five times; for 16:1 or 17:1, increase six times.

6. To cone down, that is, to reduce the field of exposure to an area less than 8 inches by 10 inches, and to maintain radiographic density, increase exposure from 20% to 60%.

7. To maintain constant radiographic density when using screens of different intensification: from medium to detail, increase exposure three and one-half times; from medium to high speed, decrease exposure approximately one half; from medium to extra fast, decrease exposure to approximately one third if kVp is less than **60;** otherwise there is no change.

REFERENCES

Characteristics and applications of x-ray grids. Cincinnati, 1968, The Liebel-Flarsheim Co.

Bloom, William L., Jr.: Medical radiographic technic, ed. 3, Springfield, Ill., 1972, Charles C Thomas, Publisher.

Fuchs, Arthur W.: Principles of radiographic exposure and processing, Springfield, Ill., 1958, Charles C Thomas, Publisher.

Longmore, T. A.: Medical photography, ed. 8, London and New York, 1969, The Focal Press.

Mees, C. E. Kenneth: The theory of the photographic process, ed. 2, New York, 1954, The Macmillan Co.

Selman, Joseph: The fundamentals of x-ray and radium physics, ed. 5, Springfield, Ill., 1972, Charles C Thomas, Publisher.

The fundamentals of radiography, ed. 11, Rochester, N.Y., 1969, Eastman Kodak Co.

Trout, E. D., Kelly, J. P., and Cathey, G. A.: The use of filters to control radiation exposure to the patient in diagnostic roentgenology, Amer. J. Roentgen. **67**:946, 1952.

QUESTIONS

1. What kind of radiation is actually responsible for the object image in the film emulsion?
2. What determines the degree of density in any part of the finished radiograph?
3. What controls contrast?
4. Explain reciprocity failure.
5. Upon what, specifically, does the exposure effect depend?
6. What extra precaution is necessary when regular film is used in cardboard holders?
7. Compare umbra and penumbra in light and shadows with definition and unsharpness in radiography.
8. Explain the circle of confusion and the relation of viewing distance to "point" diameter.
9. What is meant by the term screen speed?
10. How does the use of intensifying screens contribute to loss of definition?
11. What is meant by resolving power of the screen?
12. What principal chemical reaction occurs to change the latent into the manifest image?
13. Explain what is meant by "visibility of detail."
14. Explain how increased density in a radiograph can cause critical losses in definition.
15. Explain how the inverse square law applies to radiographic exposure; that is, radiographic density and dose to the patient.
16. In a given exposure the mAs value is 12, and

the ffd is 30 inches. What will the new mAs value be at a new ffd of 60 inches?

17. Explain why film contrast and grid ratio vary directly with each other.
18. In changing technique from a low-grid ratio to a high-grid ratio, which is preferred—increase mAs or increase kVp? Why?
19. How does the use of aluminum filters effect a reduction in the dosage given the patient?
20. What is the minimum amount of total filtration required in the primary beam?
21. How does a beam restrictor effect a decrease in secondary ray production?
22. When kVp is increased and mAs is decreased in inverse proportion, what two improvements are usually observable in the radiograph?
23. If the focal-film distance is 40 inches, and the percent of magnification is 10, what is the object-film distance in centimeters?
24. Upon what single factor of the four involved in stereoradiography does the success of stereoviewing depend?
25. For what purposes is stereoradiography employed?
26. What is the purpose of tomography?
27. What is fluoroscopy? Who performs fluoroscopy?
28. What structures of the eye perceive the low light of a fluoroscopic screen?
29. Explain both basic processes of image intensification?
30. What is the current MPD for radiologic technologists in a given week?
31. What is the MPD for these persons in any 13-week period?
32. Explain a method that you would use to determine "dose delivered to the patient" in your total evaluation of techniques on a technique chart.
33. Compare R output with increases in mAs versus increases in kVp.
34. Determine minimum wavelength in angstroms from 150 kVp (the approximate maximum voltage in radiography), and from 250 kVp (the approximate minimum voltage in therapy other than superficial).
35. What is the minimum protection in lead equivalent in a control booth for generator and tube capacities of (a) 30 to 100 kVp; (b) 100 to 150 kVp?
36. State the minimum distance between the patient and the target of the fluoroscopic tube.
37. What is the maximum rate of exposure of fluoroscopes operated at 80 kVp maximum?
38. What is the minimum source-skin distance of image intensifier equipment?
39. In fluoroscopy what is the maximum exposure rate in R per minute as measured at the tabletop?

5 • RADIATION THERAPY AND MEDICAL USES OF RADIOISOTOPES

This chapter includes minimal information on radiation therapy and the medical uses of radioisotopes. It is written to provide the student of radiologic technology with a ready source of basic information and with an understanding of the scope of these two specialties.

RADIATION THERAPY

Radiation therapy, often termed radiotherapy, may be applied from several sources; for example, x ray, radium, application, radium-beam therapy, teletherapy with radioactive cobalt (^{60}Co), and other radioactive isotopes. Radioisotopes are used also in diagnostic radiology. This section of the chapter deals with the use of x rays in therapy.

By definition, therapy is the treatment of disease. It derives from the Greek word, *therapeia,* meaning service done to the sick. X-ray therapy is applied both superficially and deeply; that is, x-ray therapy may be used to treat skin cancer, and it may be used to treat cancer deep within the body.* The ultimate purpose of using x rays in this manner is to destroy malignant growth or growths without causing permanent damage to surrounding healthy tissues. It is the responsibility and privilege of the radiologist to prescribe the therapy dose and the method(s) by which the dose is delivered. The technologist can relieve the radiologist of numerous nonlicense-requiring activities relating to x-ray therapy, especially when the technologist has basic knowledge and understanding of x-ray therapy application and its uses.

After determination of exact locus and mass or size of the lesion or tumor is made, the radiologist must next determine how many R are to be delivered to the lesion or tumor, and in what manner the dosage is to be delivered. All information relevant to planning the series of treatments is entered on the radiation field charts (Fig. 5-1, *A* to *C*). When final determination of the nature and character of the lesion or tumor is achieved, the radiologist will next proceed to develop the treatment pattern (Fig. 5-1, *D*). Among the several facets of this pattern to be developed are the many corollary items such as air dose, skin dose, depth dose, volume dose, tumor dose, integral dose and whether the dose should be applied by fractionation or protraction. (These and many other terms are defined in a subsequent section of this chapter.) When the series of therapy treatments is initiated, the exact treatment is recorded on the radiation therapy record (Fig. 5-1, *E*).

*X rays are used in treatment of other conditions such as bursitis.

Energy transfer

An in-depth treatment of radiobiology is not a goal in this text. However, information of greater scope than is offered in Chapter 3 (under the section **X rays and matter**) will aid the student's understanding of radiation therapy.

For the most part energy transfers from radiation to tissues (matter) by means of ionization. However, at least a minimal amount of the effects of radiant energy on molecules is explained as *excitation,* the moving of an orbital electron from its normal position to an orbit farther from the nucleus. Upon return of the electron to its normal position the excitation energy is emitted. Excitation energy is less than ionization energy for a specific element and orbit. Molecular absorption of excitation energy (of one of the molecule's own electrons) may cause the molecule to be more susceptible to dissociation.

In living tissues both ionization and excitation (probably) take place in the protoplasm. Assuming the foregoing statement is true (there is no reason to believe otherwise), effective ionization and/or excitation (likely) occurs either in the molecules per se, or in the solute or solvent of the whole cell.

It has been shown that the direct radiation effect is proportional to the concentration of the solute or solvent, and in dilute solutions is a minute part of the total energy dissipated per gram of solution. We recognize that the biologic effects of ionizing radiations (in some way) result from chemical changes induced by the irradiations.

Nonetheless, explanation remains difficult regarding how marked biologic effects result from amounts of radiation that produce only small degrees of chemical change. Finally, we recognize that marked biologic changes do occur from radiations in degrees more or less proportional to the administered doses.

It is readily understood from information in the preceding paragraphs that radiation therapy differs greatly from diagnostic radiology. It is also true that x-ray therapy tubes differ in construction and in operation from x-ray diagnostic tubes.

A₁

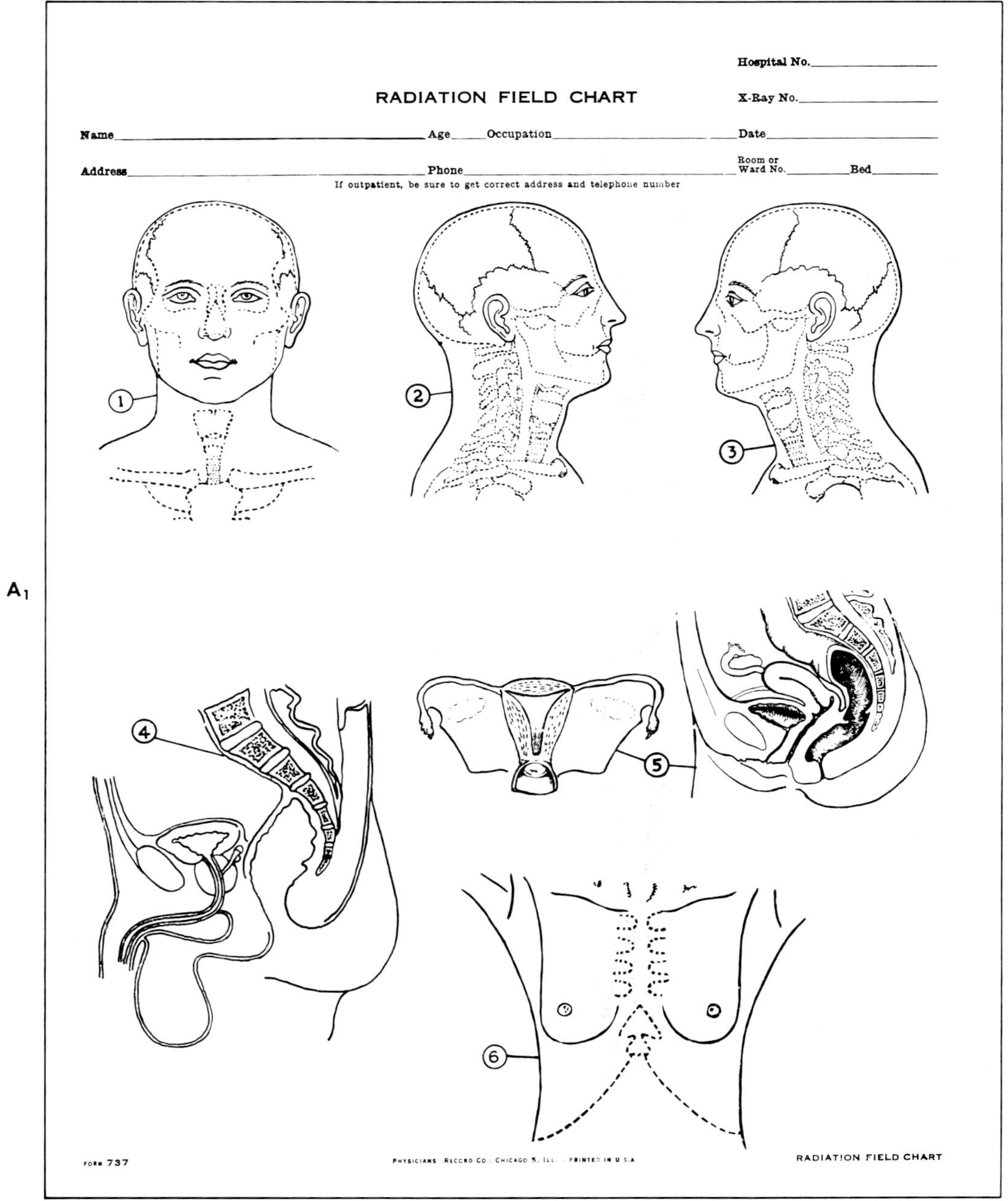
Hospital No.__________
RADIATION FIELD CHART
X-Ray No.__________
Name__________ Age____ Occupation__________ Date__________
Address__________ Phone__________ Room or Ward No._____ Bed_____
If outpatient, be sure to get correct address and telephone number

FORM 737
PHYSICIANS' RECORD CO., CHICAGO 5, ILL. - PRINTED IN U.S.A.
RADIATION FIELD CHART

Fig. 5-1. A, Radiation field chart (Form 737). *Continued.*

X-ray therapy tubes

A major difference in the operation of x-ray therapy tubes when compared with diagnostic tubes is the length of time they must be used; therapy tubes must operate continuously for rather long periods—from a few minutes to perhaps as much as an hour. Thus enormous quantities of heat are generated in the anode and must be removed. Focal spot size is relatively unimportant and may be a few millimeters or a few centimeters broad, depending on the nature of the work for which the tube is designed. All ther-

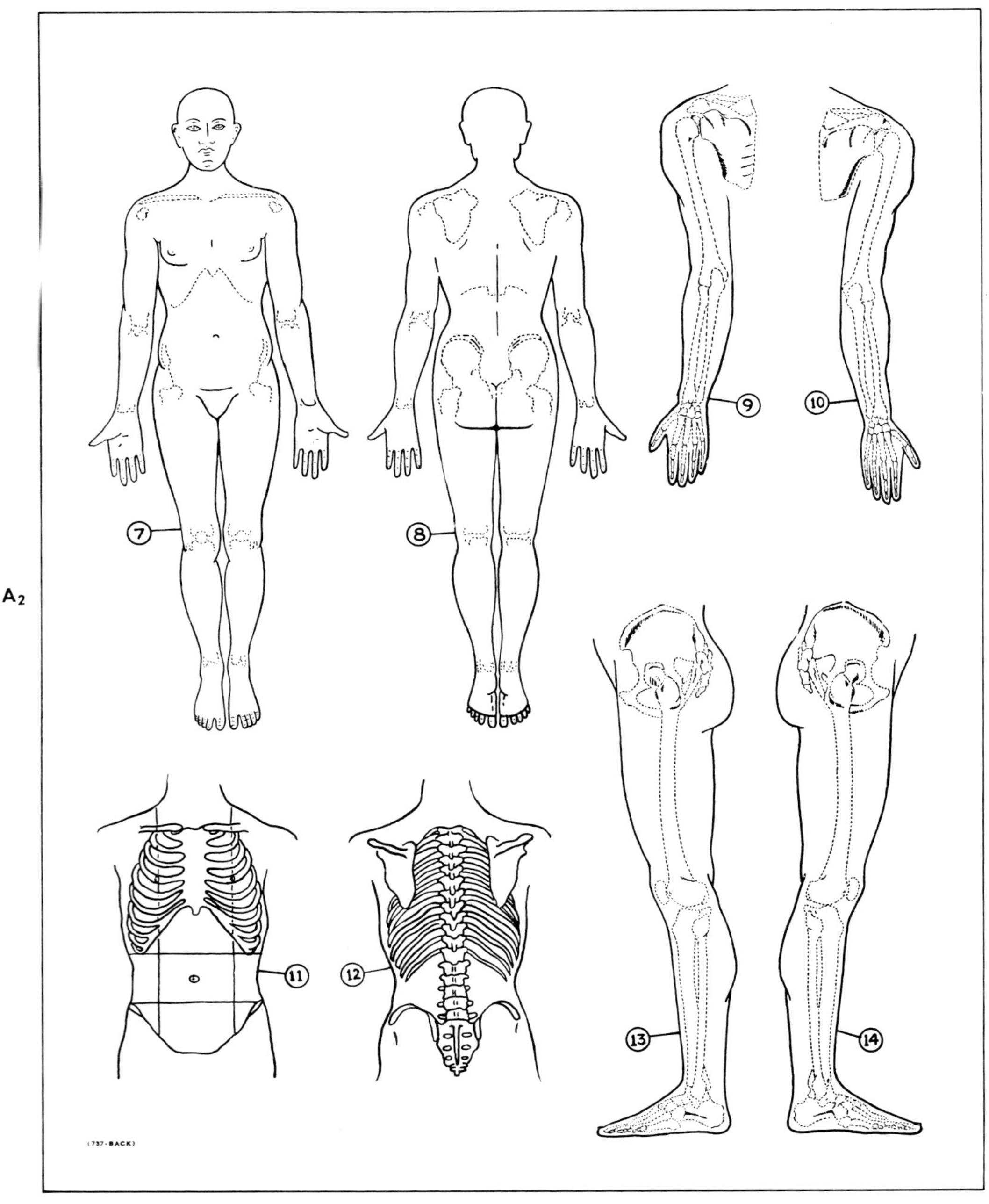

Fig. 5-1, A, cont'd. Radiation field chart (Form 737).

apy tubes operate at low values of milliamperage, usually less than 15, and at values of kilovoltage much higher than those used in diagnostic tubes.

The methods of therapy tube cooling have undergone several changes in preceding years. A common method in current use is to circulate oil under about 45 pounds pressure through the anode to absorb the heat, and then through a cold-water tank, where the heat transfers to the flowing water. Another current method of cooling employs oil somewhat differently. A large metallic core of high heat-conductivity is an integral

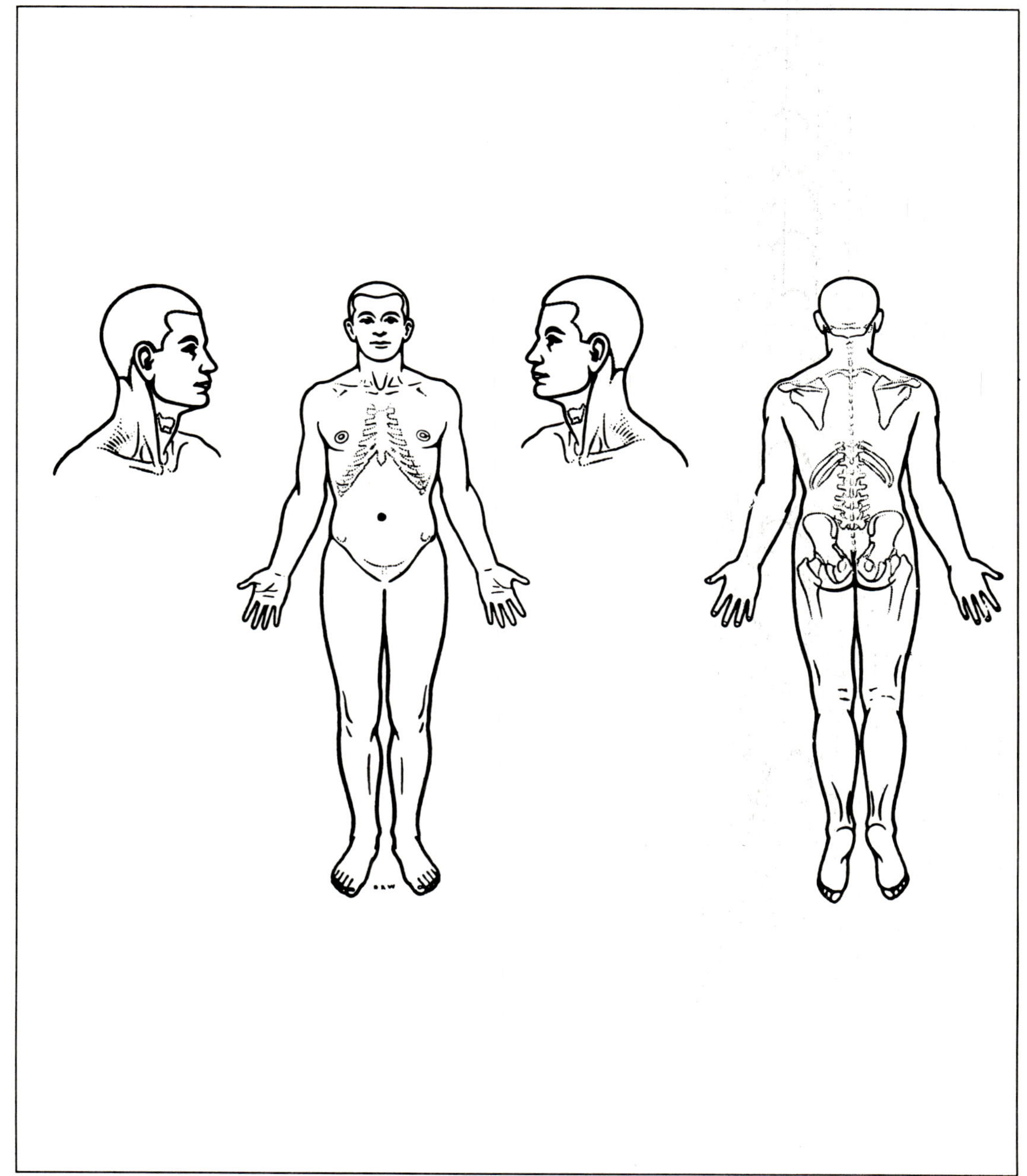

Fig. 5-1, cont'd. B, Field locations. *Continued.*

C

RADIATION THERAPY

SET-UP

PORT # | AREA | DATE

KV | FIELD SIZE | ANTICIPATED DOSE | RADIOLOGIST

TAD | TABLE | POT | TILT | AIR DOSE | METER DOSE

CALCULATIONS | FIELD DIAGRAM

Location	Off Axis	Tissue	%	Filter	Dose

COMMENTS

CALC. CHECK | TECHNICIAN

PORT # | AREA | DATE

KV | FIELD SIZE | ANTICIPATED DOSE | RADIOLOGIST

TAD | TABLE | POT | TILT | AIR DOSE | METER DOSE

CALCULATIONS | FIELD DIAGRAM

Location	Off Axis	Tissue	%	Filter	Dose

COMMENTS

CALC. CHECK | TECHNICIAN

PORT # | AREA | DATE

KV | FIELD SIZE | ANTICIPATED DOSE | RADIOLOGIST

TAD | TABLE | POT | TILT | AIR DOSE | METER DOSE

CALCULATIONS | FIELD DIAGRAM

Location	Off Axis	Tissue	%	Filter	Dose

COMMENTS

CALC. CHECK | TECHNICIAN

PORT # | AREA | DATE

KV | FIELD SIZE | ANTICIPATED DOSE | RADIOLOGIST

TAD | TABLE | POT | TILT | AIR DOSE | METER DOSE

CALCULATIONS | FIELD DIAGRAM

Location	Off Axis	Tissue	%	Filter	Dose

COMMENTS

CALC. CHECK | TECHNICIAN

PORT # | AREA | DATE

KV | FIELD SIZE | ANTICIPATED DOSE | RADIOLOGIST

TAD | TABLE | POT | TILT | AIR DOSE | METER DOSE

CALCULATIONS | FIELD DIAGRAM

Location	Off Axis	Tissue	%	Filter	Dose

COMMENTS

CALC. CHECK | TECHNICIAN

PORT # | AREA | DATE

KV | FIELD SIZE | ANTICIPATED DOSE | RADIOLOGIST

TAD | TABLE | POT | TILT | AIR DOSE | METER DOSE

CALCULATIONS | FIELD DIAGRAM

Location	Off Axis	Tissue	%	Filter	Dose

COMMENTS

CALC. CHECK | TECHNICIAN

Fig. 5-1, cont'd. C, Radiation therapy set-up.

RADIATION THERAPY

THERAPY RECORD

	DAY #	DATE	PORT #	FIELD SIZE	FILTER	DAILY AIR DOSE	TOTAL AIR DOSE	TUMOR DOSE	TUMOR DOSE	TUMOR DOSE	TUMOR DOSE	TUMOR DOSE	TUMOR DOSE	FILMS	SIG.
1															
2															
3															
4															
5															
6															
7															
8															
9															
10															
11															
12															
13															
14															
15															
16															
17															
18															
19															
20															
21															
22															
23															
24															
25															
26															
27															
28															
29															
30															
31															
32															
33															
34															
35															
36															
37															
38															
39															
40															

LATI 7 3M 1-64 TLCO

D

Fig. 5-1, cont'd. D, Radiation therapy record. (Courtesy Physicians' Record Co.)

part of the anode and extends outside the evacuated glass envelope to terminate in an oil bath where heat dissipates by means of natural convection.

Therapy tubes are designed specifically for different uses. Contact and superficial therapy require different tubes and tube construction than conventional and deep therapy require. It is also true that tubes for these therapy treatments differ in construction as well as in application.

Grenz-ray and some contact therapy tubes have the filament surrounded by a target in the form of a ring-shaped sleeve. Grenz rays are very soft x rays having electromagnetic vibrations of approximately 1.5×10^{18}/sec (2Å wavelength), thus being between (true) roentgen rays and ultraviolet rays. Grenz rays occur from voltages of 10 kV and less; contact therapy x rays occur at voltages from 40 to 60 kV. These are called "short distance" x rays because of the very short distance between the target and the skin. Since the tsd is so very short the dose rate is quite high, thus requiring a very short treatment time.

Supervoltage therapy tubes are designed to operate at voltages of one or more meV. Construction of these tubes must provide for greater (than in low-voltage tubes) kinetic energy of the bombarding electrons and for correspondingly greater insulation. Use of extremely high-voltage tubes requires generators capable of producing the high voltage. A brief discussion of the essential construction and design of cascade and Van de Graaff generators follows.

Supervoltage generators

In the decade prior to World War II initial work on high-voltage generators produced a series of 200 kVp units in four to five steps; the end result was a voltage of 800,000 to 1,000,000 (800 to 1,000 kVp). These were called cascaded or *cascade generators.* These generators were very large and cumbersome, often requiring ceiling heights of 12 feet or more. One early model produced by Philips Gloeilampenfabrieken, the forerunner of present-day North American Philips Company, Inc., produced 800 kVp and stood 8 feet high. These models required very long x-ray tubes to prevent spark-over; during operation it was necessary to apply continuous evacuation.

More recent supervoltage generators are either the alternating-current resonance-transformer type or the constant-potential electrostatic generator type. In 1933 R. J. Van de Graaff built his practical model of the latter type. In this generator the x-ray tube is mounted within the insulating column and surrounded by a series of metal rings (accelerators). Extending parallel with the tube is an endless belt that moves continuously at a speed of approximately 4,000 feet each minute. Near the lower pulley (for the belt) negative electric charges (electrons) are sprayed on the belt from a 30 kVp transformer-rectifier. These charges leave the belt near the upper pulley and spread over the inner surface of a spherical, metal electrode and move rapidly to its outer surface. When the negative charges have built up to a potential many times greater than the individual charges, the high potential is applied to the negative terminal (cathode) of the x-ray tube. The flat, water-cooled target is at the opposite (lower) end of the tube, and the electron beam passes through a series of accelerating electrodes, increasing their velocity and force as they move toward the target. The x rays radiate forward from the target (which is at right angles to the electron beam). These generators are used quite successfully in accelerating electrons, protons, and deuterons. For further descriptions the student is referred to excellent coverage of this information in numerous texts such as *Physical Foundations of Radiology* by Goodwin, Quimby, and Morgan and *Radiology Physics* by Robertson.

Despite the fact that supervoltage generators and tubes are quite compact when compared with earlier models, especially considering the enormous energies available today, these units require considerable space. Fig. 5-2, *A*, illustrates the size of supervoltage therapy equipment.

Both low voltage and supervoltage have been mentioned in relation to therapy. For practical purposes medical x rays and their corresponding wavelengths may be classified as in Table 5-1. The minimum wavelength produced by the 42 meV Betatron in Fig. 5-2 is 0.000296 Å.

Table 5-1. Medical x rays and corresponding wavelengths

Type	Voltage range	Wavelength range (Å)
Superficial therapy	5–10 kVp	2.48 –1.24
Mammography	25–45 kVp	0.496–0.2755
General diagnostic	30–150 kVp	0.413–0.08
Intermediate therapy	140 kVp	0.0885
Deep therapy	200–400 kVp	0.062–0.031
Supervoltage therapy	1 meV and over	0.0124 and less

Advantages of supervoltage x rays

We have learned previously in other chapters that greater penetration is effected with higher energy x rays. X rays of increased or greater penetration deliver a correspondingly higher percentage of depth dose at a given place under the skin. Earlier experiments with phantoms have revealed that electrons liberated in the tissues, resulting from high-energy x-ray bombardment, have a marked forward range in the tissue below the termination of the penetration. In the work of H. E. Johns it is reported that the region of maximum energy resulting from 22 meV Betatron rays is some 5 cm below the surface. In bombarding tissue (or phantom) with gamma rays from cobalt 60, the maximum

A

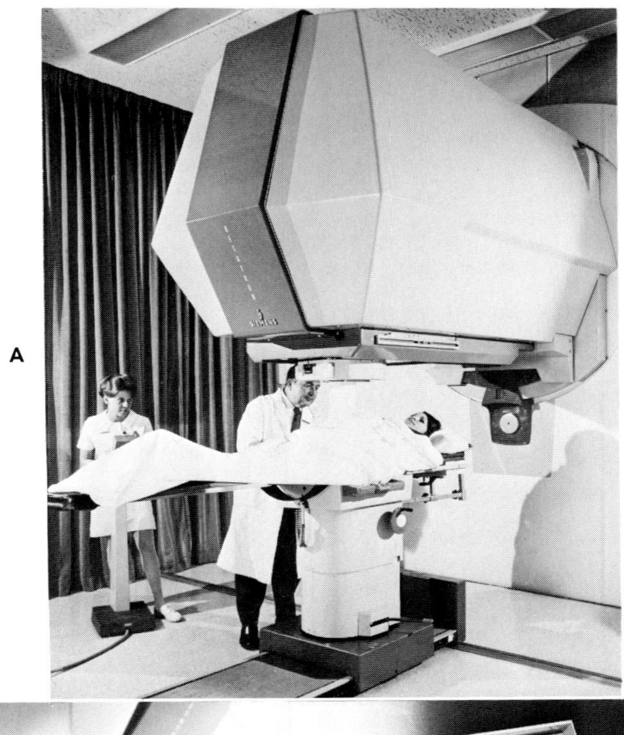

B

C

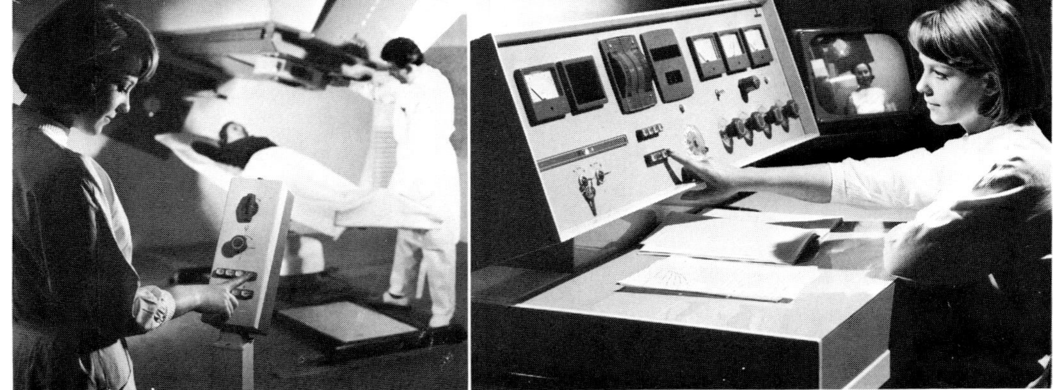

Fig. 5-2. A, 42 meV Betatron. Electron-beam energy can be varied continuously between 5 meV and 42 meV. The Betatron also delivers ultra-hard roentgen rays. Energy of the roentgen beam can also be varied, although in actual practice the 42 meV peak value is the energy of choice. **B,** Mobile table-side control for 42 meV Betatron. **C,** Control panel for 42 meV Betatron as viewed from control room. (Courtesy Siemens Corp.)

energy is at 5 to 6 mm below the skin surface. Statistics reveal that far fewer unfavorable skin reactions occur with use of supervoltage x rays and other energies than with x-ray energies used in standard therapy. Further information contained in Dr. Johns' work reveals the following: using 200 keV rays the energy absorption for bone is 300 ergs per gram per roentgen and 91 ergs per gram per roentgen for tissue; whereas using 25 meV rays the energy absorption for bone is 91 ergs per gram per roentgen and 92 ergs per gram per roentgen for muscle.

> The 42-MeV Betatron delivers both high-energy electrons and ultra-hard roentgen rays. . . . Both effective range and dynamic orientation imparted to electrons and positrons by the interaction with the tissue give rise to the build-up effect and to a dose distribution reaching its maximum depth at approximately 6 cm (in water). The surface dose is only about 20% of the dose maximum, so the dose received on the skin is very well tolerated. Nor is any systemic upset to be feared for organs and tissue which lie near the surface.
>
> The slight absorption of ultra-hard roentgen rays is reflected in the flat down-swing of the depth dose curve. At 10 cm depth the dose still accounts for about 90% of the peak value.*

From the same brochure and about the high-energy electron beam we quote the following.

> The effective range of the electrons depends on the primary energy to which they are accelerated. The higher the energy the greater the depth of penetration. As a general rule, in actual practice the effective electron beam in water or soft tissue should amount to ½ cm per MeV.
>
> In practical work the total effective range is less important than the so-called therapeutic range. It equals a 70% isodose and amounts to about ⅔ of the total range. *In consequence, the effective therapeutic range is roughly ⅓ cm per MeV.*
>
> The . . . Betatron produces an electron beam energy that can be varied continuously between 5 MeV and 42 MeV. This also allows a varying of the therapeutic range from 2 cm to 13 cm.*

Triplet production and annihilation radiation

For a very brief discussion of true pair production resulting from interaction of very high energy photons with matter, see p. 59. Additional information relating to this and other phenomena is presented here.

If the photon energy should exceed 2.04 meV, it is possible that pair production can occur in an electron field and cause the electron to recoil with considerable energy. Since this results in three high-speed particles, the process is called *triplet production.*

Normally, positrons do not exist in nature, and when produced their kinetic energy is lost or dissipated through several collisions. When a positron is without kinetic energy, it unites with an electron to form mass. The mass resulting from this union is converted into energy in the form of two gamma ray photons of 0.511 meV energy each. This process is called *annihilation radiation,* since the radiation results from the annihilation of matter.

Because pair production has nuclear involvement, probability of its occurrence depends on the nuclear charge; pair production per gram varies approximately as the Z number of the atom (material). Probability of occurrence also increases with increasing photon energy. Photoelectric effect decreases sharply with increasing energy; Compton effect decreases slowly with increasing photon energy.

With light elements, pair production is insignificant below 3 or 4 meV; it is equal to Compton absorption at 10 to 20 meV; with lead, pair production equals Compton absorption at approximately 4 meV, increasing above this energy level to account for about 98% of initial events* at 100 meV.

X-ray therapy filters

In Chapter 4 it has been stated that filters are used in diagnostic radiology primarily to afford protection to the patient and secondarily to improve radiograph quality.

Filters are used in therapy to control x-ray beam quality. The use of filters in therapy requires absolute exactness. It is necessary to measure the quality and quantity of the primary beam to determine the dose delivered to the patient. In this measurement, it is also necessary to determine the exact thickness of a given metal that will reduce the intensity of the beam to exactly one half; such a thickness is the *half-value layer (hvl).*

The materials used in therapy filters are tin, copper, aluminum, and sometimes lead. A Thoraeus filter is frequently employed in therapy. According to dosage specifications, the *Thoraeus filter consists of varying thicknesses of tin, copper, and aluminum.* Tin is usually the filter nearest the tube; *aluminum must be the external*

*From 42-MeV-Betatron, Siemens Corp., Erlangen, Germany.

*See footnote on p. 130.

Table 5-2. Materials used for measuring hvl

Voltage range	Recommended material
10 kV-10 mV	Aluminum (Al)
35 kV- 8 mV	Copper (Cu)
350 kV-3.5 mV	Lead (Pb)

filter (filter nearest the patient), since the secondary rays formed in aluminum add no energy to the x-ray beam. Supervoltage therapy may require the use of lead as a filter, in which case lead precedes tin as the filter nearest the tube.

Filtration controls the photons of energy emitted from radioactive materials in essentially the same manner as it controls x-ray photons, since both are high energy electromagnetic waves. All electromagnetic waves respond to filtration according to absorption coefficients of the absorbing layer. One millimeter of copper will absorb approximately the same quantity of energy as 10 mm of aluminum.

X-ray beam quality is expressed easily in terms of half-value layer. As recommended by the I.C.R.P.* in 1956 the preferred materials for hvl measurement are listed in Table 5-2.

Terminology and definitions

The following list of terms and definitions includes many of those in common use in most therapy departments. The list is not intended to be complete or extensive.

absorbed dose of any ionizing radiation Energy imparted to matter by ionizing particles per unit mass of irradiated material at point of interest.

absorbed dose rate Absorbed dose per unit time.

backscatter That portion of scattered radiation generated in the patient (or phantom) that radiates toward the source (of x rays) is called backscatter.

cross-fire treatment Directing two or more beams at the tumor through as many ports of entry.

depth dose (E_d) Tissue dose at d cm below the skin surface, at the same time considering the effect on the intervening tissues.

E Number of R in air at the position of the center of the field employed in the treatment.

E_0 Number of R on the skin surface at the center of the field (as above).

E_d Number of R within the body at depth d cm in the field (as above).

*I.C.R.P. stands for International Commission on Radiation Protection; N.C.R.P. stands for National Committee on Radiation Protection.

erythema A name applied to redness of the skin produced by congestion of the capillaries.

erythema dose Amount of radiant energy that, when applied to the skin, will, after a few days, cause a slight reddening. For gamma rays this dose has been stated as 1 erythema dose = 1,000 R.

exit dose Amount of radiation emerging from the body after the beam has traversed its entire thickness.

exposure dose Measure of the x-ray or gamma-ray radiation at a certain place based on its ability to produce ionization.

exposure dose rate Exposure dose per unit time.

extrapolate To project by inference into an unexplored situation from observations in an explored field on the assumption of continuity or correspondence.

extrapolation chamber A laboratory, not a clinical, instrument used for measuring accurately a limited (and variable) volume of air. Recently they have been used to measure beta-energy absorption in various metals.

field Cubic area of treatment.

fractionation Delivery of the total dose in parts at intervals.

grid therapy Longitudinal slits alternately placed in an otherwise radiopaque material, used to offer protection to tissues between the surface and a deep-seated tumor.

half-value layer The thickness of a standard material (pure metal, etc.) required to reduce the intensity of a beam of x rays (when passing through the absorber at right angles) to exactly half its original value is called the half-value layer.

integral (absorbed) dose In a given region, the total energy imparted to matter by ionizing particles in that region. The gram-rad is the established unit of the integral dose and is equal to 100 ergs.

integral dose Total energy absorbed by the body throughout the entire irradiated volume.

intensity of radiation Term used to denote dose rate; use of this term is discouraged, since intensity of radiation is the radiant energy flux density at a given point, or the energy per unit time entering a small sphere of unit cross-sectional area, centered at that place.

isodose curve Line drawn between points at different depths or distances below the surface and along the axis of the primary beam at which the dose is the same.

protraction Dose applied through continuous irradiation at a very low intensity.

rad Unit of the absorbed dose of ionizing radiation equal to an energy of 100 ergs per gram of irradiated material.

RBE Relative biologic effectiveness used in comparison of absorbed doses of radiation delivered by different types of radiation.

rem Roentgen-equivalent man. The dosage of any ionizing radiation that will cause the same amount of biological injury to human tissues as one roentgen of x-ray or gamma ray dosage is called the rem.

rep Roentgen-equivalent physical. The dosage of any ionizing radiation that will develop the same amount of energy upon absorption in human tissues as one roentgen of x-ray or gamma ray dosage is called the rep.

ripple Drop in voltage. Ripple voltage is the rising from minimum to maximum and falling from maximum to minimum of the voltage in an alternating current as diagrammed in a sine wave diagram.

roentgen International unit of x or γ (gamma) radiation. The roentgen is the quantity of x or gamma radiation such that the associated corpuscular emission per 0.001293 gram of air produces, in air, ions carrying 1 esu of quantity of electricity of either sign.

rotational therapy An extension of cross-fire treatment in which either the source of radiation or the patient is rotated in a manner to cause the central axis of the beam of rays always to pass through the region undergoing treatment.

sieve therapy Like grid therapy except that the longitudinal slits are replaced with either square or round openings.

volume dose Same as integral dose.

Knowledge and understanding of the foregoing terms will be of inestimable assistance to the technologist as he performs his or her duties in the department.

Backscatter

Backscatter is discussed briefly in Chapter 1, and is of some significance in diagnostic radiography. It is of great significance in x-ray (and other ionizing ray) therapy.

Using a scientific ionizing measuring instrument, such as a thimble chamber, placed near the tissue equivalent phantom (or patient) during exposure of the phantom shows a greater dose rate in R/min than is shown when the thimble chamber is exposed directly (away from the phantom). This increase in dose rate results from secondary rays scattering in all directions from the forward path (in the phantom) of the x rays striking the phantom. Some of the secondary radiation is *scattered back* toward the surface (point of entry), and is named *backscatter.*

Studies of the effects of scatter radiation on tissues (by Friedrich and Glasser in 1922) revealed that backscatter from the tissues below the skin caused an increase in the skin dose above the air dose at the same spot. The backscatter is small if the area treated is small; backscatter increases rapidly as the field size increases to 5 cm^2, and more slowly as the field size exceeds 100 cm^2.

X rays of low voltage do not accelerate (in tissues) secondary electrons with sufficient energy to travel far; thus backscatter is limited. However, as voltages are increased to approximately 180 kV, the skin dose increases resulting from secondary electrons from deeper and deeper layers of tissues. Above 200 kV the forward scatter increases, and backscatter decreases progressively with higher voltages.

The *surface* or *skin dose rate* is the air dose rate at a given point in the x-ray beam added to the backscatter dose rate. Backscatter is (usually) not measured separately and can be determined as a percentage of the total (dose rate) if both air dose rate and surface dose rate are known.

The radiologic technologist in the therapy department

This section treats the activities that are ethical, legal, and useful on the part of a radiologic technologist working in the therapy department. No attempt to itemize the duties and responsibilities of the certified therapy technologist is offered.

In many instances the position of radiologic technologist is filled by a female employee; however, in nearly 30 years of general radiologic technology, including radiotherapy, the authors have encountered no "problems" with female patients in therapy. However, if kindness, patience, tolerance, and general goodwill are ever needed in a radiographic department, it is readily seen that the need is greatly multiplied in a therapy department. Men can be and must be just as helpful and compassionate as can women technologists in assisting patients in therapy.

There are three ways that the technologist can be of great assistance both to the radiologist and to the patient, particularly during the procedure of "patient preparation." The technologist can *physically* assist the patient in removing street clothing and in robing in the proper attire for the therapy treatment. Next, the technologist can assist the patient onto the therapy couch, and finally the technologist can adjust the patient's position so that as little discomfort as possible is endured by the patient. Proper support with pillows, sandbags, and the like is always in order. Throughout the time of patient positioning it is advisable to be ready to make "light talk" with the patient; however, the technologist must refrain from forcing talk upon a patient and from talking about the patient's illness and other distasteful subjects.

When a patient is receiving regular treatments, the technologist should make a distinct effort to "get-to-know" the patient. After this "stage" the technologist can assist both the patient and the radiologist by making *physiologic* observations of the patient and by reporting same to the radiologist. The technologist will notice the changing condition of the patient's skin and should ask the patient if he (or she) is eating well and if food tastes good. Also, questions should be asked regarding fluid intake and output and about bowel movements. It is perfectly ethical for the technologist to inquire of the patient if he notices any nausea either during the treatment or following it. Posttherapy nausea can be aleviated to a large extent by use of certain medicines, always ordered by the radiologist or another physician.

Nearly all therapy patients are at least concerned if not outright frightened. If ever we as technologists can earn some good points on our spiritual record, we can do it by extending ourselves to help these patients. Patients either will be "resigned to accepting" what will be or will refuse to accept the final truth. It is the mark of an intelligent technologist who can, perhaps through empathy, practice good, sound *psychology* on these persons. Understanding human emotions is most important!

It goes without saying that good "housekeeping" in the therapy department is a must. Also, it is most important that odors are kept at a minimum in the therapy room. Activities that can directly relieve the radiologist of nonlicense-requiring work include having the patient's charts ready for the radiologist's perusal and having the patient in at least partial position for the treatment before the radiologist enters the therapy room. Recording the daily treatment data can be performed by the technologist if the radiologist so desires. Some radiologists prefer to do this themselves.

Above all, a cheerful attitude, neat attire, and confident movements on the part of the technologist inspire hope and confidence in the patient, and therapy patients have little enough to hope for.

Checking filters, port size, and correct entry portal should be practiced by the technologist even when the radiologist does this. Operation of the controls may be a duty delegated by the radiologist to the technologist, or the radiologist may prefer to do this. It is prudent for both the technologist and radiologist to request the patient to lie still during therapy and to explain to the patient that the slightest movement can direct the therapy beam away from the tissues to be treated.

In many instances it will be necessary to remove dressings from the area of treatment prior to therapy and to cleanse the area and apply sterile dressings after therapy. All items necessary for such activity must be in, or immediately adjacent to, the therapy room. Other procedures such as biopsies and aspirations should be anticipated and prepared for in advance.

Finally, the technologist must be the very dependable "right hand" of the radiologist. His appearance, attitude, and general helpfulness are most important to the total successful operation of the department. The well-being and "peace-of-mind" of these patients with whom we are so intimately in contact has number one priority. A technologist can upgrade or downgrade the entire departmental operation. Strive always to be a technologist who "upgrades" his department.

MEDICAL USES OF RADIOISOTOPES

HIRAM M. HUNT, Ed.D.

This section on radioisotopes deals with the more technical aspects of the medical uses of radioactive isotopes.

History

Radioactivity was discovered by A. Henri Becquerel (1852-1908) shortly after the 1895 discovery of x rays by Roentgen. Becquerel described his work with radioactive materials in the early part of 1896. Similarities between x rays and the radiation from radioactive materials were noted almost immediately. In 1899, Becquerel in France, S. Meyer and E. Von Schweidler, and F. Giesel of Germany independently discovered that radiations from radioactive substances could be deflected by a magnetic field in the same direction as are cathode rays (electrons). E. Rutherford of England discovered that there were at least two different types of radiation emitted by uranium compounds to which he assigned the terms *alpha* (α) rays and *beta* (β) rays. The beta rays were deflected by a magnetic field and were more penetrating than the alpha rays. Later Pierre and Marie Curie confirmed the fact that beta rays were negatively charged. Subsequently R. J. Strutt (later Lord Rayleigh, Fourth Baron) and W. Crookes in England showed that alpha rays were deflected by a strong magnetic field in the direction opposite to that in which beta rays were deflected. This confirmed that alpha radiation is positively charged. In 1900, P. Villard of France discovered another type of radiation from uranium compounds more penetrating than alpha or beta rays that could not be deflected by a magnetic field. Radiations of this type are now called *gamma* (γ) rays.

Fundamental information

Alpha, beta, and gamma rays are the principal radiations emitted by naturally occurring radioactive materials. Chemical separations of the elements that make up radioactive materials indicate that at least forty-two radioelements occur in nature. The majority of the naturally occurring radioelements are parts of one of three important radioactive series. A radioelement is converted to another element when alpha or beta rays are emitted, but *not when gamma rays* are emitted alone. A radioelement that converts to another element is called the *parent*, and the resulting element is called the *daughter*. The daughter may be radioactive or nonradioactive, depending on the particular parent. Nonradioactive daughters are the end product of a series. The three most important radioactive series occurring in nature are known as the actinium series, the thorium series, and the uranium series.*

Nature of the atom

The atomic nature of radioactivity was suspected at the time of its discovery and has been confirmed by many investigations. Consequently, the nature of the atom in relation to radioactivity should be reviewed. An atom is the smallest particle or unit of matter that is representative of a chemical element. Atoms are comprised of negatively charged bodies called *electrons* lying in orbits about a nucleus containing positively charged bodies called *protons* and neutrally charged bodies called *neutrons*. The term *nucleons* is used when protons and neutrons are considered together. Since charged bodies of the same sign (+, + or −, −) repel each other, it is believed that the neutrons in the nucleus, in some way, exert a force of retention upon the positively charged protons. The electrons are retained by the force of attraction between them and the positively charged protons.

The diameter of atoms is estimated to range from 1.06×10^{-8} cm to 5.70×10^{-8} cm and the order of nuclear diameters to be 10^{-12} cm. Consequently, it has been assumed that the nucleons (protons plus neutrons) are closely packed in comparison with the electron's configuration. Experimentation supports this assumption. Table 5-3 gives the known and theoretical data for the elementary atomic particles.

The number of protons in the nucleus of an atom is the atomic, or Z, number, the number of neutrons in the atomic nucleus is the N number, and the number of nucleons (protons plus neutrons) is the mass, or A, number. F. Soddy, F. Fleck, and A. S. Russell of the United Kingdom, H. N. McCoy, and W. H. Ross of the United States, and F. Fajans and W. Marckwald of Germany found, through experiment and deduction, that there were subspecies of radioelements that had different types of radioactive decay. Soddy proposed the term *isotope* be used for different species of the same element. The term isotope includes the radioactive and nonradioactive species

*Each of these series finally *decays* into one of the (four) natural isotopes of lead.

Table 5-3. Data concerning the elementary particles

Name and symbol (positive +, negative −, neutral 0)	Charge (absolute esu)	Mass (gram)	Energy (mc^2 ergs)	Atomic mass (relative $^{12}C = 12$)	Number (in 1 gram)	Diameter (cm)
Neutron n^0	0	1.67482×10^{-24}	1.5053×10^{-3}	1.0086654	5.9708×10^{23}	1.4×10^{-13}
Proton p^+	$+4.80298 \times 10^{-10}$	1.67252×10^{-24}	1.5032×10^{-3}	1.0072766	5.9790×10^{23}	1.4×10^{-13}
Electron β^-	-4.80298×10^{-10}	9.1091×10^{-28}	8.1869×10^{-7}	5.48597×10^{-4}	1.0978×10^{27}	Theoretical 5.64×10^{-13}
Positron β^+ (positive electron)	$+4.80298 \times 10^{-10}$	9.1091×10^{-28}	8.1869×10^{-7}	5.48597×10^{-4}	1.0978×10^{27}	Theoretical 5.64×10^{-13}

of the chemical elements. Subsequently, isotopes of the same chemical element were found to have the same number of protons, but different numbers of neutrons in their nuclei.

The term *nuclide* was proposed by T. P. Kohman, in the United States, for a species of atom characterized by the constituents of its nucleus. The nuclide is distinguished by the number of protons and neutrons in the nucleus of a particular atom. Nonradioactive nuclides are called *stable nuclides,* and radioactive nuclides are called *radionuclides.* The Knolls Atomic Power Laboratory, operated by the General Electric Company, publishes and revises the *Chart of the Nuclides* under the direction of Naval Reactors, United States Atomic Energy Commission. The Knolls Atomic Laboratory chart lists the Z (atomic) numbers vertically and the N (neutron) numbers horizontally. The result is that the isotopes lie in horizontal rows and nuclides having the same A number (protons plus neutrons), called isobars, lie diagonally from the upper left to the lower right. All of the common nuclear displacements that result from the emission or capture of particles by the nucleus of a nuclide may be demonstrated with the *Chart of the Nuclides.*

Rays emitted by radioactive materials are comprised of particles of matter or of discrete quantities of electromagnetic radiation called photons. Radiation particles and photons are emitted from the nuclei of unstable nuclides. The instability of nuclei may result from an excess of nucleons (protons plus neutrons), an unfavorable neutron to proton ratio, or excess of nuclear energy. The rules pertaining to the instability of nuclei are not fully understood, but no nonradioactive nuclide having more than eighty-two protons has been discovered.

Radioactivity

Alpha rays are streams of alpha particles, each of which is comprised of two protons and two neutrons, and are equivalent to the nuclei of common helium atoms. Although the energy range of alpha particles is from 4 to 10 meV (million electron volts), their relative size and the interaction of the positive charges of the protons with matter limit their penetration of air to a few centimeters. Alpha particles are ejected at speeds of from 9,000 to 20,000 miles per second and are stopped by a thin sheet of cardboard. The energy of alpha particles on penetrating matter is given up principally by ionization and excitation of the absorbing material's atoms and molecules.

Beta particles are equivalent to negatively charged electrons and are emitted as a result of an imbalance between the numbers of protons and neutrons in an atomic nucleus. Positively charged beta particles are frequently called positrons, but negatively charged beta particles are identified simply as beta particles unless the term negative beta, or negatron, is necessary for clarity. Negative beta particles are emitted when an excess neutron converts to a proton by ejecting a negative charge. Positive beta particles result when an excess proton ejects its positive charge and becomes a neutron. An alternate scheme in the case of an excess proton is for an orbital electron to be captured by the nucleus. Another electron falls into the vacancy left by the captured electron, resulting in the emission of an x ray. Beta particles have a single negative charge and a mass less than 1/7,000 that of an alpha particle. Negative beta particle energies range from a few thousand to several million electron volts. The most energetic particles can penetrate as much as 60 feet of air, but since few beta sources have energies greater than 2 meV, a distance of 25 feet is usually adequate for shielding. Beta particles cause less ionization than alpha particles, travel in straight paths for much greater distances than alpha particles, and, depending on the energy of the particles, are capable of penetrating tissues up to about 1 cm in thickness. Positively charged beta particles (positrons) are neutralized by negatively charged (common) electrons in matter by an annihilation process in which both particles are converted to electromagnetic radiation. Negatively charged beta particles, upon penetrating matter, give up their energy principally by ionizing the absorbing material's atoms and molecules and, if sufficiently energetic, in producing Bremsstrahlung (braking) radiation equivalent to x rays.

Gamma rays are electromagnetic radiations emitted from the nuclei of atoms. Gamma rays are equivalent to x rays and can only be differentiated from x rays by knowing their source. Gamma rays are usually emitted at the time beta or alpha particles are emitted, but may be emitted alone or upon the bombardment of an atomic nucleus by particles or photons. Gamma rays occasionally interact with the electrons of the atom from which they are emitted, causing displacement of the electrons with subsequent production of x rays. Gamma-ray energies run from a few thousand to several million electron volts. The penetrability of gamma rays is identical with that of x rays of equal energy, but the spectrum of radiation from a particular radionuclide will be specific, not a continuum with characteristic energies as obtained from x-ray machines. Since gamma rays are true electromagnetic waves, they travel with the speed of light; they are capable of extreme penetration and cause less ionization than do beta particles. Gamma rays are approximately 1/100 as effective in causing ionization as the beta particle and 1/10,000 as effective as the alpha particle.

Gamma rays, like all photons, are absorbed exponentially. This exponential absorption is a direct result of the nature of gamma-ray energy loss. In contrast with alpha and beta particles, gamma rays do not lose their energy continuously in small amounts; they lose their energy by absorption during interactions with matter.

The event* of a single atomic nucleus emitting a particle or photon is purely random (chance). When a large number of identical radioactive atoms is considered, it is found that the average rate of nuclear events at any one moment is proportional to the number of radioactive atoms present. This rate of nuclear events at any one moment relative to the number of radioactive atoms present is known as the *radioactive constant.* The radioactive constant is an expression of the rate at which the remaining radioactive atoms are being depleted. The depletion of the radioactive atoms means that the radioactivity is decreasing exponentially. The term *half-life* is used to indicate the time required for one half of the radioactive atoms present at any one moment to be depleted by radioactive emission. The relationship between the radioactive constant λ (lambda) and T½ (half-life) may be expressed as

$$\lambda = \frac{0.693}{T½} \text{ or } T½ = \frac{0.693}{\lambda}$$

in which 0.693 is the natural logarithm (log to the base e) of 2. For example, if a radioactive substance loses its radioactivity through the depletion of its radioactive atoms at the rate of 0.001 part per minute, the half-life will be 0.693/0.001 = 693 minutes or 11.55 hours.

The following schematic is currently used to identify useful atomic and nuclear relationships.

*Although no official change in nomenclature is in effect currently, there is strong probability that both *events* and *emissions* will be changed to *bequerels* in the near future. Other terminology changes of a similar nature are contemplated.

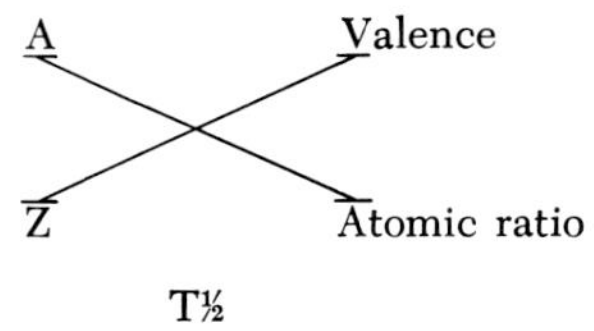

X is the chemical symbol of the element.

A is the mass number or number of nucleons (protons + neutrons).

Z is the atomic number or number of protons.

A-Z = *N* is the number of neutrons. The particular nuclide is identified by the number of protons, Z, and the number of neutrons, N.

T½ is the half-life of the particular nuclide and is expressed in seconds (s), minutes (m), hours (h), days (d), or years (y). Weeks and months are almost never used to express half-life.

Atomic ratio is the number of atoms of a particular element or number of a particular nuclide per molecule, ion, or radical.

Unless specifically needed, valence and atomic ratio are usually omitted.

The following are some examples of stable and radioactive nuclides written in schematic form:

$^{1}_{1}H$	Most prevalent, stable nuclide of hydrogen: 1 proton, no neutrons.
$^{2}_{1}H$	Less prevalent, stable nuclide of hydrogen also known as deuterium: 1 proton, 1 neutron.
$^{3}_{1}H$ — $^{-}\beta$ 12.3y	Radioactive hydrogen also known as tritium: one proton, two neutrons, 12.3 year half-life. Emits a beta particle, no gamma emission.
$^{60}_{27}Co$ — $^{-}\beta,\gamma$ 5.2y	Radioactive cobalt: 27 protons, 33 neutrons, 5.2 year half-life. Emits a beta particle and gamma rays.
$^{238}_{92}U$ — $^{++}\alpha,\gamma$ 4.51×10^{9}y	Most prevalent nuclide of natural uranium: 92 protons, 146 neutrons, 4.5 billion years half-life. Emits an alpha particle, gamma rays, and occasionally an electron.
$^{112}_{51}Sb$ — $^{+}\beta,\gamma$ 0.9m	Short-lived radioactive nuclide of antimony: 51 protons, 61 neutrons, 0.9 minute half-life. Emits a positron (positive beta).

Completing the scheme for radioactive decay by indicating the daughter product we have:

$^{3}_{1}H \rightarrow ^{3}_{2}He + ^{-}\beta$, no γ 12.3y	A neutron converts to a proton by emitting a negative charge.
$^{60}_{27}Co \rightarrow ^{60}_{28}Ni + ^{-}\beta,\gamma$ 5.2y	A neutron converts to a proton by emitting a negative charge.

${}^{238}_{92}U \rightarrow {}^{234}_{90}Th + \alpha,\gamma$ 4.5 billion y	An alpha particle consisting of 2 neutrons and 2 protons is emitted.
${}^{112}_{51}Sb \rightarrow {}^{112}_{50}Sn + {}^{+}\beta,\gamma$ 0.9m	A proton converts to a neutron by emitting a positive charge.

Like x rays, gamma rays are used extensively in therapy. Beta particles are quite limited as therapeutic agents, and alpha particles are of even less use in therapy. (However, production of alpha particles by neutron bombardment for treatment of localized tumors in such inaccessible parts of the body as the brain is being more widely accepted.)

Medical applications of radioisotopes

Artificial radioisotopes constitute much of the radioactive material used in medicine and industry. Artificial radioisotopes are obtained as fission products from nuclear reactors and nuclear explosives and by bombarding suitable targets with nuclear particles and nuclei of atoms and photons. Several hundred nuclides are available as fission products, but the number having desirable chemical properties and sufficiently long half-lives to be of possible value for medical therapy and diagnosis is probably limited to a few dozen. Some examples of artificial radioisotopes are given below:

Iodine 131, obtained as a fission product. Used in thyroid gland diagnosis and therapy.

$$ {}^{131}_{53}I \rightarrow {}^{131}_{54}Xe + {}^{-}\beta,\gamma $$

Technetium 99, obtained as the daughter product of molybdenum 99 and is used for diagnosis.

Molybdenum 99 is obtained as a fission product, but could be obtained by neutron bombardment of molybdenum 98.

$$ {}^{99}_{42}Mo \rightarrow {}^{99}_{43}Tc^{m} + {}^{-}\beta,\gamma $$
$$ {}^{99}_{43}Tc^{m} \rightarrow {}^{99}_{43}Tc + {}^{-}e,\gamma^{*} $$

Cobalt 60, obtained by neutron bombardment of cobalt 59. Used in radiographic units for therapy.

$$ {}^{59}_{27}Co + {}^{1}_{0}n \rightarrow {}^{60}_{27}Co + \gamma $$
$$ {}^{60}_{27}Co \rightarrow {}^{60}_{28}Ni + {}^{-}\beta,\gamma $$

*The "m" indicates a metastable state decaying to the more stable state technetium 99. Technetium 99 has a long half-life and therefore low activity. It has no diagnostic value and is eventually excreted. The "e" indicates the ejection of an orbital electron by the conversion of energy from a gamma ray. The γ represents the x ray that results when another electron falls into the vacancy of the ejected electron.

Gold 198, obtained by neutron bombardment of gold 197. Used in diagnosis.

$$ {}^{197}_{79}Au + {}^{1}_{0}n \rightarrow {}^{198}_{79}Au + \gamma $$
$$ {}^{198}_{79}Au \rightarrow {}^{198}_{80}Hg + {}^{-}\beta,\gamma $$

The medical applications of radioisotopes are varied, but may be considered under the broad headings of therapy and diagnosis. The basic principal of radiation therapy is the destruction of diseased or superfluous tissue. The destruction of diseased or superfluous tissue is accompanied by some damage to healthy tissue. The assumption is made in prescribing radiation therapy that the benefits will outweigh any side effects that will be experienced. The principal use of radioisotopes in diagnosis is that of tracing body functions and locating abnormalities through injection or oral administrations of radioactive substance. Radiography through the use of radioactive sources has been limited by technical difficulties.

The roentgen is the established unit of exposure to ionizing electromagnetic radiation, for example, x rays and gamma rays. Radiations other than electromagnetic radiations produce biologic effects in tissue that will vary with their type, energy, and penetration. Consequently, it is not possible to directly express the biologic effects of one radiation in terms of another. A partial solution (Table 5-4) is obtained by determining the energy deposited in tissue by a radiation and multiplying that value by a quality factor, QF, to obtain the equivalent effect that results when an identical amount of energy is deposited by x rays or gamma rays. The dose

Table 5-4. Relationships among radiation units*

Type of radiation	R	Rads	Rems (or QF)
X rays and gamma rays	1	1	1
Beta particles	—	1	1
Thermal neutrons	—	1	5
Fast neutrons	—	1	10
Alpha particles†	—	1	10–20

*From Glasstone, Samuel: Sourcebook on atomic energy, ed. 3, United States Atomic Energy Commission, Princeton, N. J., 1967, D. Van Nostrand Co., Inc., p. 743.

†The low penetrability of alpha particles prevents their being a serious external hazard. Alpha emitters incorporated in the inner tissues are very hazardous as the result of their ionizing power.

equivalent, DE, unit is the roentgen equivalent man, or Rem. The rad, equal to 100 ergs per gram of tissue, is the unit of absorbed energy.

$$\underset{\text{(Rems)}}{\text{DE}} = \underset{\text{(rads)}}{\text{Dose}} \times \underset{\text{(quality factor)}}{\text{QF}}$$

Radiation detection instruments useful for detecting x rays and gamma rays are discussed on pp. 62 to 65. Thin-walled ionization chambers, Geiger counters, and proportional counters are also used for detecting alpha and beta particles. Scintillation and semiconduction dectectors in conjunction with pulse-height spectrometers provide a means for determining the energy of a photon or radiation particle. Scintillation refers to tiny flashes of light or scintilla produced in selected solids, liquids, and gases by interaction of photons or radiation particles. Semiconduction, in relation to radiation detection, refers to the changeability of electrical conduction of selected materials that results from the interaction of a photon or radiation particle.

Neutrons, because of their lack of charge, cannot be detected by common ionization instruments. Furthermore, instruments that can detect slow neutrons may not be able to detect fast neutrons. Neutron detection is effected by nuclear reactions in selected materials that produce ionizing particles directly or by creating radioactive materials whose radiations may subsequently be detected. When the detection method will not detect fast neutrons efficiently, they may be slowed by the use of a "moderator." Materials containing hydrogen and carbon such as paraffin and many plastics are good moderators. Portable neutron-sensitive scintillation detectors may be preferable to the older neutron-sensitive ionization chambers and proportional counters in general laboratory survey work.

Some of the more commonly used radioisotopes are listed in Table 5-5, which includes, for benefit of students who are beginning studies in the medical applications of radioisotopes, some of the conditions treated or diagnosed, and some of the possible side effects.

Table 5-5. More commonly used radioisotopes

Common name	Symbol	Form		Use		Condition or structure	Side effects
		Solution	Capsule	Diagnosis	Therapy		
Iodine 131 in form of sodium iodine	^{131}I	X	X		X	Hyperthyroidism—diffuse toxic goiter and toxic nodular goiter Thyroid carcinoma and metastases Angina pectoris (through production of a hypothyroid state)	Radiation sickness Increased clinical symptoms Bone marrow depression Acute leukemia Leukemia Chromosomal abnormalities Thyroid cancer Acute thyroid crisis Blood dyscrasias including reduced hemoglobin concentration Leukopenia Thrombocytopenia Male sterility (1 case) Permanent myxedema
Rose bengal sodium iodine 131	^{131}I	X (injection)		X		Liver Gallbladder Common bile duct	Red-colored stool Possible iodine allergy
Triolein iodine 131	^{131}I	X	X	X		Malabsorption of fats from intestinal tract	

Table 5-5. More commonly used radioisotopes—cont'd

Common name	Symbol	Form		Use		Condition or structure	Side effects
		Solution	Capsule	Diagnosis	Therapy		
Oleic acid iodine 131	^{131}I	X	X	X		Differential diagnosis between mucosal defect and digestive defect	
Sodium iodide iodine 131	^{131}I		X	X		Thyroid uptake	
Liothyronine iodine 125	^{125}I	X		X		T-3 uptake Threatened abortion (probably)	
T-4 diagnostic kit	^{125}I	X (in vitro)		X		Thyroid activity (measures direct output of thyroid gland; it is a companion test to the T-3 uptake [erythrocyte uptake] test)	
Liothyronine iodine 131	^{131}I						
Sodium iodohippurate iodine 131	^{131}I	X		X		Renal function	
Gold 198	^{198}Au	X			X	Ascites Pleural effusion Prostatic carcinoma Cervical carcinoma	Nausea Vomiting Intestinal injury Chest pains Depressed leukocyte count Low-grade fever Hypoplasia of bone marrow Fibrosis All radiation sickness signs
Dilute colloidal gold 198	^{198}Au	X		X		Scintiscanning of liver, lymphatics and lymph nodes, and bones Monitoring of blood and liver	
Sodium phosphate phosphorus 32	^{32}P	X	X		X	Polycythemia vera Chronic lymphocytic leukemia Myelogenous leukemia	Aplastic anemia Leukopenia Thrombocytopenia
Colloidal phosphorus	^{32}P	X			X	Ascites Pleural effusions Prostatic tumors Bladder tumors	Aplastic anemia Leukopenia Thrombocytopenia
Technetium 99	$^{99}T^{m}_{C}$	X		X		Brain scans Detection and localization of intracranial neoplastic and nonneoplastic lesions	

ENERGY OF RADIOACTIVE PARTICLES AND PHOTONS

The electron volt (eV) is used in nuclear medicine to express the energy of the particles and photons emitted by radioactive materials. Most of the radioactive materials used in nuclear medicine have energies between 100,000 and 2,000,000 eV. The meV (million electron volts) unit is used for convenience in expressing the energies of most radioactive emissions. Following are a few examples of radioactive materials and their principal emissions:

Cobalt 60	γ 1.17 (100%)	and	1.33 meV (100%)
Cesium 137	$^{-}\beta$0.514	and	1.176 meV
Americium 243	$^{++}\alpha$ 5.28	and	5.23 meV

Problem: How much gamma energy is released by 0.1 curie of cobalt 60 in 10 minutes? (Note: cobalt 60 emits 2 photons, 1.17 meV, and 1.33 meV with 100% efficiency. One curie = 3.70×10^{10} events/second.)

Step 1:

0.1 curie $\times$ 3.7 $\times$ 10^{10} events/sec $\times$ 1.17 meV/event $\times$ 100% = 4.33 $\times$ 10^{9}

0.1 curie $\times$ 3.7 $\times$ 10^{10} events/sec $\times$ 1.33 meV/event $\times$ 100% = 4.93 $\times$ 10^{9}

4.33 $\times$ 10^{9} + 4.93 $\times$ 10^{9} = 9.26 $\times$ 10^{9} meV/sec

Step 2:

9.26 $\times$ 10^{9} meV/sec $\times$ 10^{6} eV/meV $\times$ 1.6021 $\times$ 10^{-19} joules/eV = 1.485 $\times$ 10^{-3} joules/sec

Step 3:

1.485 $\times$ 10^{-3} joules/sec $\times$ 10 min $\times$ 60 sec/min = 8.91 $\times$ 10^{-1} joules

(Note: 1 joule = 0.7376 foot-pounds = work required to raise 1 pound 0.7376 feet.)

REFERENCES

Goodwin, P. N., Quimby, E. H., and Morgan, R. H.: Physical foundations of radiology, ed. 4, New York, 1970, Harper and Row, Publishers.

Glasstone, Samuel: Sourcebook on atomic energy, ed. 3, United States Atomic Energy Commission, Princeton, N.J., 1967, D. Van Nostrand Co., Inc.

Robertson, John K.: Radiology physics, ed. 3, London, 1956, The Macmillan Co.

QUESTIONS

1. What is radiotherapy?
2. What is the purpose of radiotherapy?
3. Define the following: (a) air dose; (b) skin dose; (c) depth dose; (d) volume dose; (e) tumor dose; (f) integral dose; (g) fractionation; and (h) protraction.
4. In what way(s) does (do) therapy tubes operate differently from diagnostic x-ray tubes?
5. What was the original purpose of building very long x-ray tubes to use in conjunction with supervoltage generators?
6. When was the first model of the Van de Graaff generator built?
7. What is the wavelength in angstroms of the shortest x-ray waves produced by 200 keV of energy?
8. How deep is the penetration in tissue of wavelengths generated at 22 meV?
9. For what do the initials N.C.R.P. stand?
10. Define half-value layer.
11. For what purpose is the half-value layer used?
12. What information useful in therapy can be derived from isodose curves?
13. What is the rad?
14. Explain ripple voltage.
15. In what three ways is it possible for a radiologic technologist to offer the greatest assistance in x-ray therapy to both the patient and the radiologist?
16. Who discovered radioactivity?
17. What are the common types (kinds) of radioactive emissions?
18. When a radioelement converts to another element, the new element is called what?
19. Lead is the end product of what processes?
20. Of what is lead comprised?
21. What is a nucleon?
22. What is the diameter of atoms?
23. Define an isotope.
24. Define nuclide.
25. Explain the causes and results of radioactivity.
26. Differentiate among the following: alpha and beta particles and gamma rays?
27. What are alpha and beta rays?
28. Explain half-life.
29. Explain the process by which a neutron may change to (or become) a proton.
30. What is a joule?
31. What is the range of energies of most radioactive materials used in nuclear medicine?

6 • BONES OF THE EXTREMITIES

The normal adult human skeleton consists of 210 separate bones as they are studied radiographically. True anatomic consideration includes 206 separate bones. Table 6-1 presents the bones by section and by respective numbers and is arranged for comparison.

Radiographically the upper extremities commence with the arms as appendages from the trunk, and the lower extremities commence with the legs as appendages from the trunk. As a result it is considered that the upper extremities commence with the humeri, and that the lower extremities commence with the femora.

Anatomically these extremities commence with the corresponding bony attachments to the vertebral column. As a result it is considered that the upper extremities commence with and include the scapulas and clavicles, and that the lower extremities commence with and include the pelvic bones (ilia, ischia, and pubes). (See Figs. 6-1 and 6-2.)

Although the first bone in the upper appendage (arm) is the humerus, it is prudent to initiate studies of this extremity with the phalanges, since the thumb and fingers constitute the initial radiographic exercises.

UPPER EXTREMITY

Phalanges

The phalanges constitute the bones of the thumb and fingers. There are two phalanges in the thumb and three phalanges in each finger, making a total of fourteen phalanges on each hand. The phalanges are arranged in rows with a proximal and a distal (terminal) phalanx in the thumb, and a proximal, a middle, and a distal (terminal) phalanx in each of the four fingers. The thumb and fingers are often called manual digits: the thumb is the first digit; the index, fore- or first finger is the second digit; the middle or second finger is the third digit; the ring or third finger is the fourth digit; and the little or fourth finger is the fifth digit. (See Fig. 6-3.)

Table 6-1. Skeletal bones by section

Section	Radiographic number	Anatomic number
Upper extremities	60	64
Lower extremities	60	62
Vertebral column	24	24
Thoracic cage	25	25
Shoulder (pectoral girdle)	4	0
Pelvis (pelvic girdle)	8	2
Hyoid	1	1
Skull	22	22
Auditory ossicles	6	6
Total	210	206

Carpals and metacarpals

The carpus consists of eight bones in two rows: proximal row (from the lateral to the medial side)—scaphoid (navicular), lunate, triquetrum (triangular), and pisiform; distal row (from the lateral to the medial side)—trapezium (greater multangular), trapezoid (lesser multangular), capitate, and hamate, which has a hook-shaped process on its volar surface called the hamulus process. (See Fig. 6-3.) Articulations of the carpal bones are listed in Table 6-2 and are diagramed in Fig. 6-4. There are five metacarpals, which are numbered one through five from the lateral to the medial side. At their distal ends are the phalanges. The carpals form the wrist, the metacarpals form the hand, and the phalanges form the digits, or fingers.

Radius and ulna

The bones of the forearm are called the radius and ulna. The radius is the bone on the lateral side. It is quite small at its proximal end and quite large at its distal end. The ulna lies on the medial side and is quite large at its proximal end and small at the distal end. The radius commences at the proximal end with the head, followed by the neck and the radial tuberosity, which is inferior and medial to the head. The midportion is called the body or shaft. The distal end, which forms the greater portion of the wrist joint, has a styloid process on the lateral surface and a small notch, the ulnar notch, on the medial surface. The ulna commences proximally with the olecranon process, which con-

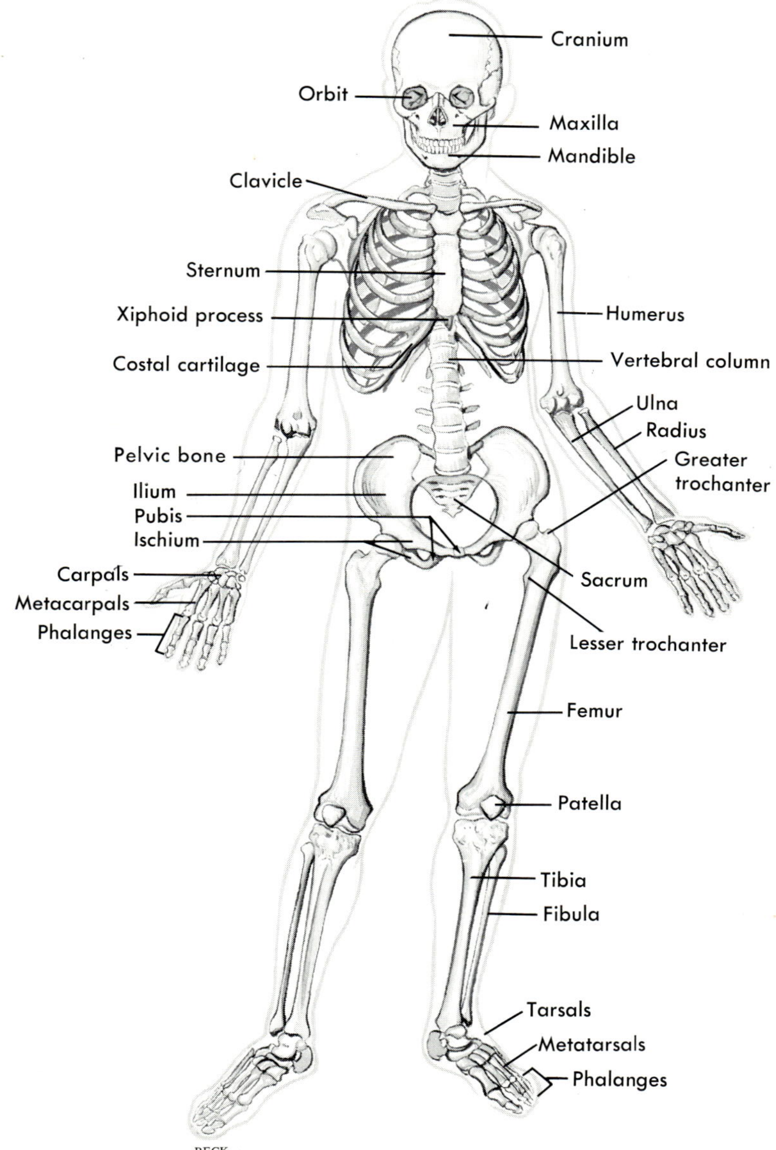

Fig. 6-1. Skeleton—anterior view. (Modified from Anthony, Catherine Parker: Textbook of anatomy and physiology, ed. 7, St. Louis, 1967, The C. V. Mosby Co.)

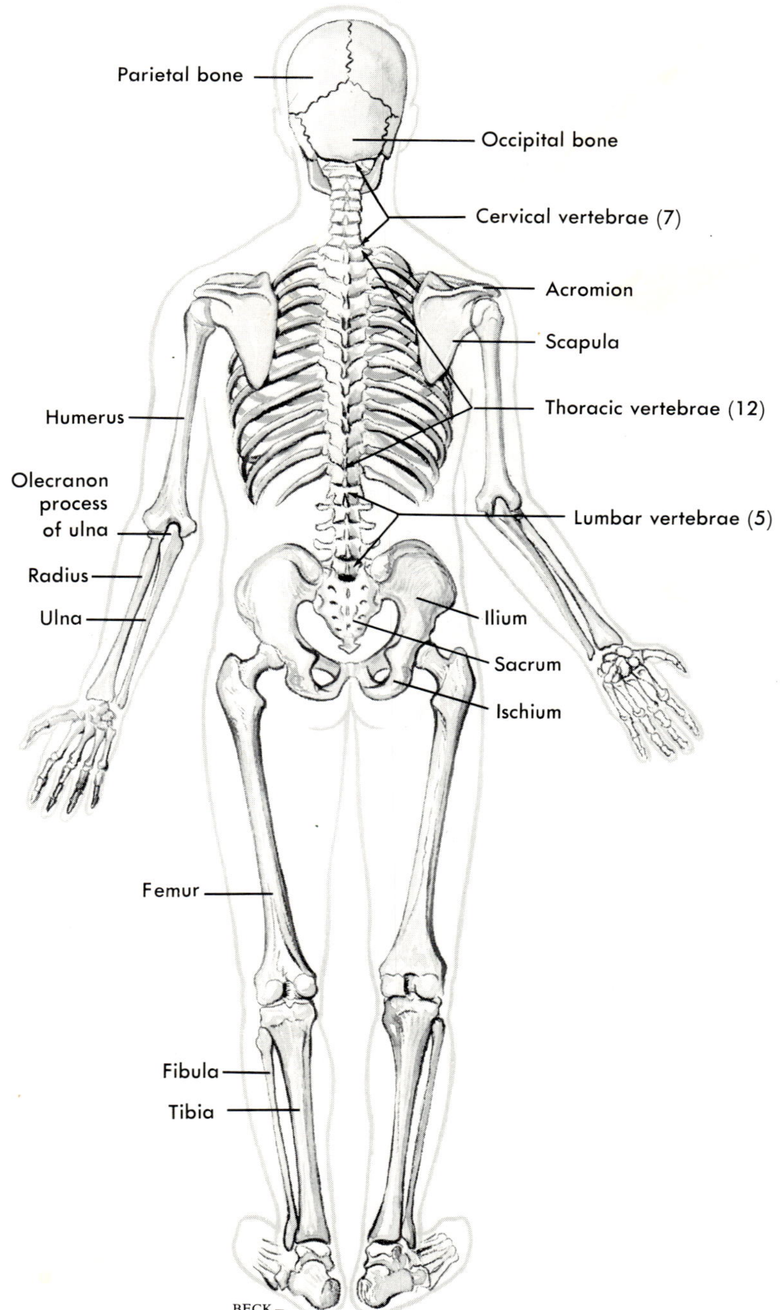

Fig. 6-2. Skeleton—posterior view. (From Anthony, Catherine Parker: Textbook of anatomy and physiology, ed. 7, St. Louis, 1967, The C. V. Mosby Co.)

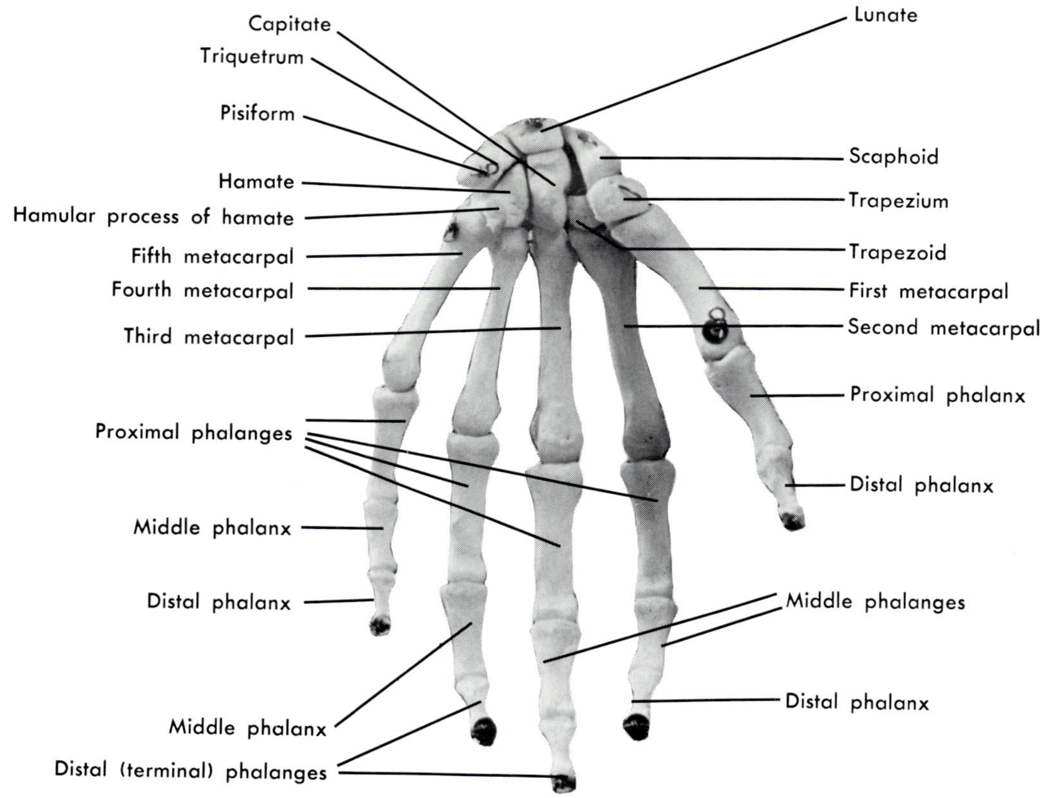

Fig. 6-3. Left-hand, palmar surface. (Note: Tufts of the terminal phalanges are obscured by the metal washers used in articulation.)

Table 6-2. Articulations of the carpus

Bone	Number of articulations	Articulations
Scaphoid	5	Radius, trapezium, trapezoid, capitate, and lunate
Lunate	5	Radius, capitate, hamate, triquetrum, and scaphoid
Triquetrum	3 and disc	Lunate, pisiform, hamate, and triangular-shaped cartilage
Pisiform	1	Triquetrum
Trapezium	4	Scaphoid, trapezoid, 1st and 2nd metacarpals
Trapezoid	4	Scaphoid, trapezium, capitate, and 2nd metacarpal
Capitate	7	Scaphoid, lunate, 2nd, 3rd, and 4th metacarpals, trapezoid, and hamate
Hamate	5	Lunate, 4th and 5th metacarpals, triquetrum, and capitate

tains, anteriorly, the semilunar notch. Inferior to the olecranon process is the coronoid process, which is anterior and superior on the anterior surface of the ulna. The radial notch is located on the lateral surface of the coronoid process. The midportion of the ulna is termed the body or shaft and terminates in the small distal end. The distal end includes the head of the ulna laterally and the styloid process medially. (See Fig. 6-5.) In the elbow joint the olecranon process of the ulna articulates with the olecranon fossa of the humerus; the coronoid process

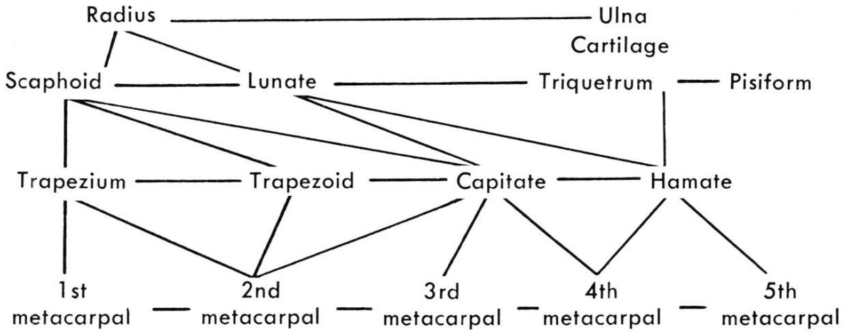

Fig. 6-4. Carpal articulations.

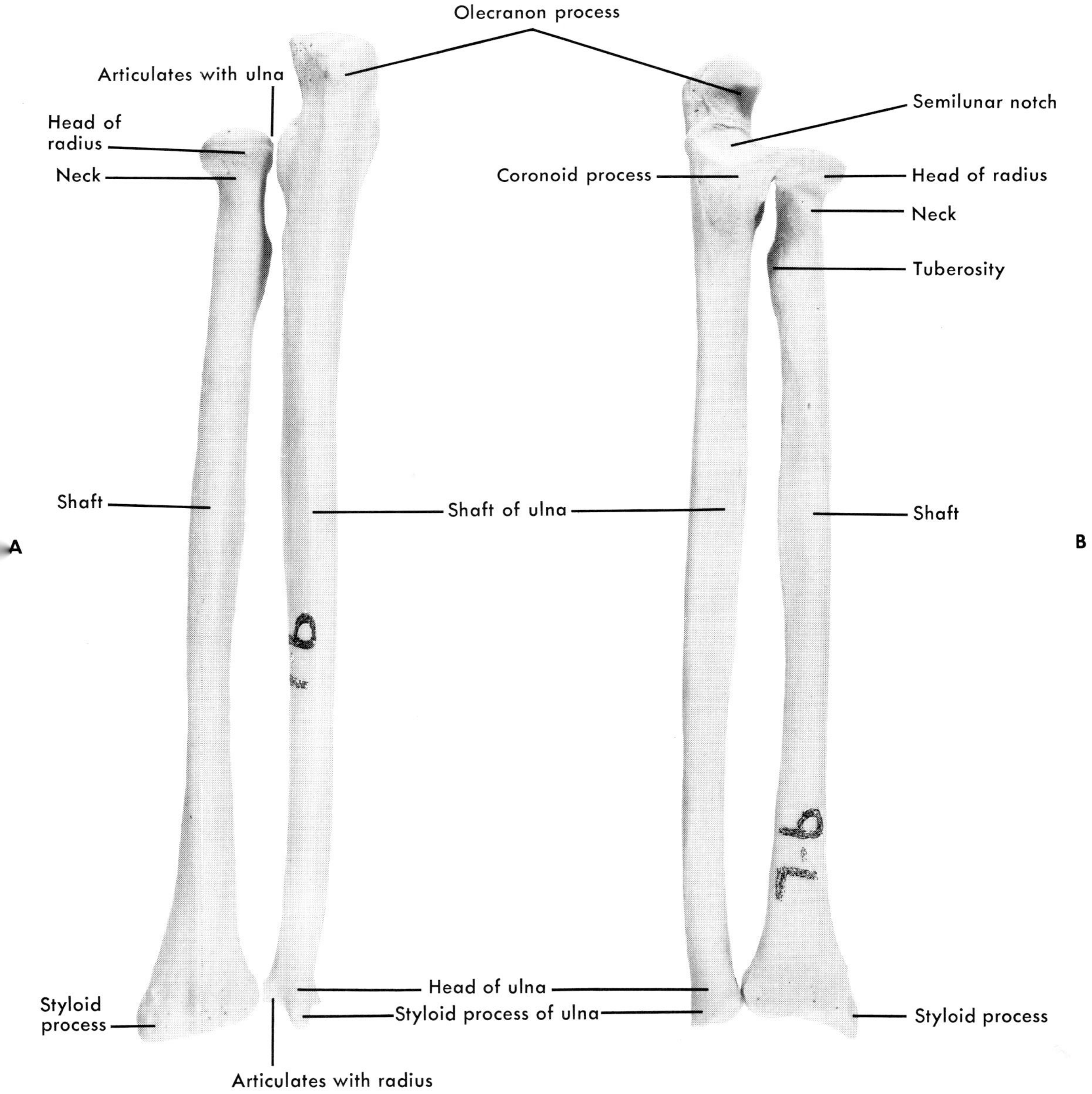

Olecranon process
Articulates with ulna
Head of radius
Neck
Shaft
A
Shaft of ulna
Styloid process
Head of ulna
Styloid process of ulna
Articulates with radius
Semilunar notch
Coronoid process
Head of radius
Neck
Tuberosity
Shaft
B
Styloid process

Fig. 6-5. Left radius and ulna. **A,** Posterior surface. **B,** Anterior surface.

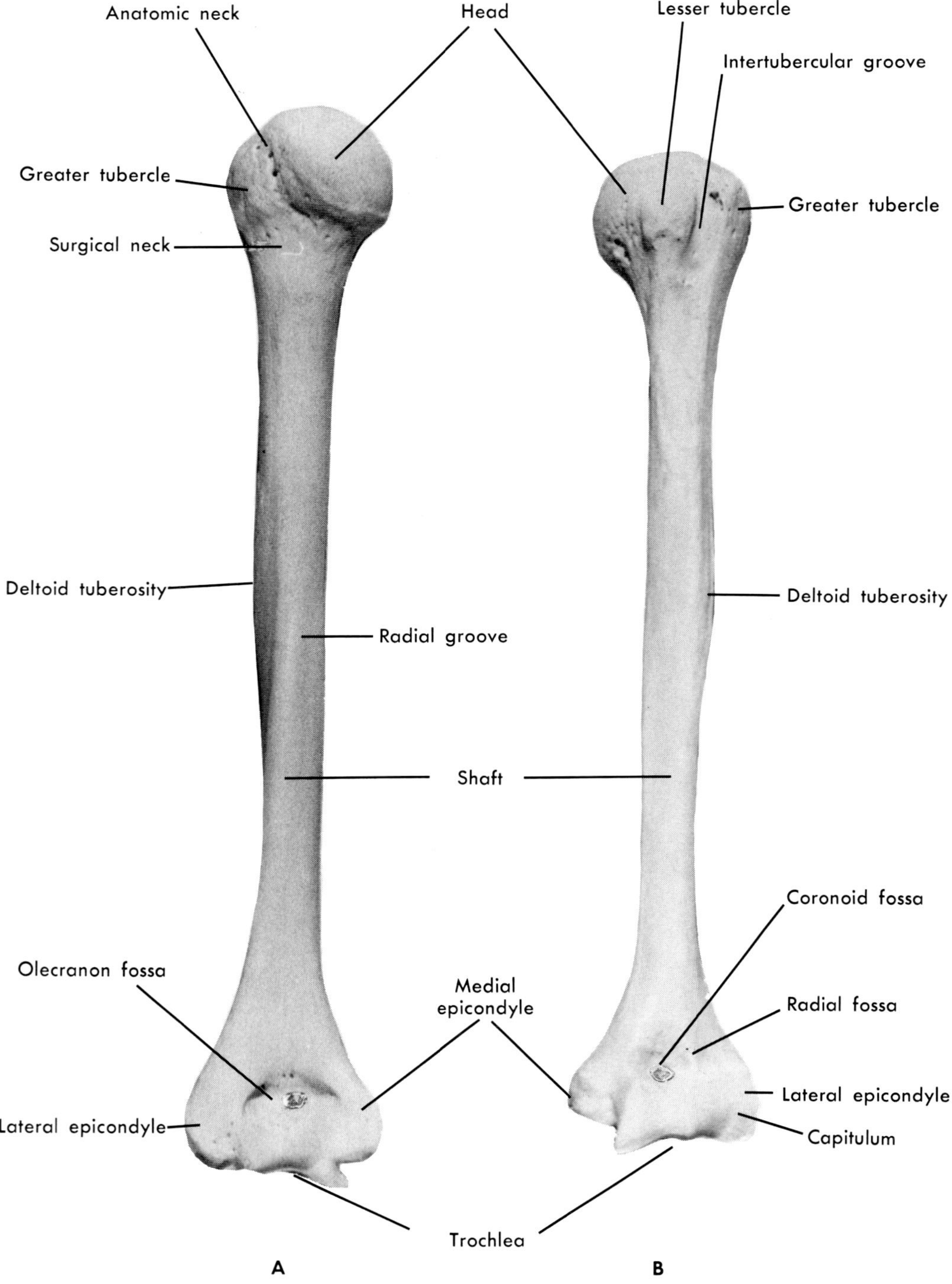

Fig. 6-6. Left humerus. **A,** Posterior surface. **B,** Anterior surface.

articulates with the coronoid fossa of the humerus; and the head of the radius articulates with the radial fossa of the humerus and with the radial notch of the coronoid process of the ulna. The distal ends of the radius and ulna articulate with each other in the ulnar notch of the radius, which is located on the medial surface of the radius. The distal end of the radius, in addition, articulates with the scaphoid and lunate of the carpus. The distal end of the ulna, in addition, articulates with a triangular-shaped cartilage.

Humerus

The upper extremity commences with the humerus, which is the long bone of the upper arm. Its proximal end consists of the head, anatomic neck, greater and lesser tubercles, intertubercular sulcus or groove, and surgical neck. The middle portion is called the body or shaft. The deltoid tuberosity is laterally located on the anterior surface of the midpart of the body. Distally and anteriorly the humerus consists of the medial epicondyle, coronoid fossa, radial fossa, and lateral epicondyle. Inferior to the coronoid fossa is the trochlea, and inferior to the radial fossa is the capitulum. Distally and posteriorly the humerus consists of the olecranon fossa, which is superior to the trochlea. (See Fig. 6-6.) The head articulates with and in the glenoid cavity of the glenoid process of the scapula in an enarthrodial or ball-and-socket type of articulation. The trochlea articulates with, and in the semilunar notch of, the ulna, and the capitulum articulates on the head of the radius. The elbow is a ginglymus or hinge joint.

LOWER EXTREMITY

Although the first bone in the lower appendage (leg) is the femur, as with the upper extremity it is logical to initiate studies of the lower extremity with the phalanges.

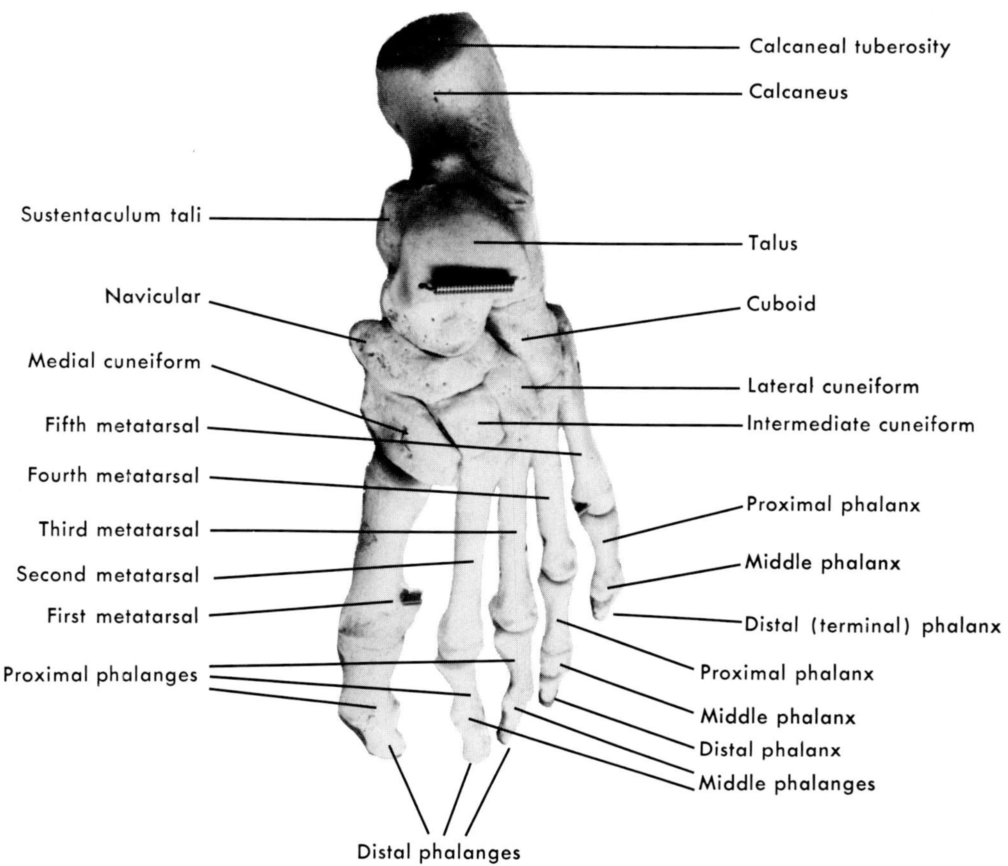

Fig. 6-7. Dorsum, left foot.

Phalanges

The phalanges of the foot constitute the bones of the toes. There are two phalanges in the first (great) toe and three phalanges in each of the remaining four toes, making a total of fourteen phalanges in each foot. The phalanges are arranged in rows with a proximal and a distal (terminal) phalanx in the first toe, and a proximal, a middle, and a distal (terminal) phalanx in each of the remaining four toes. The toes are often called the pedal digits: the first (great) toe is the first digit; the second toe is the second digit; the third toe is the third digit; the fourth toe is the fourth digit; and the fifth (little) toe is the fifth digit. (See Fig. 6-7.)

Tarsals and metatarsals

The tarsus consists of seven bones: talus, calcaneus, navicular, medial (first) cuneiform, intermediate (second) cuneiform, lateral (third) cuneiform, and cuboid. The articulations are listed in Table 6-3 and are diagramed in Fig. 6-8. There are five metatarsals, which are numbered one through five from the medial to the lateral side. At their distal ends are the phalanges. (See Fig. 6-7.) The tarsals, metatarsals, and phalanges compose the foot. The ankle articulation is that between the tibia, lateral and medial malleoli, and the talus. The phalanges, although part of the foot, comprise the toes (digits).

Table 6-3. Articulations of the tarsus

Bone	Number of articulations	Articulations
Calcaneus	2	Talus, cuboid
Talus	5	Lateral and medial malleoli, distal end of tibia, navicular, and calcaneus
Cuboid	4(5)	Calcaneus, lateral cuneiform, 4th and 5th metatarsals, and sometimes navicular
Navicular	4(5)	Medial, intermediate and lateral cuneiforms, talus, and sometimes cuboid
Medial cuneiform	4	Navicular, intermediate cuneiform, and 1st and 2nd metatarsals
Intermediate cuneiform	4	Navicular, medial and lateral cuneiforms, and 2nd metatarsal
Lateral cuneiform	6	Navicular, intermediate cuneiform, cuboid, and 2nd, 3rd, and 4th metatarsals

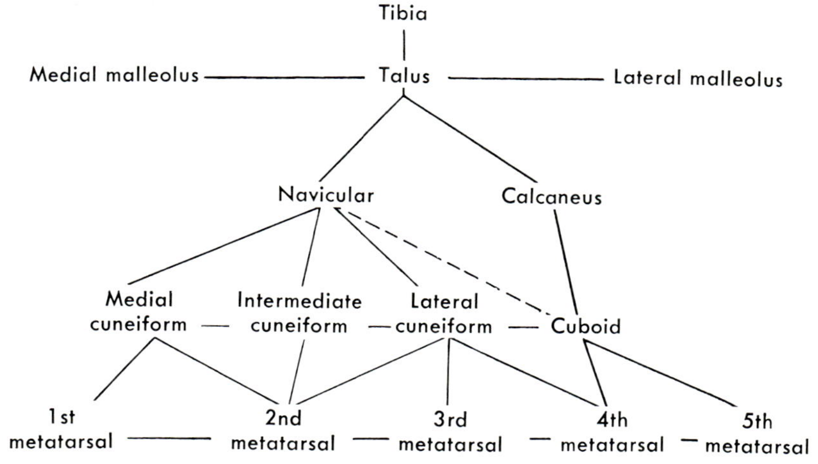

Fig. 6-8. Tarsal articulations.

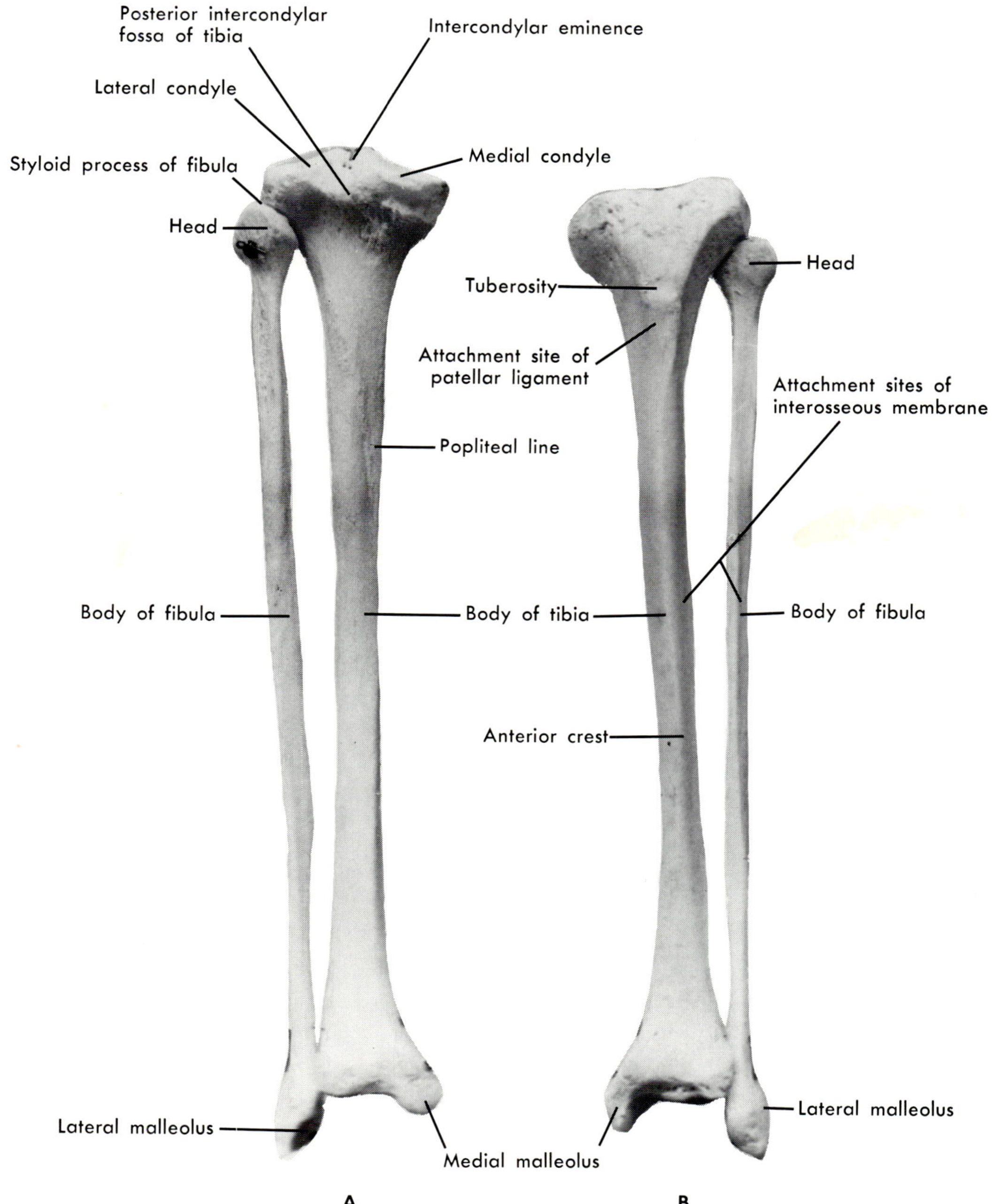

Fig. 6-9. Left tibia and fibula. **A**, Posterior surface. **B**, Anterior surface.

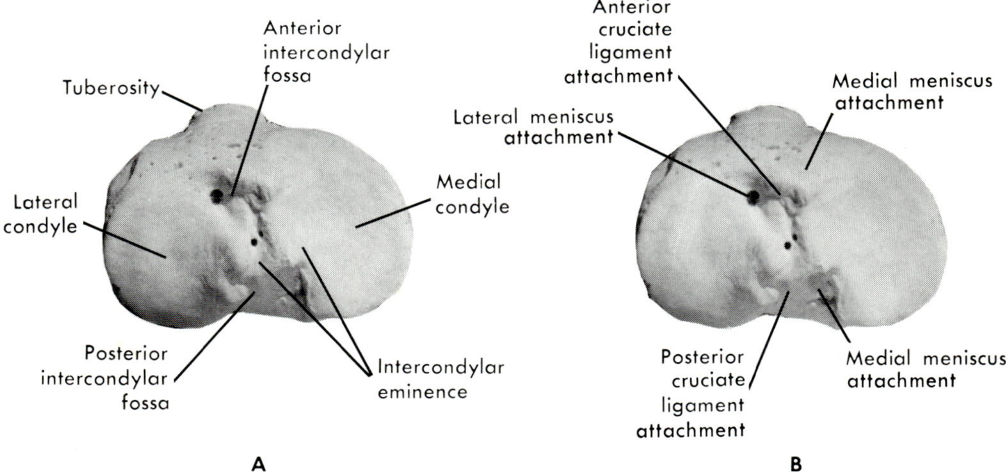

Fig. 6-10. Left tibia, proximal end. **A,** Structures. **B,** Attachment sites.

Tibia and fibula

The bones of the lower leg are the tibia and fibula. The tibia is quite large. Proximally, the tibial plateau lies between the medial and lateral condyles. This plateau is divided into the medial and lateral facets by the intercondylar eminence (spine). The intercondyloid fossae are anterior and posterior to the spine. The articular facet for the fibula is on the posterior surface of the lateral condyle. The tibial tuberosity is on the anterior surface of the tibia inferior to the plateau. The midportion of the tibia, called the body (shaft), extends into the distal end. At the distal end on the medial surface is the medial malleolus. The head of the fibula (the fibula is lateral to the tibia) has a styloid process that projects superiorly from the posterior part of it. The midpòrtion is called the body. The distal end of the fibula is called the lateral malleolus. (See Figs. 6-9 and 6-10.) Just inferior to the knee joint the head of the fibula articulates with the lateral condyle of the tibia, but the fibula does not enter into the formation of the knee joint. The distal ends of the tibia and fibula articulate with the talus.

Femur

The lower extremity commences with the femur, the long bone of the upper leg. At its proximal end are the head, anatomic neck, and greater and lesser trochanters. The intertrochanteric crest (ridge) extends obliquely between the trochanters on the posterior surface. The intertrochanteric line is on the anterior surface. It, too, lies between the trochanters. The midportion is called the body or shaft. The lateral epicondyle, lateral condyle, patellar surface, medial condyle, and medial epicondyle are located on the distal end. The intercondylar fossa is between the condyles on the posterior surface. (See Figs. 6-11 and 6-12.) The head of the femur articulates with and in the acetabulum of the pelvis, the distal end articulates with the tibia, and the patella articulates with the patellar surface.

The patella is the only sesamoid bone in the body that is essential. It is the largest of all the sesamoid bones. (See Fig. 6-13.)

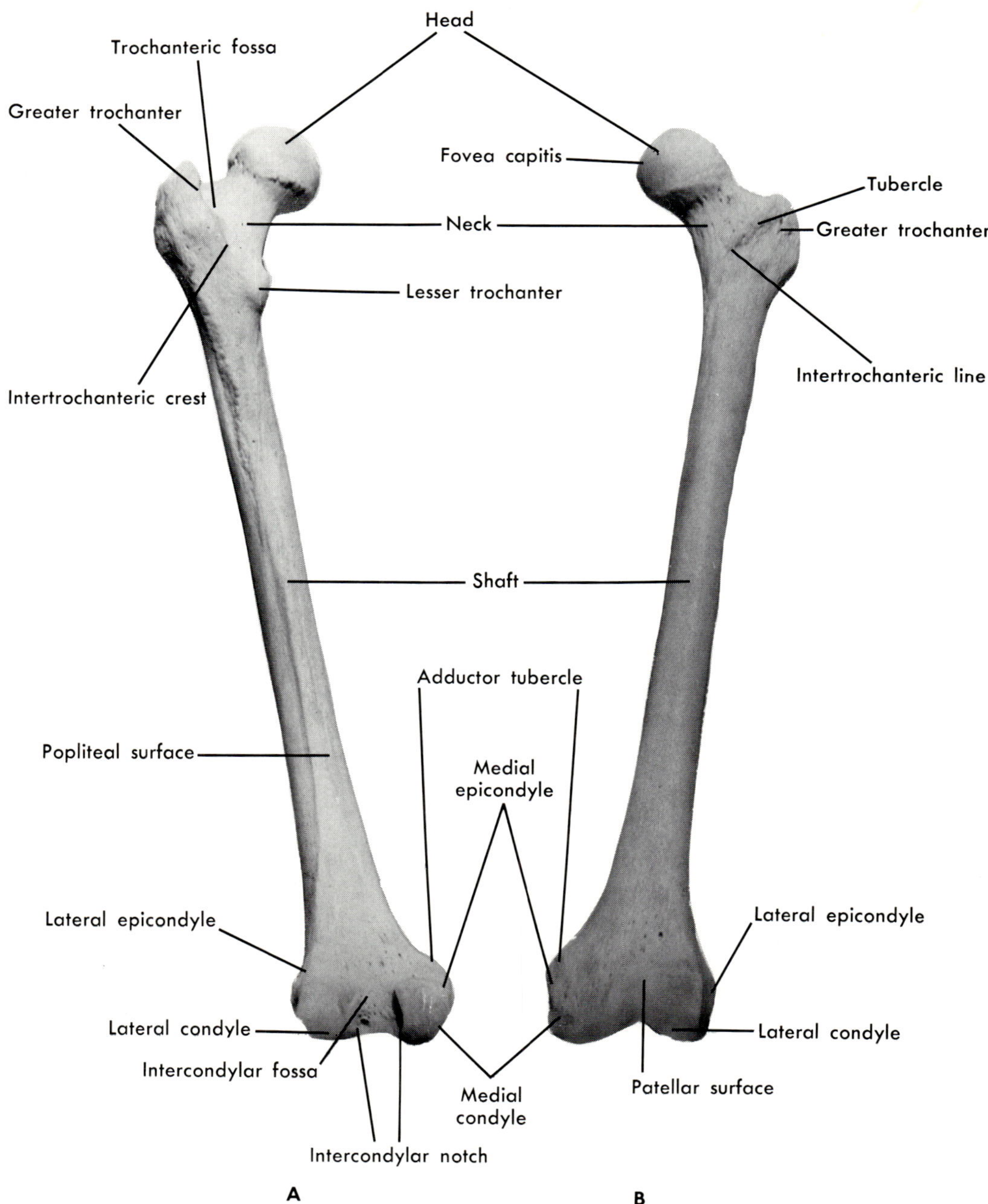

Fig. 6-11. Left femur. **A,** Posterior surface. **B,** Anterior surface.

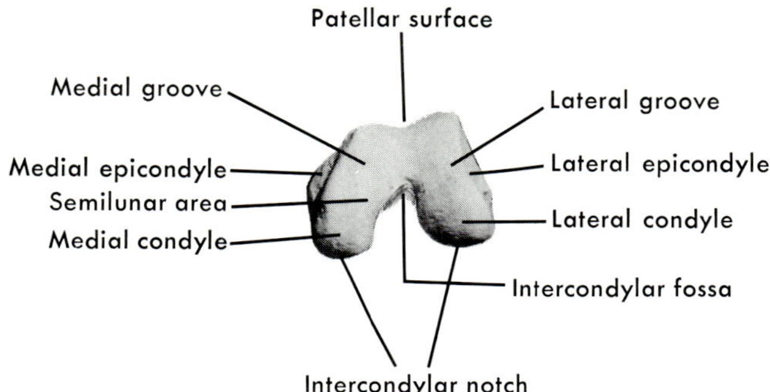

Fig. 6-12. Left femur, distal surface.

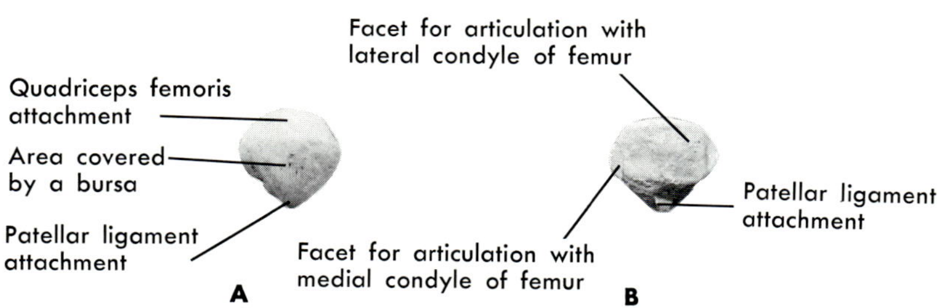

Fig. 6-13. Left patella. **A,** Anterior surface. **B,** Posterior surface.

REFERENCES

Anthony, C. P., and Kolthoff, N. J.: Textbook of anatomy and physiology, ed. 9, St. Louis, 1975, The C. V. Mosby Co.

Best, C. H., and Taylor, N. B.: The human body, New York, 1956, Henry Holt & Co., Inc.

Goss, Charles M.: Gray's anatomy, ed. 28, Philadelphia, 1966, Lea & Febiger.

Jacobi, C. A.: Textbook of anatomy and physiology in radiologic technology, ed. 2, St. Louis, 1975, The C. V. Mosby Co.

Meschan, Isadore: An atlas of anatomy basic to radiology, Philadelphia, 1975, W. B. Saunders Co.

QUESTIONS

1. Name the bones that comprise the manual digits.
2. How many of these bones are found in a normal (single) upper extremity?
3. What is the general name for all of the wrist bones?
4. How many of the wrist bones are normally found in one wrist joint?
5. Name the wrist bones beginning with the lateral surface of the proximal row, followed by those from the lateral surface in the distal row.
6. In the forearm, which is the lateral bone and which is the medial bone?
7. Which of the bones in the forearm has the head distally?
8. Describe in full the articulations of the elbow joint.
9. State the technical name of the elbow joint.
10. Describe the distal end of the bone of the upper arm.
11. Describe the origin and attachment of the biceps humeri.
12. How many bones comprise the pedal digits?
13. How many bones comprise the ankle joint?
14. How many bones in the foot and ankle are there in comparison with those comprising the wrist?
15. How many foot bones and how many hand bones are found in a single lower or upper extremity?
16. Name the larger of the bones in the lower leg.
17. Fully describe the smaller of the lower leg bones.
18. Fully describe the larger of the lower leg bones.
19. What is the name of the bone forming the kneecap?
20. Describe in detail the articulations of the knee joint.
21. What is the name of the bone of the upper leg?
22. Describe the bone of the upper leg in detail.
23. Compare the bones of the upper leg and upper arm.
24. With what does the bone of the upper arm articulate?
25. With what does the bone of the upper leg articulate?

7 • POSITIONING FOR THE EXTREMITIES

ROUTINE

The routine steps are listed as follows:

1. Know the desired position.
2. Select all factors except kilovoltage.
3. Conduct the patient into the radiographic room. If cooperation of the patient is possible, have him assume the desired position.
4. After deciding what size film to use, place the film in the film holder on the tabletop beneath the part to be radiographed. Use proper identification and *R* or *L* to denote right or left side.
5. If possible, explain to the patient what is going to be done.
6. Center the part to be radiographed to the proper film holder division.
7. Center the tube both lengthwise and crosswise to the part to be radiographed.
8. Measure the patient for thickness of the part. From the technique chart, determine the kilovoltage and select it on the control.
9. Close the primary switch and check the line voltage.
10. Give the patient instructions concerning breathing.
11. *Observe* the patient's movement *until the moment that the exposure is made.*
12. During the exposure, ascertain that the machine is delivering the desired milliamperage by watching the milliampere meter.
13. Instruct the patient to resume normal breathing.

If another view is required, select the proper factors on the control panel. Remove the exposed film (in the film holder), and replace it with the proper-sized film holder and film for the next exposure. If more than one view is to be exposed on one film, simply change the location of the lead half or third blanks and reposition the part to be radiographed. With the first exposure of a series of multiple exposures on a single film, mark the part of the anatomy that is even with the center mark of the film holder; keep this mark even with the center mark in all subsequent exposures of this series.

Be sure to complete the identification procedure. The starting factors stated for all the following techniques are for a *12:1 grid* when a Bucky is used. For table-top work, backscatter radiation can be reduced by placing a sheet of leaded rubber beneath the film holder. *Bone radiography requires the use of the small focal spot.* Extremity radiography usually requires two or more views on each film. The method of division of the film holder face is demonstrated in Fig. 7-1. In this chapter reference is made to one of these four methods of division in each set of positioning instructions.

Several devices are employed to mark or identify the radiographs. These devices include radiolucent metal plates with slots for lead numerals and letters, radiopaque plates with numbers and letters cut out in small wheels, and *flashcards* to

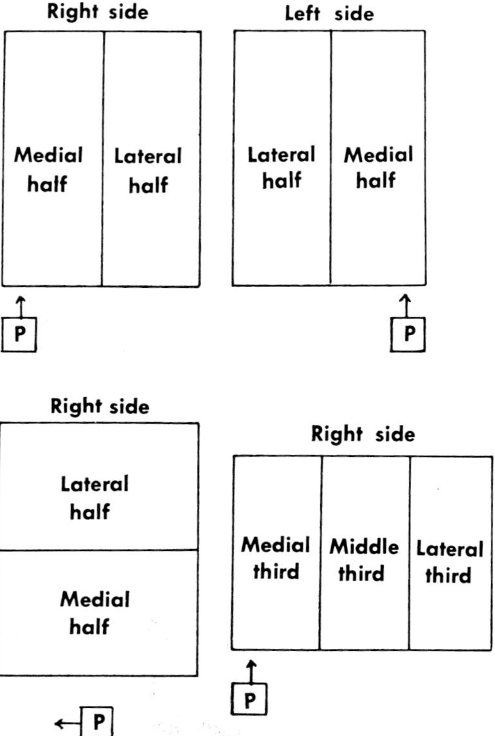

Fig. 7-1. Film holder face divisions. The square containing the letter *P* denotes the position of the patient in relation to the film on the tabletop. The arrow indicates the direction the patient faces.

be used with identifying lamps in the processing room. The last device permits a variety of data to be typed on the card and then stamped into the film emulsion. To enable use of this device, a piece of leaded tape, or other radiopaque material, is placed in one of eight positions, either on the film-holder surface or in a precut area in the intensifying screens. These positions are shown in Fig. 7-2.

It is necessary that the greatest possible protection from extraneous radiation be given both the patient and the operator. In addition to collimation of the primary beam, numerous other devices may be employed for gonadal protection. Among these are leaded rubber gloves and aprons and specially cut pieces of leaded rubber sheeting, which are available through x-ray supply houses.

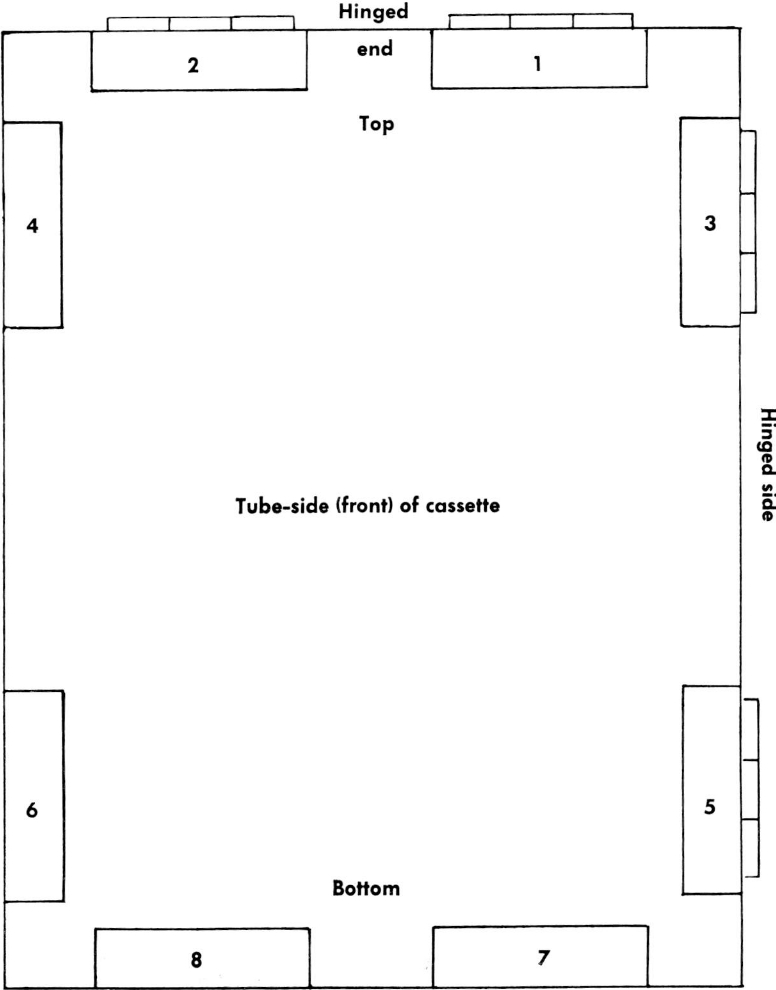

Fig. 7-2. Lead blocker positions.

Thumb—posterior (A-P), oblique, and lateral views (Figs. 7-3 to 7-5)

Film size—8″ × 10″
No-screen film holder
Crosswise
Tabletop
Collimate to cover

Technique

Factors	Screen film cassette (par)	Screen film no-screen film holder
mA	100	100
Time	0.1	0.75
mAs	10	75
Thickness in cm	2	2
kVp	44	56
Distance	40	40

Patient preparation

Remove all jewelry from the patient's hand.

Palpation point

Distal end of proximal segment.

Procedure

Posterior (A-P)—Seat the patient at the end of the table. Place the hand in internal rotation with the midposterior surface of the thumb in the center of the lateral side of the film holder.

Oblique—Place the palm flat on the film holder with the midportion of the thumb in the center of the film holder.

Lateral—Place the palm flat on the film holder with the midportion of the thumb in the center of the film holder. Flex the fingers to rotate the thumb into the true lateral position.

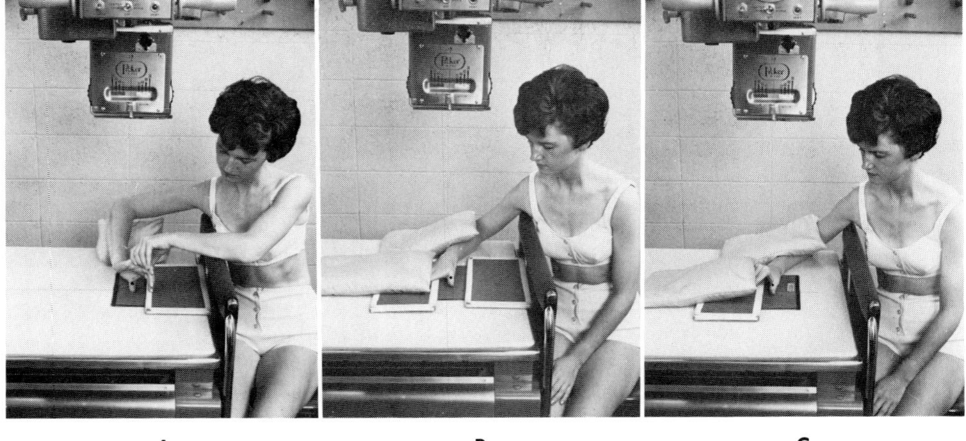

A B C

Fig. 7-3. Thumb positions. **A,** Posterior (A-P) position. **B,** Oblique position. **C,** Lateral position.

A

B

C

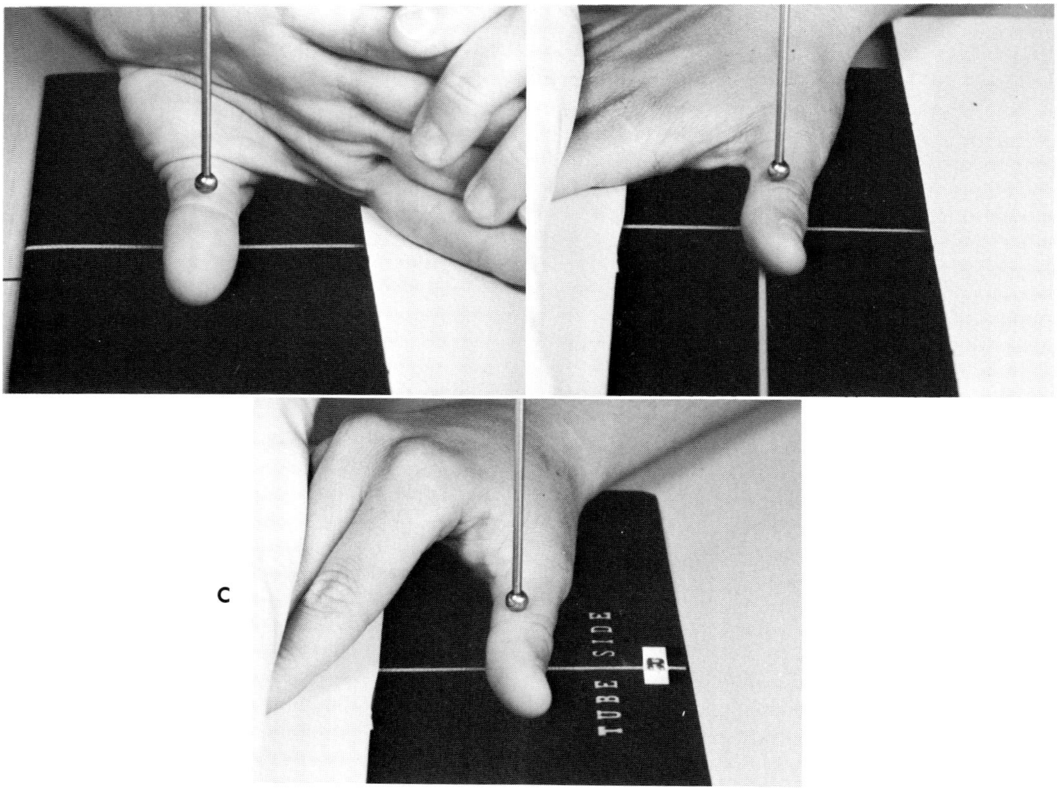

Fig. 7-4. Thumb positions. A, Posterior (A-P) position. B, Oblique position. C, Lateral position.

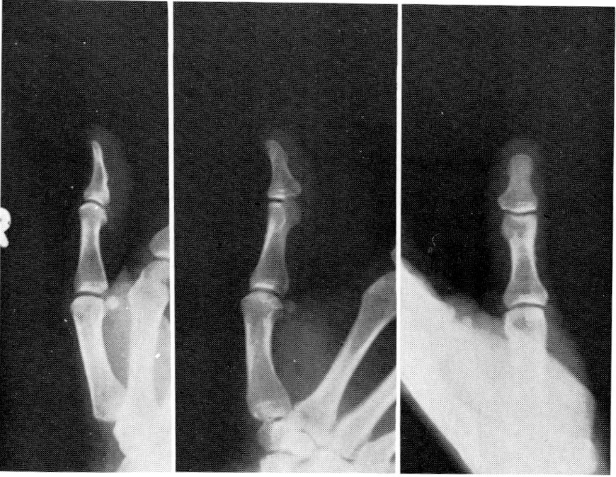

Fig. 7-5. Thumb views. Posterior (A-P), oblique, and lateral views. (Courtesy Dr. E. I. L. Cilley, Dr. T. W. Crowell, Dr. R. E. Waud, and Dr. G. H. Hoffman.)

Central ray

Direct the central ray perpendicular through the distal end of the proximal segment of the thumb to the center of each section of the film holder. Collimate to each section of film holder.

Immobilization

Posterior (A-P)—Place sandbags or sponges under the elbow. Instruct the patient to support his fingers with his other hand.

Oblique—Place sandbags on the elbow and fingertips.

Lateral—Place sandbags on the elbow and against the fingertips.

Right-left markers

Place the correct marker on the lateral view of the first metacarpal and phalanges.

Technical tips

Keep the long axis of the thumb parallel with the film to open the joint space.

Structures demonstrated

Posterior (A-P), oblique, and lateral views of the first metacarpal and phalanges.

Hand—anterior (P-A) and oblique views (Figs. 7-6 to 7-8)

Film size—10″ × 12″
No-screen film holder
Crosswise
Tabletop
Collimate to cover

Technique

Factors	Screen film cassette (par)	Screen film no-screen film holder
mA	100	100
Time	0.1	0.75
mAs	10	75
Thickness in cm	4	4
kVp	48	60
Distance	40	40

Patient preparation

Remove all jewelry, if possible.

Palpation points

Distal ends and shafts of metacarpal bones.

Procedure

Anterior (P-A)—Seat the patient at the end of the table. Place the hand in the prone position, with the fingers and thumb extended and slightly separated. Center the midshaft of the third metacarpal in the center of the medial half of the film holder.

Oblique—With the palm on the film, rotate the hand externally approximately 45 degrees. Flex and separate the fingers, and extend the thumb. Center the midshaft of the third metacarpal in the center of the lateral half of the film holder.

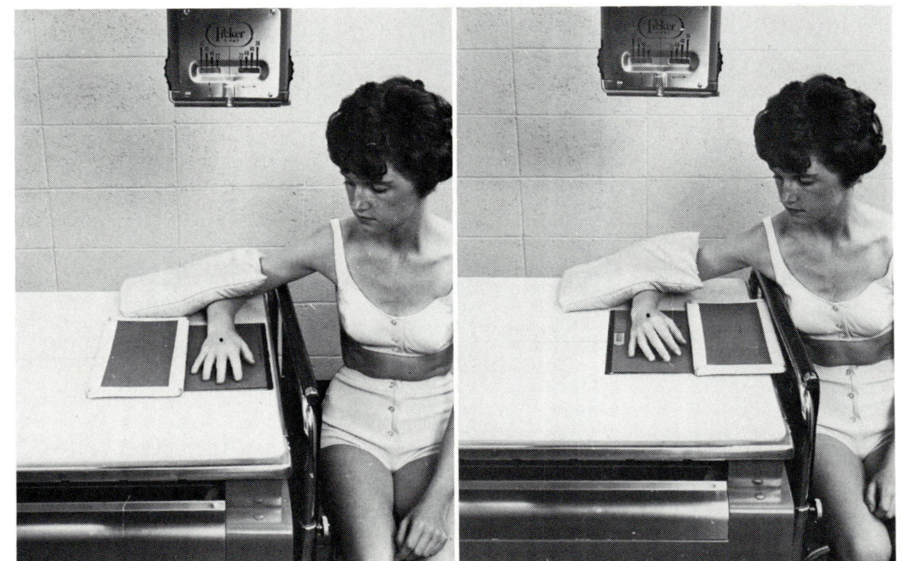

Fig. 7-6. Hand positions. **A**, Anterior (P-A) position. **B**, Oblique position.

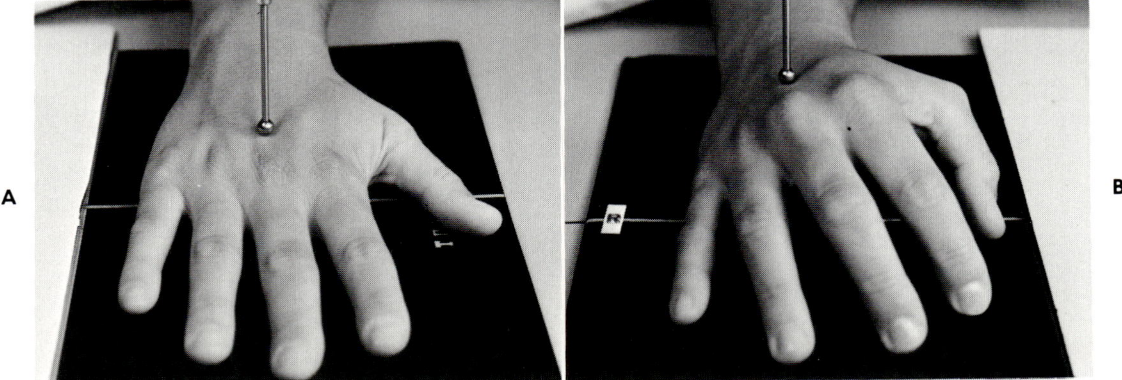

Fig. 7-7. Hand positions. **A,** Anterior (P-A) position. **B,** Oblique position.

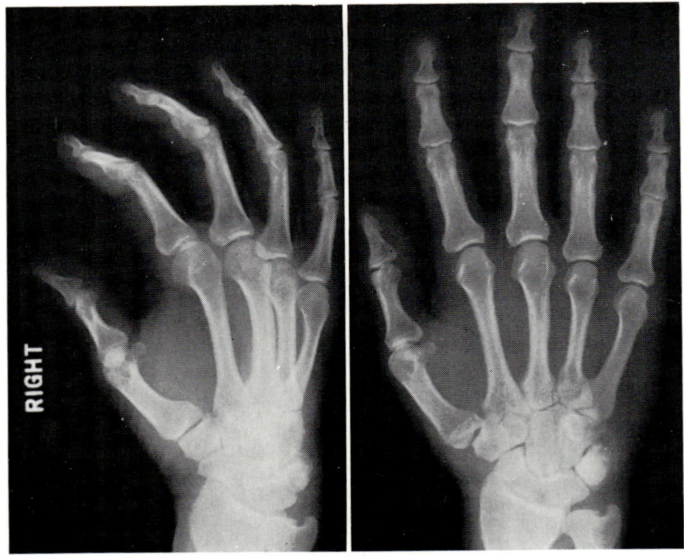

Fig. 7-8. Hand views. Anterior (P-A) and oblique views. (Courtesy Dr. E. I. L. Cilley, Dr. T. W. Crowell, Dr. R. E. Waud, and Dr. G. H. Hoffman.)

Central ray

Direct the central ray perpendicular through the midshaft of the third metacarpal to the center of each section of the film holder. Collimate to each section of film holder.

Immobilization

Place a sandbag on the forearm.

Right-left markers

Place the correct marker on the oblique view, lateral center border of the film holder.

Structures demonstrated

Anterior (P-A) and oblique views of the carpals, metacarpals, and phalanges.

Technical tips

Relax the fingers to position the long axis of the metacarpals parallel with the film surface.

Note: To demonstrate a foreign body in the hand, make exposures of the anterior (P-A) and lateral views only with a lead marker taped over the point of entry of the foreign body.

Wrist—anterior (P-A), ulnar flexion, oblique, and lateral views (Figs. 7-9 to 7-11)

Film size—10″ × 12″
No-screen film holder
Lengthwise
Tabletop
Collimate to cover

Technique

Factors	Screen film cassette (par)	Screen film no-screen film holder
mA	100	100
Time	0.1	0.75
mAs	10	75
Thickness in cm	4	4
kVp	48	60
Distance	40	40

Patient preparation

Remove all jewelry.

Palpation points

Radial and ulnar styloid processes.

Procedure

Anterior (P-A)—Seat the patient at the end of the table. Place the wrist in the prone position with the long axis of the hand in line with the forearm. Center a point halfway between the styloid processes to the center of the lower medial division of the film holder.

Ulnar flexion—Place the wrist in the prone position. Center a point halfway between the styloid processes to the center of the lower lateral division of the film holder. Hold the forearm firm, and move the hand away from the thumb side as far as possible.

Oblique—With the wrist in the prone position, rotate it externally 45 degrees. Center a point halfway between the styloid processes to the center of the upper medial division of the film holder.

Lateral—With the wrist in the prone position, rotate it externally 90 degrees so that a line through the styloid processes is perpendicular to the film holder. Ex-

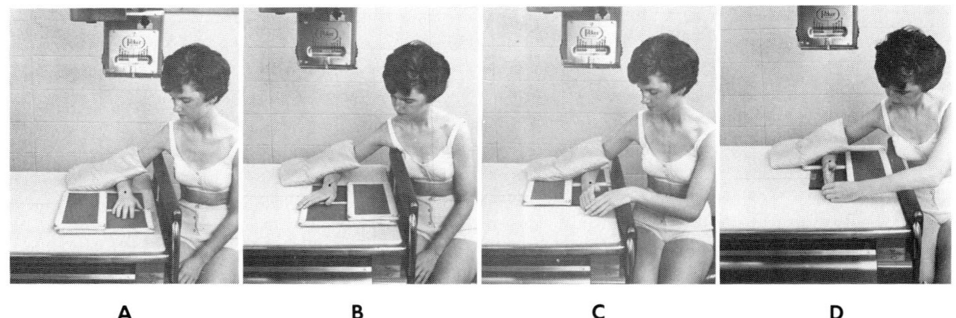

A B C D

Fig. 7-9. Wrist positions. **A,** Anterior (P-A) position. **B,** Radial deviation (ulnar flexion) position. **C,** Oblique position. **D,** Lateral position.

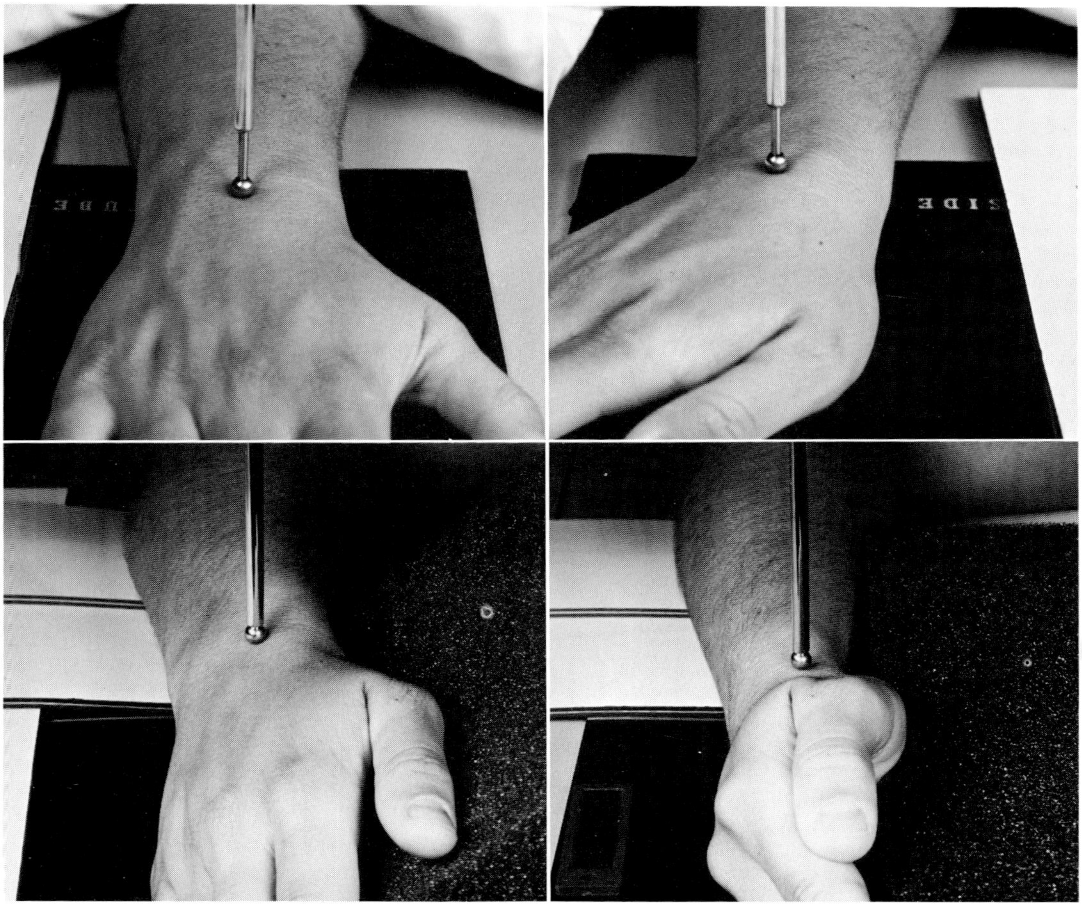

A B C D

Fig. 7-10. Wrist positions. **A,** Anterior (P-A) position. **B,** Radial deviation (ulnar flexion) position. **C,** Oblique position. **D,** Lateral position.

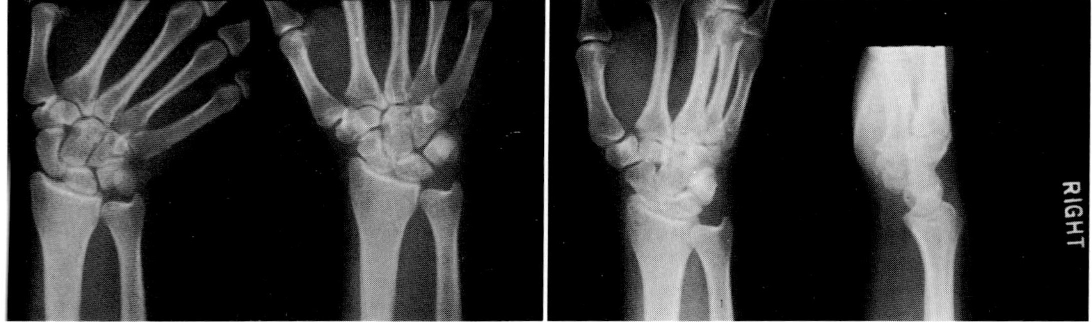

Fig. 7-11. Wrist views. Anterior (P-A), radial deviation (ulnar flexion), oblique, and lateral views. (Courtesy Dr. E. I. L. Cilley, Dr. T. W. Crowell, Dr. R. E. Waud, and Dr. G. H. Hoffman.)

tend the fingers with the thumb extended adjacent to the hand. Center the midportion of the wrist to the center of the upper lateral division of film holder.

Central ray

Direct the central ray perpendicular through the midportion of the wrist to the center of each section of the film holder. Collimate to each section of film holder.

Immobilization

Place a sandbag on the forearm. Instruct the patient to support the fingertips with the other hand.

Right-left markers

Place the correct marker on the lateral view, center border of the film holder.

Technical tips

On P-A view, relax fingers and hand to position long axis of wrist parallel with film surface.

Structures demonstrated

Anterior (P-A), oblique, and lateral views of the distal ends of the radius and ulna, the carpal bones, and the proximal ends of the metacarpals. The ulnar flexion view better demonstrates scaphoid fractures.

Forearm—posterior (A-P) and lateral views (Figs. 7-12 to 7-14)

Film size—10″ × 12″
No-screen film holder
Lengthwise
Tabletop
Collimate to cover

Technique

Factors	Screen film cassette (par)	Screen film no-screen film holder
mA	100	100
Time	0.1	0.75
mAs	10	75
Thickness in cm	5	5
kVp	50	62
Distance	40	40

Patient preparation

Remove all jewelry.

Palpation points

Radial and ulnar styloid processes; lateral and medial epicondyles of humerus.

Procedure

Posterior (A-P)—Seat the patient at the end of the table. Place the forearm in the supine position on the lateral half of the film holder with the joint nearer the injured site included on the film holder. A line through the radial and ulnar styloid processes is parallel with the film surface.

Lateral—From the posterior (A-P) position, rotate the forearm internally 90 degrees, at the same time flex the elbow 90 degrees, and rest the upper arm on the table. Place the forearm on the medial half of the film holder with the included joint in the same plane as in the posterior view. A plane through the radial and ulnar styloid processes and the humeral epicondyles is perpendicular to the film surface.

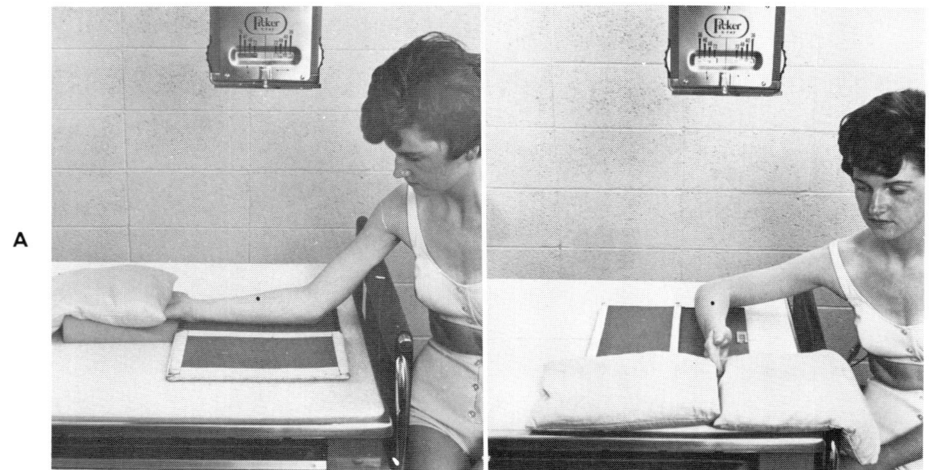

Fig. 7-12. Forearm positions. **A,** Posterior (A-P) position. **B,** Lateral position.

Fig. 7-13. Forearm positions. **A,** Posterior (A-P) position. **B,** Lateral position.

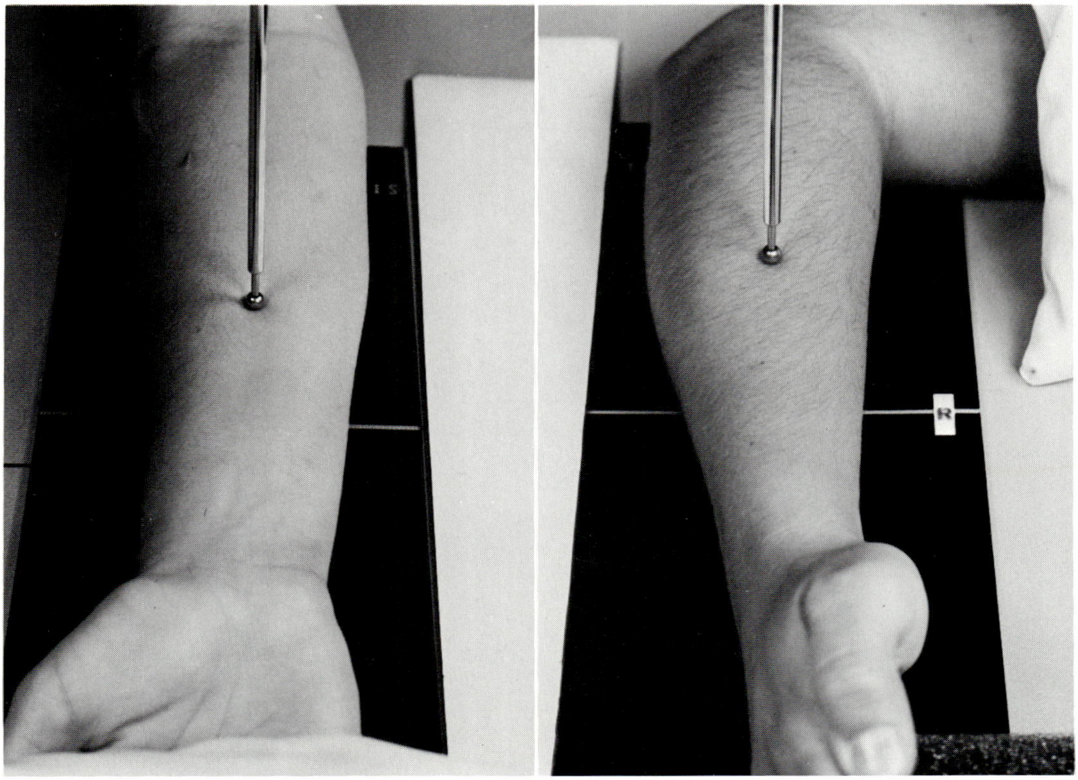

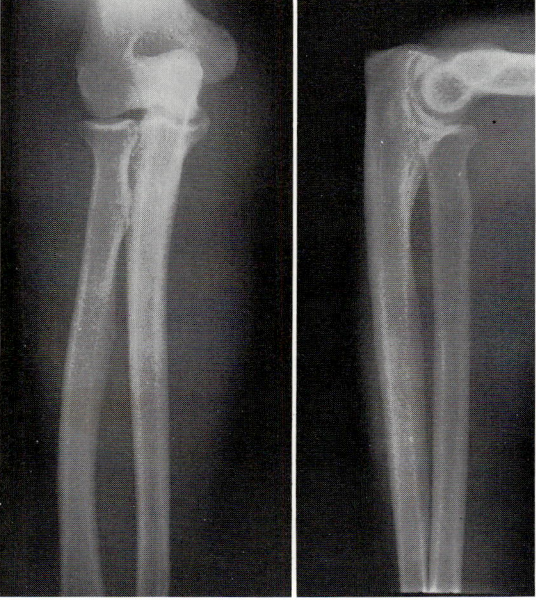

Fig. 7-14. Forearm views. Posterior (A-P) and lateral views. (Courtesy Dr. E. I. L. Cilley, Dr. T. W. Crowell, Dr. R. E. Waud, and Dr. G. H. Hoffman.)

Central ray

Direct the central ray perpendicular through the shaft of the forearm to the center of each section of the film holder. Collimate to each section of film holder.

Immobilization

Posterior (A-P)—Place a 1-inch sponge or sandbag under the hand and a heavy sandbag on the palm of the hand.

Lateral—Place sandbag on each side of the hand.

Right-left markers

Place the correct marker on the lateral view, center border of the film holder.

Technical tips

The P-A position of the hand and wrist with elbow extended presents an untrue forearm position with the radius crossing over the ulna.

Structures demonstrated

Posterior (A-P) and lateral views of the radius, ulna, and elbow, and/or wrist joints.

Elbow—posterior (A-P) and lateral views (Figs. 7-15 to 7-17)

Film size—10″ × 12″
No-screen film holder
Crosswise
Tabletop
Collimate to cover

Technique

Factors	Screen film cassette (par)	Screen film no-screen film holder
mA	100	100
Time	0.1	0.75
mAs	10	75
Thickness in cm	7	7
kVp	54	66
Distance	40	40

Patient preparation

Remove sleeve from part.

Palpation points

Radial and ulnar styloid processes; lateral and medial epicondyles of humerus.

Procedure

Posterior (A-P)—Seat the patient at the end of the table on a low stool. Place the elbow in the supine position on the lateral half of the film holder with the shoulder and elbow in the same horizontal plane. A plane through the radial and ulnar styloid processes and the humeral epicondyles is parallel with the film surface. Center the midpoint of the elbow (a point 1 inch distal to the epicondyles) to the film holder.

Lateral—From the posterior (A-P) position, rotate the elbow internally 90 degrees; at the same time flex the elbow 90 degrees, and rest the upper arm on the table. The humerus projects off the medial aspect of the film holder. A plane

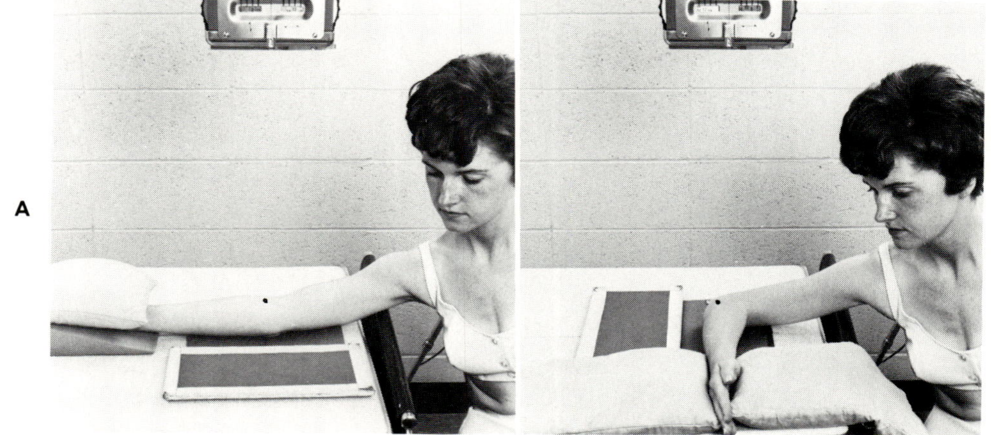

Fig. 7-15. Elbow positions. **A,** Posterior (A-P) position. **B,** Lateral position.

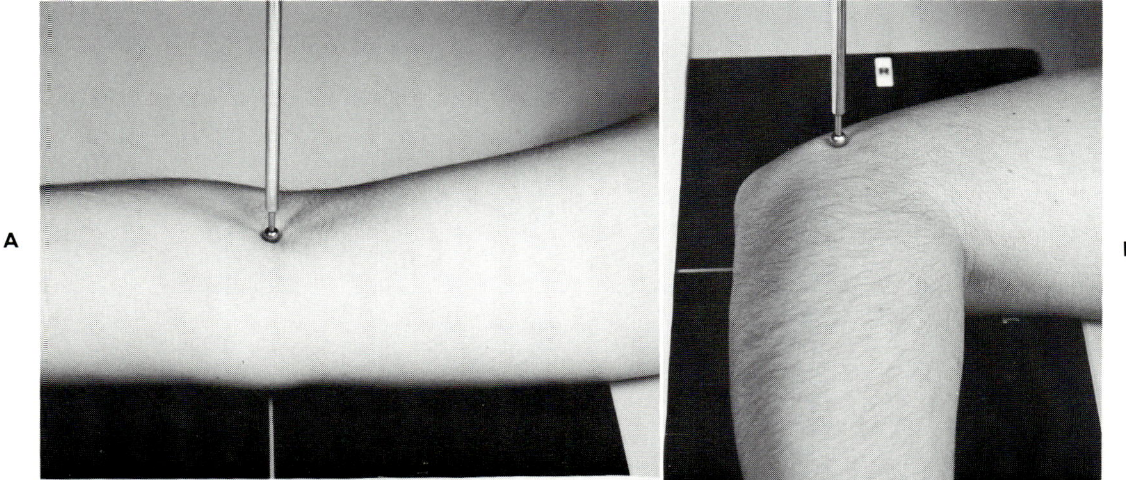

Fig. 7-16. Elbow positions. **A,** Posterior (A-P) position. **B,** Lateral position.

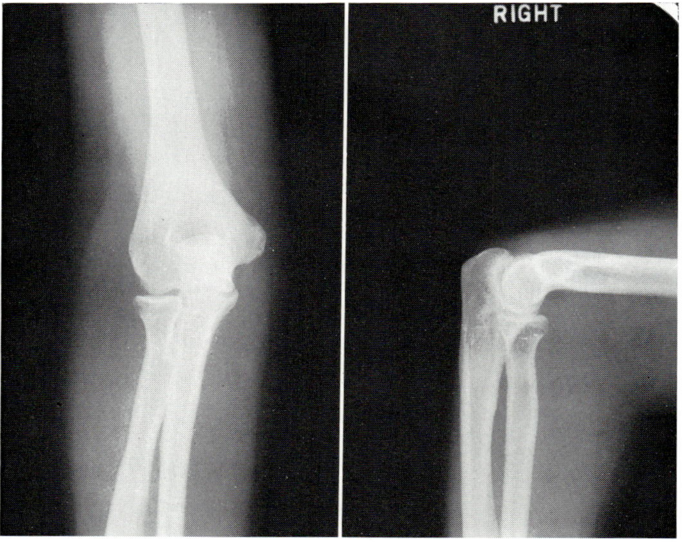

Fig. 7-17. Elbow views. Posterior (A-P) and lateral views. (Courtesy Dr. E. I. L. Cilley, Dr. T. W. Crowell, Dr. R. E. Waud, and Dr. G. H. Hoffman.)

through the radial and ulnar styloid processes and humeral epicondyles is perpendicular to the film surface. Center the midpoint of the elbow to the film holder.

Central ray

Direct the central ray perpendicular through the elbow to the center of each section of the film holder. Collimate to each section of film holder.

Immobilization

Posterior (A-P)—Place a 1-inch sponge or sandbag under the hand and a heavy sandbag on the palm of the hand.

Lateral—Place sandbags on each side of the hand.

Right-left markers

Place the correct marker on the lateral view, above the humerus, center border of the film holder.

Technical tips

In the posterior view, if the elbow cannot be extended more than 110 degrees, make two exposures: one, a posterior of the proximal forearm, and the other, a posterior of the distal humerus on one film.

Structures demonstrated

Posterior (A-P) and lateral views of the elbow joint, distal humerus, proximal radius, and ulna.

Humerus—posterior (A-P) view (Figs. 7-18 to 7-21)

Film size—10″ × 12″
Cassette or no-screen film holder
Lengthwise
Bucky or tabletop
Collimate to cover

Technique

Factors	Screen film cassette (par) Bucky	Screen film cassette (par) tabletop	Screen film no-screen film holder
mA	100	100	100
Time	0.2	0.1	0.75
mAs	20	10	75
Thickness in cm	10	10	10
kVp	66	60	72
Distance	40	40	40

Patient preparation

Remove clothing from part.

Palpation points

Lateral and medial epicondyles of humerus; acromion process of scapula.

Procedure

Place the patient in the supine position with the long axis of the humerus over the center line of the table. Rotate the arm into the supine position so that a line through the humeral epicondyles is parallel with the film surface. Include the joint nearer to the injured site, and place the edge of the cassette 2 inches beyond this joint.

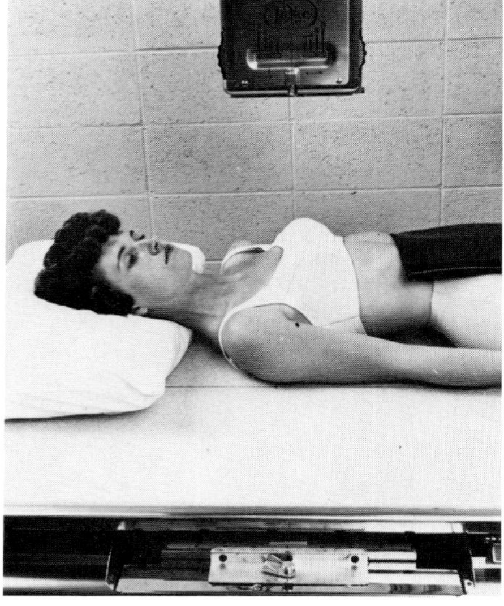

Fig. 7-18. Humerus—posterior (A-P) position, Bucky.

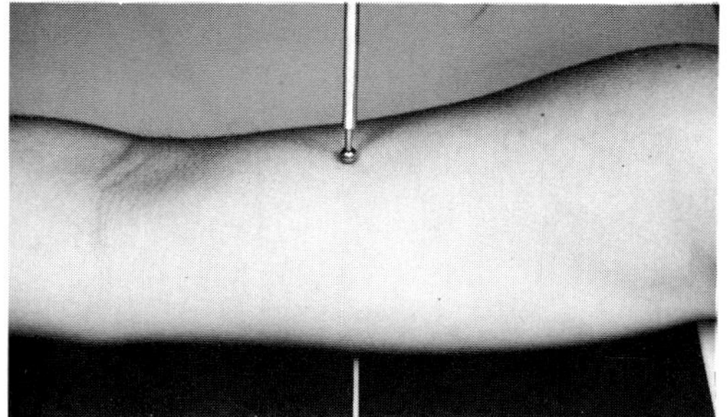

Fig. 7-19. Humerus—posterior (A-P) position, tabletop.

Central ray

Direct the central ray perpendicular through the shaft of the humerus to the center of each section of the film holder. Collimate to each section of film holder.

Immobilization

Place sandbags under and over the hand. Employ suspended respiration.

Right-left markers

Place the correct marker on the lateral side, center border of the film holder.

Technical tips

The distal humerus may best be demonstrated by seating the patient at the end of the table with his elbow extended on the tabletop and the upper arm in external rotation.

Structures demonstrated

Posterior (A-P) view of the upper two thirds or of the lower two thirds of the humerus.

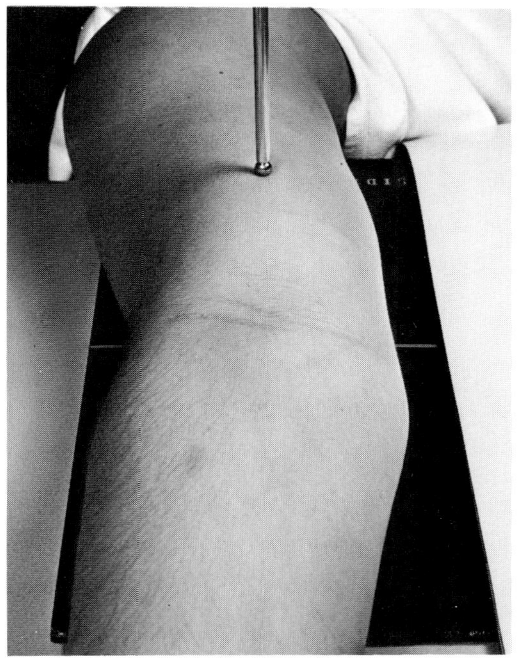

Fig. 7-20. Humerus—posterior (A-P) position, tabletop.

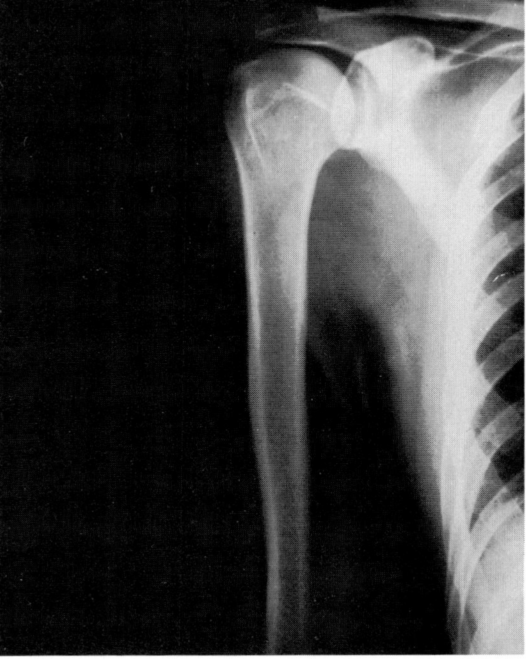

Fig. 7-21. Humerus—posterior (A-P) view. (Courtesy Dr. E. I. L. Cilley, Dr. T. W. Crowell, Dr. R. E. Waud, and Dr. G. H. Hoffman.)

Humerus—lateral view (Figs. 7-22 to 7-25)

Film size—10″ × 12″
Cassette or no-screen film holder
Lengthwise
Bucky or tabletop
Collimate to cover

Technique

Factors	Screen film cassette (par) Bucky	Screen film cassette (par) tabletop	Screen film no-screen film holder
mA	100	100	100
Time	0.2	0.1	0.75
mAs	20	10	75
Thickness in cm	10	10	10
kVp	66	60	72
Distance	40	40	40

Patient preparation

Remove clothing from part.

Palpation points

Lateral and medial epicondyles of humerus; acromion process of scapula.

Procedure

Place the patient in the supine position with the long axis of the humerus over the center line of the table. Rotate the arm internally so that a line through the humeral epicondyles is perpendicular to the film holder. Include the joint nearer to the injured site, and place the edge of the cassette 2 inches beyond this joint.

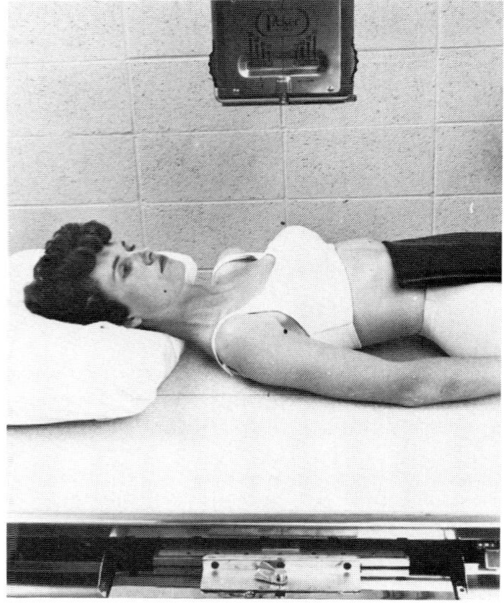

Fig. 7-22. Humerus—lateral position, Bucky.

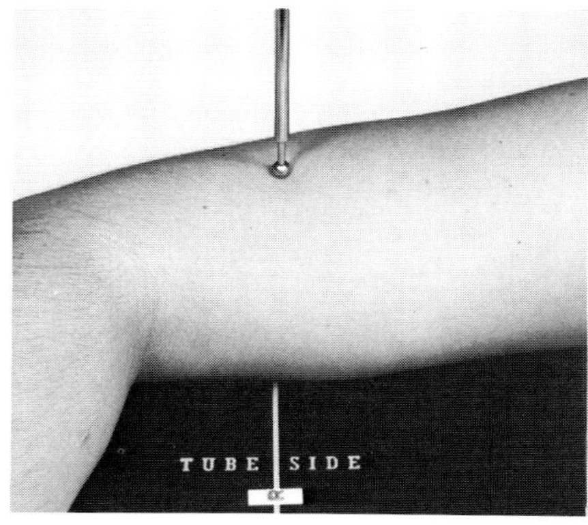

Fig. 7-23. Humerus—lateral position, tabletop.

Central ray

Direct the central ray perpendicular through the shaft of the humerus to the center of each section of the film holder. Collimate to each section of film holder.

Immobilization

Place a sandbag over the hand. Employ suspended respiration.

Right-left markers

Place the correct marker on the lateral side, center border of the film holder.

Technical tips

The distal humerus may best be demonstrated by seating the patient at the end of the table with his elbow extended on the tabletop and the upper arm in internal rotation.

Structures demonstrated

Lateral view of the upper two thirds or the lower two thirds of the humerus.

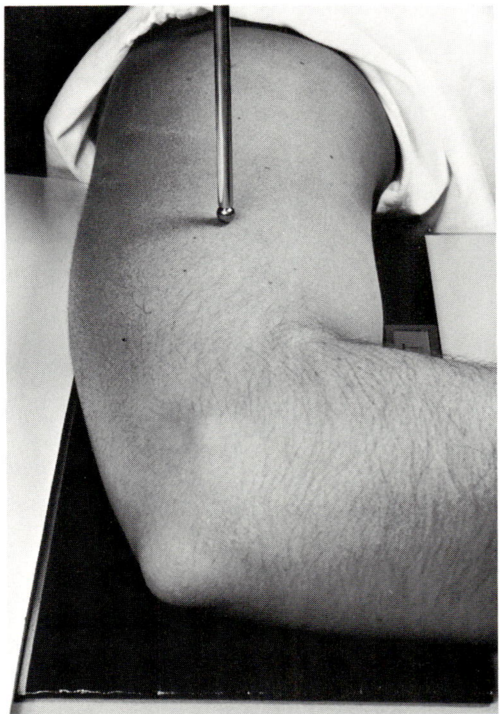

Fig. 7-24. Humerus—lateral position, tabletop.

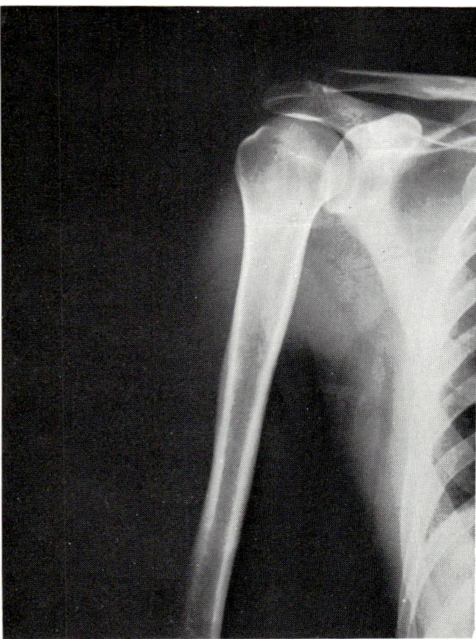

Fig. 7-25. Humerus—lateral view. (Courtesy Dr. E. I. L. Cilley, Dr. T. W. Crowell, Dr. R. E. Waud, and Dr. G. H. Hoffman.)

Toes—posterior (A-P) and oblique views (Figs. 7-26 to 7-28)

Film size—8″ × 10″
No-screen film holder
Crosswise
Tabletop
Collimate to cover

Technique

Factors	Screen film cassette (par)	Screen film no-screen film holder
mA	100	100
Time	0.1	0.75
mAs	10	75
Thickness in cm	2	2
kVp	44	56
Distance	40	40

Patient preparation

Remove shoes and socks from both feet.

Palpation points

Distal ends (heads) of metatarsal bones.

Procedure

Posterior (A-P)—Seat the patient on the table. Flex the knee, and instruct the patient to place the sole of the foot on the medial half of the film holder. Center the third toe to the center of this half of the film holder.

Oblique—From the posterior (A-P) position, rotate the foot internally 45 degrees. Center the third toe to the center of the lateral half of the film holder. Should the toes be superimposed, decrease the angle of rotation or separate the toes with small pieces of cotton, or both.

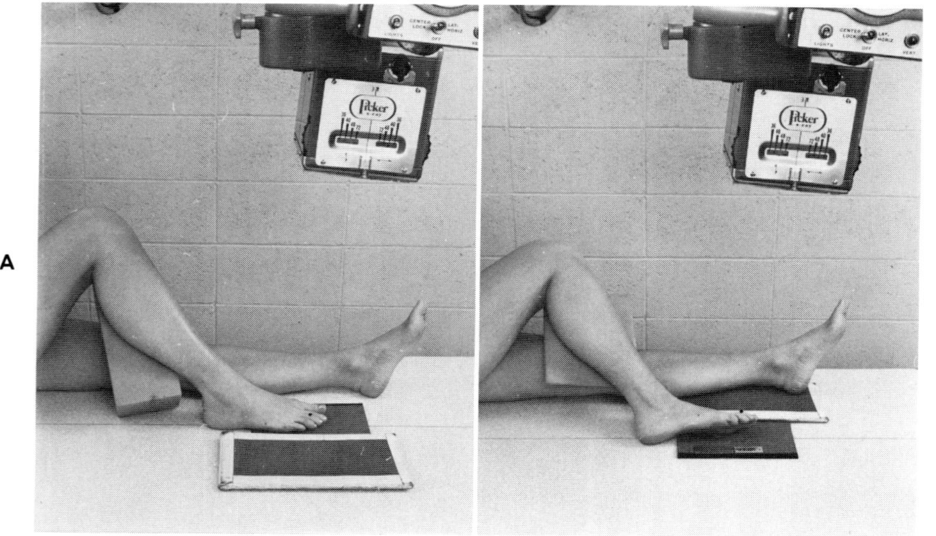

Fig. 7-26. Toe positions. **A,** Posterior (A-P) position. **B,** Oblique position.

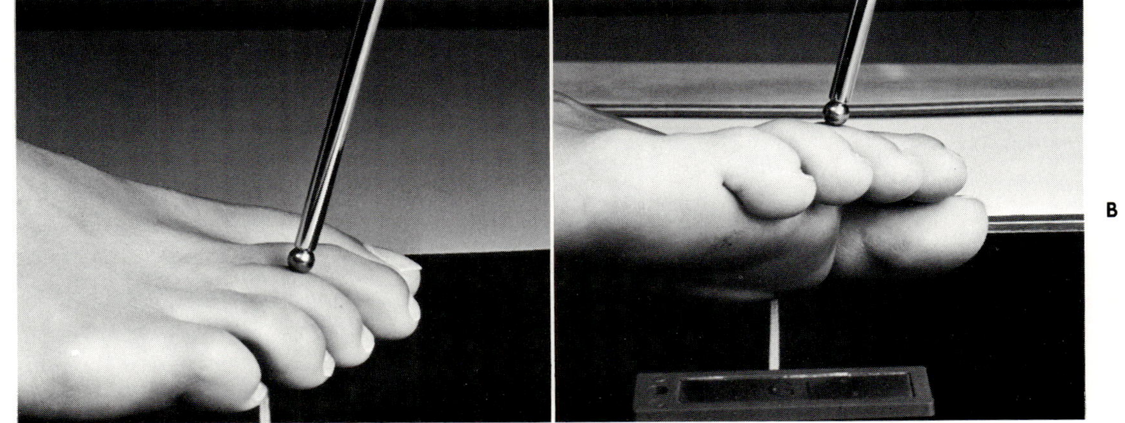

Fig. 7-27. Toe positions. **A,** Posterior (A-P) position. **B,** Oblique position.

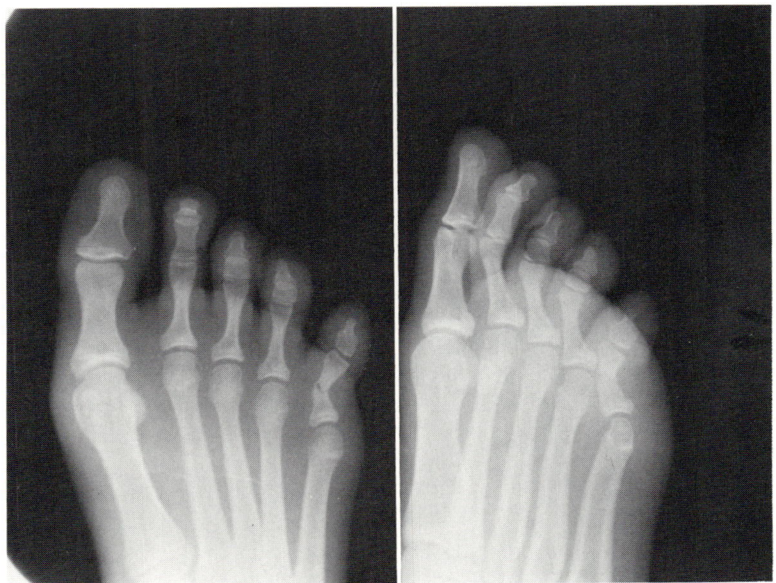

Fig. 7-28. Toe views. Posterior (A-P) and oblique views. (Courtesy Dr. E. I. L. Cilley, Dr. T. W. Crowell, Dr. R. E. Waud, and Dr. G. H. Hoffman.)

Central ray

Direct the central ray perpendicular to the long axis of the toe being examined and to each section of the film holder. Collimate to each section of film holder.

Immobilization

Posterior (A-P)—Place a large sponge between the knees or use a compression band over the foot, or both.

Oblique—Rest the opposite leg on the table, and place a sponge between the knees or use a 45-degree wedge sponge under the sole of the foot, or both.

Right-left markers

Place the correct marker on the oblique view, center border of the film holder.

Technical tips

Patient strain and motion may be reduced by placing the patient in a chair on the floor or on top of the x-ray table.

Structures demonstrated

Posterior (A-P) and oblique views of the toes and distal metatarsals.

Foot—posterior (A-P) (dorsoplantar) and oblique views (Figs. 7-29 to 7-31)

Film size—10″ × 12″
No-screen film holder
Crosswise

Tabletop
Collimate to cover

Technique

Factors	Screen film cassette (par)	Screen film no-screen film holder
mA	100	100
Time	0.1	0.75
mAs	10	75
Thickness in cm	8	8
kVp	56	68
Distance	40	40

Patient preparation

Remove shoes and socks from both feet.

Palpation point

Proximal end of third metatarsal.

Procedure

Posterior (A-P) (dorsoplantar)—Seat the patient on the table. Flex the knee, and instruct the patient to place the sole of the foot on the medial half of the film holder. Center the proximal end of the second metatarsal over the medial half of the film holder.

Oblique—From the posterior (A-P) position, rotate the foot internally 45 degrees. Center the proximal end of the fourth metatarsal over the lateral half of the film holder.

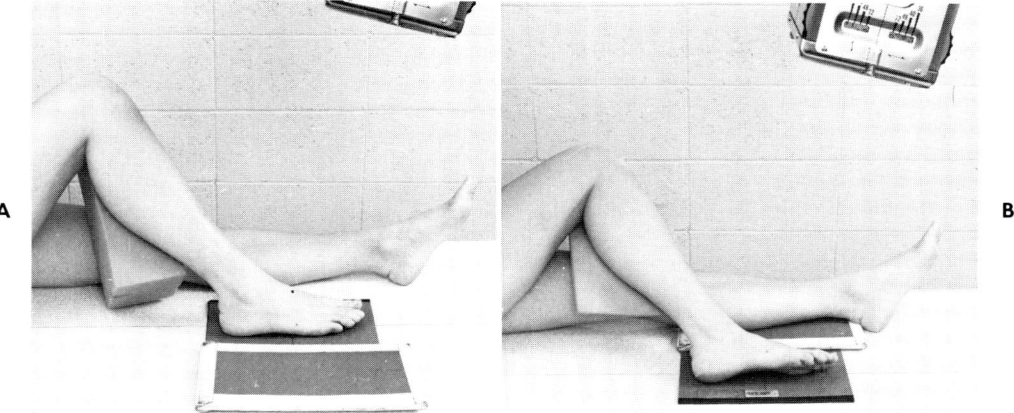

Fig. 7-29. Foot positions. **A,** Posterior (A-P) (dorsoplantar) position. **B,** Oblique position.

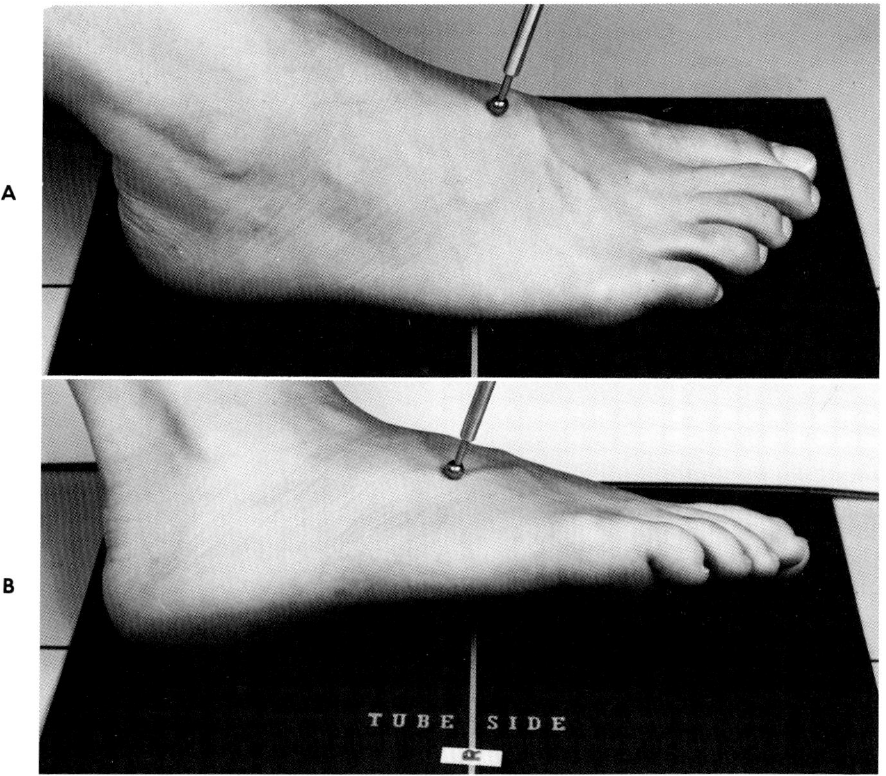

Fig. 7-30. Foot positions. **A,** Posterior (A-P) (dorsoplantar) position. **B,** Oblique position.

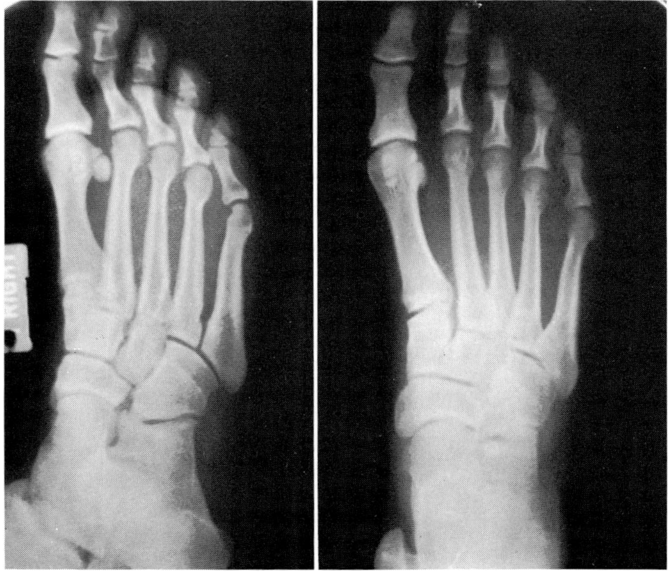

Fig. 7-31. Foot views. Posterior (A-P) (dorsoplantar) and oblique views. (Courtesy Dr. E. I. L. Cilley, Dr. T. W. Crowell, Dr. R. E. Waud, and Dr. G. H. Hoffman.)

Central ray

Direct the central ray 15 degrees cephalad or perpendicular to the long axis of the metatarsal arch through the proximal end of the third metatarsal and to the center of each half of the film holder. Collimate to each section of film holder.

Immobilization

Posterior (A-P) (dorsoplantar)—Place a large sponge between the knees or use a compression band over the foot, or both.

Oblique—Rest the opposite leg on the table, and place a sponge between the knees or use a 45-degree wedge sponge under the sole of the foot, or both.

Right-left markers

Place the correct marker on the oblique view, center border of the film holder.

Technical tips

Patient strain and motion may be reduced by placing the patient in a chair on the floor or on top of the x-ray table.

Structures demonstrated

Posterior (A-P) (dorsoplantar) and oblique views of the tarsals, metatarsals, and phalanges.

Note: Dorsoplantar and lateral *weight-bearing* views should be made when the request specifies pes-planus or pes-cavus radiographs. Dorsoplantar and lateral views should be made when the request specifies foreign body radiographs.

Calcaneus (os calcis) heel—plantodorsal (dorsal) and lateral views (Figs. 7-32 to 7-34)

Film size—8″ × 10″
No-screen film holder
Crosswise
Tabletop
Collimate to cover

Technique

Factors	Screen film cassette (par)	Screen film no-screen film holder
mA	100	100
Time	0.1	0.75
mAs	10	75
Thickness in cm	9	9
kVp	58	70
Distance	40	40

Patient preparation

Remove shoes and socks from both feet.

Palpation points

Lateral and medial malleoli; calcaneal tuberosity.

Procedure

Plantodorsal (dorsal)—Seat the patient on the table. With the legs extended, center the heel being examined on the medial half of the film holder 2½ inches past the center line. Place a strip of gauze or rubber tubing around the ball of the foot, and instruct the patient to hold the flexed foot so that the plantar surface is perpendicular to the film surface.

Lateral—From the plantodorsal (dorsal) position, rotate the leg externally so that a line through both malleoli is perpendicular to the film surface. Cross the unaffected leg over the leg being examined. Center the midpart of the calcaneus to the center of the film holder with the long axis of the foot extending off the lateral side of the film holder.

Central ray

Plantodorsal (dorsal)—Direct the central ray 45 degrees cephalad through the calcaneus to the center of each section of the film holder. Collimate to each section of film holder.

Lateral—Direct the central ray perpendicular to the calcaneus and to the center of each section of the film holder. Collimate to each section of film holder.

Immobilization

Plantodorsal (dorsal)—Place heavy sandbags over the leg and gauze strips or rubber tubing.

Lateral—Place sandbags over the leg. Support the opposite knee with large sponges or sandbags.

Right-left markers

Place the correct marker on the lateral view, bottom center border of film holder.

A C D

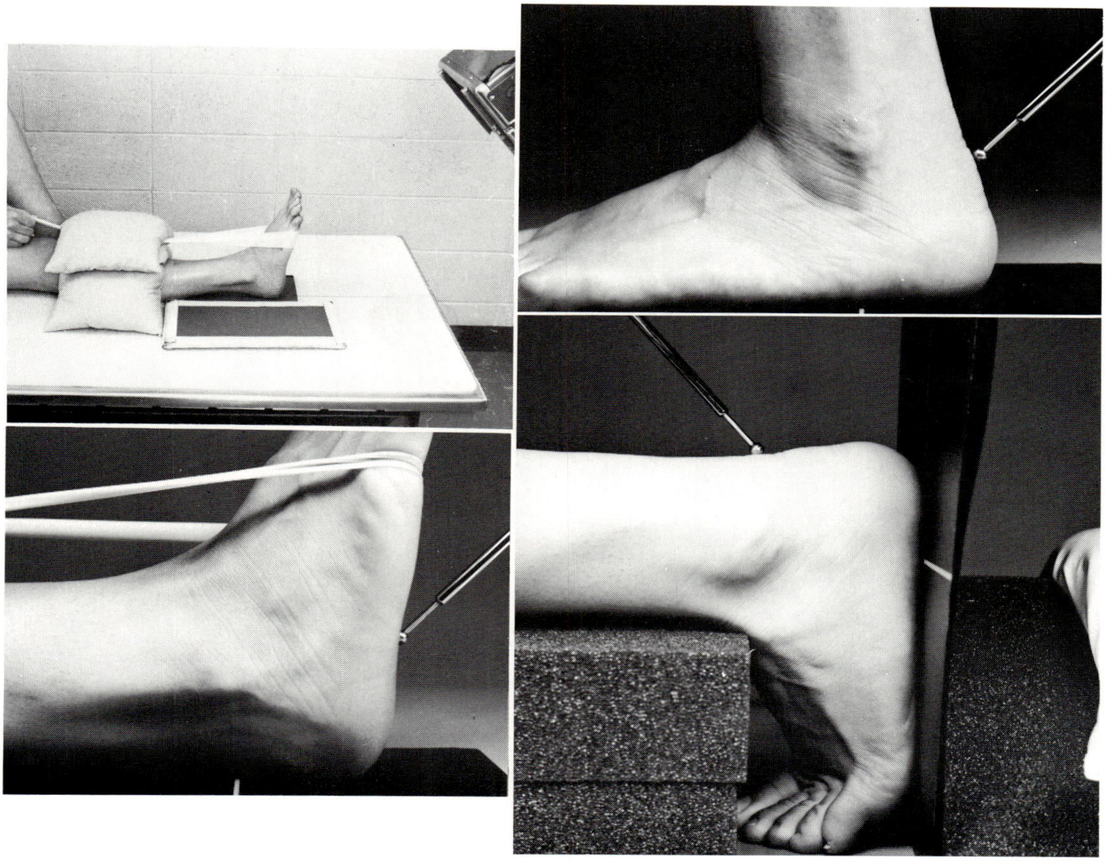

Fig. 7-32. Calcaneus (os calcis) heel positions. **A** and **B**, Plantodorsal (dorsal) positions. **C** and **D**, Dorsoplantar (plantar) positions.

A B

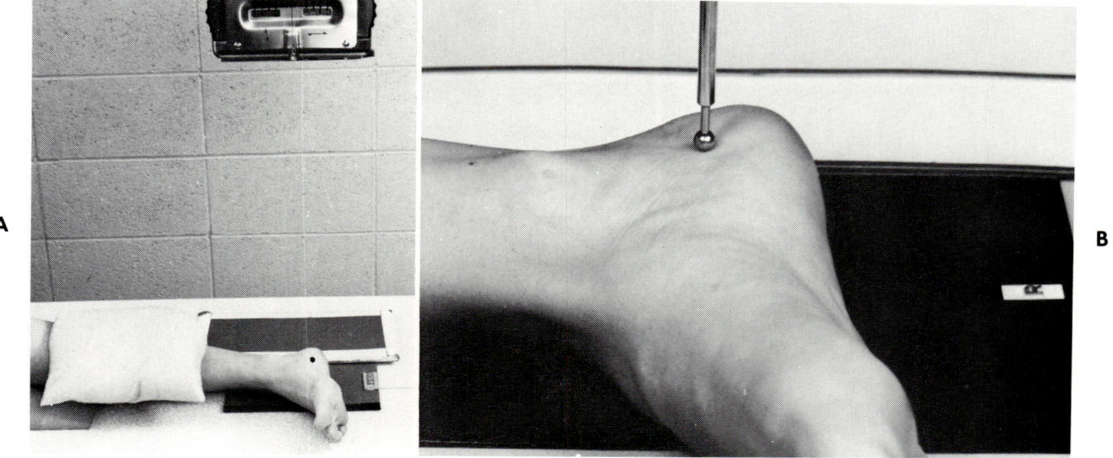

Fig. 7-33. Calcaneus (os calcis) heel positions. **A** and **B**, Lateral positions.

Technical tips

A 45-degree internal oblique plantodorsal projection will demonstrate the talocalcaneal articulation.

Structures demonstrated

Plantodorsal (dorsal)—An axial view of the calcaneus from the tuberosity to the sustentaculum tali.

Lateral—A lateral view of the body of the calcaneus.

Note: Bilateral dorsoplantar projections may be made with the patient standing on the film holder or lying prone with the vertical film holder against the plantar surfaces of both feet.

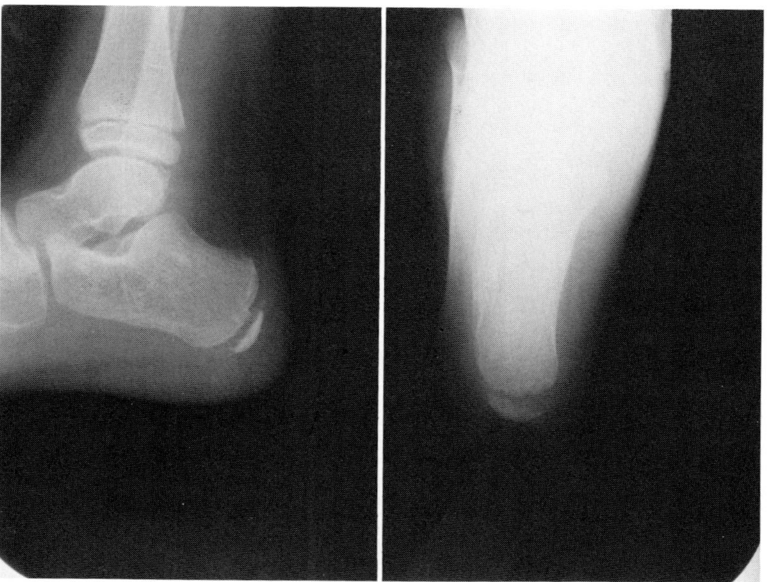

Fig. 7-34. Calcaneus (os calcis) views. Plantodorsal (dorsal) and lateral views. (Courtesy Dr. E. I. L. Cilley, Dr. T. W. Crowell, Dr. R. E. Waud, and Dr. G. H. Hoffman.)

Ankle—posterior (A-P), internal oblique, and lateral views (Figs. 7-35 to 7-37)

Film size—10″ × 12″
No-screen film holder
Crosswise
Tabletop
Collimate to cover

Technique

Factors	Screen film cassette (par)	Screen film no-screen film holder
mA	100	100
Time	0.1	0.75
mAs	10	75
Thickness in cm	9	9
kVp	58	76
Distance	40	40

Patient preparation

Remove shoes and socks from both feet.

Palpation points

Lateral and medial malleoli.

Procedure

Posterior (A-P)—Seat the patient on the table. With the leg extended, center the ankle mortise over the medial third of the film holder. The plantar surface of the foot is perpendicular to the film holder. Rotate the foot and ankle so that a line through both malleoli is parallel with the film surface.

Internal oblique—From the posterior (A-P) position, rotate the ankle internally so that a line through the malleoli forms a 45-degree angle with the film surface.

Lateral—From the posterior (A-P) position, rotate the leg externally so that a line through the malleoli is perpendicular to the film surface. Cross the unaffected leg over the leg being examined. Center the lateral malleolus to the center of the film holder with the longer axis of the foot extending off the lateral side of the film holder.

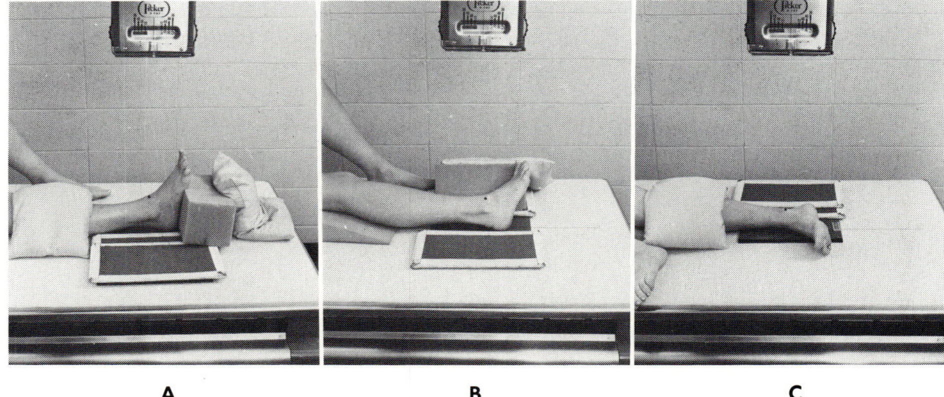

Fig. 7-35. Ankle positions. **A,** Posterior (A-P) position. **B,** Internal oblique position. **C,** Lateral position.

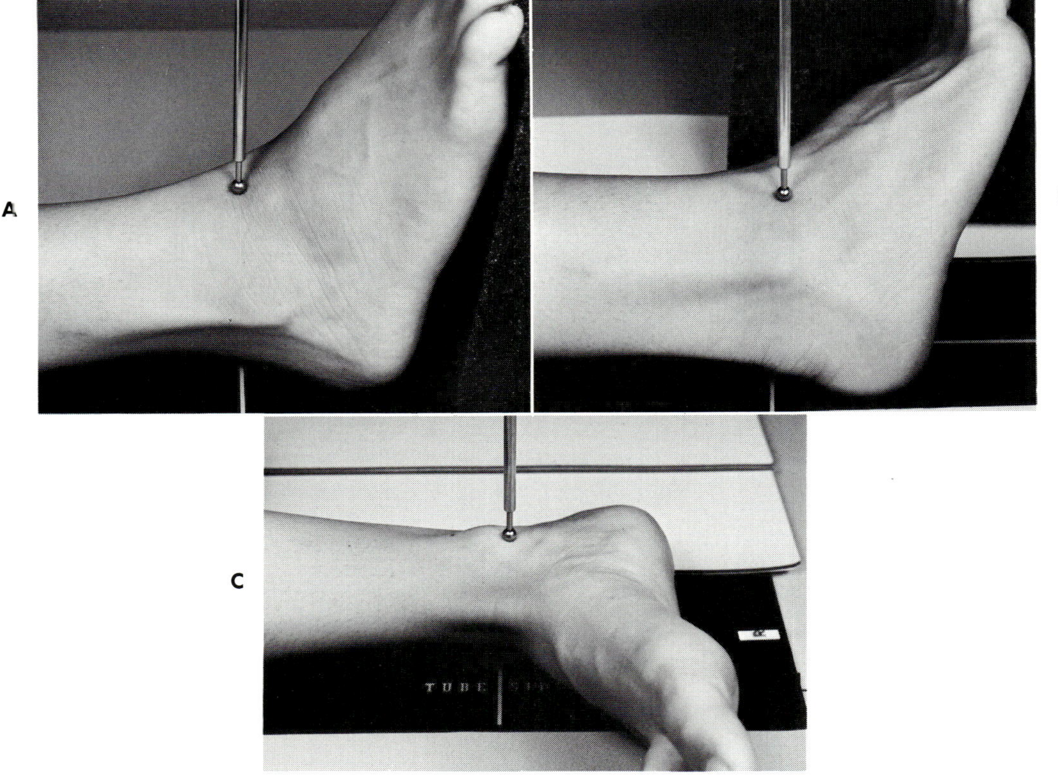

Fig. 7-36. Ankle positions. **A,** Posterior (A-P) position. **B,** Internal oblique position. **C,** Lateral position.

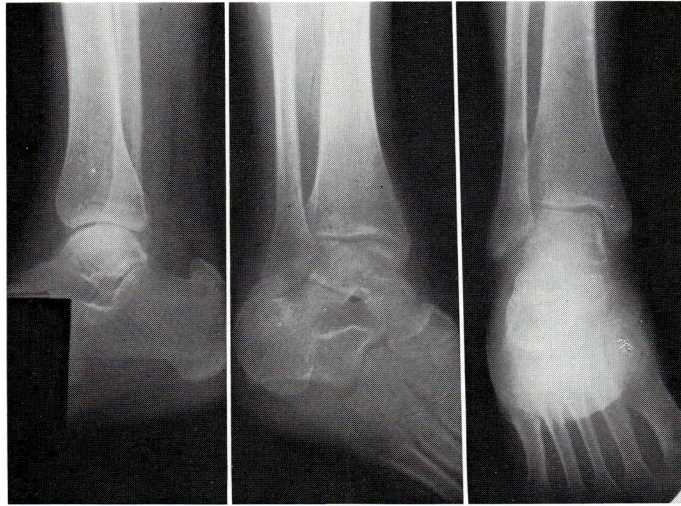

Fig. 7-37. Ankle views. Lateral, internal oblique, and posterior views. (Courtesy Dr. E. I. L. Cilley, Dr. T. W. Crowell, Dr. R. E. Waud, and Dr. G. H. Hoffman.)

Central ray

Direct the central ray perpendicular through the midportion of the ankle mortise in line with the tip of the medial malleolus to the center of each section of the film holder. Collimate to each section of film holder.

Immobilization

Place a radiolucent sponge beneath the knee. Place sandbags over the leg. Brace the plantar surface of the foot with a sponge and sandbag.

Right-left markers

Place the correct marker on the lateral view, bottom center border of the film holder.

Technical tips

For a true A-P position, the foot and ankle must be rotated internally 10 to 15 degrees.

Structures demonstrated

Posterior (A-P), internal oblique, and lateral views of the distal one third of the tibia and fibula, of the ankle mortise, and of the talus.

Ankle—posterior (A-P) forced inversion and forced eversion views (Figs. 7-38 to 7-40)

Film size—8″ × 10″
No-screen film holder
Crosswise
Tabletop
Collimate to cover

Technique

Factors	Screen film cassette (par)	Screen film no-screen film holder
mA	100	100
Time	0.1	0.75
mAs	10	75
Thickness in cm	9	9
kVp	60	72
Distance	40	40

Patient preparation

Remove shoes and socks from both feet.

Palpation points

Lateral and medial malleoli.

Procedure

Inversion—Seat the patient on the table. With the leg extended, center the ankle mortise over the medial half of the film holder. The plantar surface of the foot is perpendicular to the film holder. Rotate the ankle so that a line through both malleoli is parallel with the film surface. Invert the foot as far as possible. Place a strip of gauze around the ball of the foot and instruct the patient to hold the foot forcibly in this position.

Eversion—From the posterior (A-P) inversion position evert the foot as far as possible. Place a strip of gauze around the ball of the foot and instruct the patient to hold the foot forcibly in this position.

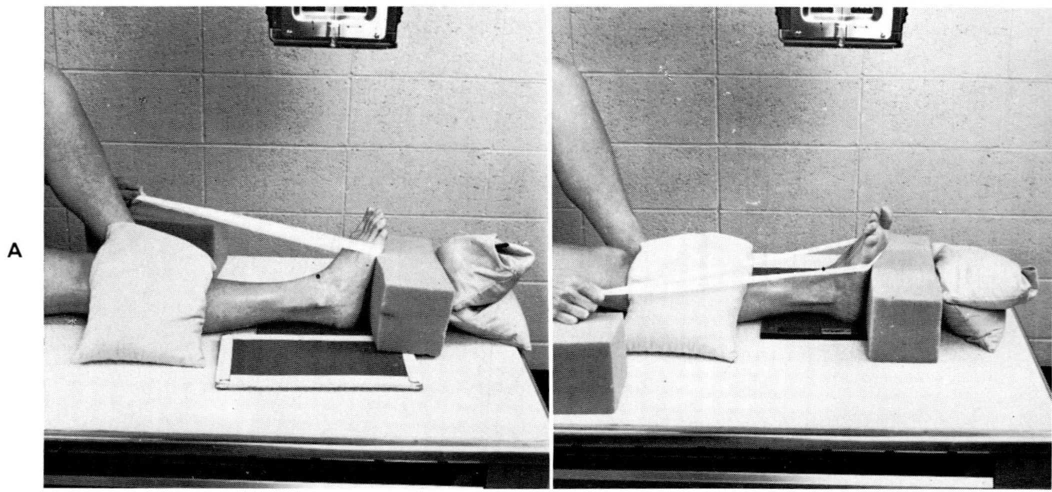

Fig. 7-38. Ankle positions. **A**, Forced inversion position. **B**, Forced eversion position.

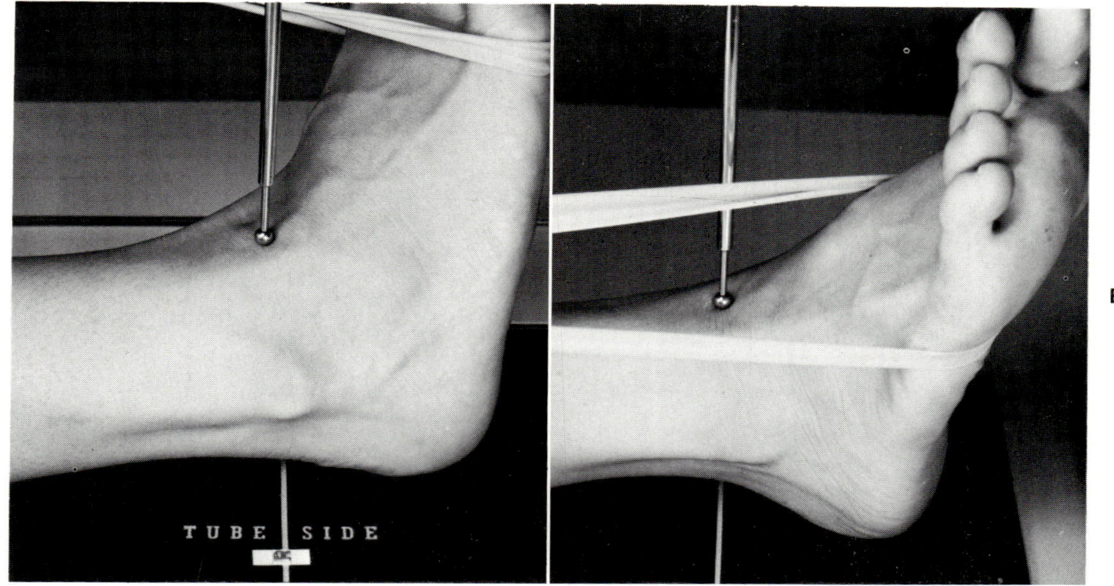

Fig. 7-39. Ankle positions. **A,** Forced inversion position. **B,** Forced eversion position.

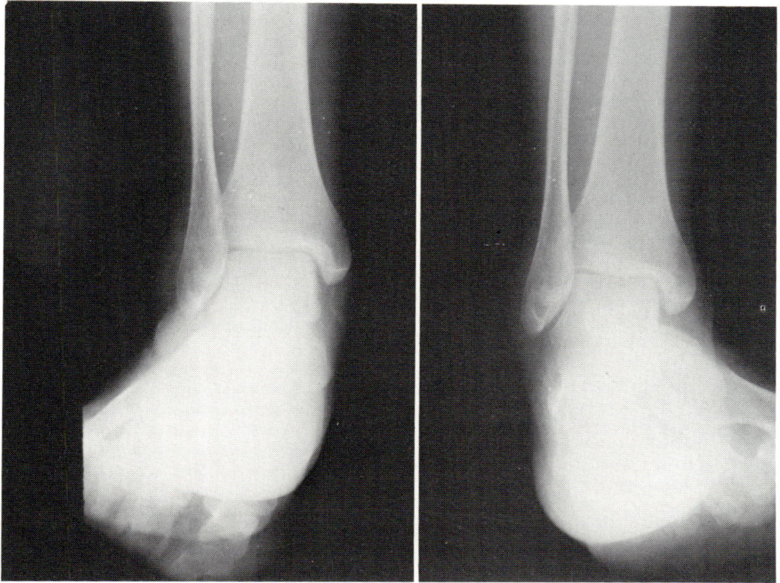

Fig. 7-40. Ankle views. Forced inversion and forced eversion views. (Courtesy Dr. E. I. L. Cilley, Dr. T. W. Crowell, Dr. R. E. Waud, and Dr. G. H. Hoffman.)

Central ray

Direct the central ray perpendicular through the midportion of the ankle mortise in line with the tip of the medial malleolus to the center of each section of the film holder. Collimate to each section of film holder.

Immobilization

Place a radiolucent sponge beneath the knee. Place heavy sandbags over the leg. Brace the plantar surface of the foot with a sponge supported by a sandbag.

Right-left markers

Place the correct marker on the eversion view, lateral side, center border of film holder.

Technical tips

Forced positions may be held in place by attaching a sandbag to the gauze sling around the foot and allowing the sandbag to hang over the side of the table.

Structures demonstrated

Inversion—An unobstructed view of the external malleolus, and medial stress on the ankle mortise.

Eversion—Lateral stress on the ankle mortise.

Note: Bilateral views should be made for comparison purposes.

Leg—posterior (A-P) and lateral views (Figs. 7-41 to 7-43)

Film size—14″ × 17″ or 7″ × 17″
Cassette
Lengthwise
Tabletop
Collimate to cover

Technique

Factors	Screen film cassette (par)
mA	100
Time	0.1
mAs	10
Thickness in cm	8
kVp	56
Distance	40

Patient preparation

Remove shoes, socks, and any other garments from both legs.

Palpation points

Lateral and medial malleoli; lateral and medial epicondyles of the femur; apex of the patella.

Procedure

Posterior (A-P)—Place the patient in the supine position on the table. With the leg extended, center the shaft of the tibia over the medial half of the film holder. Include both ankle and knee joints on the film, if possible, or the joint nearer the injured site. Rotate the epicondyles of the femur so that a line through them is parallel with the film surface.

Lateral—From the posterior (A-P) position, rotate the leg externally so that a plane through both malleoli and both femoral epicondyles is perpendicular to the film surface. Cross the unaffected leg over the leg being examined. Center the anterior two thirds of the leg to the center of the lateral half of the film holder.

Central ray

Direct the central ray perpendicular through the long axis of the leg to the center of each section of the film holder. Collimate to each section of film holder.

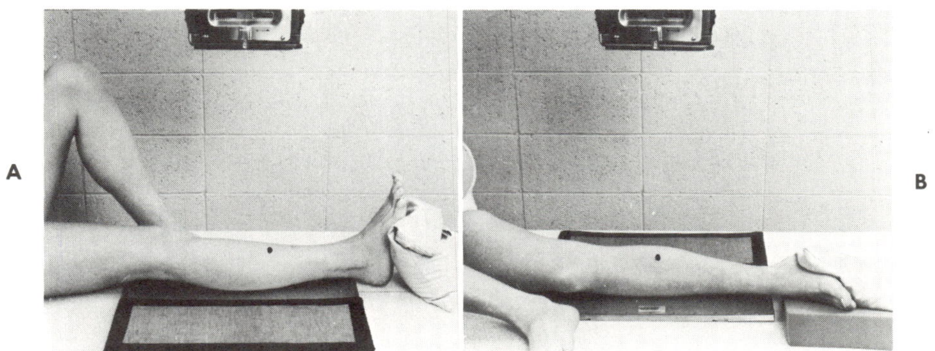

Fig. 7-41. Leg positions. **A,** Posterior (A-P) position. **B,** Lateral position.

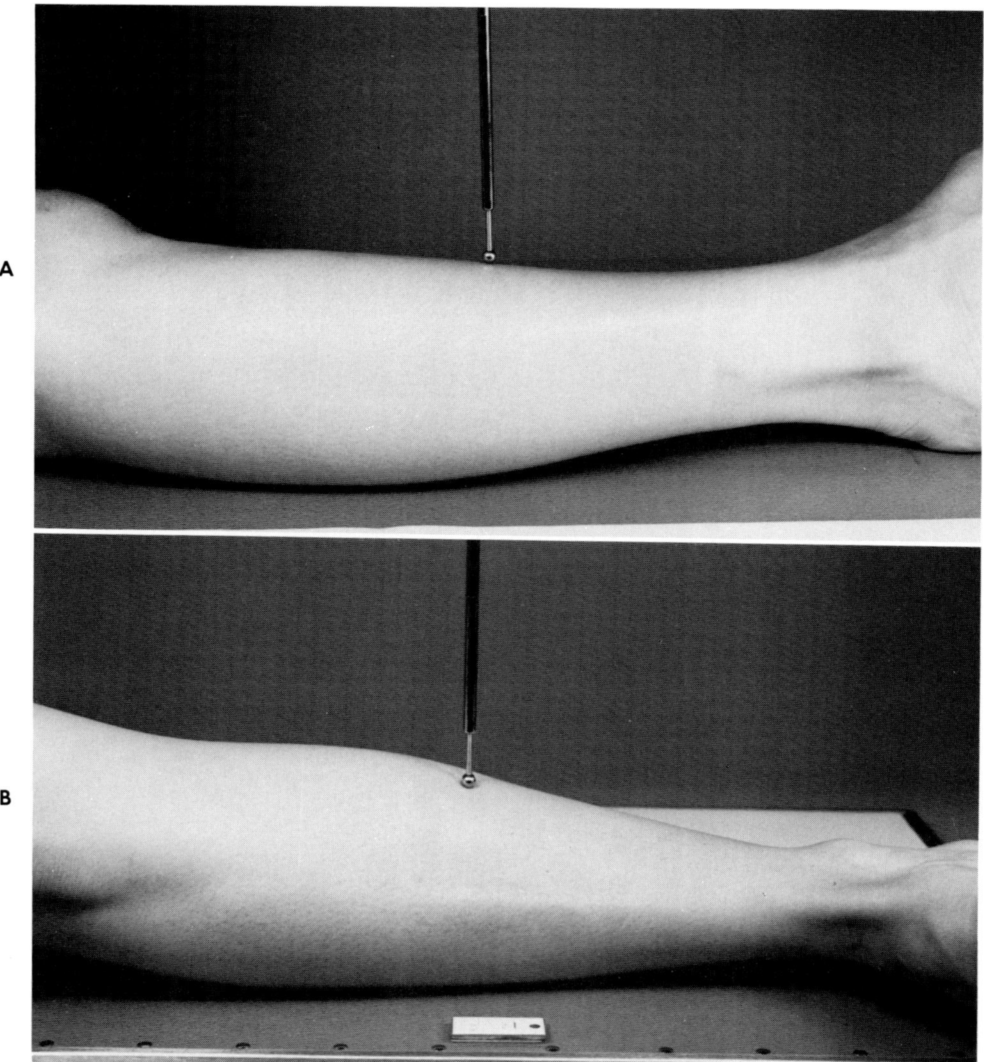

Fig. 7-42. Leg positions. **A,** Posterior (A-P) position. **B,** Lateral position.

Immobilization

Place a sandbag against the foot and a large sponge under the flexed knee.

Right-left markers

Place the correct marker on the lateral view, lateral center border of the film holder.

Technical tips

In the lateral position, have the patient rest on his forearm to reduce strain and motion.

Structures demonstrated

Posterior (A-P) and lateral views of the tibia and fibula, and of the ankle or knee joints or both.

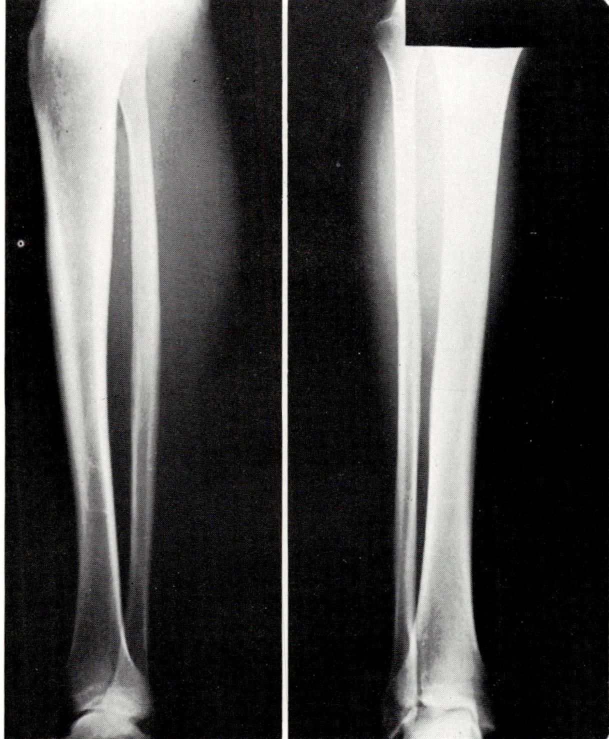

Fig. 7-43. Leg views. Posterior (A-P) and lateral views. (Courtesy Dr. E. I. L. Cilley, Dr. T. W. Crowell, Dr. R. E. Waud, and Dr. G. H. Hoffman.)

Knee—posterior (A-P) view (Figs. 7-44 to 7-46)

Film size—8″ × 10″
Cassette
Lengthwise

Tabletop
Collimate to cover

Technique

Factors	Screen film cassette (par)
mA	100
Time	0.1
mAs	10
Thickness in cm	12
kVp	62
Distance	40

Patient preparation

Remove both shoes and any garments around knee area. Provide a gown if necessary.

Palpation points

Lateral and medial epicondyles of femur; apex of patella; tibial tuberosity.

Procedure

Seat the patient on the table. With the legs extended, center the apex of the patella over the center of the film holder. Rotate the leg so that a line through both femoral epicondyles is parallel with the film surface.

Central ray

Direct the central ray 5 degrees cephalad to the center of the film holder. Collimate to film holder.

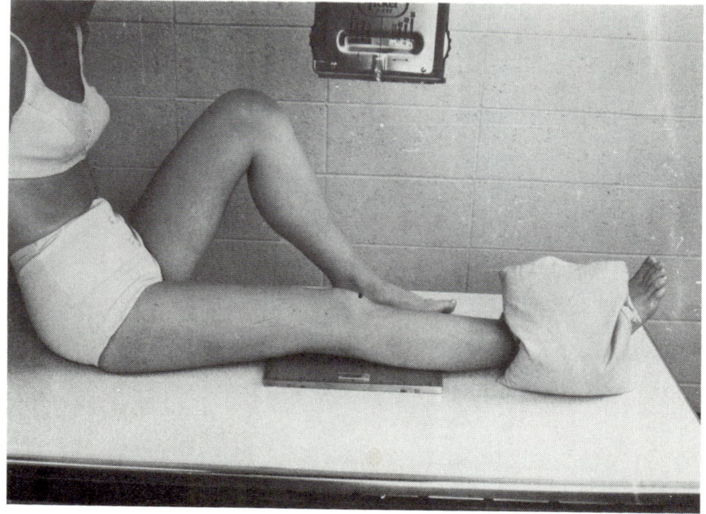

Fig. 7-44. Knee—posterior (A-P) position.

Immobilization

Place sandbags on each side of the foot and on top of the leg.

Right-left markers

Place the correct marker on the lateral center border of the film holder.

Technical tips

The apex (bottom) of the patella is directly over the knee joint.

Structures demonstrated

Posterior (A-P) view of the knee joint, patella, and intercondylar eminence.

Note: The patella or tibial tuberosity (for Osgood-Schlatter disease) is best demonstrated in P-A positions or 45-degree P-A (internal and external oblique positions).

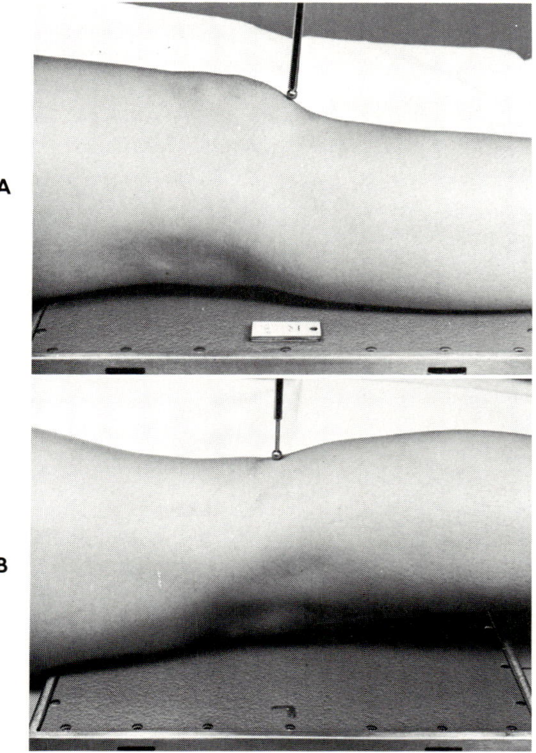

Fig. 7-45. Knee positions. **A,** Posterior (A-P) position. **B,** Anterior (P-A) position.

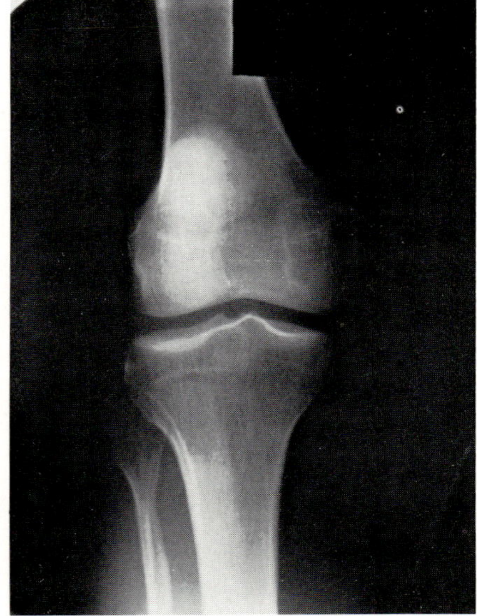

Fig. 7-46. Knee—posterior (A-P) view. (Courtesy Dr. E. I. L. Cilley, Dr. T. W. Crowell, Dr. R. E. Waud, and Dr. G. H. Hoffman.)

Knee—lateral view (Figs. 7-47 to 7-49)

Film size—8″ × 10″
Cassette
Lengthwise

Tabletop
Collimate to cover

Technique

Factors	Screen film cassette (par)
mA	100
Time	0.1
mAs	10
Thickness in cm	10
kVp	58
Distance	40

Patient preparation

Remove both shoes and any garments around the knee area. Provide a gown if necessary.

Palpation points

Lateral and medial epicondyles of the femur; apex of the patella; tibial tuberosity.

Procedure

Place the patient on the table with the side of the leg being examined down. Cross the opposite leg over the leg being examined. Flex the injured leg 45 degrees and center the midpart of the knee ½ inch below the medial epicondyle to the center of the film holder. The shaft of the femur should extend off the superior midcenter of the film holder. The shaft of the tibia should bisect the

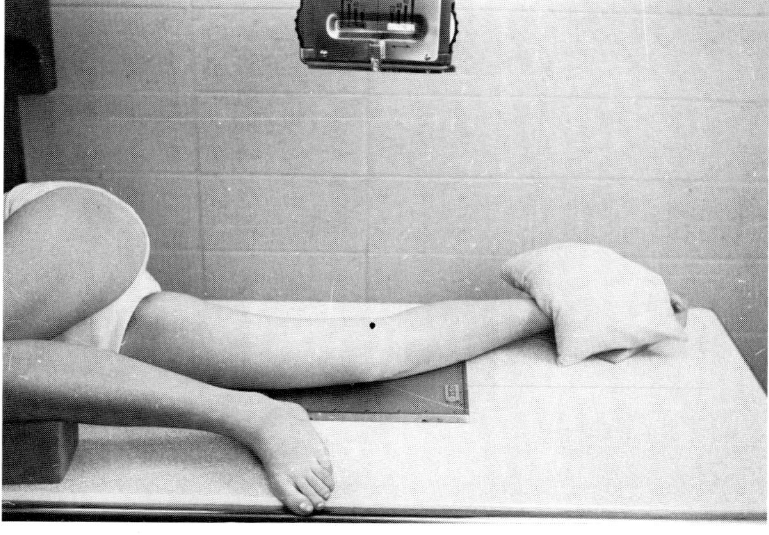

Fig. 7-47. Knee—lateral position.

lower posterior angle of the film holder. Rotate the leg so that a line through both femoral epicondyles is perpendicular to the film surface.

Central ray

Direct the central ray perpendicular through the knee to the center of the film holder. Collimate to film holder.

Immobilization

Place a wedge sponge or sandbag under the foot and a sandbag over the ankle and leg. Place a large sponge under the opposite knee for support.

Right-left markers

Center the correct marker on the inferior border of the film holder below the patella.

Technical tips

For correct superimposition of femoral condyles, keep the long axis of the femur and the tibia parallel with the film.

Structures demonstrated

Lateral view of the distal femur, patella, proximal tibia, and fibula.

Note: For supine or prone patients, make lateral to medial projections on a vertical film holder placed between the patient's knees.

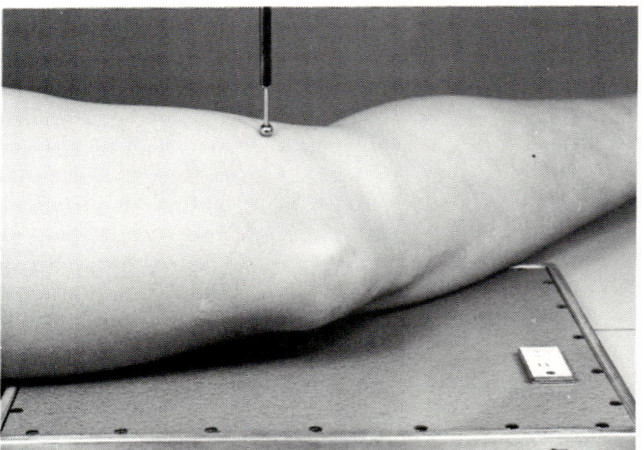

Fig. 7-48. Knee—lateral position.

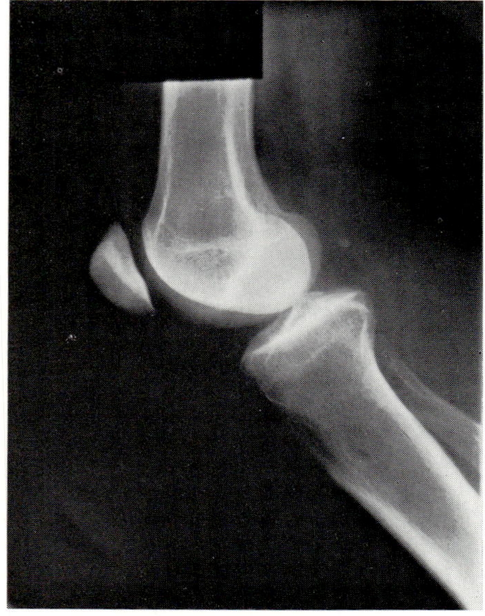

Fig. 7-49. Knee—lateral view. (Courtesy Dr. E. I. L. Cilley, Dr. T. W. Crowell, Dr. R. E. Waud, and Dr. G. H. Hoffman.)

Knee—notch (intercondylar) view (Figs. 7-50 to 7-52)

Film size—8″ × 10″
Cassette or no-screen film holder
Lengthwise
Tabletop
Extension cone (fully extended)

Technique

Factors	Screen film cassette (par)	Screen film no-screen film holder
mA	100	100
Time	0.1	0.75
mAs	10	75
Thickness in cm	13	13
kVp	66	78
Distance	40	40

Patient preparation

Remove both shoes and any garments around the knee area. Provide a gown if necessary.

Palpation points

Lateral and medial epicondyles of the femur; apex of the patella.

Procedure

Place the patient on the table in the kneeling position with both feet extended over the end of the table. Center the apex of the patella to the center of the film holder. Position the body so that the long axis of both the femur and tibia are in the same plane. Instruct the patient to lean forward so the shaft of the femur will form a 25-degree angle with the central ray.

Central ray

Direct the central ray perpendicular through the knee to the center of the film holder.

Immobilization

Place wedge sponges under both ankles and a sponge under the opposite knee to alleviate discomfort.

Right-left markers

The correct marker is burned in the superior center border of the film over the cone field after the exposure is made.

Technical tips

Place elderly patients in a kneeling position on a bench at the end of the table, with the thorax resting on the tabletop.

Structures demonstrated

Anterior (P-A) views of the intercondylar fossa, joint space between the femur and tibia, tibial plateau, and intercondylar eminence.

Note: For supine patients, place a curved or flexible film holder beneath the posterior surface of the knee (flexed 115 degrees) and reverse the central ray angle through the notch to the film holder.

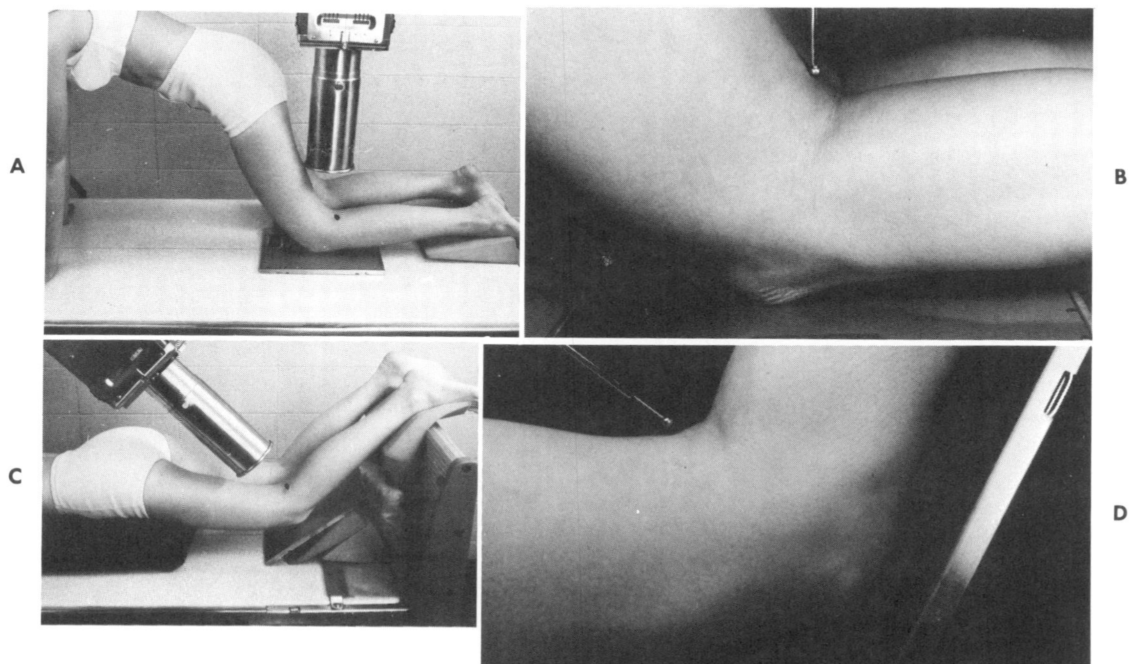

Fig. 7-50. Knee—notch (intercondylar) position. A and B, Normal notch position. C and D, Variation of normal notch position.

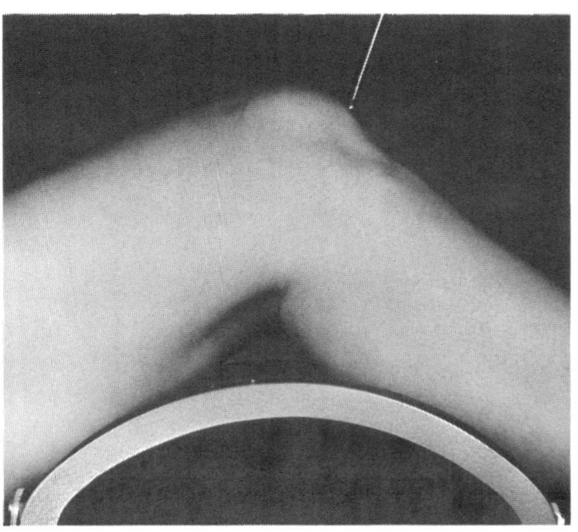

Fig. 7-51. Knee—notch (intercondylar) posterior (A-P) position.

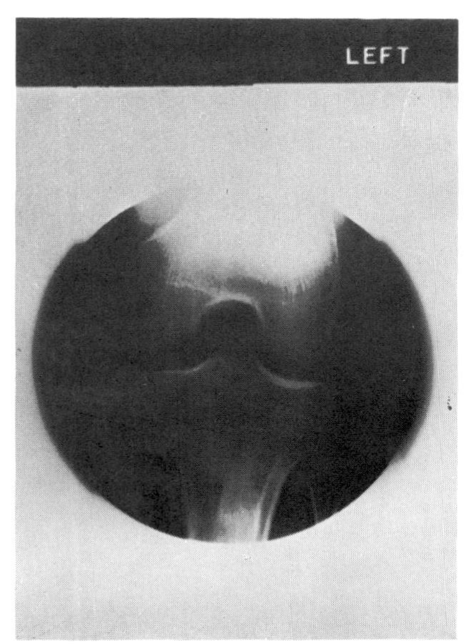

Fig. 7-52. Knee—notch (intercondylar) view. (Courtesy Dr. E. I. L. Cilley, Dr. T. W. Crowell, Dr. R. E. Waud, and Dr. G. H. Hoffman.)

Knee—patella—tangential view (Figs. 7-53 to 7-55)

Film size—8″ × 10″
Cassette or no-screen film holder
Lengthwise
Tabletop
Extension cone (fully extended)

Technique

Factors	Screen film cassette (par)	Screen film no-screen film holder
mA	100	100
Time	0.1	0.75
mAs	10	75
Thickness in cm	13	13
kVp	66	78
Distance	40	40

Patient preparation

Remove both shoes and any garments around the knee area. Provide a gown if necessary.

Palpation points

Lateral and medial epicondyles of the femur; patellar body and apex.

Procedure

Place the patient in the prone position. Flex the knee slowly so that the long axis of the tibia forms a 60-degree angle with the femur. Center the cassette under the patella. Place a gauze strip around the ankle and extend the gauze over the shoulder; instruct the patient to hold the gauze securely.

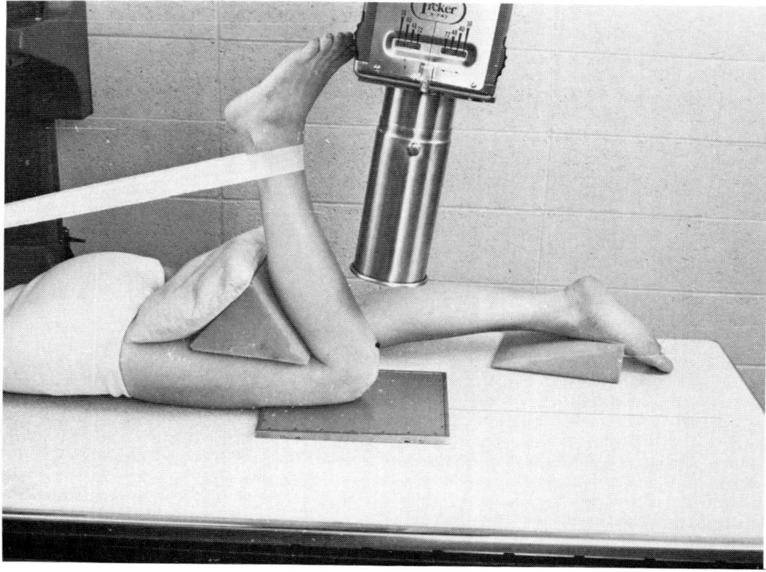

Fig. 7-53. Knee—patella, tangential position.

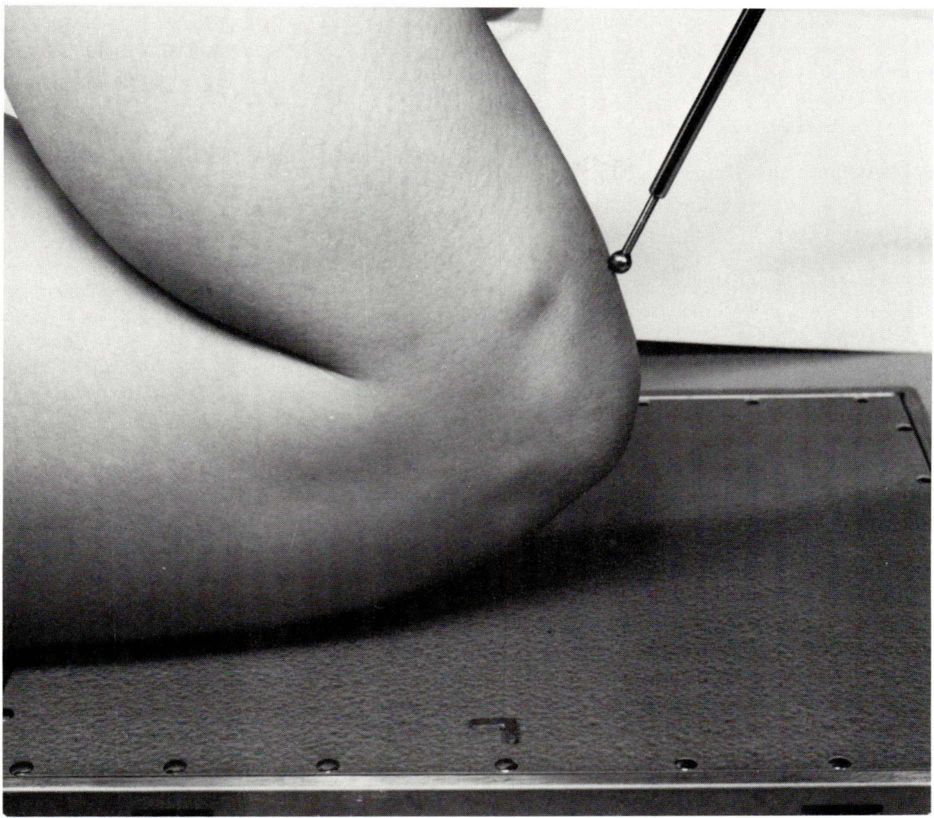

Fig. 7-54. Knee—patella, tangential position.

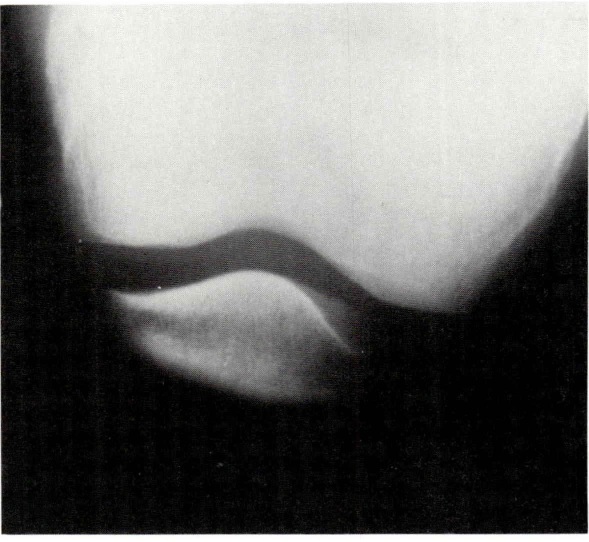

Fig. 7-55. Knee—patella, tangential view. (Courtesy Dr. Frank S. Cavallaro and Valley Hospital, Las Vegas, Nevada.)

Central ray

Direct the central ray 10 degrees cephalad through the patella to the center of the film holder.

Immobilization

Place sandbags over the femur. Place a wedge sponge in the back of the knee to support the leg. The gauze strip around the ankle should complete the immobilization.

Right-left markers

The correct marker is burned in the superior center border of the film holder over the cone field after the exposure is made.

Technical tips

The long axis of the tibia is located in the anterior one third of the leg.

Structures demonstrated

Axial views of the patella and patellar surface of the femur.

Note: For supine patients, have the patient support the film holder parallel with the femur over the anterior knee (flexed 60 degrees) and reverse the central ray angle through the patella to the film holder.

Femur—posterior (A-P) view (Figs. 7-56 to 7-58)

Film size—14″ × 17″ or 7″ × 17″	*Bucky*
Cassette	*Collimate to cover*
Lengthwise	

Technique

Factors	Screen film cassette (par) Bucky	Screen film cassette (par) tabletop
mA	100	100
Time	0.7	0.1
mAs	70	10
Thickness in cm	16	16
kVp	66	72
Distance	40	40

Patient preparation

Remove shoes and garments from waist to knee. Provide a gown.

Palpation points

Lateral and medial epicondyles and greater trochanter of the femur; apex of the patella.

Procedure

Place the patient in the supine position with the legs fully extended. Center the long axis of the femur over the center line of the table. Rotate the leg so that a line through both femoral epicondyles is parallel with the film surface. Include the joint nearer to the injured site. For the upper femur, place the superior edge of the cassette 3 inches above the greater trochanter. For the lower femur, place the inferior edge of the cassette 2 inches below the apex of the patella.

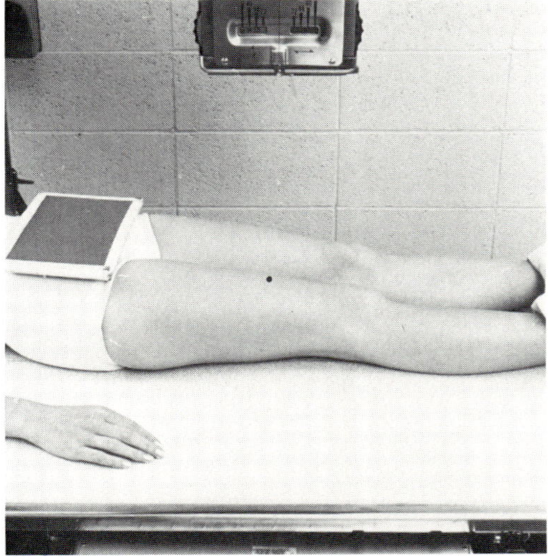

Fig. 7-56. Femur—posterior (A-P) position.

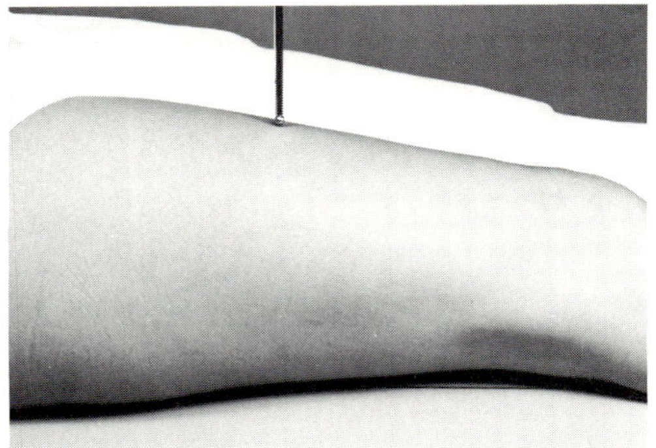

Fig. 7-57. Femur—posterior (A-P) position.

Central ray

Direct the central ray perpendicular through the shaft of the femur to the center of the film holder. Collimate to film holder.

Immobilization

Place sandbags on each side of the foot. Employ suspended expiration.

Right-left markers

Place the correct marker on the lateral center border of the film holder.

Technical tips

Keep the long axis of the femur parallel with the film by placing a radiolucent sponge beneath the posterior knee.

Structures demonstrated

Posterior (A-P) views of the femur, hip, and/or knee joints.

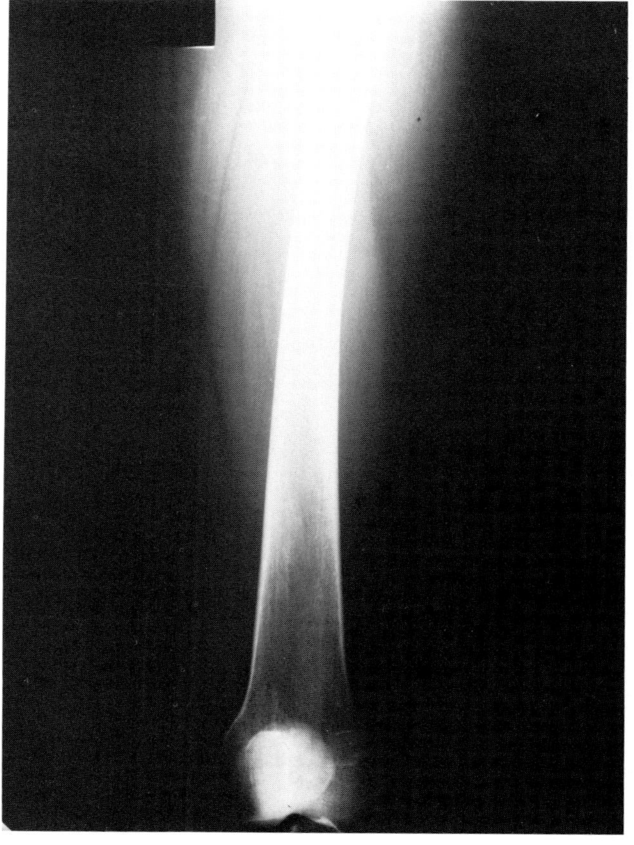

Fig. 7-58. Femur—posterior (A-P) view. (Courtesy Dr. E. I. L. Cilley, Dr. T. W. Crowell, Dr. R. E. Waud, and Dr. G. H. Hoffman.)

Femur—lateral view (Figs. 7-59 to 7-61)

Film size—14" × 17" or 7" × 17"
Cassette
Lengthwise
Bucky
Collimate to cover

Technique

Factors	Screen film cassette (par) Bucky	Screen film cassette (par) tabletop
mA	100	100
Time	0.7	0.1
mAs	70	10
Thickness in cm	16	16
kVp	66	72
Distance	40	40

Patient preparation

Remove shoes and garments from wait to knee. Provide a gown.

Palpation points

Lateral and medial epicondyles and greater trochanter of the femur; apex of the patella.

Procedure

Place the patient in a lateral recumbent position on the side being examined. Flex the opposite knee and cross it over the affected leg as far as possible. Center the long axis of the femur over the center line of the table. Rotate the body so that a line through both femoral epicondyles is perpendicular to the film surface. Place the inferior edge of the cassette 2 inches below the apex of the patella.

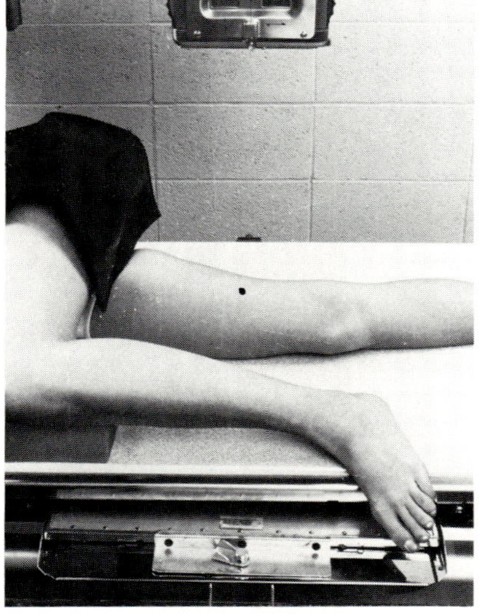

Fig. 7-59. Femur—lateral position.

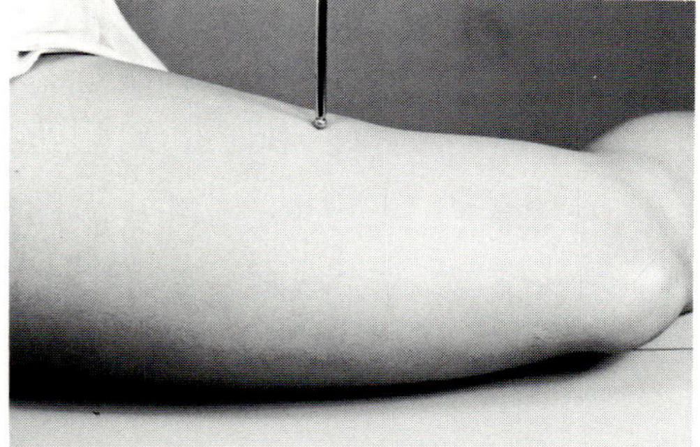

Fig. 7-60. Femur—lateral position.

Central ray

Direct the central ray perpendicular through the shaft of the femur to the center of the film holder. Collimate to film holder.

Immobilization

Place a sponge under the foot, and sandbags on the leg of the affected side. Place a large sponge under the opposite knee for support.

Right-left markers

Place the correct marker on the anterior center border of the film holder.

Technical tips

Adjust technique as necessary to compensate for an increased thickness of the proximal thigh.

Structures demonstrated

Lateral views of the lower two thirds of the femur, knee joint, and patella.

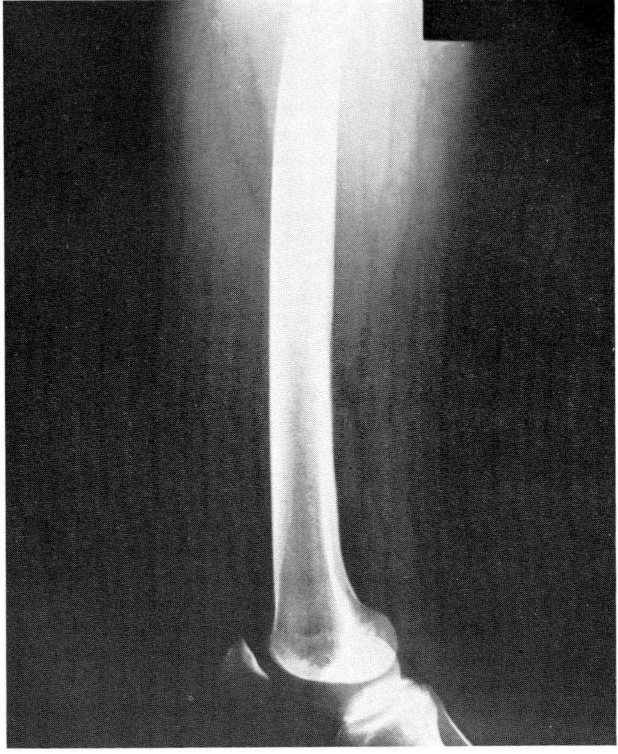

Fig. 7-61. Femur—lateral view. (Courtesy Dr. E. I. L. Cilley, Dr. T. W. Crowell, Dr. R. E. Waud, and Dr. G. H. Hoffman.)

QUESTIONS

1. What is the name of the prominent projection that can be felt at the inner margin of the elbow?
2. In the anteroposterior view of the knee, what central ray angle and direction must be used to better visualize the joint space?
3. What degree of angulation must you use to obtain an oblique view of the right hand?
4. Describe the routine procedure for the left wrist.
5. What view does one obtain with the patient prone and the affected knee fully flexed with the patella at right angles to the film?
6. Describe the view to best visualize the talofibular articulation.
7. Describe the radiographic procedure for the right elbow.
8. Name the radiographic procedure when the central ray is perpendicular to the film and the leg and ankle is rotated medially 45 degrees.
9. Name the radiographic position that would best demonstrate the radial head.
10. Describe the radiographic procedure for the anteroposterior humerus.
11. In addition to weight-bearing views, when is it essential to include a "lateral view" in a routine foot series?
12. What is the normal degree of central ray angulation in the routine dorsoplantar view of the foot?
13. Name the major palpation points used in the lateral view of the left ankle.
14. Which maneuver is used to better demonstrate the scaphoid bone in the routine radiographic procedure of the wrist?
15. Describe the radiographic position to best demonstrate the longitudinal arch of the foot.
16. Describe the normal anatomic position.
17. Give three names of the radiographic position that best demonstrates the intercondylar fossa (or notch) of the femur.
18. Describe the radiographic procedure for Jones' view of the patella.
19. Describe the radiographic procedures for weight-bearing views of both feet.

8 • BONES OF THE TRUNK

VERTEBRAL COLUMN

The vertebral column consists of twenty-four true vertebrae and nine other segments. It is divided into five sections: the *cervical,* seven vertebrae, the first of which is called the *atlas* and the second the *axis;* the *thoracic,* twelve vertebrae; the *lumbar,* five vertebrae; the *sacrum,* five segments that are fused together; and the *coccyx,* from three to five segments, with an average of four. A lateral projection of the vertebral column demonstrates four distinct curves; the cervical, anteriorly convex; the thoracic, anteriorly concave; the lumbar, anteriorly convex; and the sacrum and coccyx, anteriorly concave. (See Fig. 8-1.)

Since the x rays radiate from the target in an arc limited in degrees by the tube port and the cone or diaphragm, it is often useful to take advantage of the natural spinal curvatures for radiography. Since the anterior curvatures of the thoracic spine and sacrococcygeal region are concave, a posterior projection permits the x rays to pass between the vertebral bodies and demonstrate the intervertebral spaces. Because the anterior curvatures of the cervical and lumbar regions are convex, the best separation of the vertebral bodies in these regions results from anterior projections. It is necessary either to obtain prior permission to change routine or to inform the physician who reads the radiographs of any changes from routine in the positions used.

Common aspects of all vertebrae

Two distinct portions are found in each vertebra: anteriorly, the *body,* and posteriorly, the *neural,* or vertebral, *arch.* These parts enclose the *spinal foramen.** The neural arch is composed of the two *pedicles* and the two *laminae.* Seven processes extend from the neural arch: four articular, two transverse, and one spinous. One of the functions of the vertebrae is the formation of a column that supports the entire body. Since each vertebra articulates closely with the one immediately above and the one immediately below it, the spinal foramina join together to form the *spinal canal,* which protects the spinal cord *(medulla spinalis);* this is another function of the spine. The spinal nerves and branches, along with the nutrient vessels, pass through the *intervertebral foramina,* which are bilateral between each two vertebrae.

Body. The body is round and is the largest single part. The superior and inferior surfaces are flat and rough, and their margins form a distinct rim.

Pedicles. There are two strong pedicles located bilaterally and posteriorly on each body. They project from the junction of the posterior and lateral surfaces. The *vertebral notches* are the depressions that are superior and inferior to the pedicles. The intervertebral foramen is formed by the inferior vertebral notch of the body of the vertebra above joining the superior vertebral notch of the body of the vertebra below.

Laminae. The laminae extend posteriorly and medially from the pedicles. The spinal foramen is closed posteriorly by their midline fusion.

Processes. There are seven processes common to all typical vertebral bodies.

SPINOUS PROCESS. The spinous process, which can be palpated, projects posteriorly and inferiorly from the fusion of the laminae.

ARTICULAR PROCESSES. The pedicles join the laminae bilaterally to form parts of the neural arch. From these junctions extend the two superior and two inferior articular processes. The superior articular surfaces extend posteriorly and the inferior articular surfaces extend anteriorly. The superior facet of the body of the vertebra below articulates with the inferior facet of the body of the vertebra above.

TRANSVERSE PROCESSES. The juncture of the laminae with the pedicles is below the base of the superior articular process and above the base of the inferior articular process. From this site extend the transverse processes.

Cervical vertebrae

The cervical vertebrae are quite small and are the only vertebrae that contain a foramen

*The spinal foramen is also called the vertebral foramen.

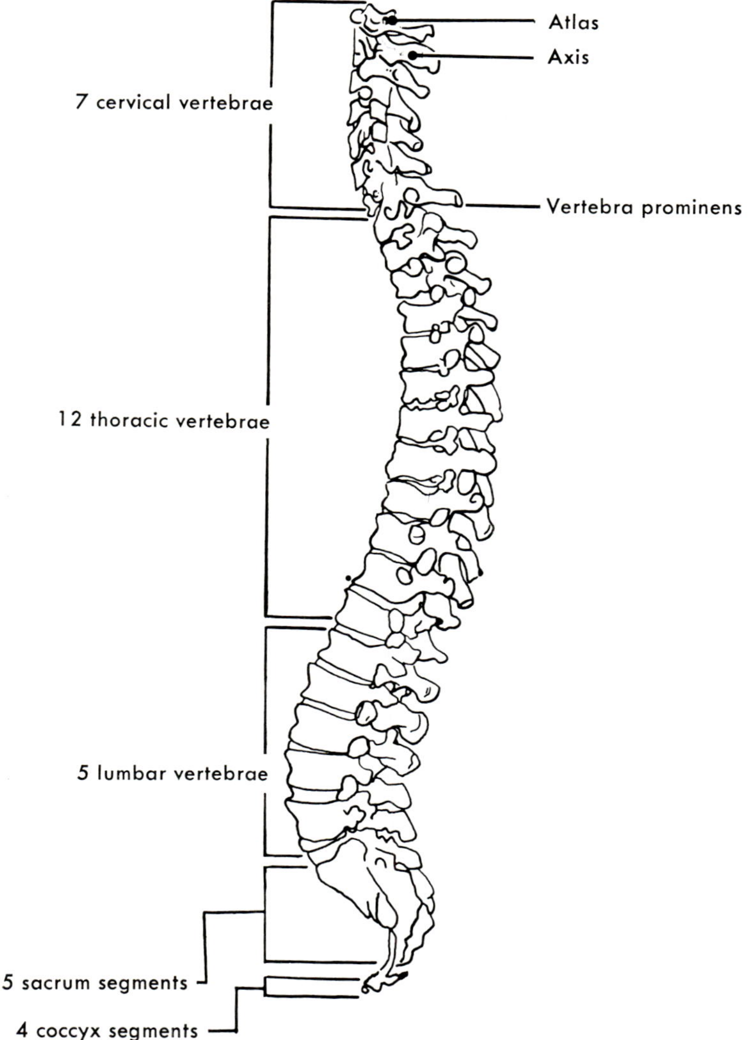

Fig. 8-1. Spine, lateral view.

in each transverse process (called *transverse foramina*). There is uniqueness in the structure of three of the cervical vertebrae, the first, second, and seventh. The second through the seventh have two superior and two inferior articular facets, one spinous process, and two transverse processes.

First cervical vertebrae (atlas). The head articulates in a forward and backward "rocking" motion upon the ring-shaped atlas (first cervical vertebra), which has no body. In prenatal life the body of the first cervical vertebra fuses with that of the second (axis), forming a superior projection *(odontoid process)* of the axis. The first cervical vertebra has no spinous process. Two lateral masses separate its anterior and posterior arches. In the center of the posterior margin of the anterior arch there is an articular surface with which the odontoid process (dens) articulates. The posterior arch presents a posterior tubercle instead of a spinous process. The superior articular facets articulate with the occipital condyles, and the inferior articular facets articulate with the superior articular facets of the axis. (See Fig. 8-2.)

Second cervical vertebra (axis). The axis is

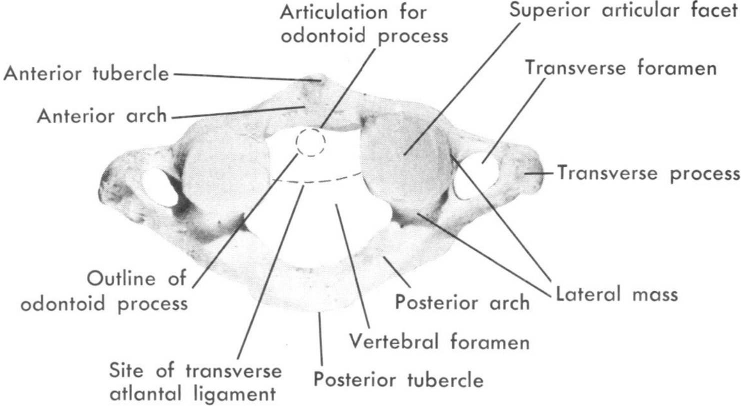

Fig. 8-2. Atlas, superior surface.

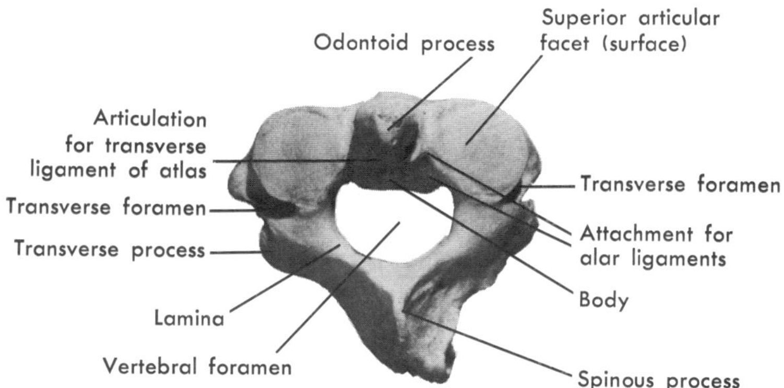

Fig. 8-3. Axis, posterosuperior surface.

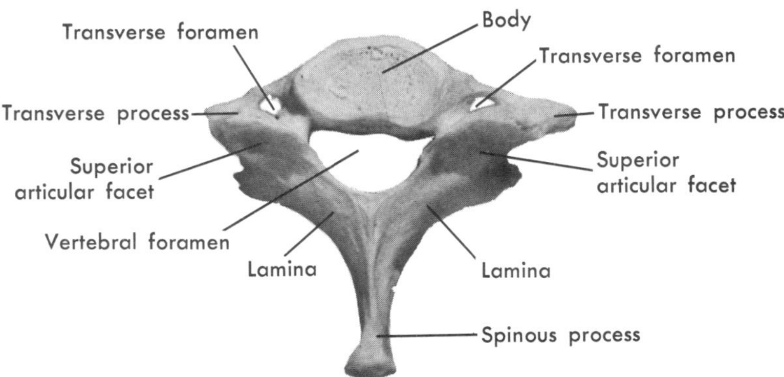

Fig. 8-4. Vertebra prominens, superior surface.

unique in that it supports the odontoid process *(dens epistropheus)*, which enables rotation of the atlas. (See Fig. 8-3.)

Seventh cervical vertebra. The most prominent spinous process of all the sections is on the seventh cervical vertebra. For this reason this vertebra is called the *vertebra prominens.* The posterior end of the spinous process of the seventh cervical vertebra is usually bifurcated, although this condition is nonexistent in the spinous processes of the other cervical vertebra. The transverse processes are larger in this vertebra than in the other cervical vertebrae. (See Fig. 8-4.)

Thoracic vertebrae

The thoracic vertebrae are larger than the cervical vertebrae. They become progressively larger from the first through the twelfth. The *costal* (rib) *facets* are found only on these vertebrae. From the first through the tenth there are additional facets that articulate with the rib tubercles. The differences of articulation in the thoracic vertebral bodies are as follows:

1. The first pair of ribs articulates with the costotransverse facet and the costovertebral facet of the first thoracic vertebra. The second pair of ribs articulates with the costotransverse facet and the upper costal facet of the second thoracic vertebra and the lower costal facet of the first.
2. The third pair of ribs articulates with the costotransverse facet and the upper costal facet of the third thoracic vertebra and the lower costal facet of the second.
3. The first through the eighth thoracic ver-

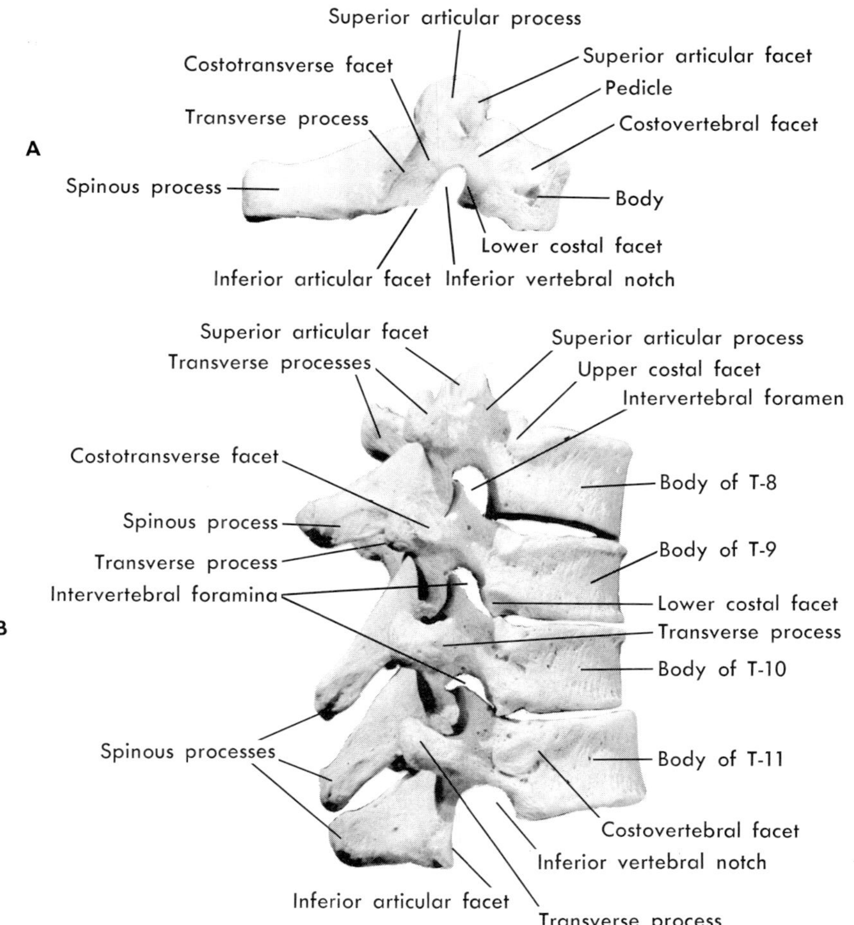

Fig. 8-5. Thoracic vertebrae, lateral surfaces. **A,** First thoracic vertebra. **B,** Eighth, ninth, tenth, and eleventh thoracic vertebrae.

tebrae have two rib articulations on each side of each vertebra.

4. The ninth and tenth thoracic vertebrae are slightly different in that the ninth pair of ribs articulates with a costotransverse facet and a costovertebral facet of the ninth thoracic vertebra, and the tenth pair of ribs articulates with a costotransverse facet and a costovertebral facet of the tenth thoracic vertebra. The eleventh and twelfth thoracic vertebrae have no costotransverse facets, only costovertebral facets on each side.

Throughout the vertebral column the superior articular facets of a body articulate with the inferior articular facets of the body above. This type of articulation is a true *apophyseal articulation;* an apophysis is an outgrowth (process) that has never been entirely separated from a bone. Each vertebral body (centrum) articulates with the intervertebral disks, the spongelike fibrocartilages located between each two vertebral bodies. (See Fig. 8-5.)

Lumbar vertebrae

The lumbar vertebrae are remarkably larger than the thoracic. The transverse processes are more prominent radiographically, although they are longer and more slender than are those of the other sections. The transverse processes of the first three lumbar vertebrae are truly horizontal, whereas those of the last two are inclined somewhat superiorly. The thickness of the fifth lumbar vertebra (anteriorly) accounts for the prominence of the *lumbosacral articulation.* Its spinous process is smaller and its transverse processes are thicker. The inferior articular facets are spaced farther apart. The fifth lumbar body frequently presents a condition termed *spina bifida occulta.** The articulations of the lumbar vertebrae are the same as those of the thoracic except that there are no rib articulations. (See Fig. 8-6.) The one very important articulation, called the lumbosacral joint, is that of the last lumbar vertebra with the sacrum.

Sacrum and coccyx

In very young children the sacrum and coccyx (nine segments) are distinct and separate. The proximal five fuse and constitute the sacrum. The distal four, which do not usually fuse, constitute the coccyx. At times the coccyx may consist of three or five segments.

Sacrum. The sacrum is large and resembles a triangle whose base is proximal and apex is distal. It is inferior to the fifth lumbar vertebra, between the ilia. It forms the superior and posterior parts of the pelvic cavity. Superiorly it articulates with the inferior surface of the last (usually fifth) lumbar vertebra, forming the lumbosacral joint. Inferiorly it articulates with the coccyx, forming the sacrococcygeal joint. Bilaterally its articulations form the right and left *sacroiliac joints.* In radiographic examinations the sacrum and coccyx are considered as parts of the pelvis and not true vertebrae. Anatomically the sacrum and coccyx are considered as parts of the vertebral column. The first sacral segment has articular facets that articulate with the inferior articular facets of

*A spina bifida occulta, determined by radiography because it is not visible externally, is a bony defect of the covering of the spinal cord without protrusion of the cord or meninges.

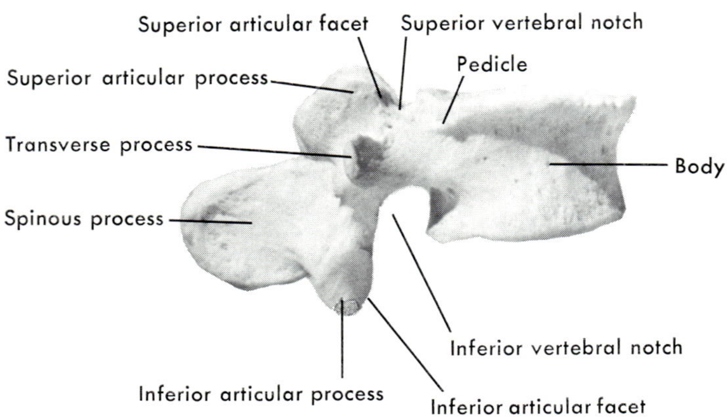

Fig. 8-6. Fourth lumbar vertebra, lateral surface.

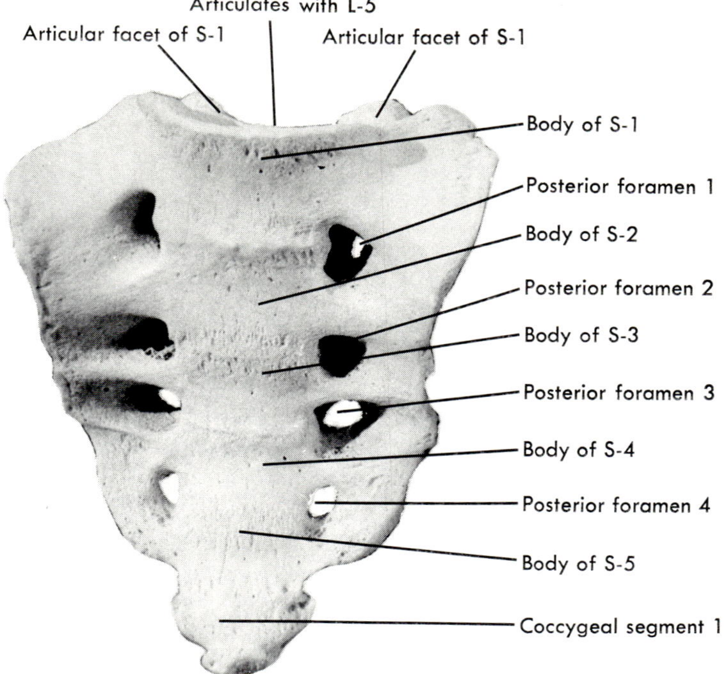

Fig. 8-7. Sacrum, dorsal surface.

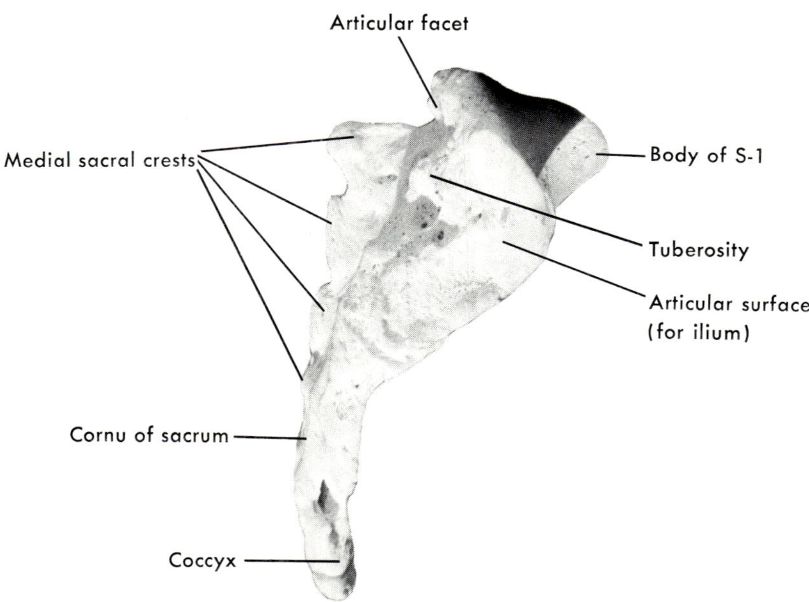

Fig. 8-8. Sacrum and coccyx, lateral surface.

the last lumbar vertebra. The concave pelvic surface of the sacrum presents four transverse ridges that are in line with the early articulations of the five segments. The anterior sacral foramina are bilateral at the ends of these ridges. The spinal canal exists in most of the sacrum and contains the sacral nerves. The walls of the spinal canal contain the anterior and posterior sacral foramina. (See Fig. 8-7.)

Coccyx. None of the coccygeal segments has pedicles, laminae, or spinous processes. The proximal segment is the largest of these segments and is usually separate. The remaining segments become progressively smaller in size and are frequently fused. The apex of the coccyx is rounded, sometimes bifid, and frequently displaced to either side. (See Fig. 8-8.)

THORACIC CAGE

Radiographically the bones of the thoracic cage present essentially the same, or at least similar, problems in penetration. These bones include the clavicles, sternum, scapulae, and ribs. (See Fig. 8-9.)

Clavicle

The anterosuperior portion of the shoulder girdle is formed by the clavicle. This bone is shaped somewhat like a shallow S. It is slightly superior to the first rib anteriorly and is very nearly horizontal. It is easily palpated. The clavicle extends from the sternum, medially, to the acromion process of the scapula, laterally. As previously mentioned, it presents two curves: convex anteriorly and medially and concave anteriorly and laterally. It forms the *sternoclavicular articulation,* or joint, in its articulation with the manubrium of the sternum, and the *acromioclavicular articulation,* or joint, in its articulation with the acromion process of the scapula. In addition to the medial articulation with the sternum, it articulates medially and inferiorly with the cartilage of the first rib. Cancellous tissue makes up most of the clavicle. It is the last bone of the body to ossify. It is ossified from two centers, a medial and a lateral for the body, and one center for the sternal end. The first two centers are primary, and the latter is secondary. The clavicle is not completely ossified until about the twenty-fifth year of life.

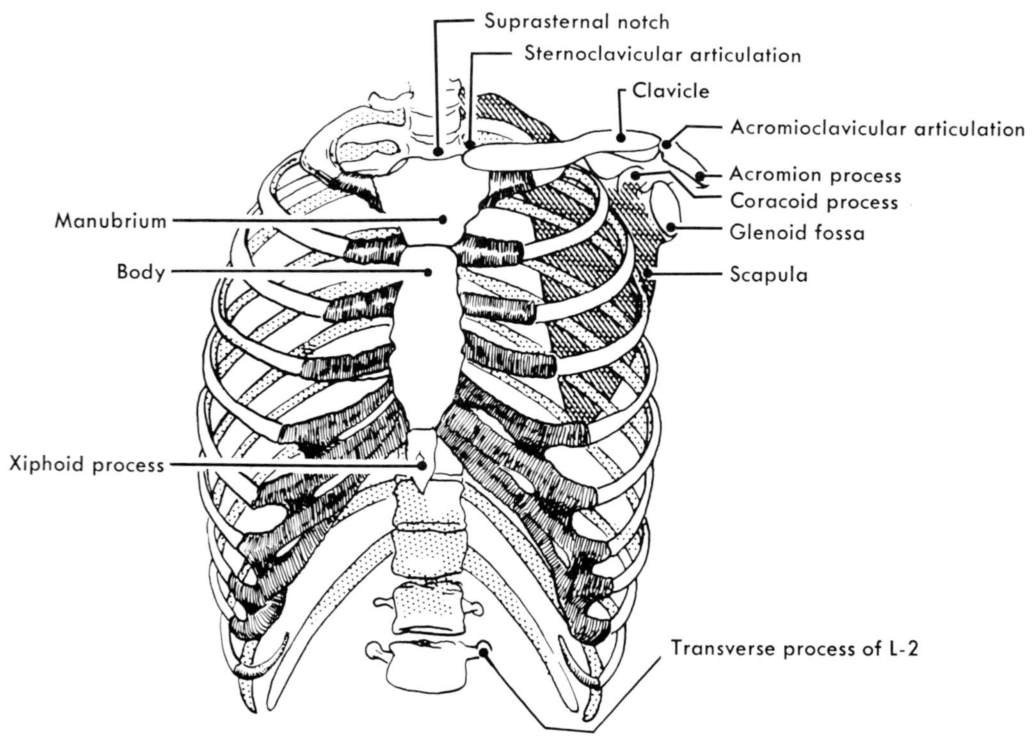

Fig. 8-9. Thoracic cage, anterior view.

Sternum

The sternum, or breastbone, consists of three parts: proximally, the *manubrium*, or handle; medially, the *body*, or gladiolus; and distally, the *xiphoid process*, or ensiform cartilage. It lies between the anterior ends of the first seven ribs in the anterior wall of the thoracic cavity. It is thin and flat and is composed chiefly of cancellous tissue. True bone forms the outer layer. The manubrium is the thickest part of the sternum. The xiphoid process does not completely ossify and is usually entirely cartilaginous until late in life. Superiorly on the manubrium and between the sternoclavicular articulations is the *sternal notch*. In addition to the articulations with the clavicles, the manubrium has five other articular surfaces: inferiorly, one for the body; bilaterally on each side and inferior to the sternoclaviculars, two for the first costal cartilages; bilaterally on each side and inferiorly, two for the second costal cartilages. The body articulates superiorly with the manubrium and inferiorly with the xiphoid process. The second rib articulates in the angle formed by the junction of the body and manubrium. The body articulates with the second through the seventh ribs on both sides. These articulations are with the costal cartilages. The xiphoid process articulates superiorly with the body and slightly with the seventh rib cartilage on each side. It usually ends in a rather sharp point but may be bifid or angled to either side.

Scapula

The scapula, or shoulder blade, is located posteriorly, superiorly, and laterally in relation to the thoracic cage. Together with the clavicle, it forms the *shoulder girdle*. The scapula is a flat bone. The three borders with the three angles form a triangle. The *spine* of the scapula is on the posterior surface and extends obliquely upward from the junction of the proximal and mid-thirds of the vertebral border and across the lateral angle. The scapula has a base, which is the superior border, and an apex, which is inferior to the body. The three borders are as follows: the vertebral, or medial; axillary, or lateral; and superior, or base. The three angles are as follows: the medial, at the junction of the vertebral and superior borders; the inferior (apex), at the junction of the vertebral and axillary borders; and the lateral (head of the scapula), at the junction of the axillary and superior borders. The lateral angle contains a shallow fossa called the *glenoid fossa,* which is the articular surface for the head of the humerus. The spine of the scapula extends beyond the lateral angle and curves forward over the glenoid cavity, terminating in a process called the *acromion*. The acromion process articulates with the lateral end of the clavicle. The *coracoid process* is quite thick and is attached to the neck of the scapula. It extends in a generally ventral or anterior direction from the scapula.

Ribs

There are usually twelve pairs of ribs; however, there may be an additional pair of ribs, either on the last cervical body or on the first lumbar body. Sometimes there are only eleven pairs. The first seven pairs articulate with the sternum and vertebral column; these are called *true ribs*. The eighth, ninth, and tenth pairs articulate posteriorly with the vertebral column and anteriorly with the cartilage of the rib above; the latter are called *false ribs*. The eleventh and twelfth pairs are not attached anteriorly and are the *floating,* or vertebral, *ribs*. Radiographically the ribs must be considered in two groups: those above the diaphragm and those below the diaphragm. Each rib has a posterior, or vertebral end, and an anterior, or sternal end, which are separated by the body. The major articulation of each rib is with the thoracic vertebra of the same number. In addition to a head, each rib has a neck and a tubercle. A rib extends obliquely downward to the midaxillary line, from which point it continues downward and anteriorly to its anterior (sternal) articulation. The spaces between each two ribs are called the intercostal spaces.

PELVIS

Anatomically the pelvis consists of two bones, the pelvic (innominate) bones. Each pelvic bone is composed of three bones that are solidly fused: the *ilium*, the *ischium*, and the *pubis*. They are fused in the *acetabulum* (hip socket), which is the articular fossa for the head of the femur. (See Figs. 8-10 and 8-11.)

Ilium

The ilium is composed of a body and a wing (ala). The body is inferior, near the acetabulum. The wing is quite large and extends upward, laterally and medially. It forms the lateral boundary of the pelvis and derives its name from its relation with the flank. In general outline the crest of the ilium is convex and rough. The thickened anterior and posterior parts terminate

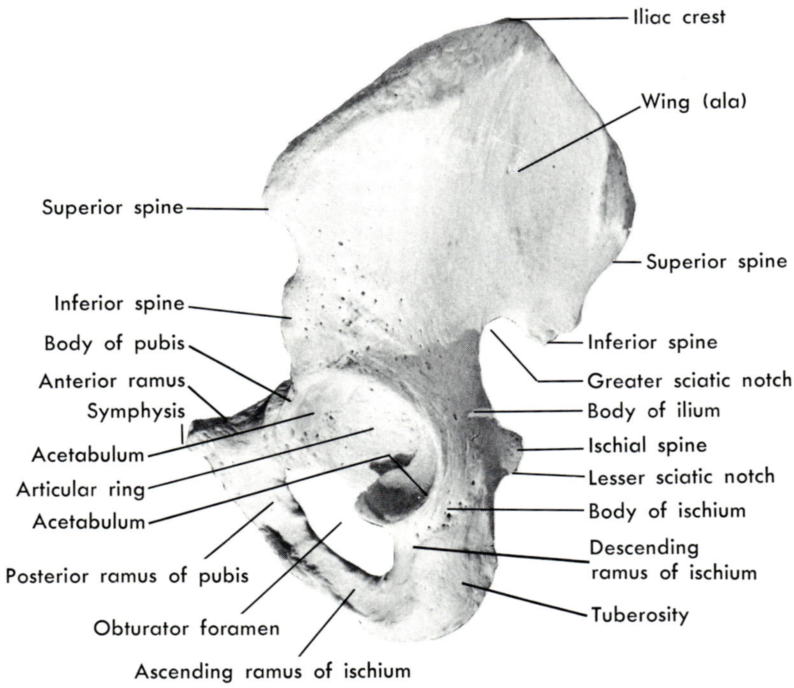

Fig. 8-10. Left pelvic (innominate) bone, lateral surface.

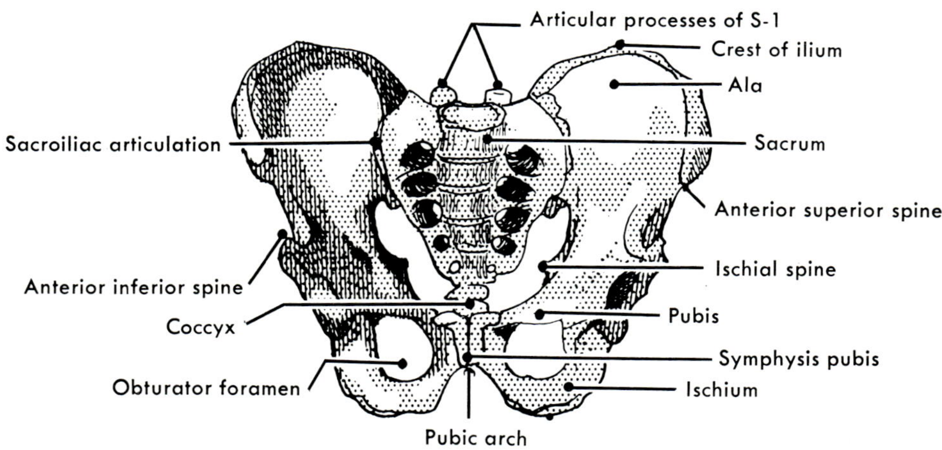

Fig. 8-11. Male bony pelvis, anterior view.

in the *anterior* and *posterior superior iliac spines.* The *anterior* and *posterior inferior iliac spines* are separated from the superior iliac spines by a distinct notch. The anterior superior iliac spine is an important landmark radiographically.

Ischium

The ischium is the most inferior and the strongest bone of the pelvis. It extends inferiorly from the acetabulum, forming a large tuberosity, and then continues and curves anteriorly, where it forms, with the pubis, the *obturator foramen.* The ishium consists of a *body,* a *superior ramus,* and an *inferior ramus.* The superior and inferior rami join below the obturator foramen. On the inferior surface of this junction is the *ischial tuberosity.* The superior ramus descends posteriorly from the acetabulum to its junction with the inferior ramus, while the inferior ramus ascends anteriorly from this junction. The *ischial spine*, an important radiographic landmark in posterior projections of the pelvis, projects medially from the posterior border of the body.

Pubis

The pubis lies medially and inferiorly to the acetabulum. It articulates with the opposite pubis in the midsagittal plane, forming the *symphysis pubis*. It forms the anterior portion of the pelvis. The pubis consists of a body and two rami. From its junction with the inferior ramus of the ischium, the *inferior ramus* of the pubis ascends to its junction with the *superior ramus*.

Acetabulum

The acetabulum is formed by the fusion of the bodies of the ilium, ischium, and pubis. The pubis forms only one fifth, whereas the remainder is formed equally by the ilium and the ischium. The pubis is medial, the ilium is superior, and the ischium is inferior.

Obturator foramen

The obturator foramen is bounded as follows: superiorly, by the superior ramus of the pubis; medially and anteriorly, by the union of the superior and inferior rami of the pubis; laterally and posteriorly, by the superior ramus of the ischium; and inferiorly, by inferior rami of the ischium and pubis.

REFERENCES

Anthony, C. P., and Kolthoff, N. J.: Textbook of anatomy and physiology, ed. 9, St. Louis, 1975, The C. V. Mosby Co.

Goss, Charles M.: Gray's anatomy, ed. 28, Philadelphia, 1966, Lea & Febiger.

Jacobi, C. A.: Textbook of anatomy and physiology in radiologic technology, ed. 2, St. Louis, 1975, The C. V. Mosby Co.

Meschan, Isadore: An atlas of anatomy basic to radiology, Philadelphia, 1975, W. B. Saunders Co.

QUESTIONS

1. Describe the natural curvatures of the vertebral column.
2. Describe the ideal position of the patient during radiography in which to take advantage of the natural curve of a particular section of the vertebral column.
3. What items are common to all vertebral bodies?
4. What vertebral segments replace bodies?
5. Why are the above called (properly) segments instead of bodies?
6. Through what part of a vertebral body does the spinal cord pass?
7. What structures of a vertebral body fuse to form the spinous process?
8. Name the processes and corresponding numbers of a typical vertebra.
9. Describe the origin, formation, and location of the dens epistropheus.
10. Describe the articulations of the seventh right rib.
11. What purpose is served by the intervertebral foramina?
12. What is an apophyseal articulation?
13. Define a spina bifida. Differentiate between this and a spina bifida occulta.
14. Differentiate between the true, false, and floating ribs.
15. Describe and give the proper name of the shoulder blade.
16. What forms the collarbone? What are its articulations?
17. What are the names and parts of the breastbone?
18. What bones form the pelvis?
19. State the boundaries of the obturator foramen.
20. What bones and parts form the hip joint?

9 • POSITIONING FOR THE TRUNK

ROUTINE

The routine steps are as follows:

1. Know the desired position.
2. Select all factors except kilovoltage.
3. Conduct the patient into the radiographic room. If cooperation of the patient is possible, have him assume the desired position.
4. After deciding what size film to use, place the film in the Bucky tray. Use proper identification and an *R* or *L* to denote the right or left side.
5. If possible, explain to the patient what is going to be done.
6. Use the center of the cone or tube as a guide to center the patient crosswise on the table.
7. Center the film holder or the tube (the selection depends on the radiographic position) to the part being radiographed.
8. If the patient is centered with the tube, then center the film holder to the tube. If the film holder is centered to the patient, then center the tube to the center of the film holder.
9. Measure the patient for the thickness of the part, and, from the technique chart, determine the kilovoltage and select the proper kilovoltage on the control panel.
10. Close the primary switch, and check the line voltage.
11. Double check the Bucky switch.
12. Give the patient proper breathing instructions.
13. *Observe movement of the patient until the moment that the exposure is made.*
14. During the exposure, ascertain that the machine is delivering the desired milliamperage by watching the milliampere meter.
15. Instruct the patient to resume normal breathing.

If another view is required, select the proper factors on the control panel at this time, remove the exposed film (in the casette), and replace with the proper-sized film and film holder for the next exposure. Then repeat the same routine steps. The starting factors stated for all the following techniques are for a 12:1 grid when a Bucky is used. These technique factors generally will produce high-contrast radiographs. If high-kilovoltage technique is employed, corresponding and appropriate changes in steps 2 and 9 are to be made.

Cervical spine—posterior (A-P) view (Figs. 9-1 and 9-2)

Film size—8″ × 10″
Cassette
Lengthwise
Bucky
Collimate to cover

Technique

Factors	Screen film cassette (par) Bucky
mA	100
Time	0.5
mAs	50
Thickness in cm	14
kVp	62
Distance	40

Patient preparation

Remove all garments down to the shoulders. Remove dentures, hairpins, and jewelry around the cervical area. Provide a gown for female patients.

Palpation points

Angle of the mandible; thyroid cartilage; vertebra prominens.

Procedure

Place the patient in the supine position with the midline of the body over the center line of the table. The midsagittal plane of the head is perpendicular to the tabletop. Elevate the chin so that a line from the upper occlusal plane to the base of the occiput is perpendicular to the tabletop.

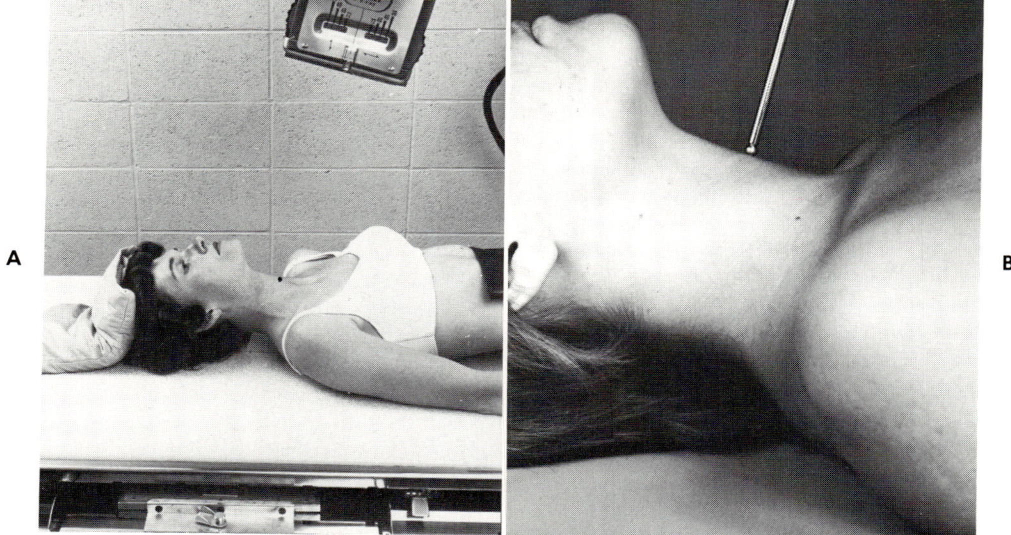

Fig. 9-1. Cervical spine. **A** and **B**, Posterior (A-P) positions.

Central ray

Direct the central ray 15 degree cephalad through the thyroid cartilage to the center of the film holder. Collimate to film holder.

Immobilization

If necessary, brace both sides of the cranium with sandbags. Place sponges under the knees. Employ suspended expiration.

Right-left markers

Place the *R* marker on the right side, center border of the film holder.

Technical tips

Decrease the central ray angle to demonstrate the upper intervertebral spaces. Increase the central ray angle to demonstrate the lower intervertebral spaces.

Structures demonstrated

Posterior (A-P) views of the lower five cervical bodies, the corresponding intervertebral spaces, the transverse processes, the interpedicular spaces, and the upper two or three thoracic bodies.

Note: To demonstrate cervical ribs, direct the central ray perpendicular through the seventh cervical vertebra to the center of a 10″ × 12″ film holder.

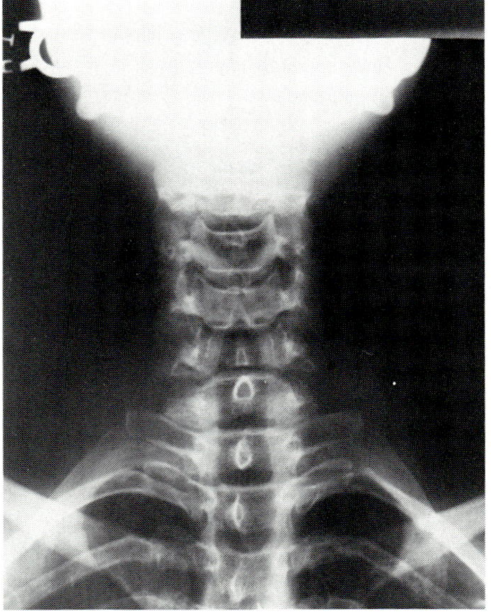

Fig. 9-2. Cervical spine—posterior (A-P) view. (Courtesy Dr. Frank S. Cavallaro and Valley Hospital, Las Vegas, Nevada.)

Cervical spine—posterior (A-P) atlas and axis (open-mouth) view (Figs. 9-3 and 9-4)

Film size—8″ × 10″
Cassette
Lengthwise
Bucky
Extension cone (fully extended)

Technique

Factors	Screen film cassette (par) Bucky
mA	100
Time	0.5
mAs	50
Thickness in cm	14
kVp	66
Distance	40

Patient preparation

Remove dentures and hairpins over the occipital area.

Palpation point

Base of occiput.

Procedure

Place the patient in the supine position with the midline of the body over the center line of the table. The midsagittal plane of the head is perpendicular to the tabletop. Elevate the chin so that a line from the upper occlusal plane to the base of the occiput is perpendicular to the tabletop. Insert a sterile 1½-inch cork between the patient's jaws.

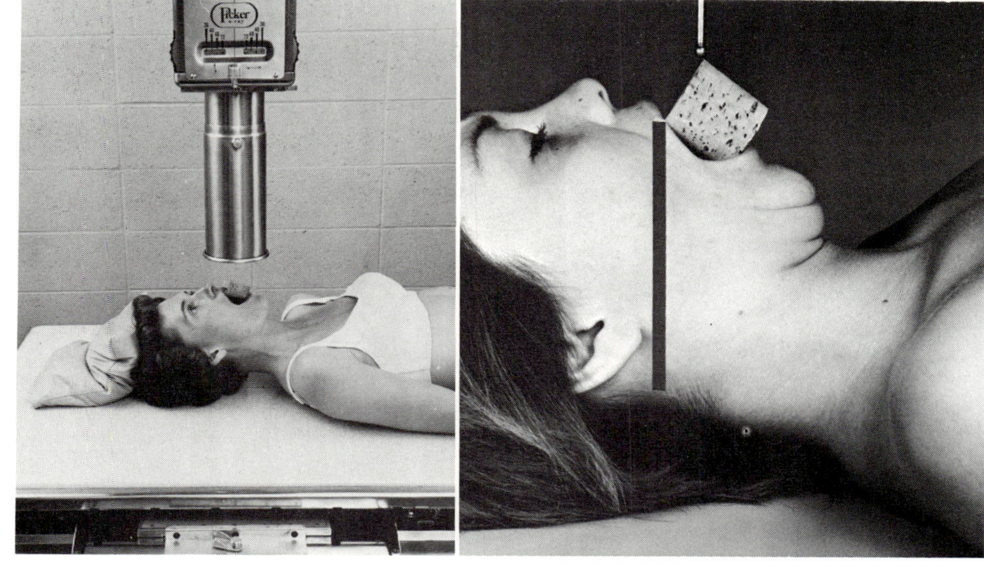

Fig. 9-3. Cervical spine. **A** and **B,** Atlas and axis (open-mouth) positions.

Central ray

Direct the central ray ½ inch inferior to and parallel with the upper occlusal plane to the center of the film holder.

Immobilization

Place sandbags against the vertex of the cranium. Employ suspended expiration.

Right-left markers

Burn the *R* marker in the superior border of the right side of the film holder above the cone field after the exposure is made.

Technical tips

For patients with short stocky necks, elevate the occiput slightly with a radiolucent sponge to aid in vertical alignment.

Structures demonstrated

Posterior (A-P) views of the atlas and axis through the open mouth.

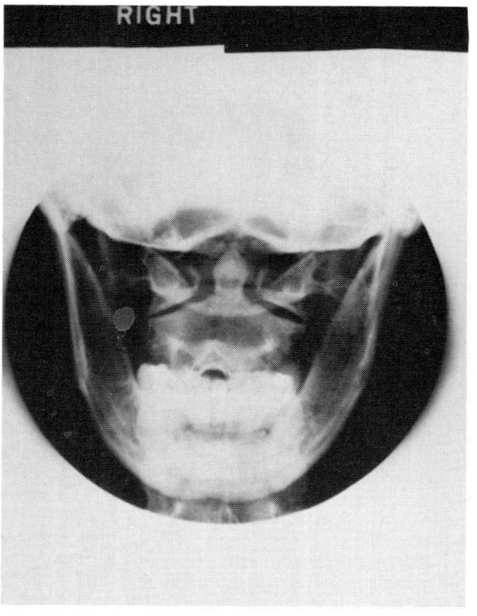

Fig. 9-4. Cervical spine—atlas and axis (open-mouth) view. (Courtesy Dr. E. I. L. Cilley, Dr. T. W. Crowell, Dr. R. E. Waud, and Dr. G. H. Hoffman.)

Cervical spine—lateral view (Figs. 9-5 and 9-6)

Film size—10″ × 12″
Cassette
Lengthwise
Erect film holder
Collimate to cover

Technique

Factors	Screen film cassette (par)
mA	100
Time	0.3
mAs	30
Thickness in cm	12
kVp	66
Distance	72

Patient preparation

Remove all garments down to the shoulders. Remove dentures, hairpins, and jewelry around the cervical area. Provide a gown for female patients.

Palpation points

Angle of the mandible; thyroid cartilage; vertebra prominens.

Procedure

Place the patient in a lateral position, either sitting or standing, with one shoulder against an erect film holder. Have the patient keep his back straight and shoulders relaxed, then place a sandbag in each hand to hold the shoulders down. The midsagittal plane of the head and body is parallel with the film surface. Elevate the chin, and place the top of the cassette 2 inches above the external auditory meatus.

A

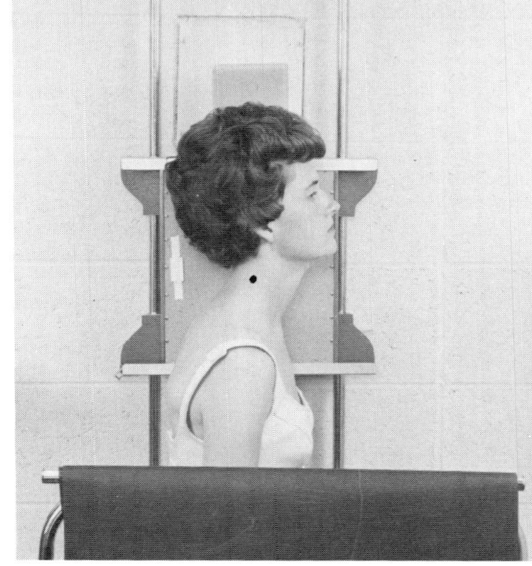

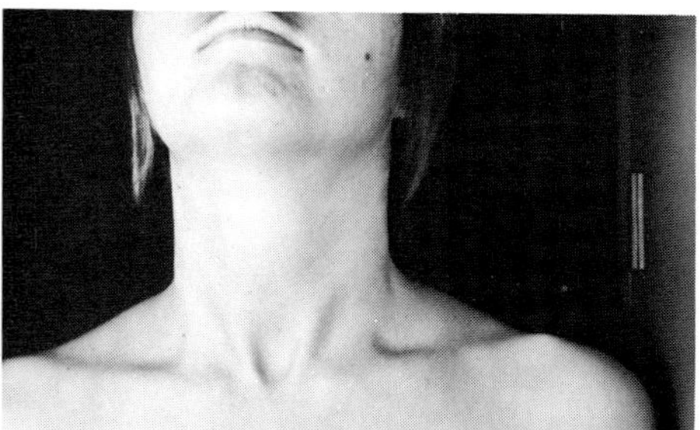

B

Fig. 9-5. Cervical spine. A and B, Lateral positions.

Central ray

Direct the central ray perpendicular through the cervical spine to the center of the film holder. Collimate to film holder.

Immobilization

Place a radiolucent sponge between the head and the film holder. Use a compression band if necessary. Employ suspended expiration.

Right-left markers

Place the correct marker on the posterior center border of the film holder.

Technical tips

Because the patient will always move slightly after suspending respiration, delay the exposure approximately 2 seconds.

Structures demonstrated

Lateral views of the cervical bodies, interspaces, lower apophyseal articulations, and spinous processes.

Note: For supine patients, elevate the head and place a vertical film holder parallel with the cervical spine. If possible, use a 72-inch focal-film distance to compensate for increased object-film distance.

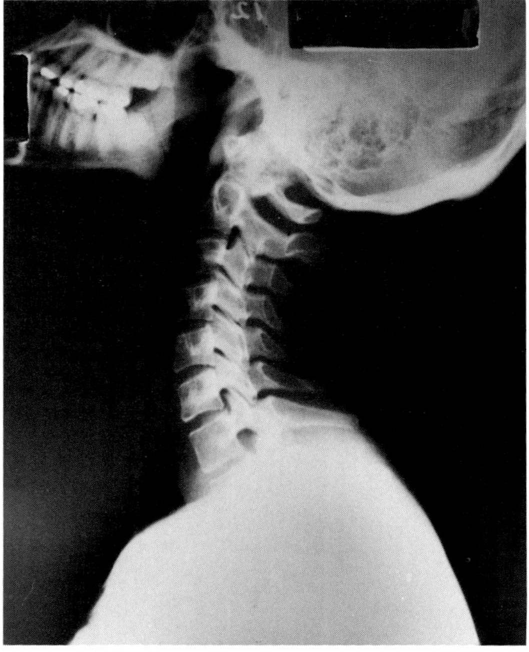

Fig. 9-6. Cervical spine—lateral view. (Courtesy Dr. Frank S. Cavallaro and Valley Hospital, Las Vegas, Nevada.)

Cervical spine—posteroanterior-oblique (L.A.O.-R.A.O.) view (Figs. 9-7 and 9-8)

Film size—8″ × 10″
Cassette
Lengthwise
Bucky
Collimate to cover

Technique

Factors	Screen film cassette (par)
mA	100
Time	0.6
mAs	60
Thickness in cm	14
kVp	66
Distance	40

Patient preparation

Remove all garments down to the shoulders. Remove dentures, hairpins, and jewelry around the cervical area. Provide a gown for female patients.

Palpation points

Base of occiput; vertebra prominens.

Procedure

Place the patient in the prone position. Elevate the side opposite the one being examined so that the midsagittal plane of the head and body forms a 45-degree angle with the tabletop. Flex the knee and elbow of the elevated side for support. Align the long axis of the spine over the center line of the table.

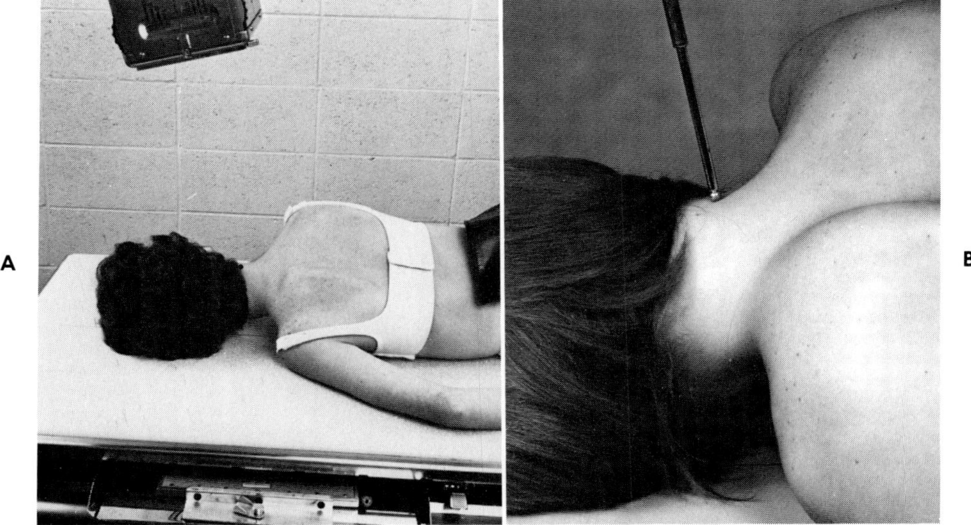

Fig. 9-7. Cervical spine. **A** and **B,** Posteroanterior-oblique (L.A.O.) positions.

Central ray

Direct the central ray 15 degrees caudad through the fourth cervical vertebra to the center of the film holder. Collimate to film holder.

Immobilization

Place wedge sponges under the head and flexed knee. A compression band may be used across the patient's head for additional support. Employ suspended expiration.

Right-left markers

Place the correct marker on the posterior center border of the film holder.

Technical tips

Extend the neck to eliminate the possibility of superimposing the mandibular angle over the vertebral bodies.

Structures demonstrated

Oblique view of the cervical spine, which demonstrates the intervertebral foramina of the side nearest the film; oblique view of the vertebral bodies.

Note: Both oblique views are usually made for comparison. Erect patients may be positioned 45 degrees right posterior oblique and 45 degrees left posterior oblique with a 15-degree cephalad angle and a 72-inch focal-film distance to compensate for the increased object-film distance.

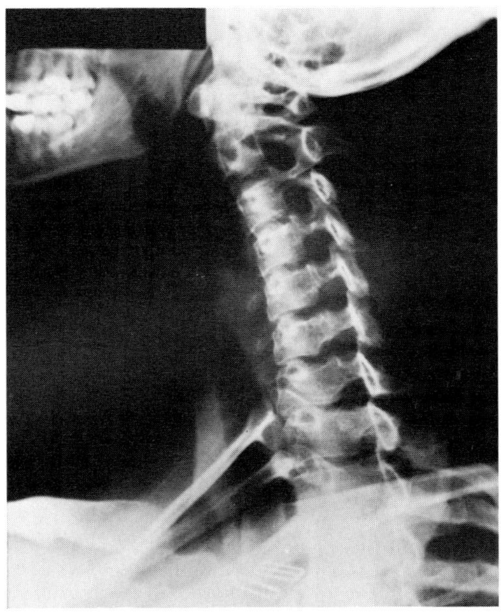

Fig. 9-8. Cervical spine—posteroanterior-oblique (L.A.O.) view. (Courtesy Dr. E. I. L. Cilley, Dr. T. W. Crowell, Dr. R. E. Waud, and Dr. G. H. Hoffman.)

Thoracic spine—posterior (A-P) view (Figs. 9-9 to 9-11)

Film size—14″ × 17″ or 7″ × 17″
Cassette
Lengthwise
Bucky
Collimate to cover

Technique

Factors	Screen film cassette (par)
mA	100
Time	1.0
mAs	100
Thickness in cm	20
kVp	66
Distance	40

Patient preparation

Remove all garments down to the waist. Provide a gown for female patients.

Palpation point

Vertebra prominens.

Procedure

Place the patient in the supine position. Center the midline of the body over the center line of the table. Extend the arms at the sides of the body. Grasp the patient by the ankles and pull gently to straighten the spine. Place the top of the cassette 3 inches above the vertebra prominens (spinous process of the seventh cervical vertebra).

Central ray

Direct the central ray perpendicular through the long axis of the thoracic spine to the center of the film holder. Collimate to film holder.

Immobilization

Place large sponges or sandbags under both knees for comfort. Employ suspended inspiration.

A
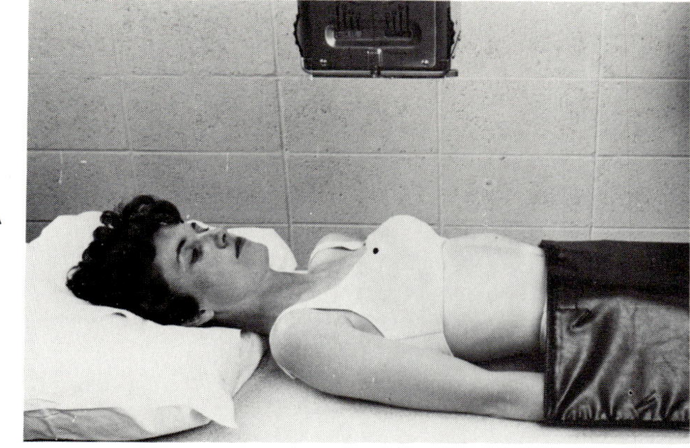
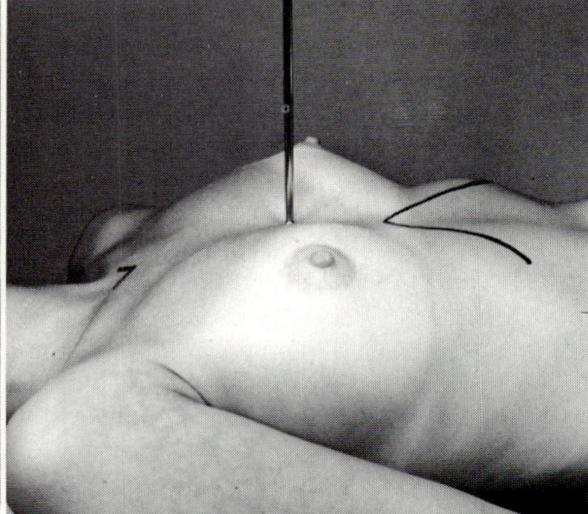
B

Fig. 9-9. Thoracic spine. **A** and **B**, Posterior (A-P) positions.

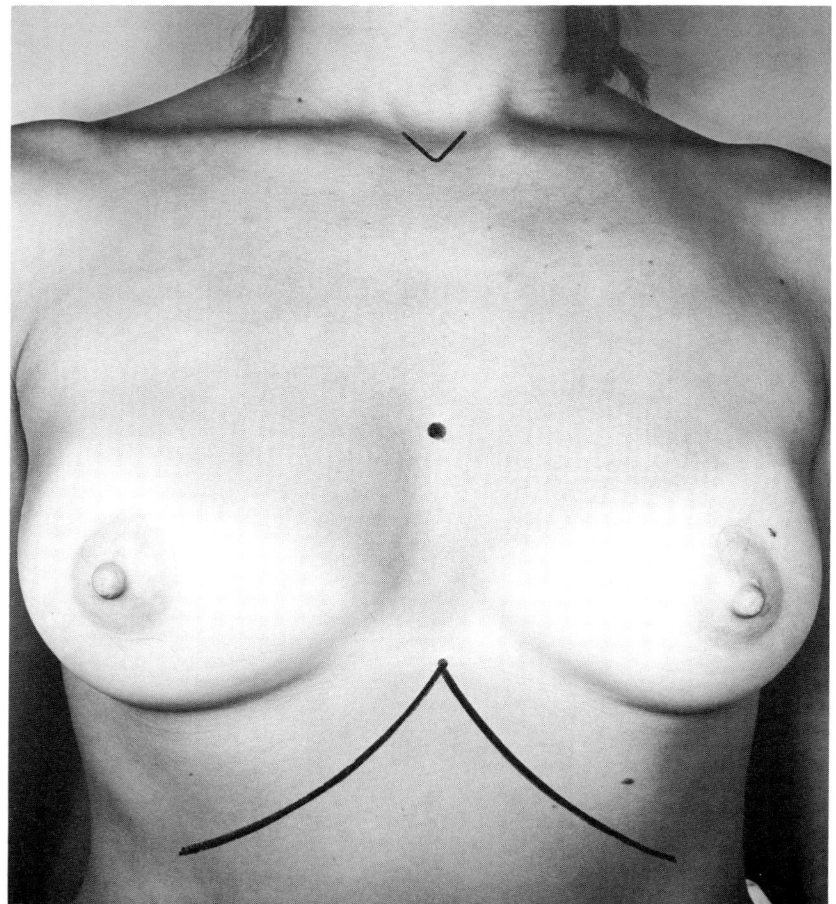

Fig. 9-10. Thoracic spine—posterior (A-P) position.

Right-left markers

Place the *R* marker on the right lateral center border of the film holder.

Technical tips

For more uniform radiographic density, use $\frac{1}{10}$ mm added copper filter internally plus an increase of 10 kVp.

Structures demonstrated

Posterior (A-P) views of the thoracic bodies, of the corresponding interpedicular spaces, and generally of the intervertebral spaces.

Note: The *heel effect* is most effective in this view. Position the patient with his head at the anode end of the x-ray tube.

For posture radiographs, place the patient in the anteroposterior erect position with the body weight distributed equally on both feet.

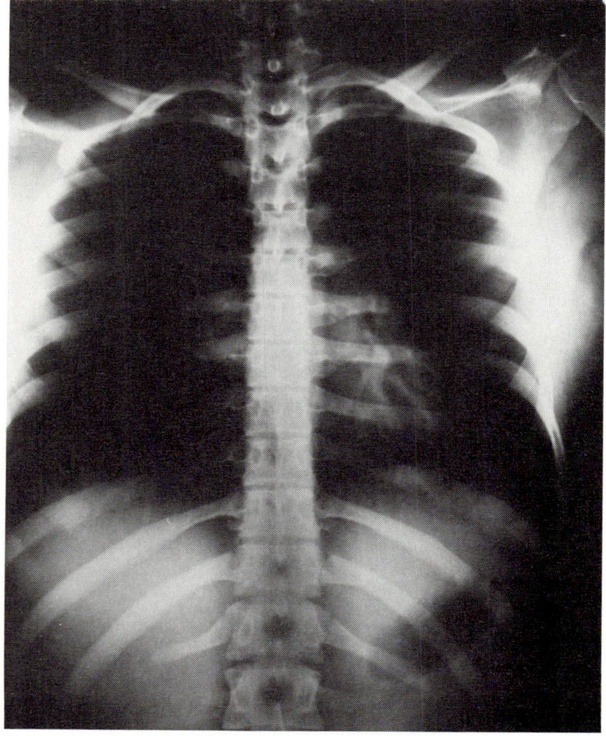

Fig. 9-11. Thoracic spine—posterior (A-P) view. (Courtesy Dr. E. I. L. Cilley, Dr. T. R. Crowell, Dr. R. E. Waud, and Dr. G. H. Hoffman.)

Thoracic spine—lateral view (Figs. 9-12 and 9-13)

Film size—14″ × 17″ or 7″ × 17″	*Bucky*
Cassette	*Collimate to cover*
Lengthwise	

Technique

Factors	Screen film cassette (par)
mA	100
Time	1.0
mAs	100
Thickness in cm	32
kVp	70
Distance	40

Patient preparation

Remove all garments down to the waist. Provide a gown for female patients.

Palpation points

Vertebra prominens; spinous processes of the thoracic vertebrae.

Procedure

Place the patient in a lateral recumbent position. Flex the hips and knees for support. Center the midaxillary plane of the body over the center line of the table. Flex the bottom elbow and place the forearm under the pillow. Flex the top elbow and place the forearm above the head with the hand grasping the edge of the table. Rotate the body into the true lateral position.

Central ray

Direct the central ray perpendicular to the long axis of the spine and through the sixth thoracic body to the center of the film holder. Collimate to film holder.

Immobilization

Place a sponge or sandbag between the knees. Place a compression band over the pelvis. Employ suspended inspiration.

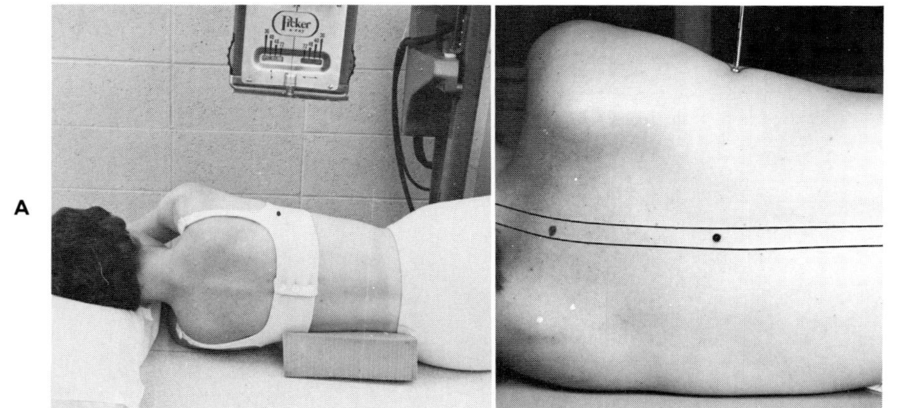

Fig. 9-12. Thoracic spine. **A** and **B**, Lateral positions.

Right-left markers

Place the correct marker on the anterior center border of the film holder.

Technical tips

A slight lateral concavity or "sagging" of the thoracic spine is beneficial in demonstrating intervertebral spaces, which are parallel to the divergent rays.

Structures demonstrated

Lateral views of the thoracic bodies, the corresponding interspaces, and intervertebral foramina.

Note: The upper three thoracic vertebrae are not demonstrated in this view.

To better demonstrate the upper lateral thoracic vertebrae, employ the rapid, shallow breathing technique with low milliamperage for a longer time (25 mA for 6 seconds).

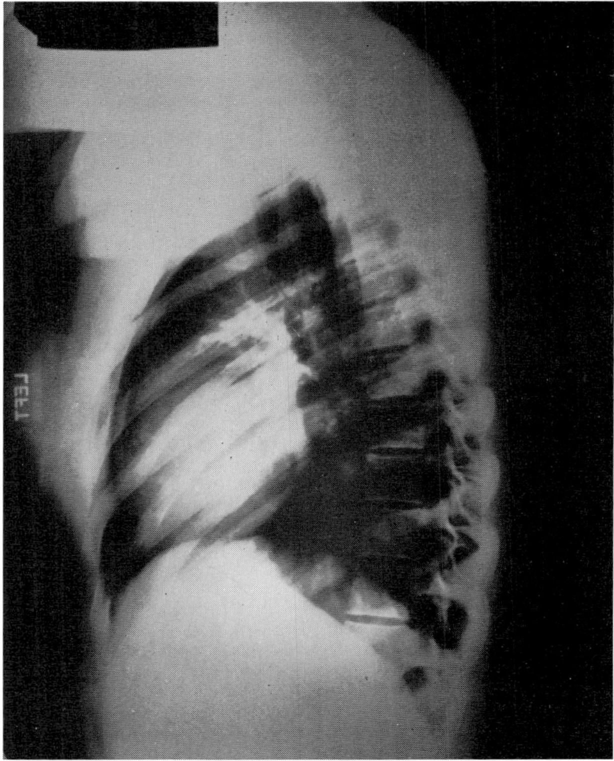

Fig. 9-13. Thoracic spine—lateral view. (Courtesy Dr. E. I. L. Cilley, Dr. T. W. Crowell, Dr. R. E. Waud, and Dr. G. H. Hoffman.)

Thoracic spine—upper oblique view (Figs. 9-14 and 9-15)

Film size—10″ × 12″
Cassette
Lengthwise
Bucky
Collimate to cover

Technique

Factors	Screen film cassette (par)
mA	100
Time	0.6
mAs	60
Thickness in cm	30
kVp	78
Distance	40

Patient preparation

Remove all garments down to the waist. Provide a gown for female patients.

Palpation points

Manubrium; vertebra prominens.

Procedure

Place the patient in lateral position, either sitting or standing, with one shoulder against an erect Bucky. The midsagittal plane of the head and body is parallel with the film surface. Flex the elbow nearer to the film; at the same time raise the arm and rotate that shoulder anteriorly as far as possible without rotating the thorax. Place the opposite hand on the hip; relax this shoulder and rotate it posteriorly as far as possible. Center the midportion of the cervicothoracic spine over the center line of the Bucky.

Central ray

Direct the central ray perpendicular through a point at the level of the manubrium to the center of the film holder. Collimate to film holder.

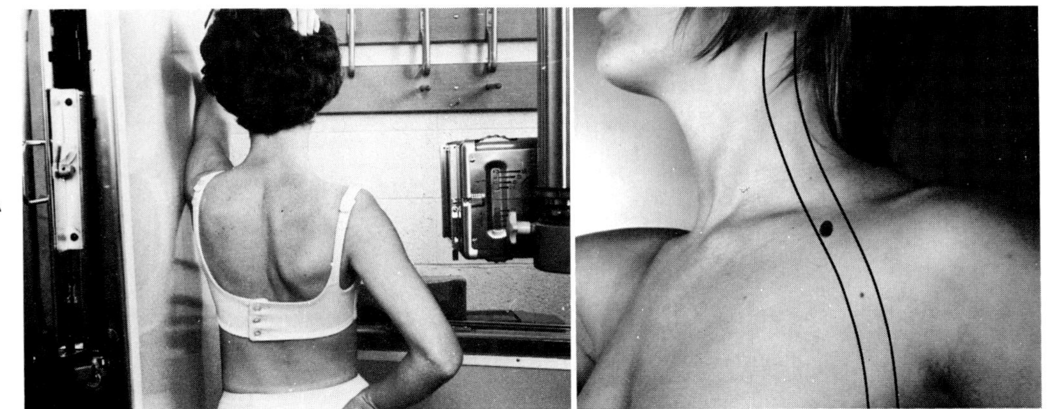

Fig. 9-14. Thoracic spine—upper oblique positions. **A,** Left oblique. **B,** Right oblique.

Immobilization

Place a large sponge between the patient's head and the film holder. A compression band may be employed around the abdomen. Employ suspended expiration.

Right-left markers

Place the correct marker on the anterior center border of the film holder.

Technical tips

For more uniform radiographic density, use $\frac{1}{10}$ mm added copper filter internally plus an increase of 10 kVp.

Structures demonstrated

Semilateral view of the upper thoracic and lower cervical vertebrae between the humeral heads; this view demonstrates the apophyseal articulations and the intervertebral spaces.

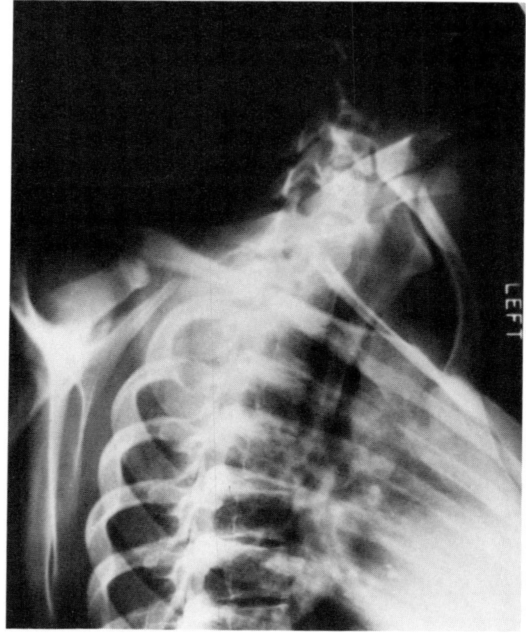

Fig. 9-15. Thoracic spine—upper oblique view. (Courtesy Dr. E. I. L. Cilley, Dr. T. W. Crowell, Dr. R. E. Waud, and Dr. G. H. Hoffman.)

Lumbar spine—posterior (A-P) view (Figs. 9-16 to 9-18)

Film size—14″ × 17″
Cassette
Lengthwise
Bucky
Collimate to cover

Technique

Factors	Screen film cassette (par)
mA	100
Time	1.0
mAs	100
Thickness in cm	20
kVp	66
Distance	40

Patient preparation

Remove all clothing except shoes and socks. Provide a gown for the patient.

Palpation point

Crest of ilium.

Procedure

Place the patient in the supine position with the midline of the body over the center line of the table. Grasp the patient by the ankles and pull gently to straighten the spine. Flex both knees a minimum of 6 inches and support them with sponges. Rotate the ankles internally into a true posterior (A-P) position. Center the film holder to the crest of the ilium.

Central ray

Direct the central ray perpendicular to the center of the film holder. Collimate to film holder.

Immobilization

Place sandbags on the lateral sides of the ankles. A compression band may be used across large abdomens. Employ suspended expiration.

Right-left markers

Place the *R* marker on the right lateral center border of the film holder.

Technical tips

Increased knee flexion will aid in relaxation of the normal lumbar curve.

Structures demonstrated

Posterior (A-P) views of the lumbar bodies, the associated interspaces, the interpedicular spaces, the laminae, the transverse processes, the pelvis, and femoral heads; axial views of the spinous processes.

Note: For thin patients, a posteroanterior projection will better demonstrate the intervertebral spaces.

A

B

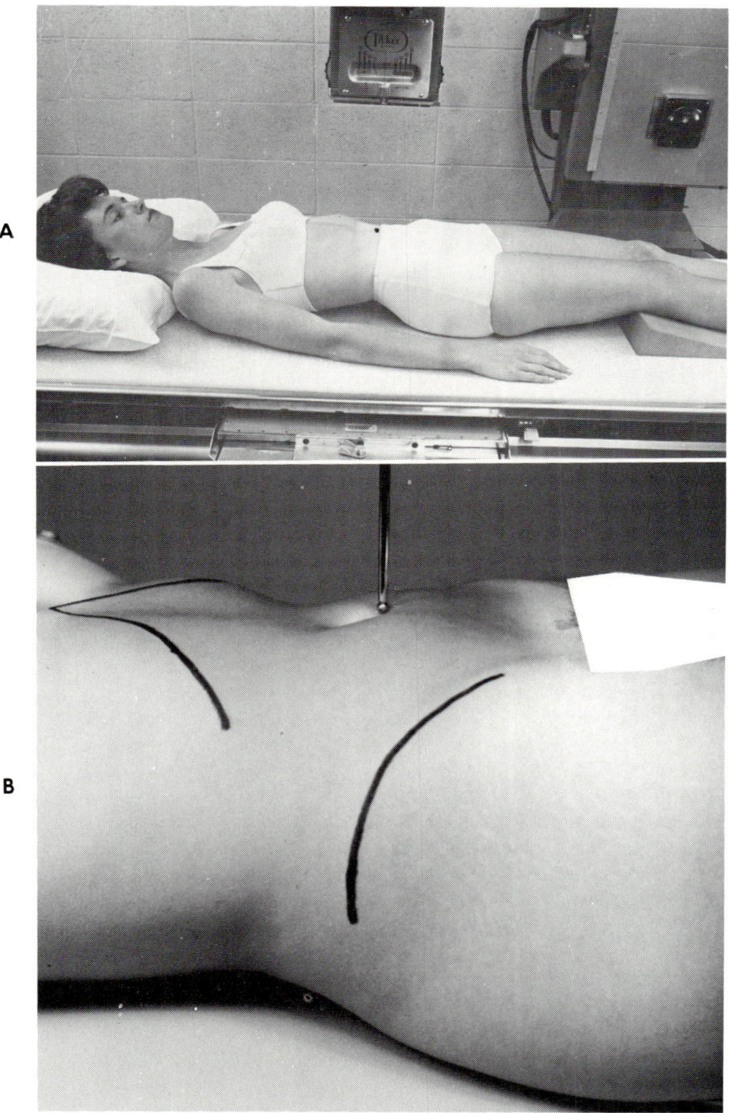

Fig. 9-16. Lumbar spine. **A** and **B,** Posterior (A-P) positions.

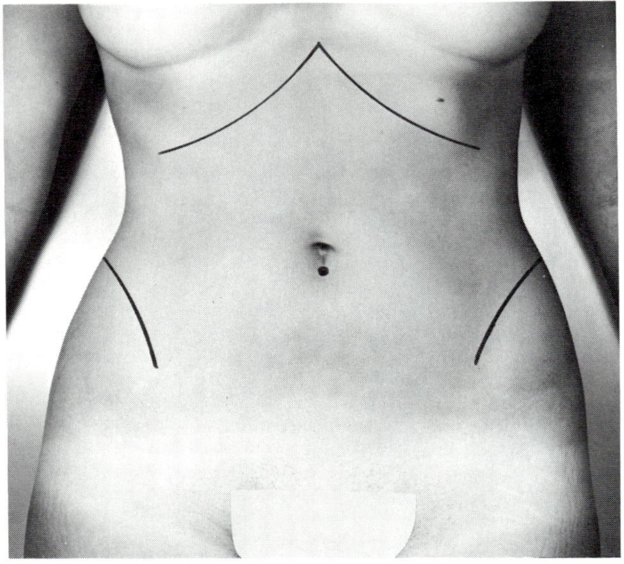

Fig. 9-17. Lumbar spine—posterior (A-P) position.

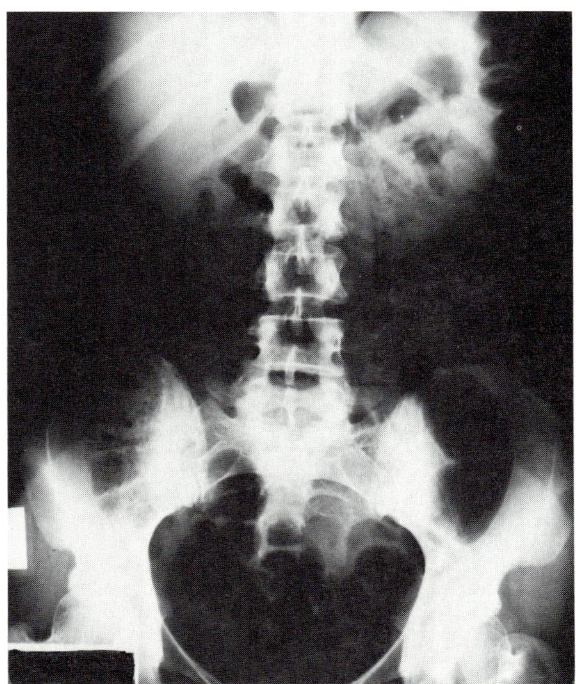

Fig. 9-18. Lumbar spine—posterior (A-P) view. (Courtesy Scottsdale Memorial Hospital, Scottsdale, Arizona.)

Lumbar spine—upper lateral view (Figs. 9-19 and 9-20)

Film size—10″ × 12″
Cassette
Lengthwise
Bucky
Collimate to cover

Technique

Factors	Screen film cassette (par)
mA	100
Time	2.75
mAs	275
Thickness in cm	28
kVp	76
Distance	40

Patient preparation

Remove all clothing except shoes and socks. Provide a gown for the patient.

Palpation points

Crest of the ilium; spinous processes of the lumbar vertebrae.

Procedure

Place the patient in the lateral recumbent position. Flex the hips and knees for support. Align the long axis of the spine over the center line of the table (4 inches anterior to the posterior surface). Flex the bottom elbow and place the forearm under the pillow. Flex the top elbow and place the forearm above the head with the hand grasping the edge of the table. Rotate the body into a true lateral position.

Central ray

Direct the central ray perpendicular through a point 4 inches superior to the crest of the ilium to the center of the film holder. Collimate to film holder.

Immobilization

Place a sponge or sandbag between the knees. Place a compression band over the pelvis. Employ suspended expiration.

Right-left markers

Place the correct marker on the anterior center border of the film holder.

Technical tips

A slight lateral concavity or "sagging" of the lumbar spine is beneficial in demonstrating intervertebral spaces. Excessive sagging will produce "wedging" of the vertebral bodies and decrease diagnostic quality.

Structures demonstrated

Lateral views of the lower thoracic and the lumbar bodies, the corresponding interspaces, the intervertebral foramina, and the spinous processes.

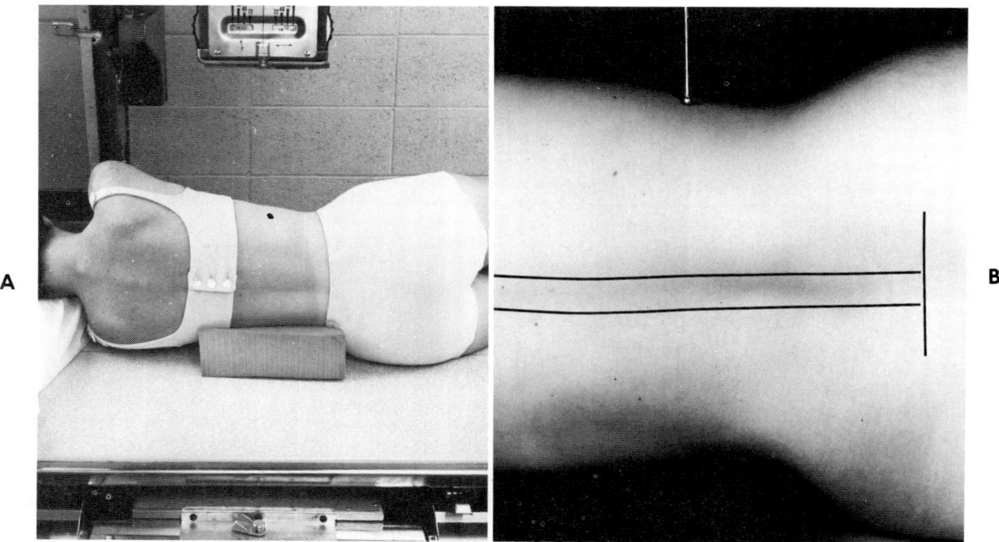

Fig. 9-19. Lumbar spine. A and B, Upper lateral positions.

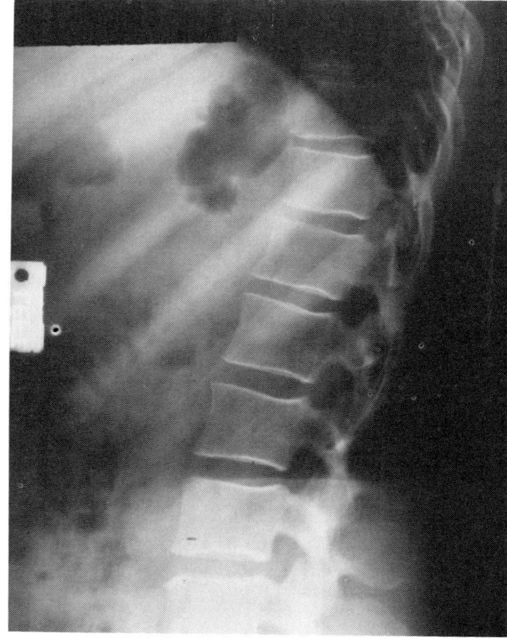

Fig. 9-20. Lumbar spine—upper lateral view. (Courtesy Dr. E. I. L. Cilley, Dr. T. W. Crowell, Dr. R. E. Waud, and Dr. G. H. Hoffman.)

Lumbar spine—lateral lumbosacral view (Figs. 9-21 and 9-22)

Film size—10″ × 12″
Cassette
Lengthwise
Bucky
Collimate to cover

Technique

Factors	Screen film cassette (par)
mA	100
Time	3.0
mAs	300
Thickness in cm	32
kVp	82
Distance	40

Patient preparation

Remove all clothing except shoes and socks. Provide a gown for the patient.

Palpation points

Crest of the ilium; spinous processes of the lumbar vertebrae.

Procedure

Place the patient in the lateral recumbent position. Flex the hips and knees for support. Align the long axis of the spine over the center line of the table (4 inches anterior to the posterior surface). Flex the bottom elbow and place the forearm under the pillow. Flex the top elbow and place the forearm above the head with the hand grasping the edge of the table. Rotate the body into a true lateral position.

Central ray

Direct the central ray perpendicular 1½ inches inferior to and parallel with a line between the crests of the ilia, through the lumbosacral junction to the center of the film holder. Collimate to film holder.

Immobilization

Place a sponge or sandbag between the knees. Place a compression band over the pelvis. Employ suspended expiration.

Right-left markers

Place the correct marker on the anterior center border of the film holder.

Technical tips

Most patients will require a caudad central ray angle for this view.

Structures demonstrated

Lateral views of the lumbar bodies, the lumbar interspaces, the intervertebral foramina, the spinous processes, the lumbosacral junction, and the sacrum.

Note: For suspected spondylolisthesis, make an erect lateral view utilizing the above procedure. Sacral depressions are unreliable landmarks for consistent accuracy.

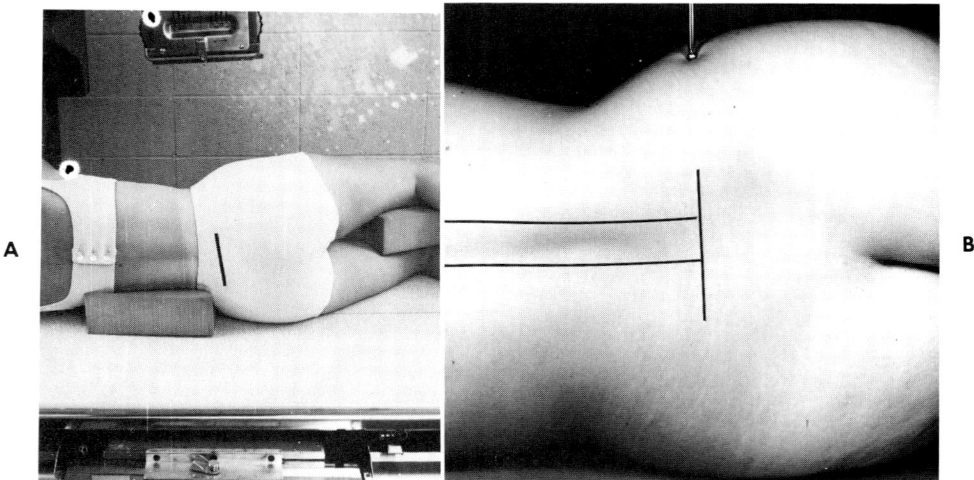

Fig. 9-21. Lumbar spine. A and B, Lumbosacral region, lateral positions.

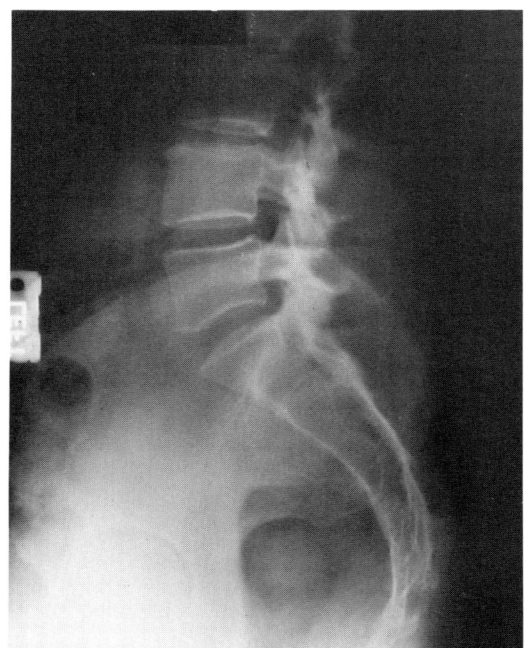

Fig. 9-22. Lumbar spine–lumbosacral region, lateral view. (Courtesy Dr. E. I. L. Cilley, Dr. T. W. Crowell, Dr. R. E. Waud, and Dr. G. H. Hoffman.)

Lumbar spine—anterior (P-A) oblique (L.A.O.-R.A.O.) view (Figs. 9-23 and 9-24)

Film size—10″ × 12″
Cassette
Lengthwise
Bucky
Collimate to cover

Technique

Factors	Screen film cassette (par)
mA	100
Time	1.5
mAs	150
Thickness in cm	28
kVp	74
Distance	40

Patient preparation

Remove all clothing except shoes and socks. Provide a gown for the patient.

Palpation points

Crest of the ilium; spinous processes of the lumbar vertebrae.

Procedure

Place the patient in the prone position. Elevate the side being examined so that the midsagittal plane of the body forms a 35-degree angle with the tabletop. Flex the knee and elbow of the elevated side for support. Center a line on the elevated side that is 1 inch lateral to the long axis of the spine over the center line of the table. Center the film holder to the top of the iliac crest.

Central ray

Direct the central ray perpendicular to the center of the film holder. Collimate to film holder.

Immobilization

Place a wedge sponge under the flexed knee. Employ suspended expiration.

Right-left markers

Place the correct marker on the elevated side, lateral center border of the film holder.

Technical tips

Increase the body rotation 10 degrees if the lower apophyseal joints are non-visualized.

Structures demonstrated

Oblique view of the lumbar vertebrae demonstrating the apophyseal joints of the elevated side.

Note: Both oblique views are usually made for comparison.

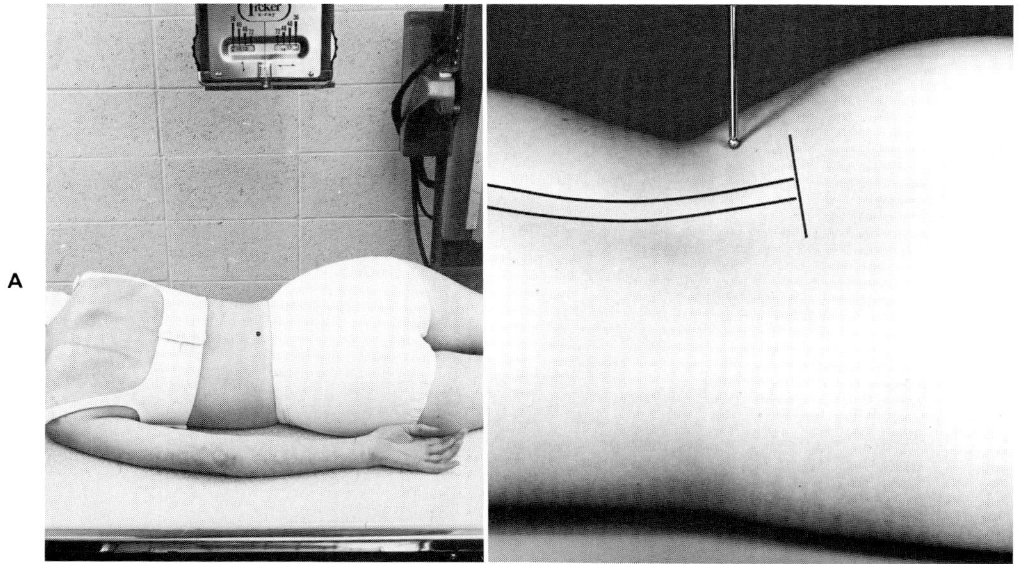

Fig. 9-23. Lumbar spine. **A** and **B,** Left anterior oblique (L.A.O.) positions.

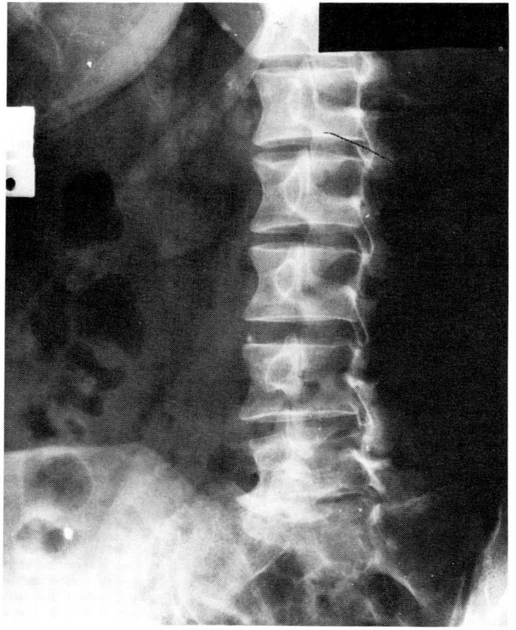

Fig. 9-24. Lumbar spine–left anterior oblique (L.A.O.) view. (Courtesy Dr. E. I. L. Cilley, Dr. T. W. Crowell, Dr. R. E. Waud, and Dr. G. H. Hoffman.)

Lumbar spine—posterior (A-P) lumbosacral articulation view (Figs. 9-25 and 9-26)

Film size—8″ × 10″
Cassette
Lengthwise
Bucky
Extension cone (fully extended)

Technique

Factors	Screen film cassette (par)
mA	100
Time	1.25
mAs	125
Thickness in cm	22
kVp	70
Distance	40

Patient preparation

Remove all garments from the waist down. Provide a gown for the patient.

Palpation point

Symphysis pubis.

Procedure

Place the patient in the supine position with the midline of the body over the center line of the table. Grasp the patient by the ankles and pull gently to straighten the spine. Flex the knees 90 degrees, placing the feet flat on the table. Brace the feet with sandbags.

Central ray

Direct the central ray 15 degrees cephalad to enter a point 4 inches above the symphysis pubis, through the lumbosacral spine to the center of the film holder.

Immobilization

Place sandbags on the lateral sides of the ankles. A compression band may be used across large abdomens. Employ suspended expiration.

Right-left markers

Burn the *R* marker in the superior border of the right side of the film holder above the cone field after the exposure is made.

Technical tips

To assist in palpation, the symphysis pubis is in the transverse line with the greater trochanter of the femur.

Structures demonstrated

Posterior (A-P) views of the lumbosacral structures and interspaces.

Note: The degree of central ray angulation will be governed somewhat by the physical stature and sex of the patient.

For prone patients, reverse the central ray angle, centering to the spinous process of the fifth lumbar vertebra.

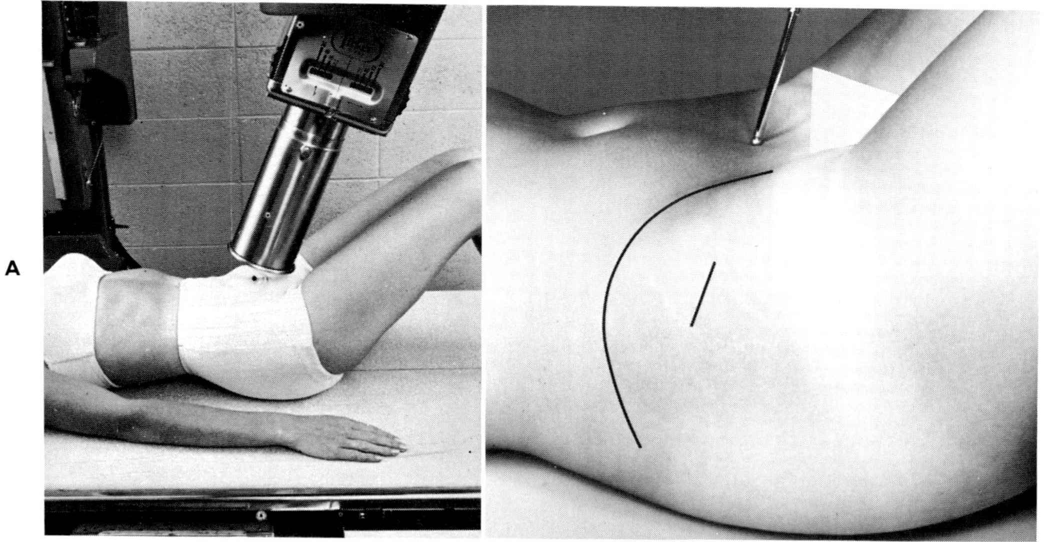

Fig. 9-25. Lumbar spine. **A** and **B,** Lumbosacral articulation, posterior (A-P) positions.

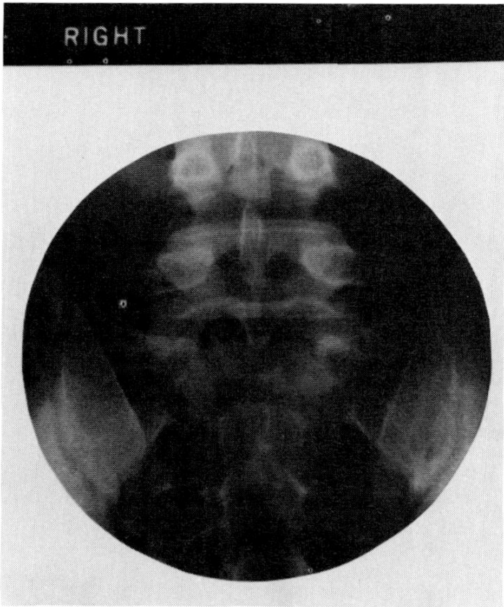

Fig. 9-26. Lumbar spine—lumbosacral articulation, posterior (A-P) view. (Courtesy Dr. E. I. L. Cilley, Dr. T. W. Crowell, Dr. R. E. Waud, and Dr. G. H. Hoffman.)

Pelvis—posterior (A-P) view (Figs. 9-27 and 9-28)

Film size—14″ × 17″
Cassette
Crosswise
Bucky
Collimate to cover

Technique

Factors	Screen film cassette (par)
mA	100
Time	1.0
mAs	100
Thickness in cm	20
kVp	66
Distance	40

Patient preparation

Remove all clothing from the waist down except shoes and socks. Provide a gown for the patient.

Palpation points

Symphysis pubis; crest of the ilium; greater trochanter of the femur.

Procedure

Place the patient in the supine position with the midline of the body over the center line of the table. Grasp the patient by the ankles and pull gently to straighten the spine. Flex the knees approximately 6 inches and support them with sponges. Rotate the ankles internally into a true posterior (A-P) position. Center a point midway between the crest of the ilium and the greater trochanter to the center of the film holder.

Central ray

Direct the central ray perpendicular to the center of the film holder. Collimate to film holder.

Immobilization

Place sandbags on the lateral sides of the ankles. A compression band may be used across large abdomens. Employ suspended expiration.

Right-left markers

Place the *R* marker on the right lateral center border of the film holder.

Technical tips

To assist in palpation, the symphysis pubis is in the transverse line with the greater trochanter of the femur.

Structures demonstrated

Posterior (A-P) views of the pelvic girdle and the head, neck, and trochanters of each femur.

Note: To better demonstrate the symphysis pubis, make an anterior (P-A) view of the pelvis.

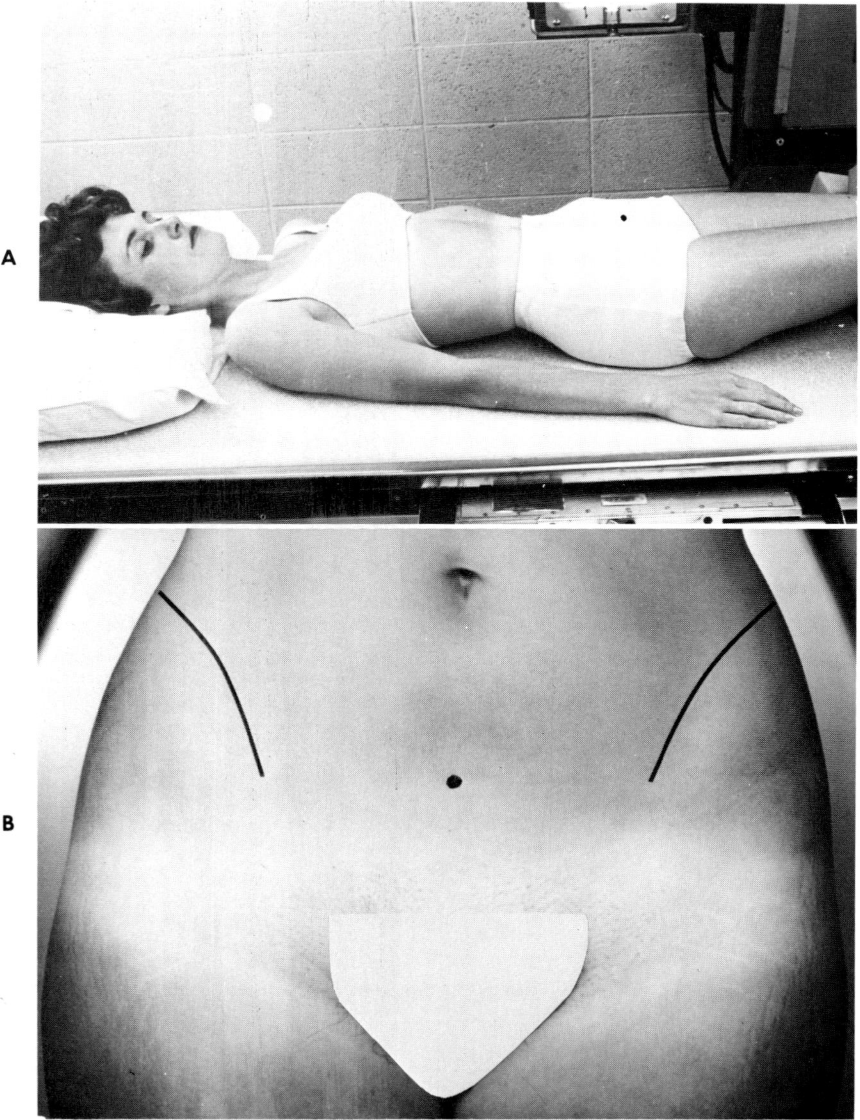

Fig. 9-27. Pelvis. **A** and **B,** Posterior (A-P) positions.

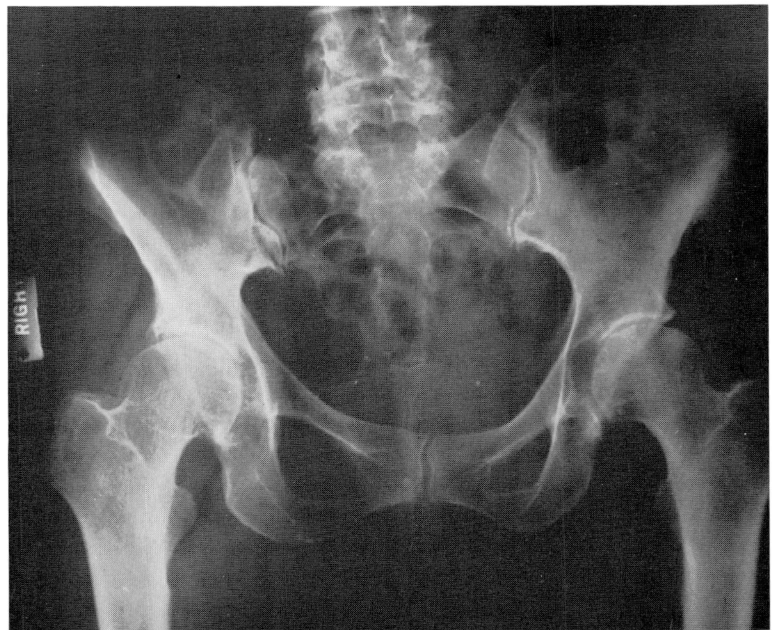

Fig. 9-28. Pelvis—posterior (A-P) view. (Courtesy Dr. E. I. L. Cilley, Dr. T. W. Crowell, Dr. R. E. Waud, and Dr. G. H. Hoffman.)

Sacrum—posterior (A-P) view (Figs. 9-29 to 9-31)

Film size—10″ × 12″
Cassette
Lengthwise

Bucky
Collimate to cover

Technique

Factors	Screen film cassette (par)
mA	100
Time	1.0
mAs	100
Thickness in cm	20
kVp	66
Distance	40

Patient preparation

Remove all clothing from the waist down except shoes and socks. Provide a gown for the patient.

Palpation points

Symphysis pubis; anterior superior iliac spinous processes; greater trochanter of the femur.

Procedure

Place the patient in the supine position with the midline of the body over the center line of the table. Grasp the patient by the ankles and pull gently to straighten the spine. Flex the knees approximately 6 inches and support them with sponges.

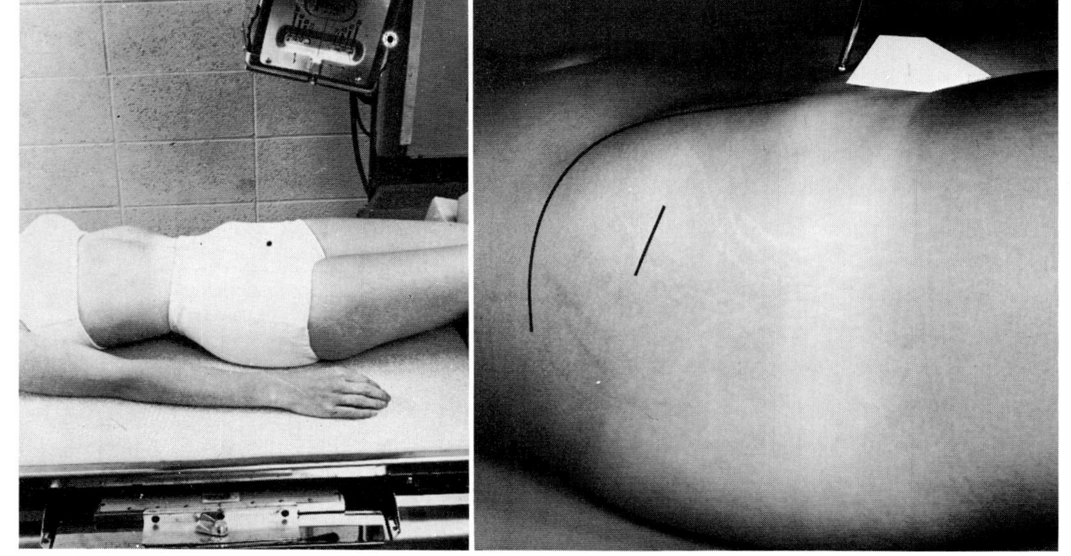

Fig. 9-29. Sacrum. **A** and **B,** Posterior (A-P) positions.

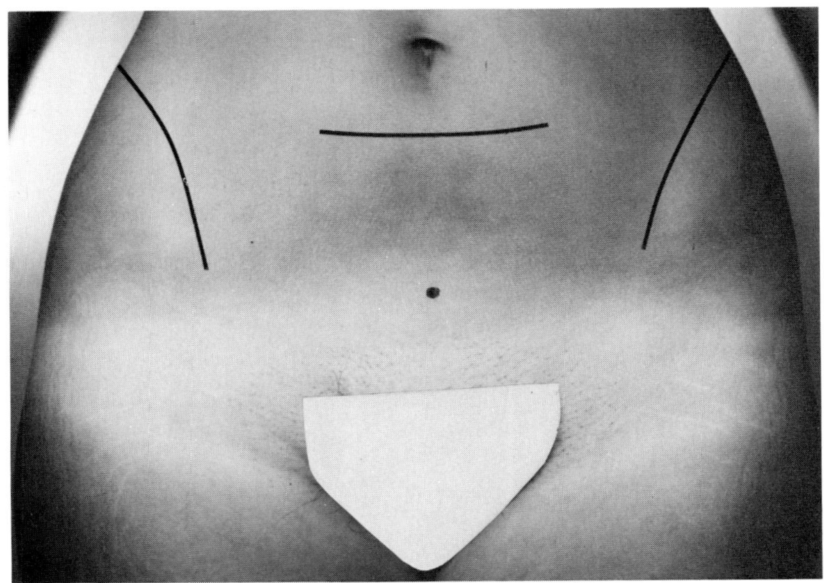

Fig. 9-30. Sacrum—posterior (A-P) view.

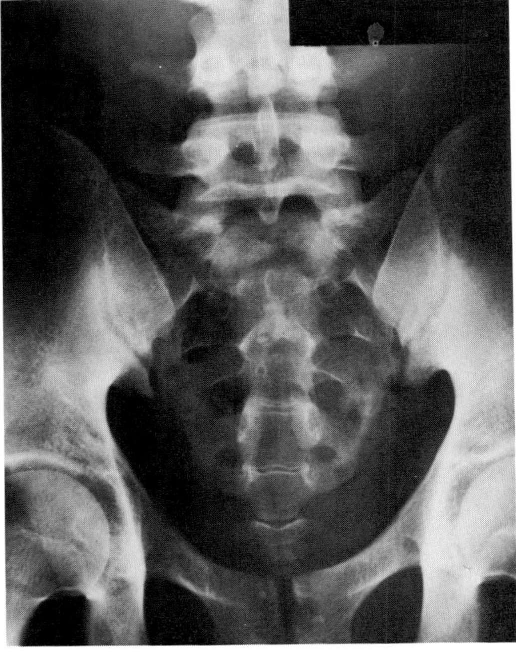

Fig. 9-31. Sacrum—posterior (A-P) view. (Courtesy Dr. E. I. L. Cilley, Dr. T. W. Crowell, Dr. R. E. Waud, and Dr. G. H. Hoffman.)

Central ray

Direct the central ray 15 degrees cephalad to enter a point 2½ inches above the symphysis pubis, to the center of the film holder. Collimate to film holder.

Immobilization

A compression band may be used across large abdomens. Employ suspended expiration.

Right-left markers

Place the *R* marker on the right lateral center border of the film holder.

Technical tips

Improved radiographic quality results when the patient is requested to void his urine prior to the examination.

Structures demonstrated

Posterior (A-P) views of the sacrum, the lumbosacral junction, and the sacro-iliac joints.

Note: For prone patients, angle the central ray 15 degrees caudad, centering to a point 3 inches inferior to a line connecting the iliac crests.

Sacrum—lateral view (Figs. 9-32 and 9-33)

Film size—10″ × 12″
Cassette
Lengthwise
Bucky
Collimate to cover

Technique

Factors	Screen film cassette (par)
mA	100
Time	2.5
mAs	250
Thickness in cm	30
kVp	80
Distance	40

Patient preparation

Remove all clothing from the waist down except shoes and socks. Provide a gown for the patient.

Palpation points

Anterior superior iliac spines.

Procedure

Place the patient in a lateral recumbent position. Flex the hips and knees for support. Align the long axis of the sacrum over the center line of the table (2 inches anterior to the posterior surface). Flex the bottom elbow and place the forearm under the pillow. Flex the top elbow and place the forearm above the head with the hand grasping the edge of the table. Rotate the body into a true lateral position. Center the film holder to the level of the anterior superior iliac spines.

Central ray

Direct the central ray perpendicular to the center of the film holder. Collimate to film holder.

Immobilization

Place sponges or sandbags between the knees and ankles. Place a compression band over the pelvis. Employ suspended expiration.

Right-left markers

Place the correct marker on the anterior center border of the film holder.

Technical tips

For more uniform radiographic density, use an aluminum wedge filter or $\frac{1}{10}$ mm added copper filter internally plus an increase of 10 kVp.

Structures demonstrated

Lateral views of the sacrum and coccyx, and of the lumbosacral junction.

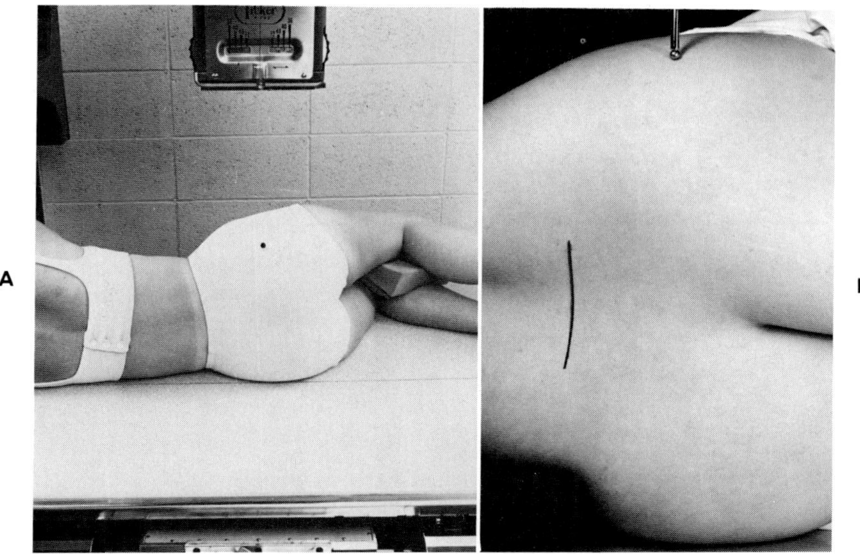

Fig. 9-32. Sacrum. **A** and **B,** Lateral positions.

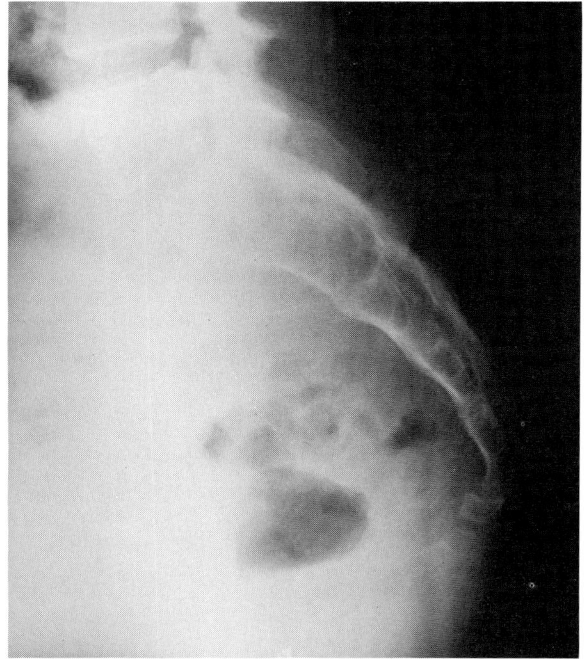

Fig. 9-33. Sacrum—lateral view. (Courtesy Scottsdale Memorial Hospital, Scottsdale, Arizona.)

Coccyx—posterior (A-P) view (Figs. 9-34 and 9-35)

Film size—8″ × 10″
Cassette
Lengthwise
Bucky
Extension cone (fully extended)

Technique

Factors	Screen film cassette (par)
mA	100
Time	1.0
mAs	100
Thickness in cm	22
kVp	70
Distance	40

Patient preparation

Remove all clothing from the waist down except shoes and socks. Provide a gown for the patient.

Palpation points

Symphysis pubis; greater trochanter of the femur.

Procedure

Place the patient in the supine position with the midline of the body over the center line of the table. Grasp the patient by the ankles and pull gently to straighten the spine. Flex the knees approximately 6 inches and support them with sponges.

Central ray

Direct the central ray 15 degrees caudad to enter a point 2½ inches above the symphysis pubis, to the center of the film holder.

Immobilization

A compression band may be used across large abdomens. Employ suspended expiration.

Right-left markers

Burn the *R* marker in the superior border of the right side of the film holder above the cone field after the exposure is made.

Technical tips

Improved radiographic quality results when the patient is requested to void urine and evacuate any intestinal contents prior to the examination.

Structures demonstrated

Posterior (A-P) view of the coccyx.

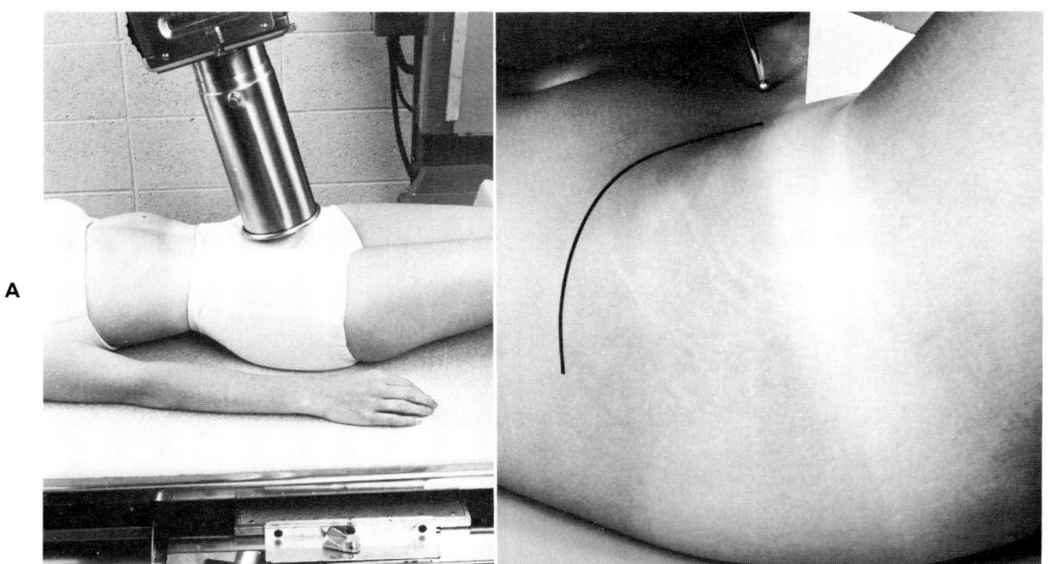

Fig. 9-34. Coccyx. **A** and **B**, Posterior (A-P) positions.

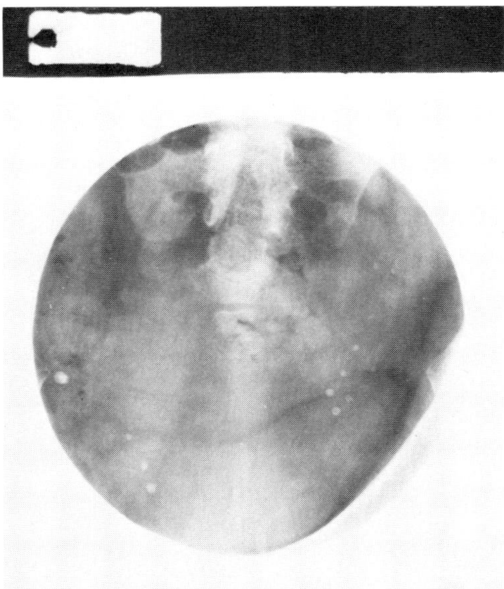

Fig. 9-35. Coccyx—posterior (A-P) view. (Courtesy Dr. E. I. L. Cilley, Dr. T. W. Crowell, Dr. R. E. Waud, and Dr. G. H. Hoffman.)

Coccyx—lateral view (Figs. 9-36 and 9-37)

Film size—8″ × 10″
Cassette
Lengthwise

Bucky
Extension cone (fully extended)

Technique

Factors	Screen film cassette (par)
mA	100
Time	2.5
mAs	250
Thickness in cm	30
kVp	80
Distance	40

Patient preparation

Remove all clothing from the waist down except shoes and socks. Provide a gown for the patient.

Palpation points

Posterior surface of the coccyx; greater trochanter of the femur.

Procedure

Place the patient in a lateral recumbent position. Flex the hips and knees for support. Align the long axis of the sacrum and coccyx over the center line of the table (2 inches anterior to the posterior surface of the sacrum). Flex the bottom elbow and place the forearm under the pillow. Flex the top elbow and place the forearm above the head with the hand grasping the edge of the table. Rotate the body into a true lateral position.

Central ray

Direct the central ray perpendicular through a point 1 inch superior to the greater trochanter to the center of the film holder.

Immobilization

Place sponges or sandbags between the knees and ankles. Place a compression band over the pelvis. Employ suspended expiration.

Right-left markers

Burn the left or right marker in the superior center border of the film holder after the exposure is made.

Technical tips

Use the smallest collimator opening possible and a minimum distance of 40 inches to compensate for the increased object-film distance.

Structures demonstrated

Lateral views of the coccyx and lower sacrum.

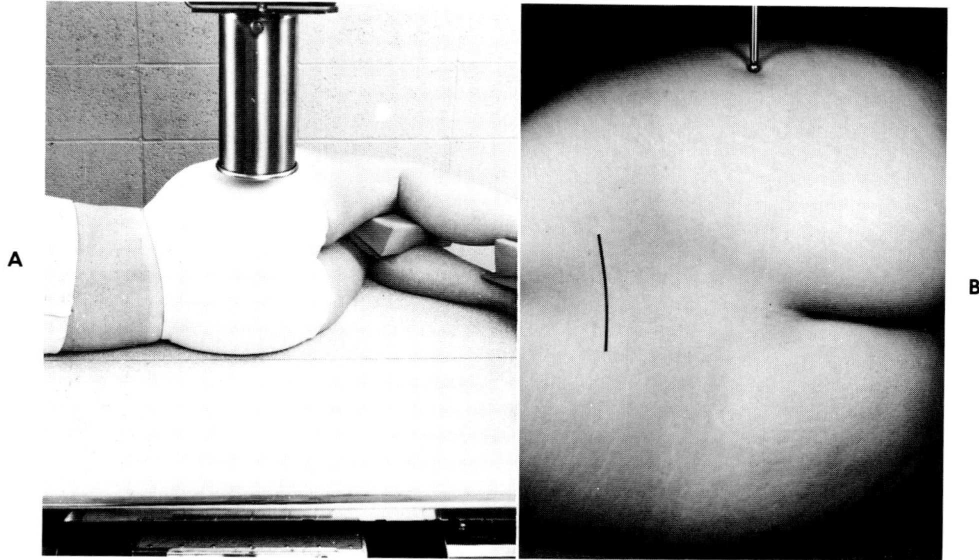

Fig. 9-36. Coccyx. **A** and **B,** Lateral positions.

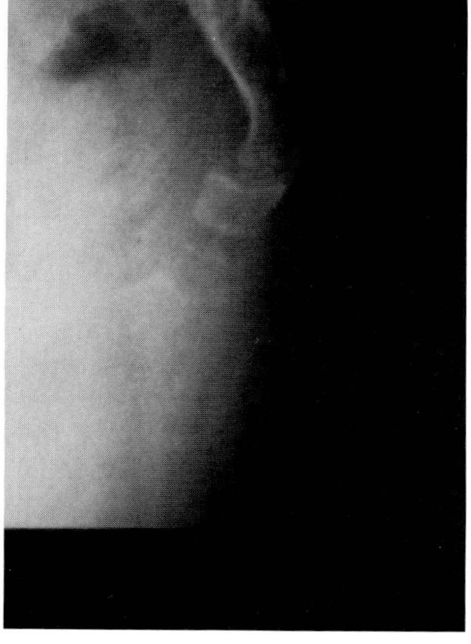

Fig. 9-37. Coccyx—lateral view. (Courtesy Scottsdale Memorial Hospital, Scottsdale, Arizona.)

Hip—posterior (A-P) (unilateral) view (Figs. 9-38 and 9-39)

Film size—10″ × 12″
Cassette
Lengthwise
Bucky
Collimate to cover

Technique

Factors	Screen film cassette (par)
mA	100
Time	1.0
mAs	100
Thickness in cm	20
kVp	66
Distance	40

Patient preparation

Remove all clothing from the waist down except shoes and socks. Provide a gown for the patient.

Palpation points

Symphysis pubis; anterior superior iliac spine.

Procedure

Place the patient in the supine position. Locate the hip joint as follows: at right angles bisect a line between the anterior superior iliac spine and the symphysis pubis; select a point on the bisecting line 2 inches inferior to the first line; center this point over the center line of the table. Rotate the ankles internally into a true posterior (A-P) position.

Central ray

Direct the central ray perpendicular through the located point to the center of the film holder. Collimate to film holder.

Immobilization

Place sandbags on each side of the foot and ankle. Employ suspended expiration.

Right-left markers

Place the correct marker in the superior lateral border of the film holder.

Technical tips

To locate the femoral head and neck, select points 2½ inches and 3 inches, respectively, inferior to the bisected line.

Structures demonstrated

Posterior (A-P) views of the femoral head, anatomic and surgical necks, and trochanters, all in relationship to the acetabulum.

Note: For children under 12 years of age, the radiographic request may be for views of both hips for comparison; this examination should be performed employing a single exposure on a film of suitable size placed crosswise with the pelvis. *Be sure to employ gonadal protection.*

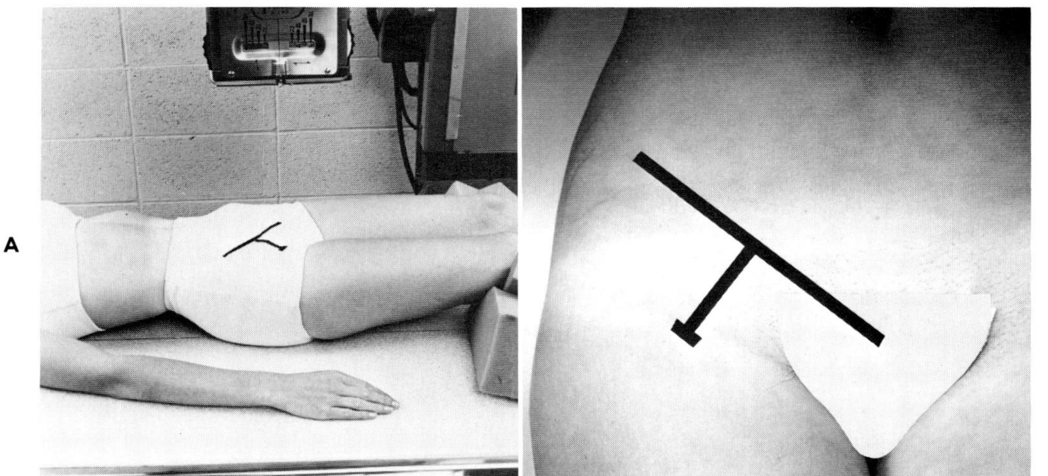

Fig. 9-38. Hip. **A** and **B**, Posterior (A-P) positions.

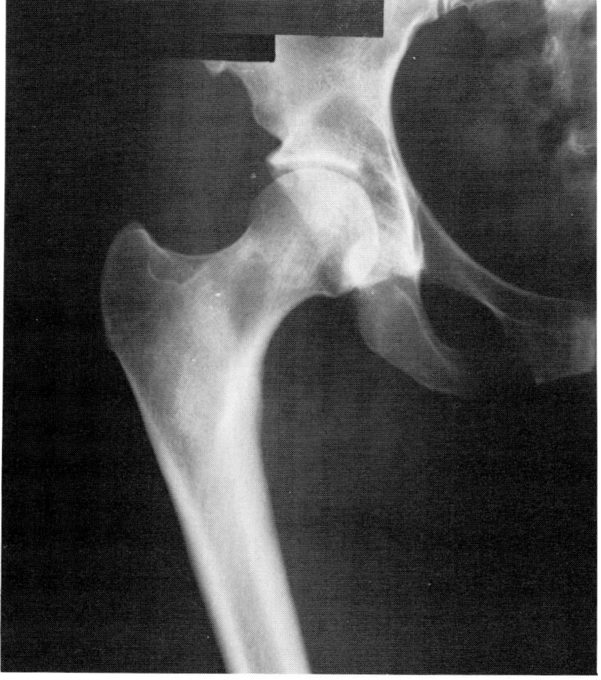

Fig. 9-39. Hip—posterior (A-P) view. (Courtesy Dr. E. I. L. Cilley, Dr. T. W. Crowell, Dr. R. E. Waud, and Dr. G. H. Hoffman.)

Hip—lateral (unilateral) "frog" view (Figs. 9-40 to 9-42)

Film size—10″ × 12″
Cassette
Crosswise
Bucky
Collimate to cover

Technique

Factors	Screen film cassette (par)
mA	100
Time	1.0
mAs	100
Thickness in cm	20
kVp	66
Distance	40

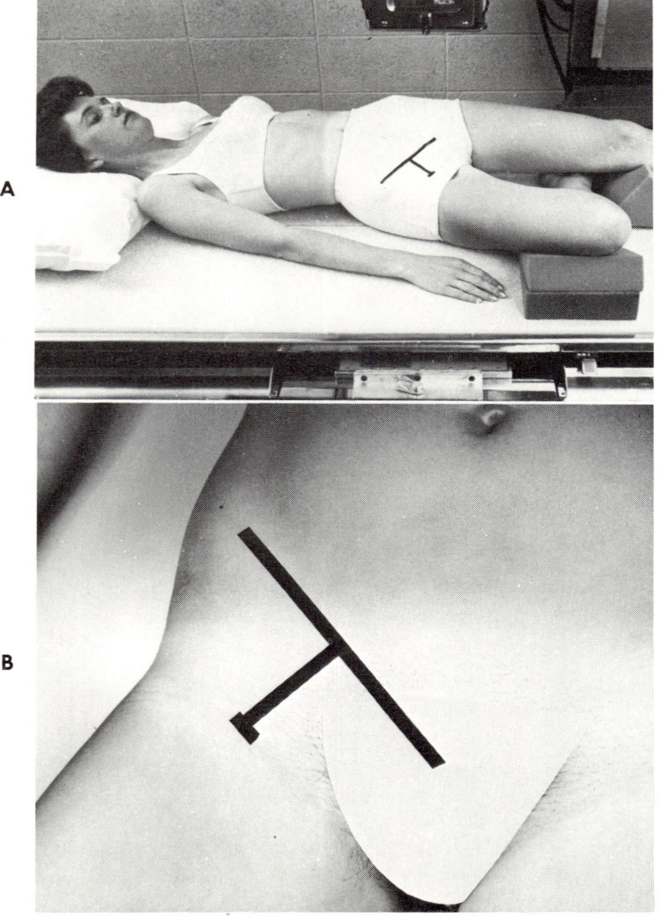

Fig. 9-40. Hip. **A** and **B,** Unilateral (frog) positions.

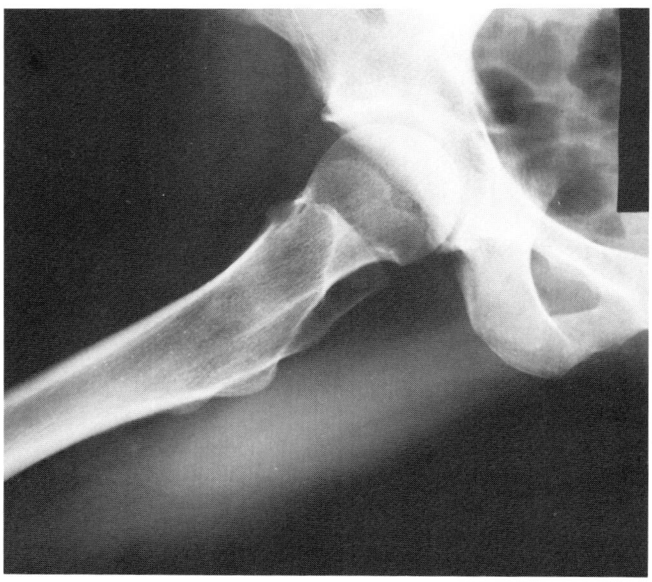

Fig. 9-41. Hip—unilateral (frog) view. (Courtesy Dr. E. I. L. Cilley, Dr. T. W. Crowell, Dr. R. E. Waud, and Dr. G. H. Hoffman.)

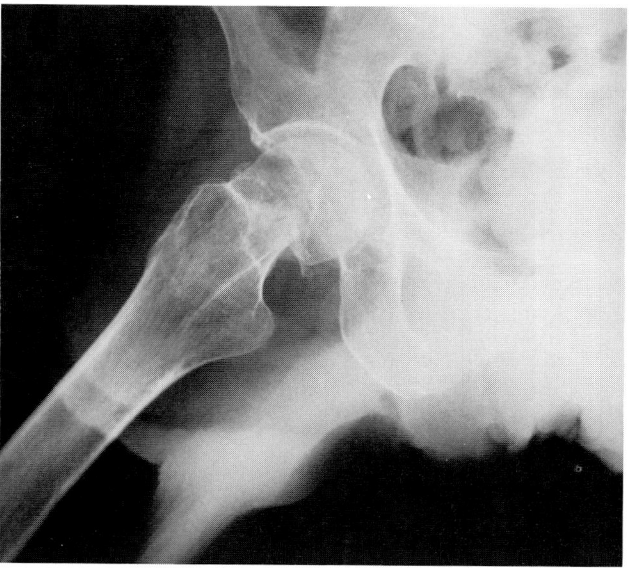

Fig. 9-42. Hip—unilateral (frog) view. (Courtesy Scottsdale Memorial Hospital, Scottsdale, Arizona.)

Patient preparation

Remove all clothing from the waist down except shoes and socks. Provide a gown for the patient.

Palpation points

Symphysis pubis; anterior superior iliac spine.

Procedure

Place the patient in the supine position. Locate the hip joint as follows: at right angles bisect a line between the anterior superior iliac spine and the symphysis pubis; select a point on the bisecting line 2 inches inferior to the first line; center this point over the center line of the table. Flex the knee 90 degrees, and abduct it as far as possible, turning the foot on its lateral side.

Central ray

Direct the central ray perpendicular through the located point to the center of the film holder. Collimate to film holder.

Immobilization

Place a sponge or sandbag under the lateral side of the flexed knee, and a heavy sandbag on top of the foot. Employ suspended expiration.

Right-left markers

Place the correct marker in the superior lateral border of the film holder.

Technical tips

A reduction in technique from the anteroposterior hip view is usually necessary for this view.

Structures demonstrated

Lateral views of the femoral head, anatomic and surgical necks, and the trochanters in relationship to the acetabulum.

Note: For children under 12 years of age, the radiographic request may be for views of both hips for comparison; this examination should be performed employing a single exposure on a film of suitable size placed crosswise with the pelvis, and with both hips in the position described above (frog position). *Be sure to employ gonadal protection.*

Hip—translateral view (Figs. 9-43 to 9-45)

Film size—8″ × 10″
Cassette
Lengthwise

Grid cassette
Extension cone (fully extended)

Technique

Factors	Screen film cassette (par)
mA	100
Time	1.75
mAs	175
Thickness in cm	22
kVp	68
Distance	40

Patient preparation

Remove all clothing from the waist down. Provide a gown for the patient.

Palpation points

Symphysis pubis; anterior superior iliac spine; iliac crest.

Procedure

Place the patient in the supine position on a cushion or pillows to elevate the body. Fully extend the leg to be examined; rotate the ankle internally into a true posterior (A-P) position. Flex the opposite knee to form an arch, and place the foot on an elevated support. Place the cassette on edge and brace its superior edge against the body above the crest of the ilium with a sandbag. The cassette face is parallel with a perpendicular plane that bisects a line between the anterior superior iliac spine and the symphysis pubis.

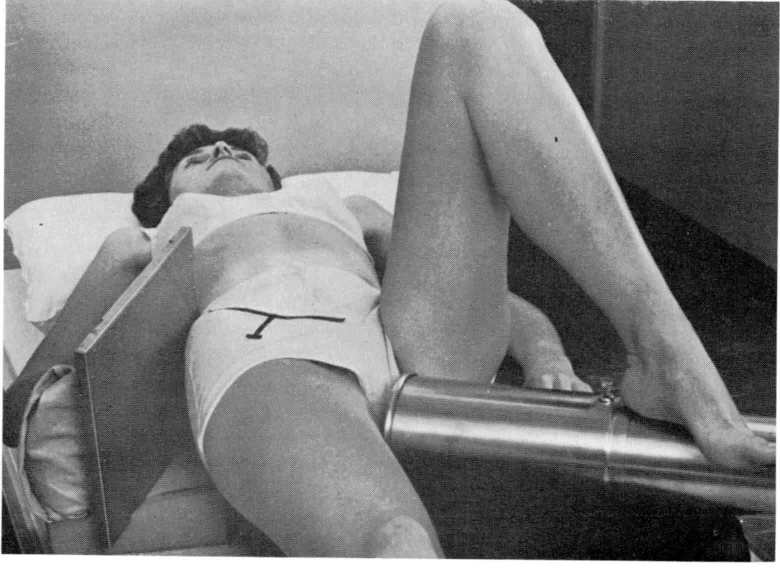

Fig. 9-43. Hip—translateral position.

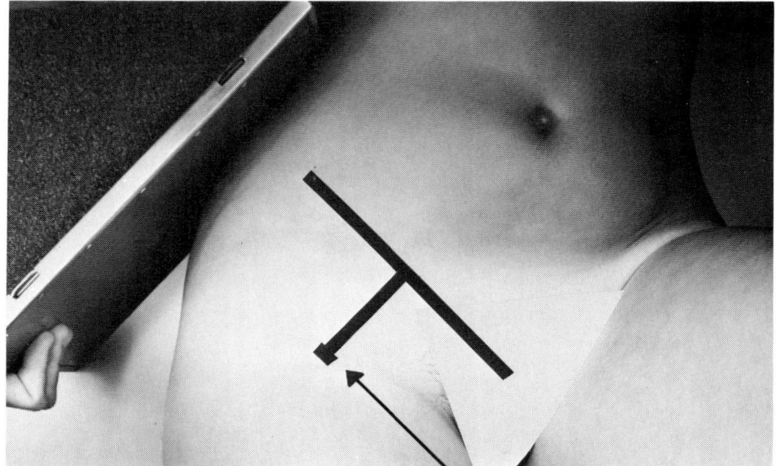

Fig. 9-44. Hip—translateral position.

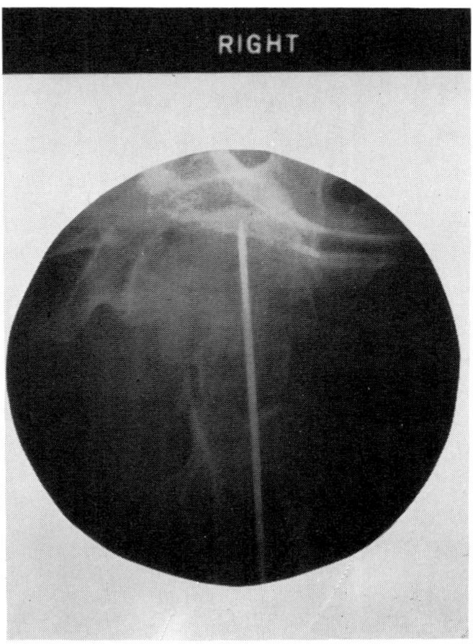

Fig. 9-45. Hip—translateral view. (Courtesy Dr. E. I. L. Cilley, Dr. T. W. Crowell, Dr. R. E. Waud, and Dr. G. H. Hoffman.)

Central ray

In a horizontal plane direct the central ray perpendicular under the flexed knee through the greater trochanter to the center of the film holder.

Immobilization

Place sandbags on each side of the foot. Employ suspended expiration.

Right-left markers

Burn the correct marker in the superior center border of the film holder above the cone field after the exposure is made.

Technical tips

If the patient cannot flex the opposite knee, have him abduct that thigh and hang the leg over the table edge.

Structures demonstrated

Lateral views of the femoral head, anatomic neck, and trochanters. This examination results in minimum discomfort to the patient.

Shoulder—posterior (A-P) view, external rotation (Figs. 9-46 and 9-47)

Film size—10″ × 12″
Cassette
Crosswise
Bucky
Collimate to cover

Technique

Factors	Screen film cassette (par) Bucky	Screen film cassette (par) tabletop
mA	100	100
Time	0.2	0.1
mAs	20	10
Thickness in cm	14	14
kVp	74	68
Distance	40	40

Patient preparation

Remove all garments down to the waist. Provide a gown for female patients.

Palpation points

Coracoid process of the scapula; humeral epicondyles.

Procedure

Place the patient in the supine position. Center the coracoid process over the center line of the table. Elevate the opposite shoulder 6 inches and support it with a sandbag. Rotate the entire arm externally so that a line through the humeral epicondyles is parallel with the tabletop.

Central ray

Direct the central ray perpendicular through the coracoid process to the center of the film holder. Collimate to film holder.

Immobilization

Place one sandbag under, and a second on top of, the hand. Employ suspended expiration.

Right-left markers

Place the correct marker on the superior center border of the film holder.

Technical tips

The external rotation view will demonstrate the humeral head projected medially.

Structures demonstrated

Posterior (A-P) views of the bony structures of the shoulder in the true anatomic position.

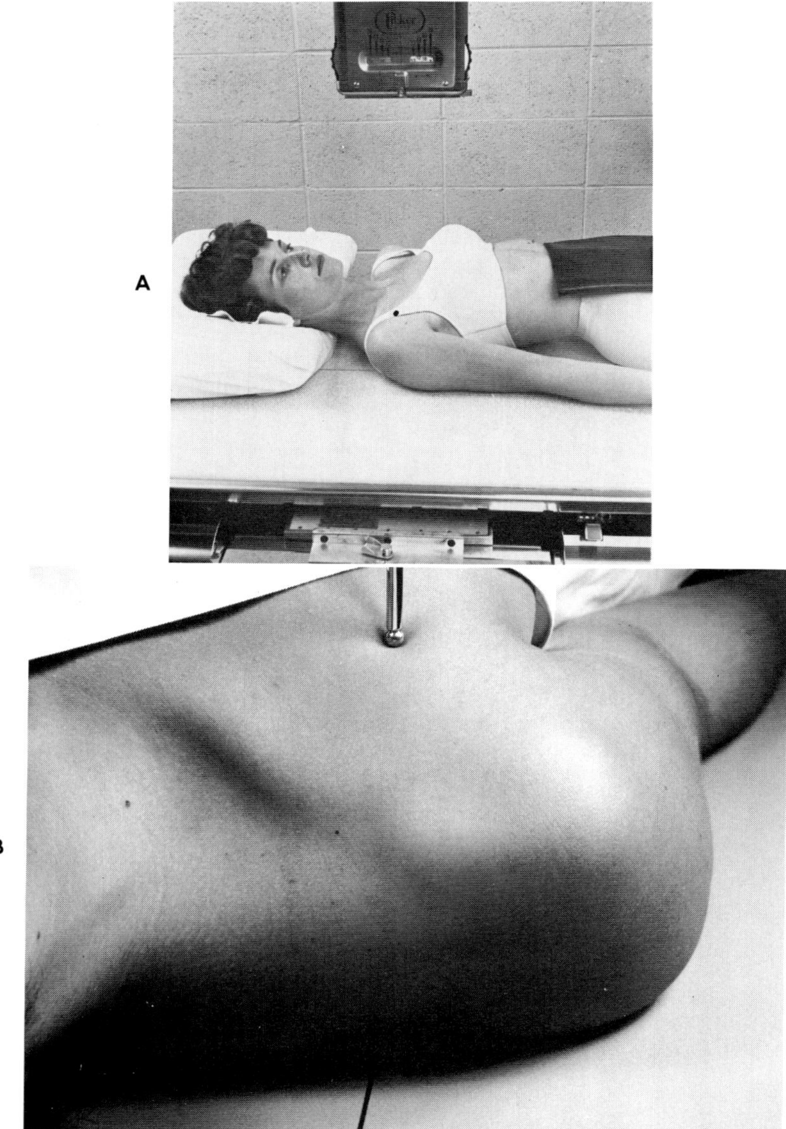

Fig. 9-46. Shoulder. A and B, Posterior (A-P) positions, external rotation.

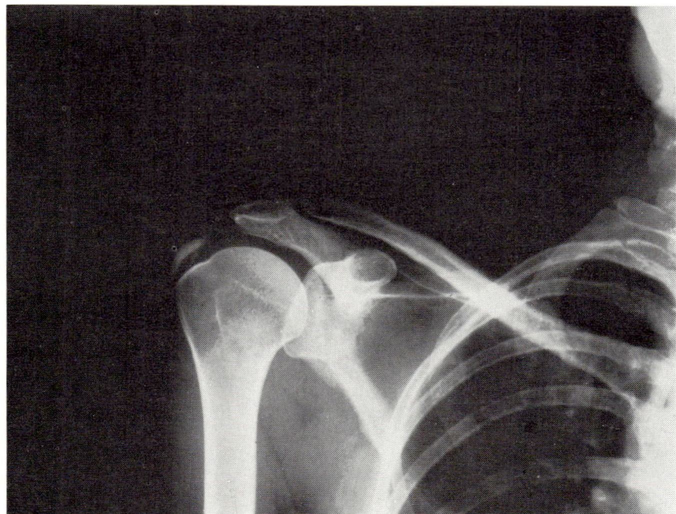

Fig. 9-47. Shoulder—posterior (A-P) view, external rotation. (Courtesy Dr. E. I. L. Cilley, Dr. T. W. Crowell, Dr. R. E. Waud, and Dr. G. H. Hoffman.)

Shoulder—posterior (A-P) view, internal rotation (Figs. 9-48 and 9-49)

Film size—10″ × 12″
Cassette
Crosswise

Bucky
Collimate to cover

Technique

Factors	Screen film cassette (par) Bucky	Screen film cassette (par) tabletop
mA	100	100
Time	0.2	0.1
mAs	20	10
Thickness in cm	14	14
kVp	74	68
Distance	40	40

Patient preparation

Remove all garments down to the waist. Provide a gown for female patients.

Palpation points

Coracoid process of the scapula; humeral epicondyles.

Procedure

Place the patient in the supine position. Center the coracoid process over the center line of the table. Elevate the opposite shoulder 6 inches and support it with a sandbag. Rotate the entire arm internally so that a line through the humeral epicondyles is perpendicular to the tabletop.

Central ray

Direct the central ray perpendicular through the coracoid process to the center of the film holder. Collimate to film holder.

Immobilization

Place a sandbag on top of the hand. Employ suspended expiration.

Right-left markers

Place the correct marker on the superior center border of the film holder.

Technical tips

The internal rotation view will demonstrate the humeral head projected posteriorly.

Structures demonstrated

Posterior (A-P) views of the bony structures of the shoulder and of the lateral humerus in relationship to the glenoid cavity.

Note: Both internal and external rotation views of the shoulder should be made in routine examinations, particularly on patients with suspected bursitis.

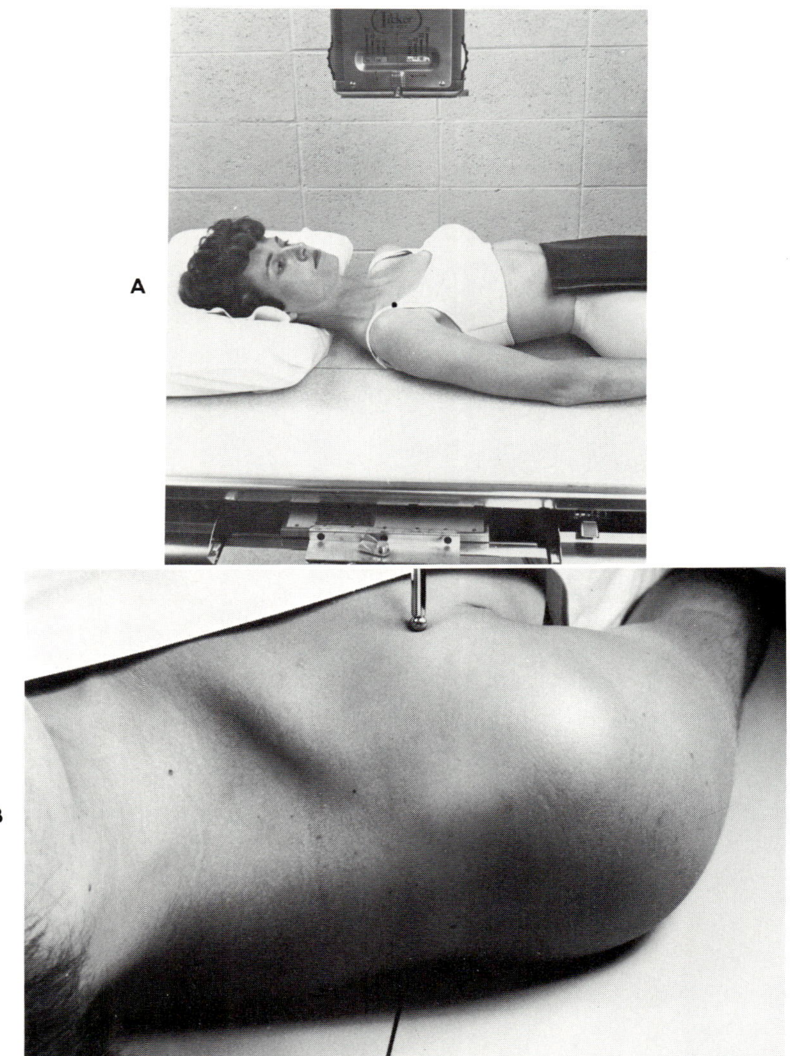

Fig. 9-48. Shoulder. **A** and **B**, Posterior (A-P) positions, internal rotation.

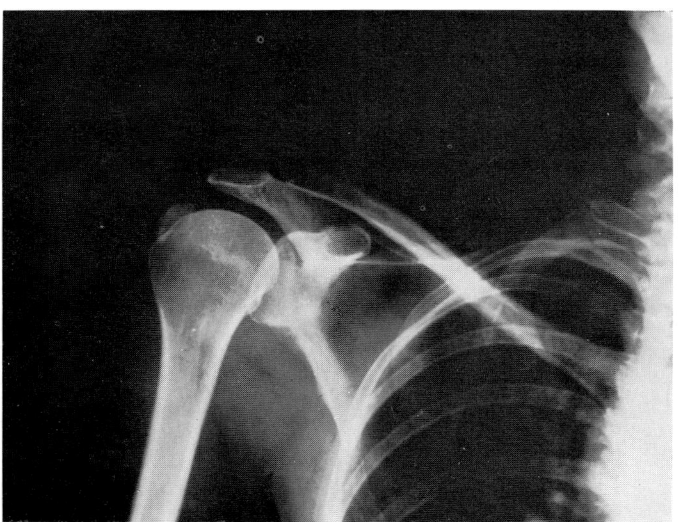

Fig. 9-49. Shoulder—posterior (A-P) view, internal rotation. (Courtesy Dr. E. I. L. Cilley, Dr. T. W. Crowell, Dr. R. E. Waud, and Dr. G. H. Hoffman.)

Shoulder—lateral view through the thorax (Figs. 9-50 and 9-51)

Film size—10″ × 12″	*Bucky (erect)*
Cassette	*Collimate to cover*
Lengthwise	*(Rapid shallow breathing technique)*

Technique

Factors	Screen film cassette (par)
mA	25
Time	6
mAs	150
Thickness in cm	32
kVp	78
Distance	40

Patient preparation

Remove all garments down to the waist. Provide a gown for female patients.

Palpation points

Greater tubercle and surgical neck of the humerus; sternum; spinous processes of the thoracic vertebrae.

Procedure

Place the patient in the erect position, either sitting or standing, with the shoulder being examined against the erect Bucky or grid. Flex this elbow, and rest the palm of the hand against the anterior chest. Place the opposite forearm on top of the head. Rotate the body so that the humerus being radiographed is midway between the sternum and the vertebral column.

Central ray

Direct the central ray 10 degrees cephalad through the surgical neck of the humerus to the center of the film holder. Collimate to film holder.

Immobilization

Use a compression band around the thorax. Employ rapid shallow breathing during the radiographic exposure.

Right-left markers

Place the correct marker on the anterior side, center border of the film holder.

Technical tips

In this position the surgical neck of the humerus is on the same plane as the spinous process of the fourth thoracic vertebra.

Structures demonstrated

Lateral views of the humeral head, neck, and the upper one third of the shaft projected through the thorax.

Note: This view should be made for all patients with suspected fractures, immobilized fractures, or hanging casts involving the proximal humerus.

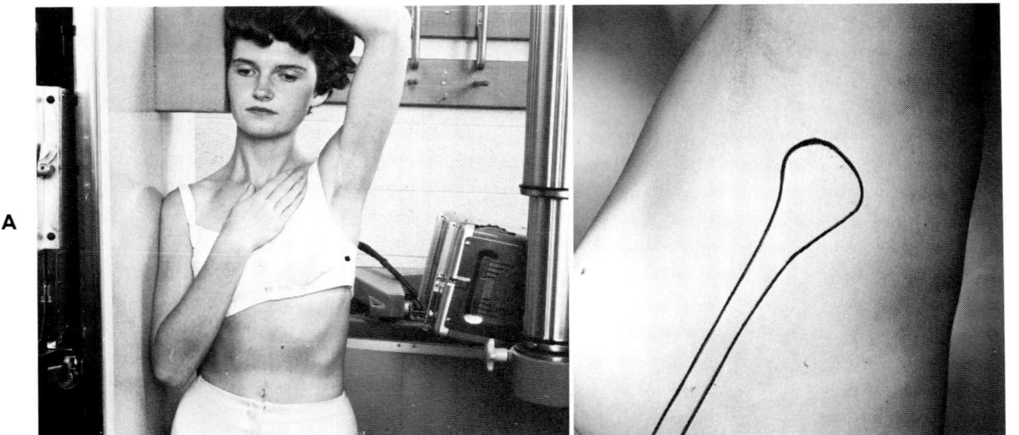

Fig. 9-50. Shoulder. **A** and **B**, Lateral (through the thorax) positions.

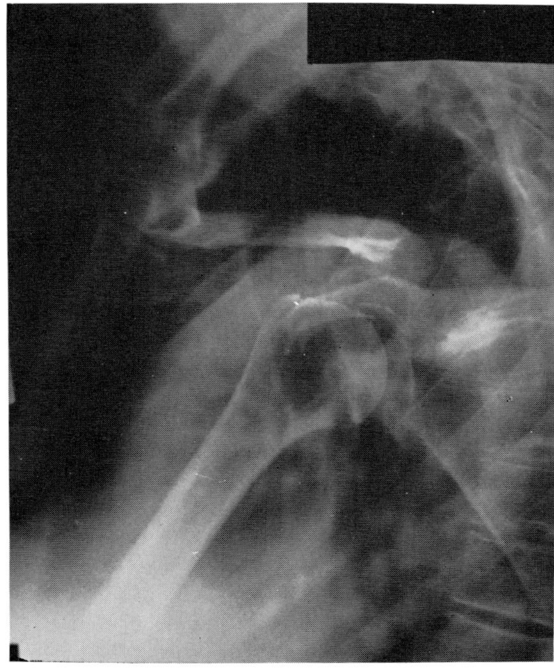

Fig. 9-51. Shoulder—lateral (through the thorax) view. (Courtesy Dr. E. I. L. Cilley, Dr. T. W. Crowell, Dr. R. E. Waud, and Dr. G. H. Hoffman.)

Clavicle—anterior (P-A) view (Figs. 9-52 and 9-53)

Film size—10″ × 12″
Cassette
Crosswise

Bucky
Collimate to cover

Technique

Factors	Screen film cassette (par) Bucky	Screen film cassette (par) tabletop
mA	100	100
Time	0.2	0.1
mAs	20	10
Thickness in cm	14	14
kVp	74	68
Distance	40	40

Patient preparation

Remove all garments down to the waist. Provide a gown for female patients.

Palpation points

Acromioclavicular articulation; sternoclavicular articulation; shaft of the clavicle.

Procedure

Place the patient in the prone or anterior (P-A) erect position with the arms extended down the body. Extend the chin and rest it on the table. Center the midshaft of the clavicle over the center line of the table.

Central ray

Direct the central ray 10 degrees caudad through the clavicle to the center of the film holder. Collimate to film holder.

Immobilization

A compression band may be used across the chest. Employ suspended expiration.

Right-left markers

Place the correct marker on the superior center border of the film holder.

Technical tips

To better demonstrate the sternal end of the clavicle, elevate the side being examined 5 to 10 degrees.

Structures demonstrated

Anterior (P-A) view of the entire clavicle.

Note: For supine patients, angle the central ray 10 degrees cephalad.

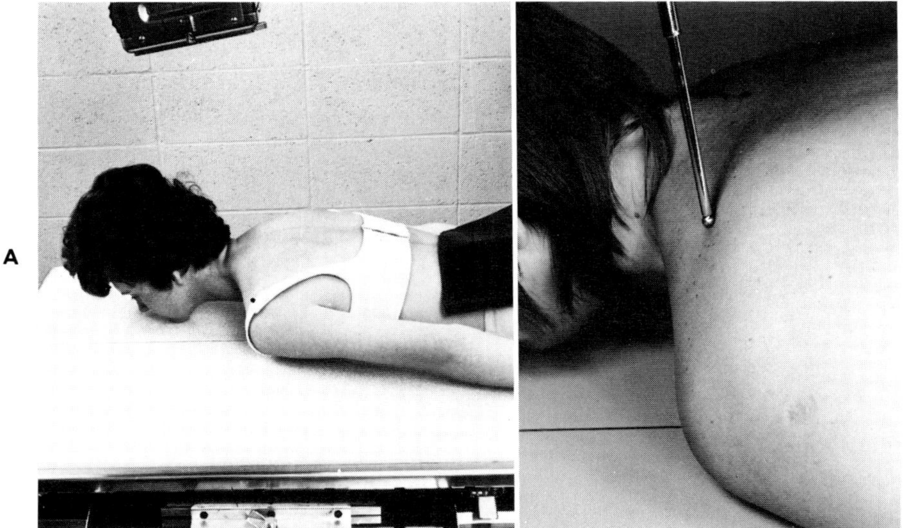

Fig. 9-52. Clavicle. **A** and **B**, Anterior (P-A) positions.

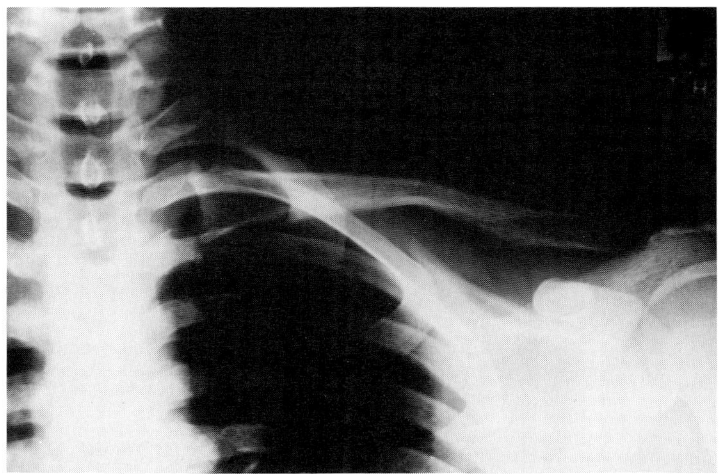

Fig. 9-53. Clavicle—anterior (P-A) view. (Courtesy Scottsdale Memorial Hospital, Scottsdale, Arizona.)

Clavicle—anterior (P-A) view, sternoclavicular articulations (Figs. 9-54 and 9-55)

Film size—8″ × 10″
Cassette
Crosswise
Bucky
Collimate to cover

Technique

Factors	Screen film cassette (par)
mA	100
Time	0.6
mAs	60
Thickness in cm	21
kVp	78
Distance	40

Patient preparation

Remove all garments down to the waist. Provide a gown for female patients.

Palpation points

Sternoclavicular articulations; shaft of the clavicle; manubrium.

Procedure

Place the patient in the prone or anterior (P-A) erect position with the arms extended down the body. Extend the chin and rest it on the table. Center the midsagittal plane of the body over the center line of the table.

Central ray

Direct the central ray perpendicular through the third thoracic vertebra to the center of the film. Collimate to film holder.

Immobilization

A compression band may be used across the chest. Employ suspended expiration.

Right-left markers

Place the *R* marker in the right superior border of the film.

Technical tips

To emphasize the inferior portion of the sternoclavicular articulations, place the forearms above the head.

Structures demonstrated

Anterior (P-A) view of the sternoclavicular joints.

Note: For acromioclavicular separation, make unilateral anteroposterior erect views of each shoulder while the patient is holding a 5-pound sandbag in each hand. Center the horizontal central ray through each acromioclavicular joint.

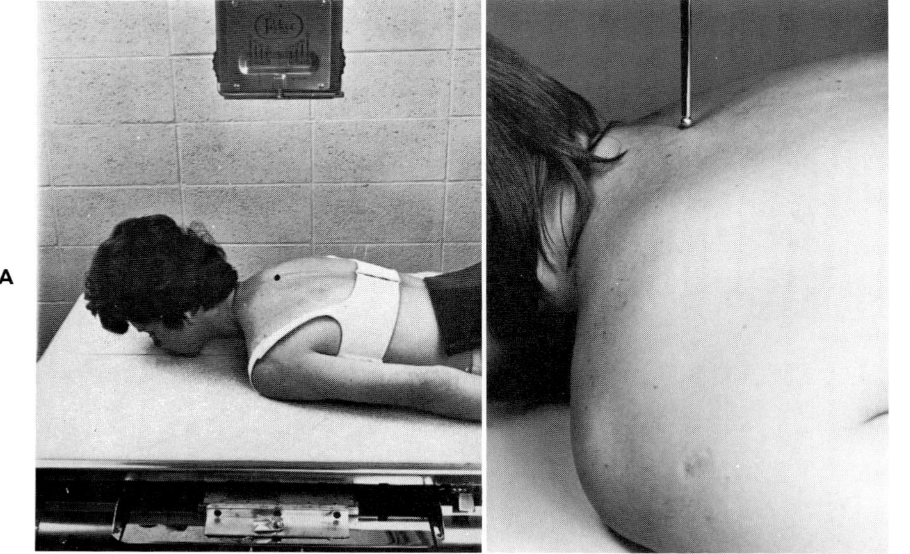

Fig. 9-54. Clavicle. **A** and **B,** Anterior (P-A) positions, sternoclavicular articulations.

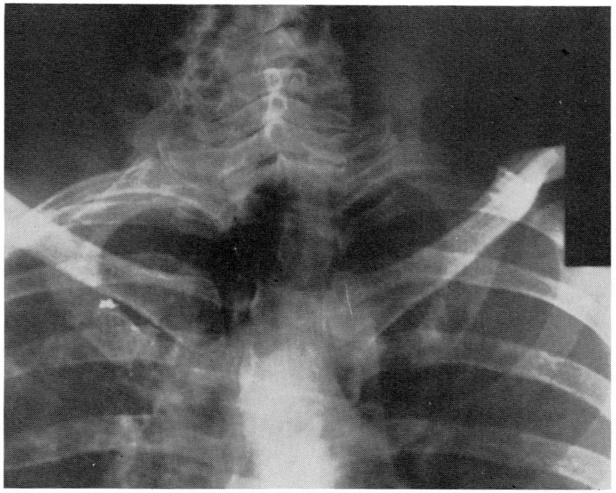

Fig. 9-55. Clavicle—anterior (P-A) view, sternoclavicular articulations. (Courtesy Dr. E. I. L. Cilley, Dr. T. W. Crowell, Dr. R. E. Waud, and Dr. G. H. Hoffman.)

Clavicle—anterior (P-A) oblique view, sternoclavicular articulation (Figs. 9-56 and 9-57)

Film size—8″ × 10″
Cassette
Lengthwise
Bucky
Extension cone (fully extended)

Technique

Factors	Screen film cassette (par)
mA	100
Time	0.6
mAs	60
Thickness in cm	21
kVp	78
Distance	40

Patient preparation

Remove all garments down to the waist. Provide a gown for female patients.

Palpation points

Sternoclavicular articulations; shaft of the clavicle; manubrium.

Procedure

Place the patient in the prone or anterior (P-A) erect position. Elevate the side opposite the one being examined so that the midsagittal plane of the head and body forms a 45-degree angle with the tabletop. When the patient is prone, flex the knee and the elbow of the elevated side for support. Align the joint being examined over the center line of the table.

Central ray

Direct the central ray perpendicular through the sternoclavicular articulation to the center of the film holder.

Immobilization

Place a sponge or sandbag under the flexed knee. Employ suspended expiration.

Right-left markers

Burn the correct marker in the superior center border of the film holder above the cone field after the exposure is made.

Technical tips

The sternoclavicular articulation is on the same transverse plane as the spinous process of the third thoracic vertebra.

Structures demonstrated

Anterior (P-A) oblique views of the sternoclavicular articluation and of the manubrium.

Note: Both right and left views should be made for comparison.

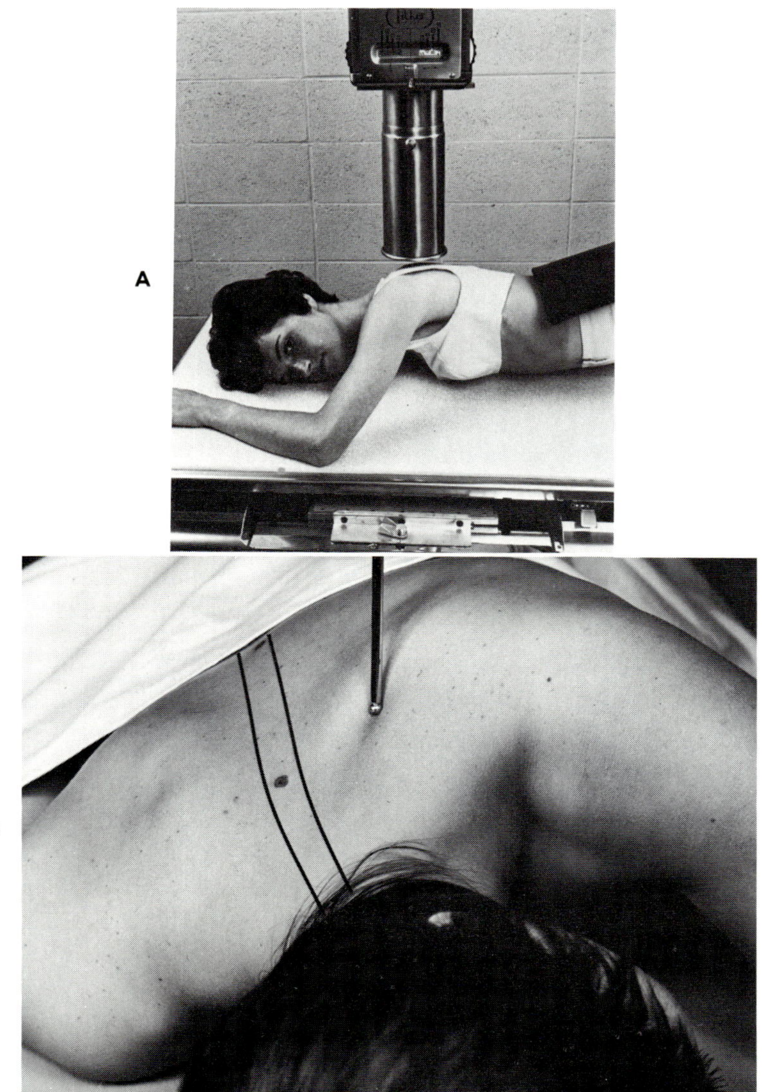

Fig. 9-56. Clavicle. **A** and **B,** Anterior (P-A) oblique positions, sternoclavicular articulation.

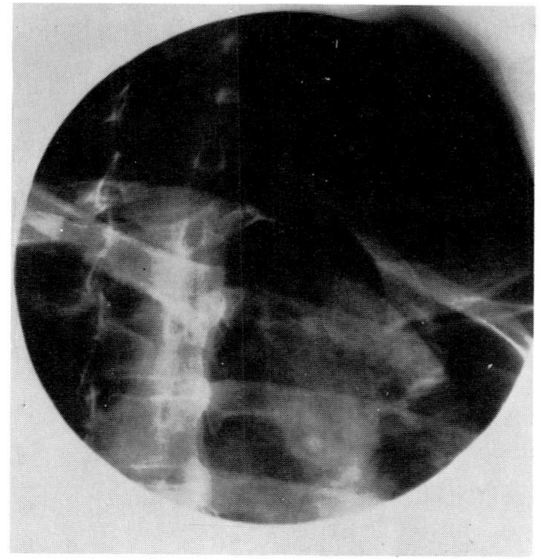

Fig. 9-57. Clavicle—anterior (P-A) oblique view, sternoclavicular articulation. (Courtesy Dr. E. I. L. Cilley, Dr. T. W. Crowell, Dr. R. E. Waud, and Dr. G. H. Hoffman.)

Sternum—anterior (P-A) oblique view (Figs. 9-58 to 9-60)

Film size—10″ × 12″
Cassette
Lengthwise

Bucky
Collimate to cover
(Rapid shallow breathing technique)

Technique

Factors	Screen film cassette (par)
mA	25
Time	1.0
mAs	25
Thickness in cm	25
kVp	82
Distance	30

Patient preparation

Remove all garments down to the waist. Provide a gown for female patients.

Palpation points

Manubrium and xiphoid processes of the sternum.

Procedure

Place the patient in the prone position. Elevate the left side of the body approximately 30 degrees and flex the left knee and elbow for support. Align the long axis of the sternum over the center line of the table. Place a wedge sponge under the elevated thoracic cage. Instruct the patient to extend the left arm down the body and simultaneously relax the left shoulder and roll it anteriorly.

A

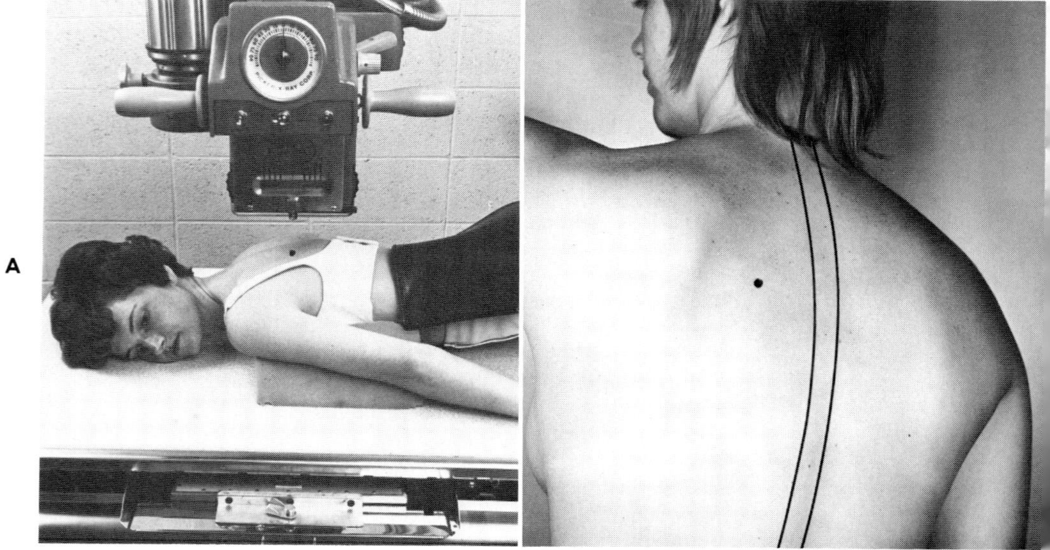

Fig. 9-58. Sternum. **A** and **B,** Anterior (P-A) oblique positions.

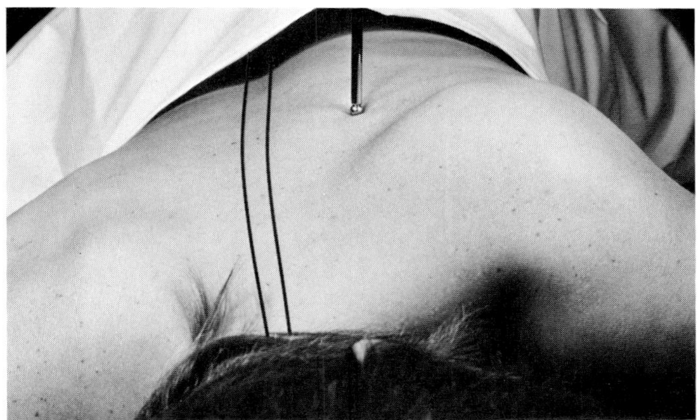

Fig. 9-59. Sternum—anterior (P-A) oblique position.

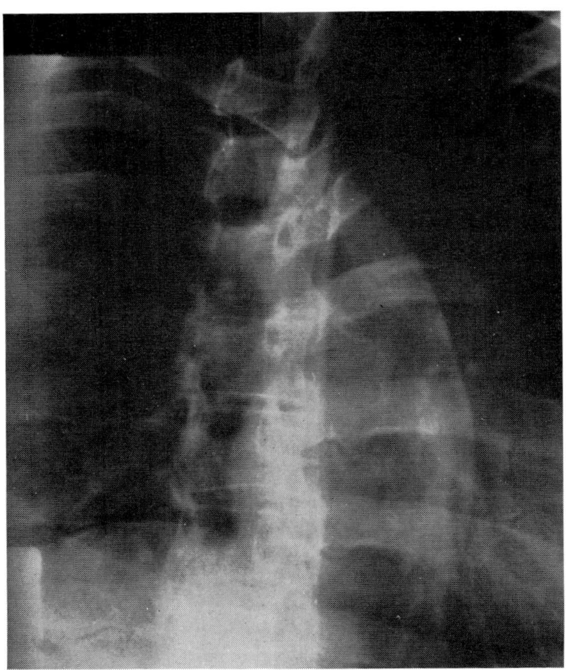

Fig. 9-60. Sternum—anterior (P-A) oblique view. (Courtesy Dr. E. I. L. Cilley, Dr. T. W. Crowell, Dr. R. E. Waud, and Dr. G. H. Hoffman.)

Central ray

Direct the central ray perpendicular through a point halfway between the manubrium and xiphoid process to the center of the film holder. Collimate to film holder.

Immobilization

Place a wedge sponge or a sandbag under the flexed knee. A compression band may be used across the thoracic cage. Employ rapid shallow breathing during the radiographic exposure.

Right-left markers

Place the *L* marker on the left lateral center border of the film holder.

Technical tips

For left anterior oblique position, reduce the kVp 4 kilovolts.

Structures demonstrated

Anterior (P-A) oblique view of the sternum.

Note: A short focal-film distance with the rapid shallow breathing technique will blur out surrounding structures.

Sternum—lateral view (Figs. 9-61 and 9-62)

Film size—10″ × 12″
Cassette
Lengthwise
Bucky (erect)
Collimate to cover

Technique

Factors	Screen film cassette (par)
mA	100
Time	0.6
mAs	60
Thickness in cm	30
kVp	80
Distance	40

Patient preparation

Remove all garments down to the waist. Provide a gown for female patients.

Palpation points

Manubrium and xiphoid processes of the sternum.

Procedure

Place the patient in a lateral erect position, either standing or sitting. Place the arms behind the back and clasp the hands together. Relax the shoulders and roll them posteriorly. Align the long axis of the sternum over the center line of the table.

Central ray

Direct the central ray perpendicular through a point halfway between the manubrium and the xiphoid process to the center of the film holder. Collimate to film holder.

Immobilization

Place a compression band around the patient's body. Employ suspended inspiration.

Right-left markers

Place the correct marker on the anterior center border of the film holder.

Technical tips

Measurements for technique should be made transversely across the entire anterior chest wall.

Structures demonstrated

Lateral view of the sternum.

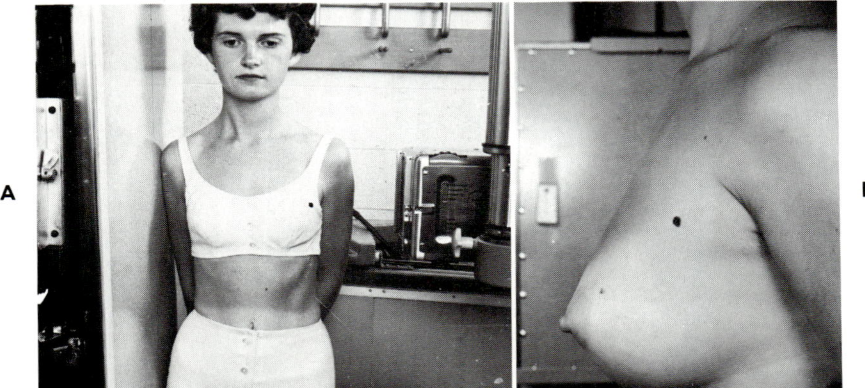

Fig. 9-61. Sternum. **A** and **B,** Lateral positions.

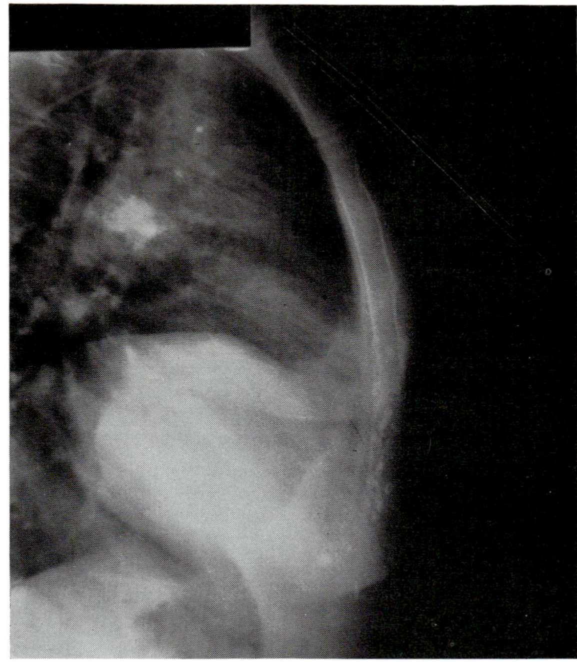

Fig. 9-62. Sternum—lateral view. (Courtesy Dr. E. I. L. Cilley, Dr. T. W. Crowell, Dr. R. E. Waud, and Dr. G. H. Hoffman.)

Scapula—posterior (A-P) view (Figs. 9-63 and 9-64)

Film size—10″ × 12″
Cassette
Lengthwise

Bucky
Collimate to cover

Technique

Factors	Screen film cassette (par)
mA	100
Time	0.3
mAs	30
Thickness in cm	16
kVp	76
Distance	40

Patient preparation

Remove all garments down to the waist. Provide a gown for female patients.

Palpation points

Acromion process, spine, and apex of the scapula; spinous processes of the thoracic vertebrae.

Procedure

Place the patient in the supine position. Center a point halfway between the midline of the body and the lateral border of the shoulder over the center line of the table. Extend the arm at the side of the body with the palm up.

Central ray

Direct the central ray perpendicularly to enter a point halfway between the top of the shoulder and the apex of the scapula, to the center of the film holder. Collimate to film holder.

Immobilization

Place one sandbag under and a second on top of the hand. Employ suspended inspiration.

Right-left markers

Place the correct marker on the lateral center border of the film holder.

Technical tips

To better demonstrate the axillary border of the scapula being radiographed, place that forearm over the head.

Structures demonstrated

Posterior (A-P) views of the scapula and lateral clavicle.

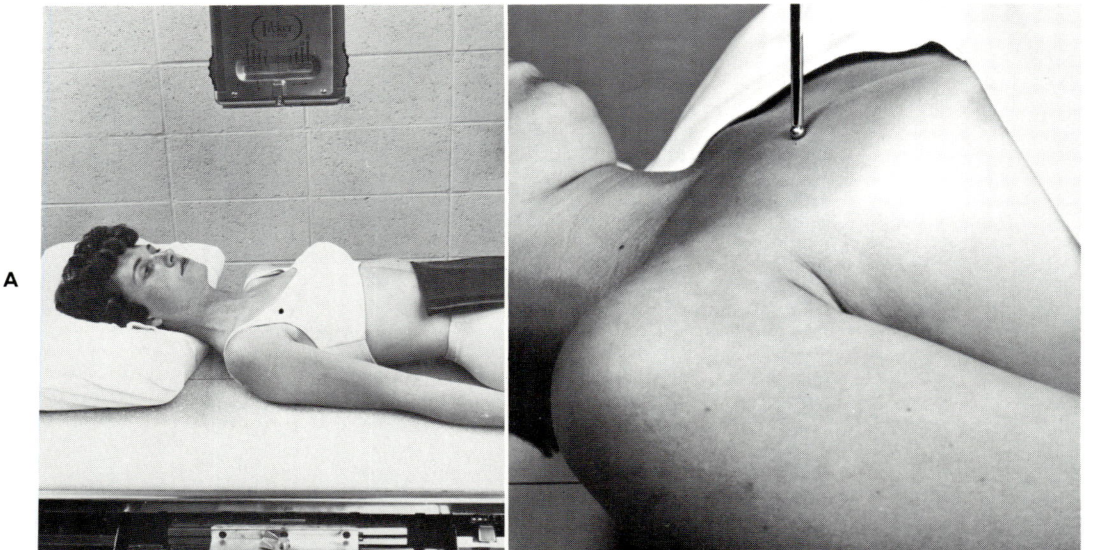

Fig. 9-63. Scapula. **A** and **B,** Posterior (A-P) positions.

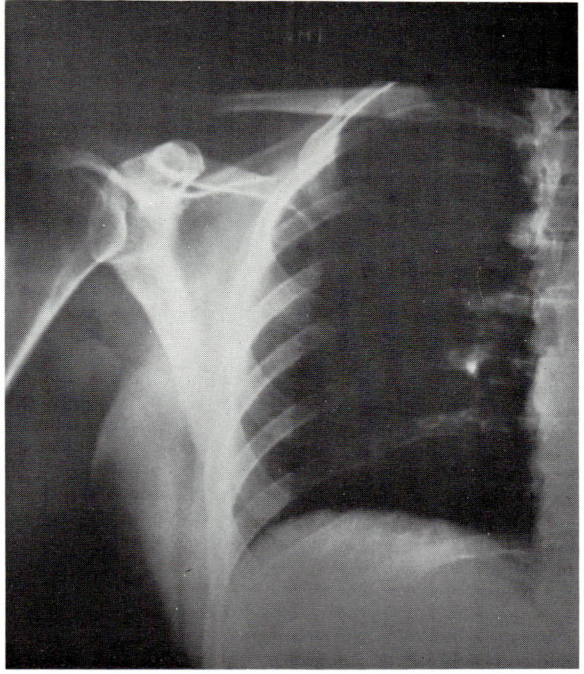

Fig. 9-64. Scapula—posterior (A-P) view. (Courtesy Dr. E. I. L. Cilley, Dr. T. W. Crowell, Dr. R. E. Waud, and Dr. G. H. Hoffman.)

Scapula—lateral view (Figs. 9-65 and 9-66)

Film size—10″ × 12″
Cassette
Lengthwise
Bucky (erect)
Collimate to cover

Technique

Factors	Screen film cassette (par)
mA	100
Time	0.6
mAs	60
Thickness in cm	16
kVp	78
Distance	40

Patient preparation

Remove all garments down to the waist. Provide a gown for female patients.

Palpation points

Acromion process, spine, and apex of the scapula; spinous processes of the thoracic vertebrae.

Procedure

Place the patient in an erect position, either sitting or standing, with the shoulder being examined against the erect Bucky. Flex the elbow nearer to the film and place the arm behind the patient with the back of hand against the posterior ribs. Instruct the patient to grasp the edge of the table with the opposite hand and to roll the opposite shoulder anteriorly. Rotate the body slightly to align the flat surface of the scapula so that it is perpendicular to and over the center line of the upright Bucky.

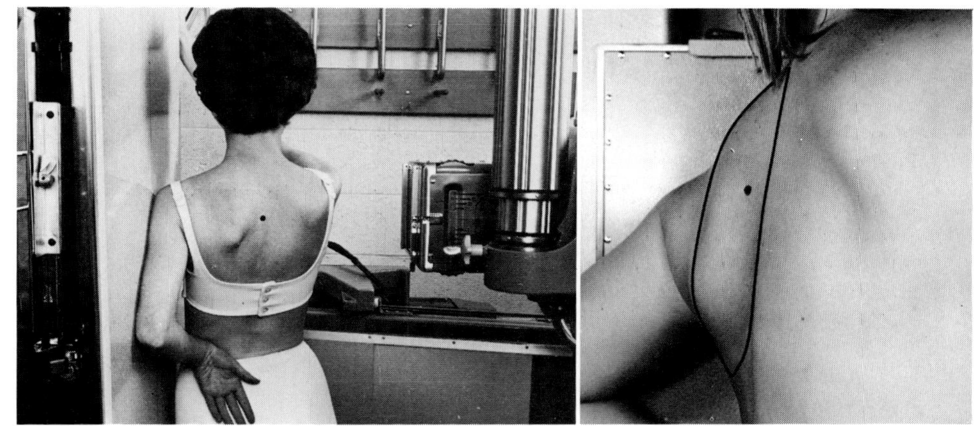

Fig. 9-65. Scapula. **A** and **B,** Lateral positions.

Central ray

Direct the central ray perpendicularly to enter a point halfway between the top of the shoulder and the apex of the scapula, to the center of the film holder. Collimate to film holder.

Immobilization

A compression band may be placed around the patient's lower thoracic region. Employ suspended expiration.

Right-left markers

Place the correct marker on the anterior center border of the film holder.

Technical tips

For uniform radiographic density, use 1/10 mm copper filter internally plus an increase of 10 kVp.

Structures demonstrated

Lateral view of the scapula projected away from the rib cage.

Note: For supine patients, elevate the side being examined 25 degrees, placing the forearm over the head; align the central ray perpendicularly through the midscapula to the center of the film holder.

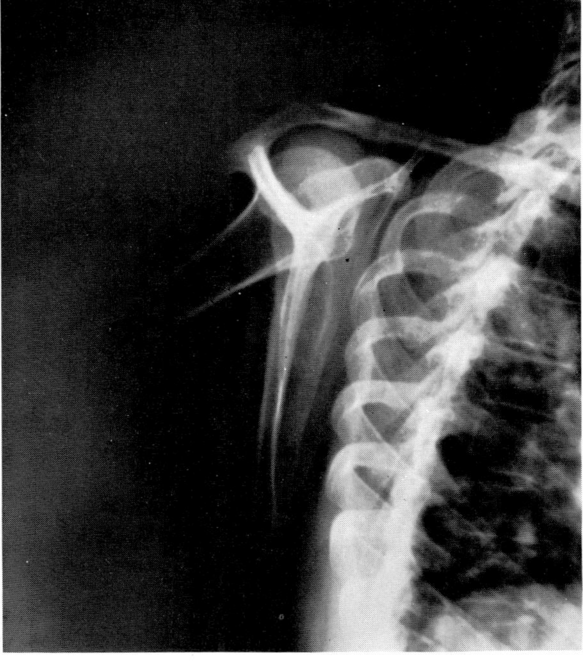

Fig. 9-66. Scapula—lateral view. (Courtesy Dr. E. I. L. Cilley, Dr. T. W. Crowell, Dr. R. E. Waud, and Dr. G. H. Hoffman.)

Ribs—posterior (A-P) or anterior (P-A) view above the diaphragm (Figs. 9-67 and 9-68)

Film size—14″ × 17″
Cassette
Crosswise
Bucky
Collimate to cover

Technique

Factors	Screen film cassette (par)
mA	100
Time	0.4
mAs	40
Thickness in cm	20
kVp	70
Distance	40

Patient preparation

Remove all garments down to the waist. Provide a gown for female patients.

Palpation points

Vertebra prominens; lateral ribs.

Procedure

Place the patient either in the prone or the supine position with the side being examined nearer the table. Center the midline of the body over the center line of the table. Extend both arms down the sides of the body. Align the top of the cassette 2 inches above the vertebra prominens (seventh cervical vertebra).

Central ray

Direct the central ray perpendicular to the center of the film holder. Collimate to film holder.

Immobilization

Employ suspended expiration.

Right-left markers

Place the *R* marker on the right lateral center border of the film holder.

Technical tips

Complete expiration will produce lung-tissue concentration and provide for more uniform object density.

Structures demonstrated

Posterior (A-P) or anterior (P-A) view of the upper two thirds of the bilateral rib cage.

Note: Make erect views if the patient has any difficulty in assuming the positions described previously.

For patients measuring less than 19 cm, use chest positioning, microline grid, and optimum kVp chest technique.

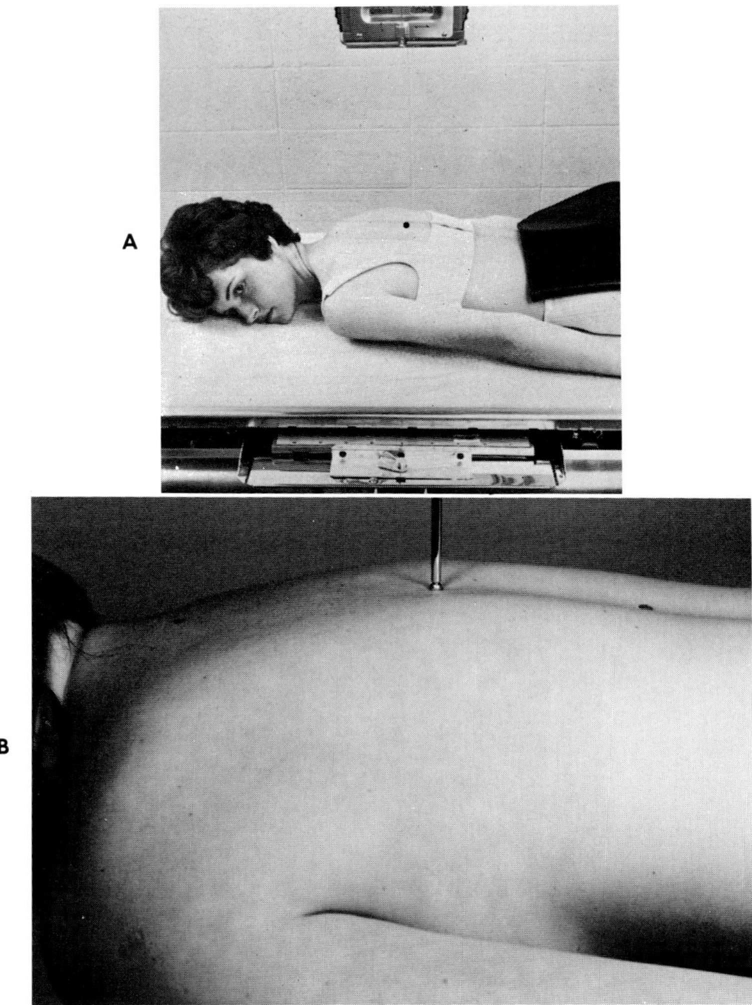

Fig. 9-67. Ribs. **A** and **B,** Anterior (P-A) positions, above the diaphragm.

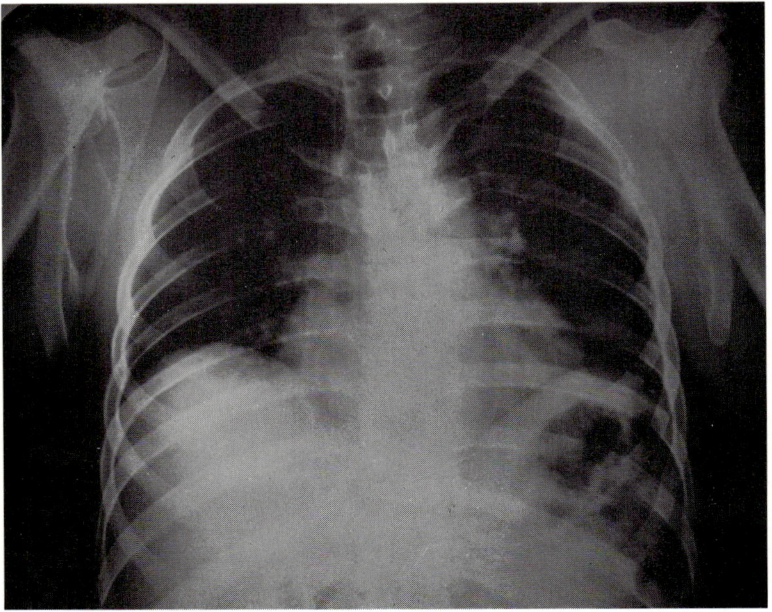

Fig. 9-68. Ribs—anterior (P-A) view, above the diaphragm. (Courtesy Dr. E. I. L. Cilley, Dr. T. W. Crowell, Dr. R. E. Waud, and Dr. G. H. Hoffman.)

Ribs—anterior (P-A) oblique (L.A.O.-R.A.O.) view (Figs. 9-69 and 9-70)

Film size—14″ × 17″
Cassette
Lengthwise
Bucky
Collimate to cover

Technique

Factors	Screen film cassette (par)
mA	100
Time	0.4
mAs	40
Thickness in cm	23
kVp	76
Distance	40

Patient preparation

Remove all garments down to the waist. Provide a gown for female patients.

Palpation points

Vertebra prominens; lateral ribs.

Procedure

Place the patient in the prone position. Elevate the side being examined 35 degrees, and flex the elbow and knee for support. Center a point midway between the spine and the lateral margin of the ribs of the side being examined over the center line of the table. Align the top of the film holder with the vertebra prominens (seventh cervical vertebra).

Central ray

Direct the central ray perpendicular to the center of the film holder. Collimate to film holder.

Immobilization

Employ suspended expiration.

Right-left markers

Place the correct marker on the anterior center border of the film holder.

Technical tips

Complete expiration will produce lung-tissue concentration and provide for more uniform object density.

Structures demonstrated

Axillary view of the unilateral rib cage.

Note: Make erect views if the patient has any difficulty in assuming the positions described previously.

For patients measuring less than 19 cm, use chest positioning, microline grid, and optimum kVp chest technique.

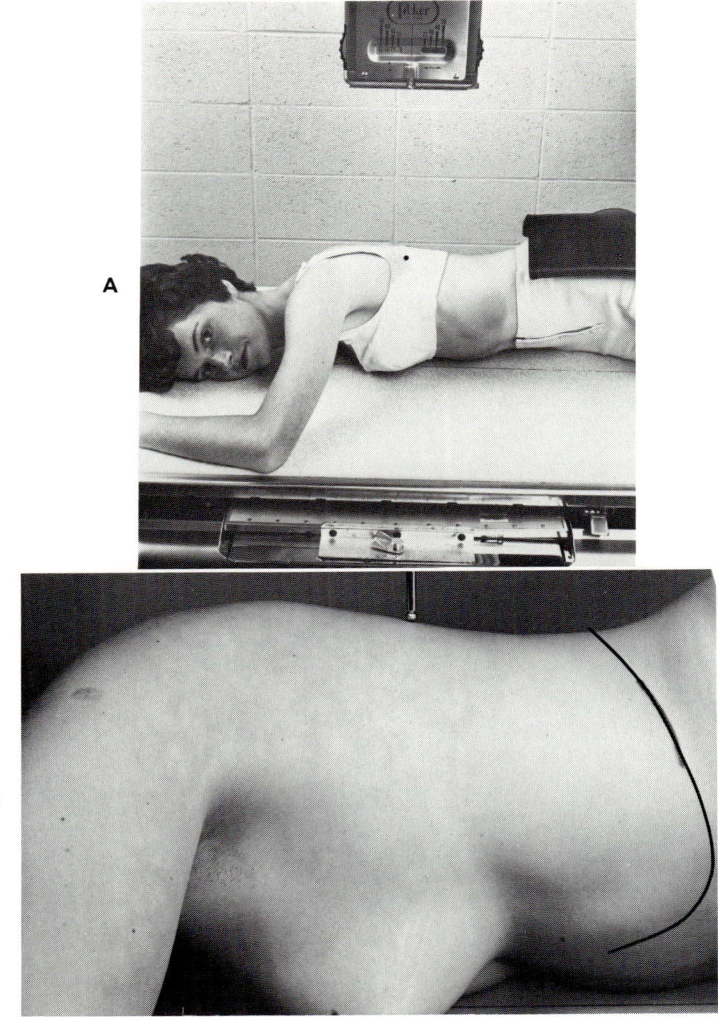

Fig. 9-69. Ribs. **A** and **B,** Anterior (P-A) oblique (R.A.O.) positions.

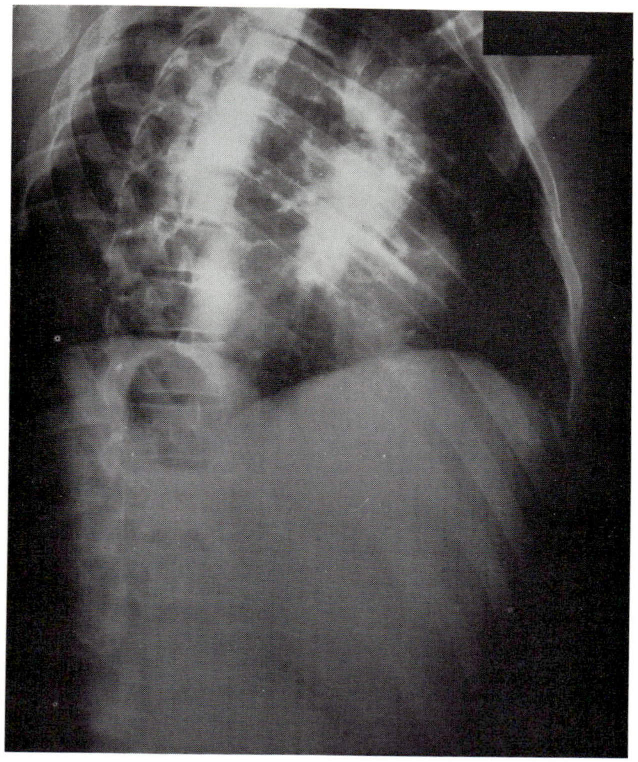

Fig. 9-70. Ribs—anterior (P-A) oblique (R.A.O.) view. (Courtesy Dr. E. I. L. Cilley, Dr. T. W. Crowell, Dr. R. E. Waud, and Dr. G. H. Hoffman.)

Ribs—posterior (A-P) or anterior (P-A) view below the diaphragm (Figs. 9-71 and 9-72)

Film size—14″ × 17″
Cassette
Crosswise
Bucky
Collimate to cover

Technique

Factors	Screen film cassette (par)
mA	100
Time	0.5
mAs	50
Thickness in cm	22
kVp	78
Distance	40

Patient preparation

Remove all garments down to the waist. Provide a gown for female patients.

Palpation points

Iliac crest; lateral ribs.

Procedure

Place the patient in either the prone or the supine position with the side being examined nearer the table. Extend the arms down the sides of the body. Align the bottom of the cassette with the iliac crest.

Central ray

Direct the central ray perpendicular to the center of the film holder. Collimate to film holder.

Immobilization

Employ suspended expiration.

Right-left markers

Place the *R* marker on the right lateral center border of the film holder.

Technical tips

Complete expiration will produce lung-tissue concentration and provide for more uniform object density.

Structures demonstrated

Posterior (A-P) or anterior (P-A) view of the lower two thirds of the bilateral rib cage.

Note: Make erect views if the patient has any difficulty in assuming the positions described above.

For patients measuring less than 19 cm, use chest positioning, microline grid, and optimum kVp chest technique.

A

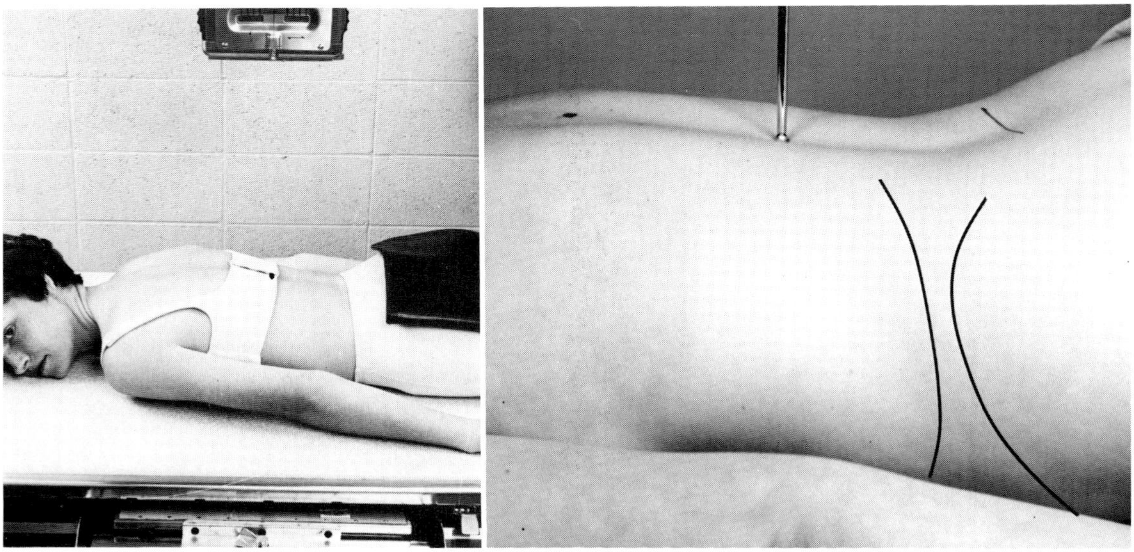

B

Fig. 9-71. Ribs. **A** and **B**, Anterior (P-A) positions, below the diaphragm.

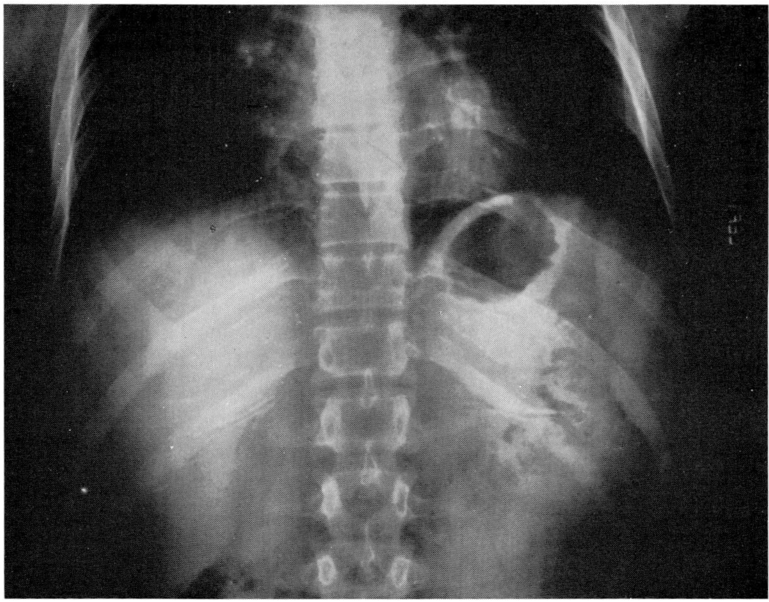

Fig. 9-72. Ribs—anterior (P-A) view, below the diaphragm. (Courtesy Dr. E. I. L. Cilley, Dr. T. W. Crowell, Dr. R. E. Waud, and Dr. G. H. Hoffman.)

Chest—anterior (P-A) view (Figs. 9-73 and 9-74)

Film size—14″ × 17″
Cassette
Lengthwise
Erect film holder
Collimate to cover

Technique

Factors	Screen film cassette (par)
mA	300
Time	$0.0\overline{33}$
mAs	10
Thickness in cm	22
kVp	64
Distance	72

Patient preparation

Remove all garments down to the waist. Provide a gown for female patients.

Palpation points

Acromion processes; lateral ribs; apex of the scapula.

Procedure

Place the patient in the erect position with the anterior surface of the chest against the cassette. Center the midline of the body over the center line of the film holder. Align the top of the cassette 3 inches above the acromion processes. Elevate the chin so that it rests on top of the film holder. Place the backs of the hands on the hips. Roll the shoulders anteriorly as far as possible.

Central ray

Direct the central ray horizontally, perpendicular to the center of the film holder. Collimate to film holder.

Immobilization

A compression band may be used across the thoracic cage. Employ deep suspended inspiration.

Right-left markers

Place the *L* marker in the left superior corner of the film holder.

Technical tips

The spinous process of the seventh thoracic vertebra is on the same plane as the apex of the scapula and the midportion of the lung field.

Structures demonstrated

Anterior (P-A) views of the lungs, heart, and the rib structures above the diaphragm.

Note: For heart series, make a routine chest series; include the patient's weight, height, and age on the protocol.

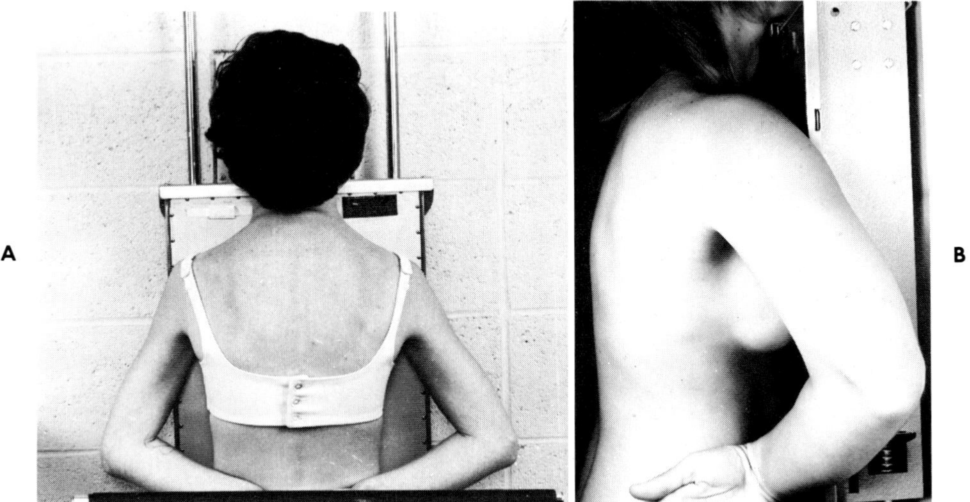

Fig. 9-73. Chest. A and B, Anterior (P-A) positions.

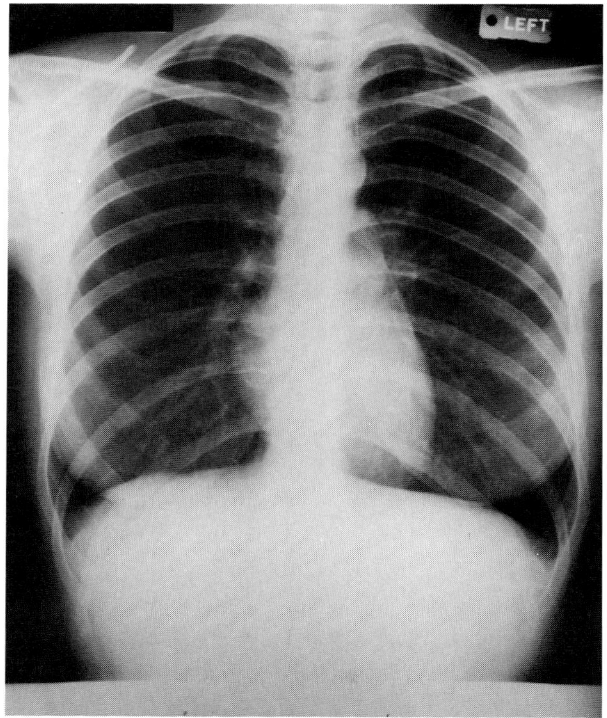

Fig. 9-74. Chest—anterior (P-A) view. (Courtesy Dr. E. I. L. Cilley, Dr. T. W. Crowell, Dr. R. E. Waud, and Dr. G. H. Hoffman.)

Chest—lateral view (Figs. 9-75 and 9-76)

Film size—14″ × 17″
Cassette
Lengthwise
Erect film holder
Collimate to cover

Technique

Factors	Screen film cassette (par)
mA	300
Time	$0.0\overline{66}$
mAs	20
Thickness in cm	30
kVp	74
Distance	72

Patient preparation

Remove all garments down to the waist. Provide a gown for female patients.

Palpation points

Acromion processes; posterior ribs; sternum.

Procedure

Place the patient in the erect position with the lateral surface of the chest against the cassette. Center the midaxillary line of the body over the center line of the film holder. Align the top of the cassette 3 inches above the acromion process. Cross the arms over the head and rest the forearms on top of the head. Rotate the body into a true lateral position.

Central ray

Direct the central ray horizontally, perpendicular to the center of the film holder. Collimate to film holder.

Immobilization

Brace the shoulder against the cassette. A compression band may be used across the thoracic cage. Employ deep suspended inspiration.

Right-left markers

Place the correct marker in the left superior corner of the film holder.

Technical tips

Holding the breath on the second inspiration will ensure a greater area of lung visualization.

Structures demonstrated

Lateral views of both lungs superimposed, heart and aorta, and the midthoracic spine.

Note: Make a left lateral view unless otherwise directed.

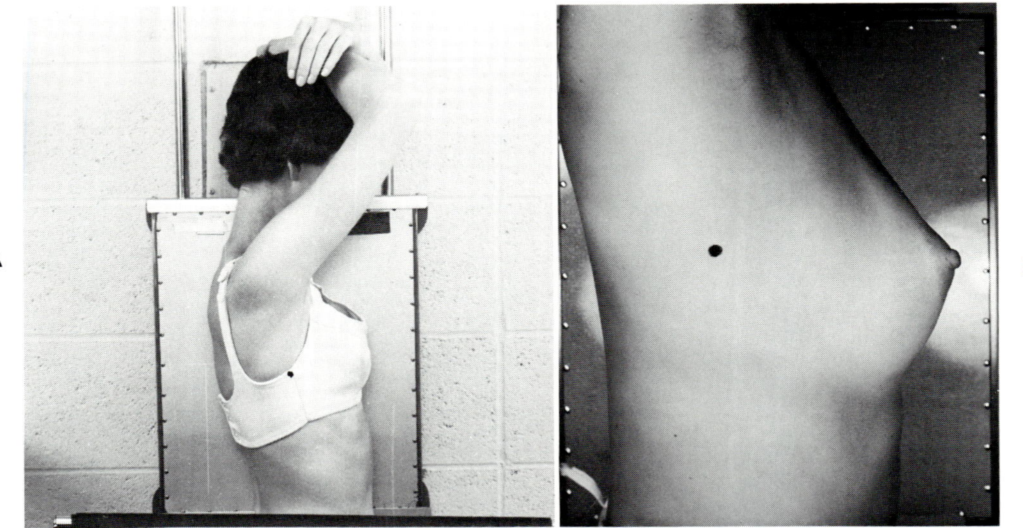

Fig. 9-75. Chest. A and B, Lateral positions.

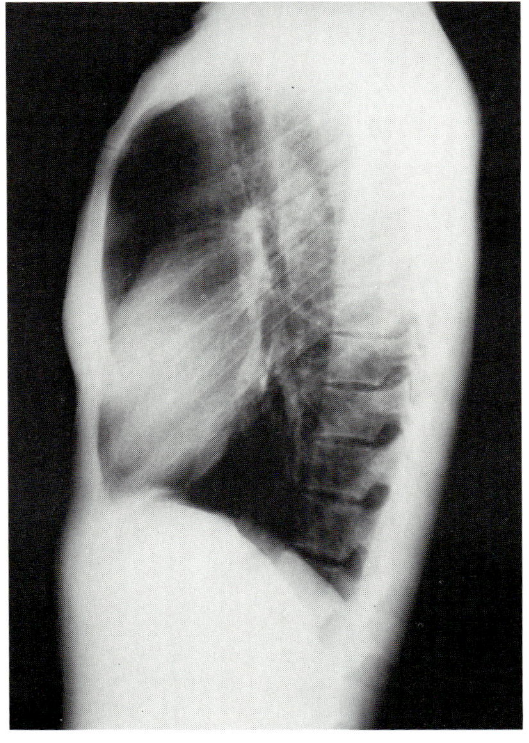

Fig. 9-76. Chest–lateral view. (Courtesy Scottsdale Memorial Hospital, Scottsdale, Arizona.)

Chest—anterior (P-A) oblique view (Figs. 9-77 to 9-79)

Film size—14″ × 17″
Cassette
Lengthwise
Erect film holder
Collimate to cover

Technique

Factors	Screen film cassette (par)
mA	300
Time	$0.0\overline{33}$
mAs	10
Thickness in cm	26
kVp	70
Distance	72

Patient preparation

Remove all garments down to the waist. Provide a gown for female patients.

Palpation points

Acromion processes; lateral ribs; spinous processes of the thoracic vertebrae.

Procedure

Place the patient in the erect position with the anterior surface of the chest against the cassette. Align the top of the cassette 3 inches above the acromion process. Rotate the side of the chest being examined away from the cassette 45 degrees; flex that elbow and place the hand on top of the film holder. Flex the opposite elbow and place the hand on the hip. Align a point midway between the spine and the lateral margin of the side of the chest being examined over the center line of the film holder.

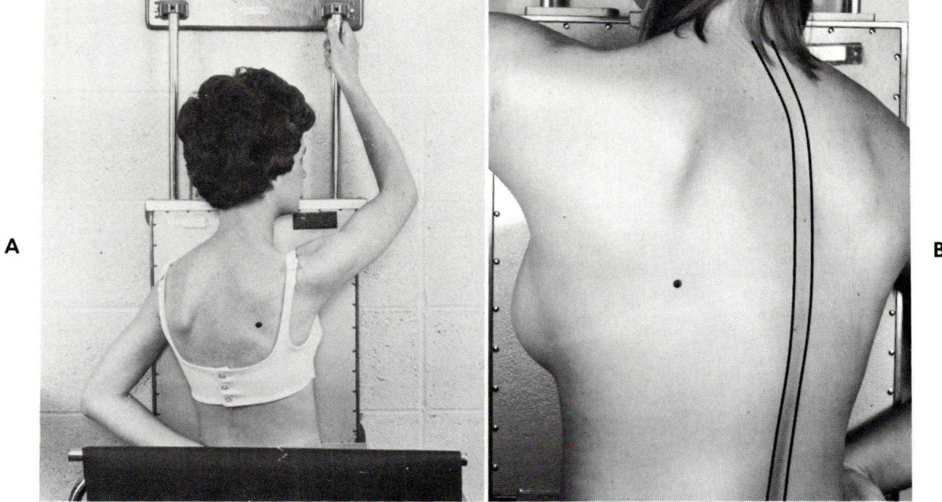

Fig. 9-77. Chest—left anterior oblique positions. **A,** L.A.O. **B,** R.A.O.

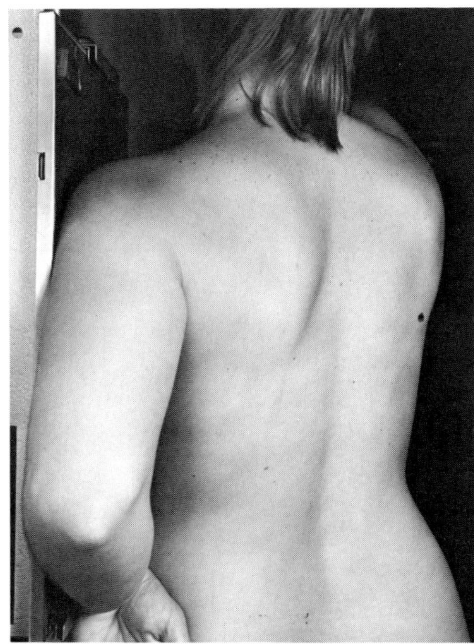

Fig. 9-78. Chest—left anterior oblique (L.A.O.) position.

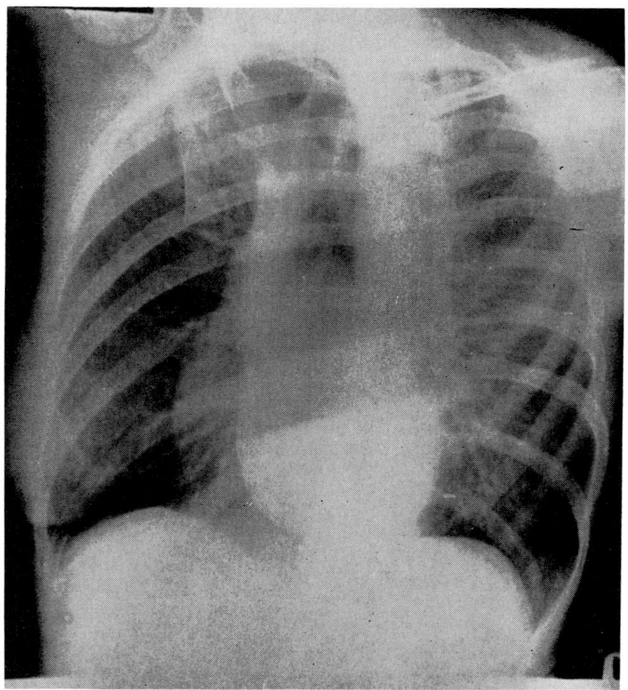

Fig. 9-79. Chest—left anterior oblique (L.A.O.) view. (Courtesy Dr. E. I. L. Cilley, Dr. T. W. Crowell, Dr. R. E. Waud, and Dr. G. H. Hoffman.)

Central ray

Direct the central ray horizontally, perpendicular to the center of the film holder. Collimate to film holder.

Immobilization

A compression band may be used across the thoracic cage. Employ deep suspended inspiration.

Right-left markers

Place the *L* marker in the left superior corner of the film holder.

Technical tips

Holding the breath on the second inspiration will ensure a greater area of lung visualization.

Structures demonstrated

Right anterior oblique—maximum view of the left lung field, the trachea, and entire right bronchial tree; left atrium and both ventricles of the heart. When filled with barium sulfate, the esophagus is well demonstrated in this view.

Left anterior oblique—maximum view of the right lung field, the trachea, and left bronchial tree.

Note: For supine patients, elevate the side opposite the one being radiographed 45 degrees. Use a 72-inch focal-film distance if possible.

Chest—apical lordotic view (Figs. 9-80 and 9-81)

Film size—14″ × 17″
Cassette
Lengthwise
Erect film holder
Collimate to cover

Technique

Factors	Screen film cassette (par)
mA	300
Time	$0.0\overline{33}$
mAs	10
Thickness in cm	26
kVp	70
Distance	72

Patient preparation

Remove all garments down to the waist. Provide a gown for female patients.

Palpation points

Acromion processes; lateral ribs; sternum.

Procedure

Place the patient in the erect posterior (A-P) position 1 foot in front of the erect film holder. Align the top of the cassette 2 inches above the acromion processes. Place the backs of the hands on the hips, and roll the shoulders anteriorly as far as possible. Instruct the patient to lean backward and rest the tops of his shoulders against the cassette. Center the median line of the body over the center line of the film holder.

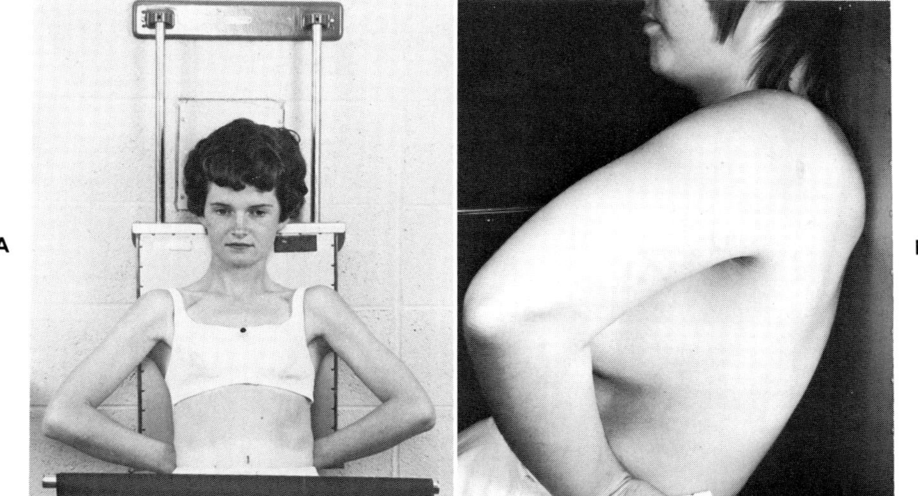

Fig. 9-80. Chest. **A** and **B**, Apical lordotic positions.

Central ray

Direct the central ray horizontally, perpendicular to the center of the film holder. Collimate to film holder.

Immobilization

Employ deep suspended inspiration.

Right-left markers

Place the *R* marker in the left superior border of the film holder.

Technical tips

If the patient is incapable of assuming complete extension for this position, angle the central ray 10 degrees cephalad.

Structures demonstrated

Semiaxial view of the lungs visualizing the apices.

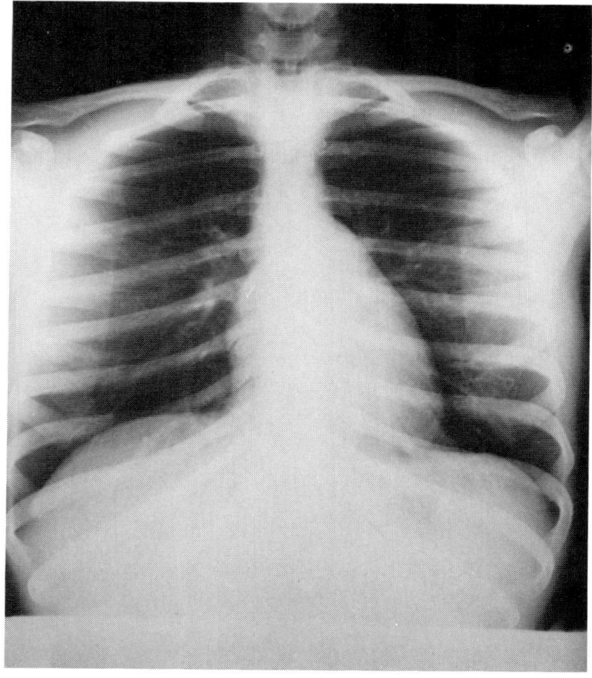

Fig. 9-81. Chest—apical lordotic view. (Courtesy Dr. E. I. L. Cilley, Dr. T. W. Crowell, Dr. R. E. Waud, and Dr. G. H. Hoffman.)

QUESTIONS

1. Describe the radiographic position that best demonstrates the right intervertebral foramina.
2. Explain why a slight lateral concavity (or sagging) of the thoracic spine in the lateral projection is found to be beneficial.
3. Name two radiographic positions that will best demonstrate the left intervertebral foramina.
4. In sternum radiography, what procedure is used to blur out the shadows of the overlying pulmonary markings?
5. Describe the radiographic procedure to best demonstrate the anteroposterior projection of the atlas and axis.
6. Name an articulation that is best demonstrated in a true left anterior oblique projection of the lumbar spine.
7. Define the term "kyphosis."
8. Which vertebrae are least defined in a routine lateral projection of the thoracic spine?
9. Which vertebrae have facets for articulation with the ribs?
10. For an anteroposterior projection of the sacrum describe how you locate the point of entry for the central ray.
11. Describe the radiographic procedure for a transthoracic projection of the upper right humerus.
12. In radiography, what do the initials R.P.O. stand for?
13. Explain the purpose for taking a routine apical lordotic radiograph of the chest.
14. Name two major palpation points used to help localize the hip joint.
15. Where is the film holder centered in the routine posteroanterior projection of the ribs above the diaphragm?
16. Define the term "laterally recumbent."
17. Explain the purpose for using a 72″ focal-film distance when taking a lateral cervical radiograph.
18. Define the term "lateral decubitus."
19. What term is used to describe a lateral curvature of the spinal column?
20. Name the centering point used in the anteroposterior projection of the thoracic spine.
21. What position is used to best demonstrate the right intervertebral foramina of the cervical spine?
22. In a normal anteroposterior view of the cervical spine, what is the angle and degree of the central ray?
23. What numbered vertebra is located at the same level as the sternal angle?
24. What numbered vertebrae are located at the same level as the umbilicus?
25. What is the total amount of tube shift for stereoscopic projections of the posteroanterior chest?
26. Locate the central ray centering point in a lateral lumbosacral projection.
27. Locate the centering point for the normal anteroposterior projection of the cervical spine.
28. Describe the radiographic procedure that best demonstrates the left cervical apophyseal articulations.
29. Describe the radiographic procedure for the anteroposterior projection of the coccyx.
30. With the patient in the supine position, describe what takes place in the lumbar region when increased knee flexion is used.

10 • BONES OF THE SKULL

CRANIAL BONES

The superior surface of the skull is oval or circular in appearance. Frequently, variations of these types occur. The average skull is *mesocephalic.* A wide skull is *brachycephalic.* The transverse diameter of a brachycephalic skull is more than eight tenths of its anteroposterior diameter. An elongated skull is *dolichocephalic.* Dolicho- is a combining form meaning long or narrow. From the superior aspect, the calvarium shape is described by use of the *cephalic index.* The cephalic index is obtained by dividing the maximum breadth by the maximum length and multiplying by 100. A cephalic index of 75.9 or less indicates a dolichocephalic skull, whereas a cephalic index of 81 or more indicates a brachycephalic skull.

There are three sutures on the superior surface of the skull: *coronal,* at the junction of the frontal with the parietal bones; *sagittal,* between the parietal bones and at right angles to the coronal and lambdoidal sutures; and *lambdoidal,* at the junction of the occipital and the parietal bones and paralleling the coronal suture in direction.

The upper part of the skull, *calvarium** (skullcap), includes parts of four bones and all of two bones: the squama of the occipital, frontal, and temporal bones, and all of the two parietal bones. The cranial case includes eight bones: one frontal, two parietal, two temporal, one occipital, one sphenoid, and one ethmoid. The cranial floor includes parts of six bones: the sphenoid, ethmoid, both temporals, the occipital, and frontal.

Frontal bone

Two parts make up the frontal bone. The horizontal *(orbital)* part lies between the nasal cavity and the eye orbits. The *squama* curves toward its perimeter from the anterior portion of the orbital part. The *frontal eminences* are on the anterior surface of the squama, above the *supraorbital ridges* and bilateral to the midsagittal line. The *glabella* is raised and smooth and is located between the *superciliary arches.* The frontal bone articulates inferiorly with both nasal bones, forming a suture, the midpoint of which is called the *nasion.* The frontal processes of the maxillae and the nasal bones all lie above the nasal process, which terminates in the *nasal spine.* The supraorbital margin is the line of demarcation between the squama and the orbital portion. (See Figs. 10-1 and 10-2.) The *ethmoidal notch* is between the orbital plates and contains the *cribriform plate* of the ethmoid bone. The superior surfaces of the eye orbits are the orbital plates. The *frontal sinus* is directly behind the glabella and is usually separated into two parts by a septum. The frontal sinus and the squama are demonstrated radiographically by the use of the frontal-ethmoidal (modified Caldwell) and lateral sinus views. The frontal bone articulates with the ethmoid bone, sphenoid bone, both maxillae, both zygomatic bones, both parietal bones, both nasal bones, and both lacrimal bones.

Ethmoid bone

The ethmoid bone occupies the space surrounded by the frontal bone, the maxillae, and the sphenoid bone. The cribriform plate is horizontal between the orbital plates of the frontal bone. The *perpendicular plate* forms the major portion of the *nasal septum.* The *laminae papyraceae,* on the lateral surfaces of the two *lateral masses,* articulate in the eye orbit in the space surrounded by the maxillae, palatine bones, lacrimal bones, sphenoid bone, and frontal bone. The *crista galli* extends superiorly above the cribriform plate. The *ethmoid cells* are in the superior concha. The cells and the ethmoid bone are demonstrated radiographically by the use of the frontal-ethmoidal (modified Caldwell) and lateral sinus views. The ethmoid bone articulates with the frontal bone, sphenoid bone, both sphenoidal conchae, both nasal bones, both maxillae, both palatine bones, both lacrimal bones, vomer, and both inferior nasal turbinate bones.

Sphenoid bone

The sphenoid bone occupies the space in the floor of the cranium anterior to the occipital and

*The calvarium is that portion of the skull lying above a plane extending through the supraorbital ridges anteriorly and the superior nuchal lines (of the occipital bone) posteriorly.

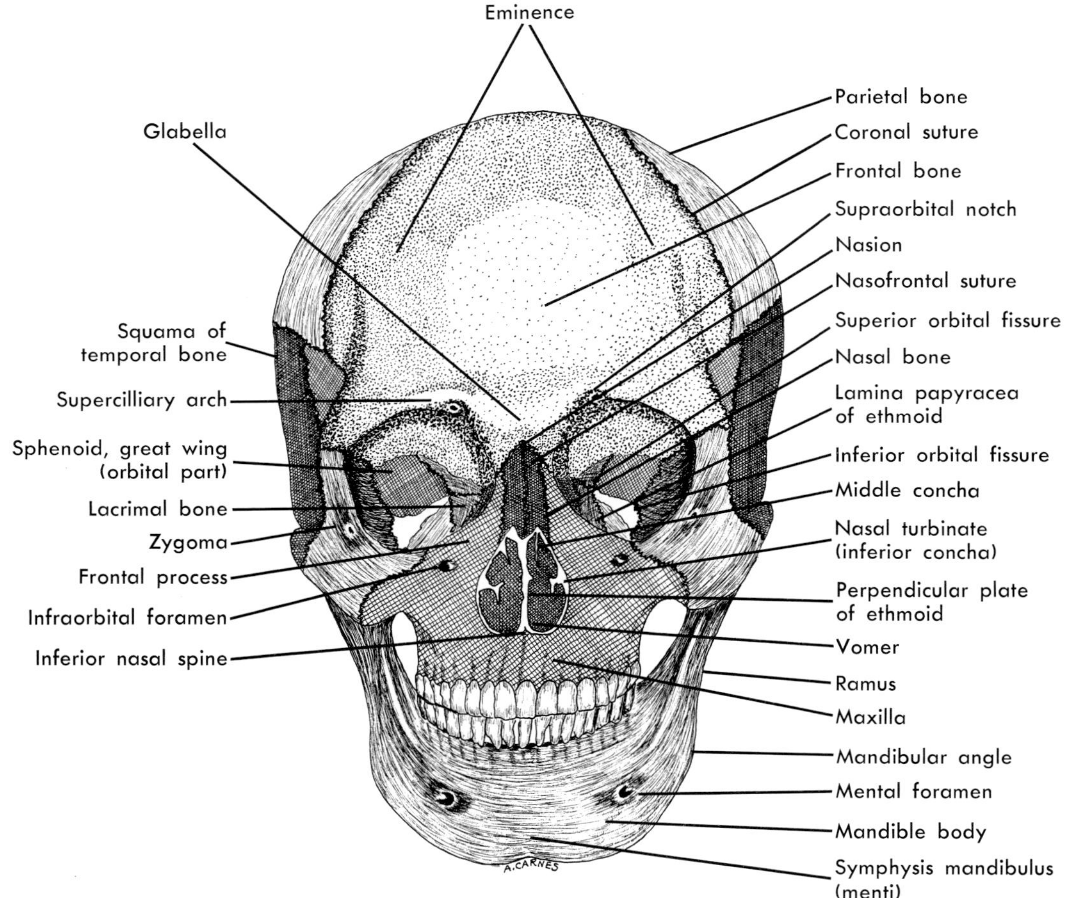

Fig. 10-1. Skull, anterior aspect.

temporal bones and posterior to the frontal bone and ethmoid bone. It is irregularly shaped. From its body project two *great wings,* two *small wings,* and two *pterygoid processes.* (See Figs. 10-3 to 10-5). The body is hollow. A septum divides this space into the *sphenoidal sinuses,* which are inferior to the *sella turcica.** The sella turcica is the saddle-shaped part of the sphenoid bone that contains the pituitary gland. The cribriform plate of the ethmoid bone articulates with the *ethmoid spine,* which extends above the body. The chiasmatic groove is posterior to the ethmoid spine in a smooth, raised part and is anterior to the *tuberculum sellae.* The sella turcica is directly behind and below the tuberculum sellae. It is bounded anteriorly by the *middle* and *anterior clinoid processes* and posteriorly by the dorsum sellae, which terminates superiorly in the *posterior clinoid process.* The *petrosal process* is inferior to the *dorsum sellae.* The apex of the *petrous portion* of the temporal bone articulates with the petrosal process. The *clivus* is posterior to the dorsum sellae and articulates posteriorly with the basilar part of the occipital bone. The perpendicular plate of the ethmoid bone articulates posteriorly with the sphenoidal crest, which joins the *rostrum* of the sphenoid bone. The lower lateral margins of the anterior surface form parts of the eye orbits. Between the alae of the vomer is the sphenoidal rostrum. On both sides a portion of the lateral wall of the skull is formed by a part of the greater wing of the sphenoid. This portion occupies the space between the temporal and frontal bones and between the parietal and zygomatic bones. The *spina angularis* is an inferior projec-

*Other names for the sella turcica are the pituitary fossa and the hypophyseal fossa.

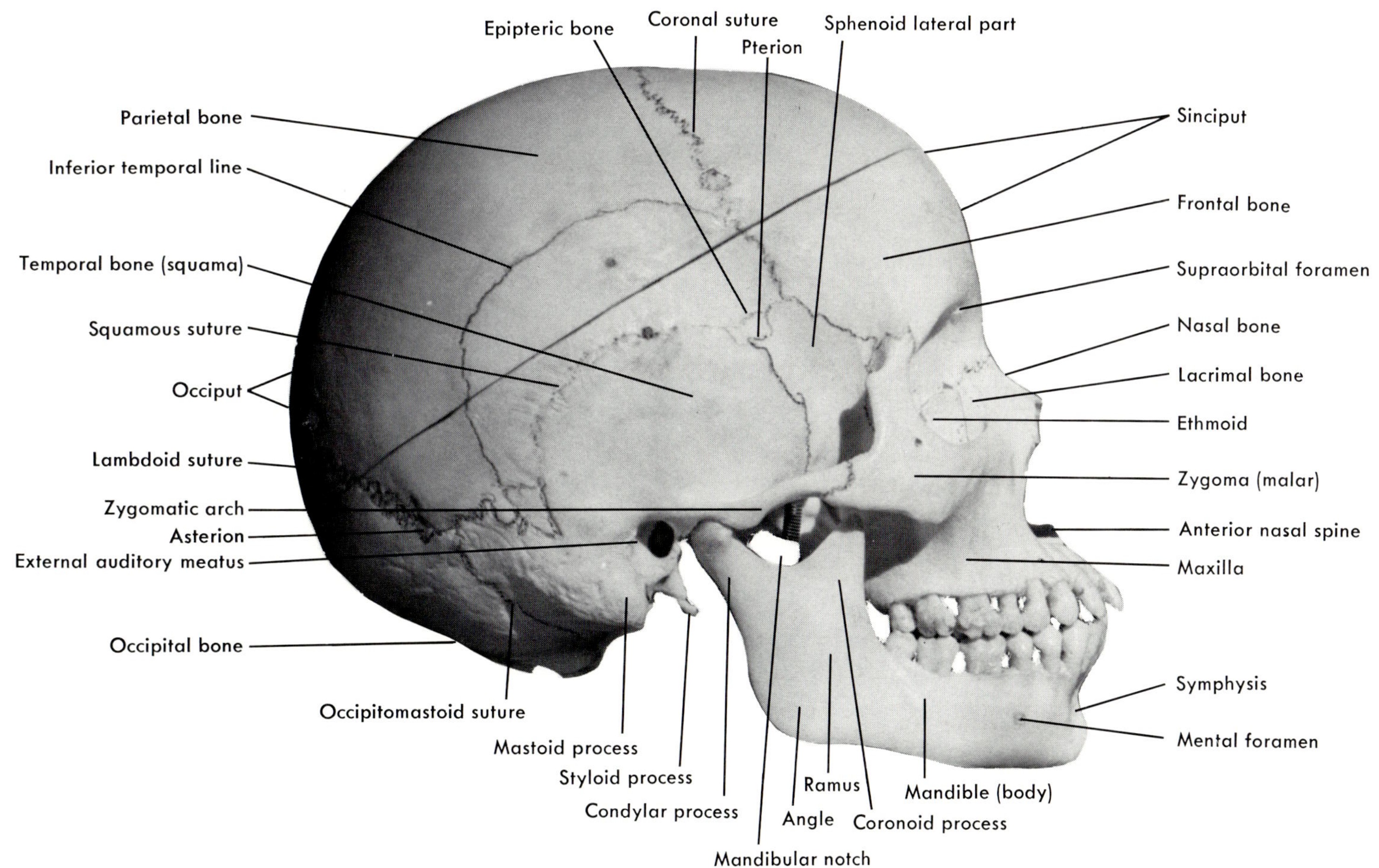

Fig. 10-2. Skull, lateral surface.

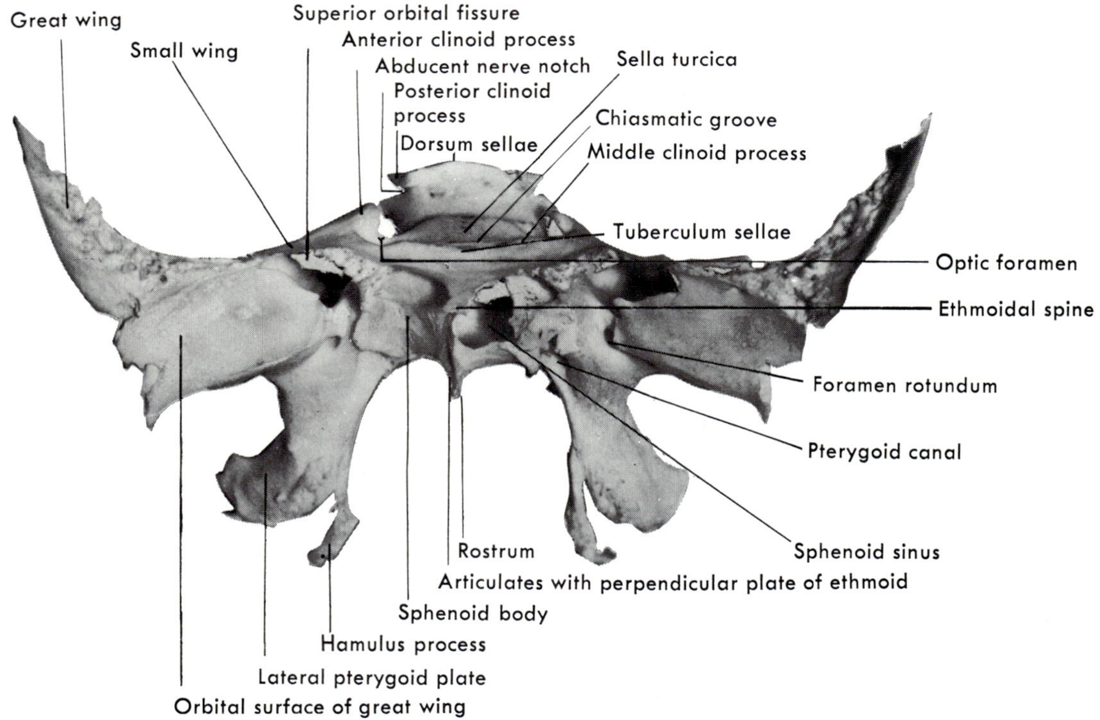

Fig. 10-3. Sphenoid, supero-oblique aspect. (Courtesy Clay-Adams, Inc.)

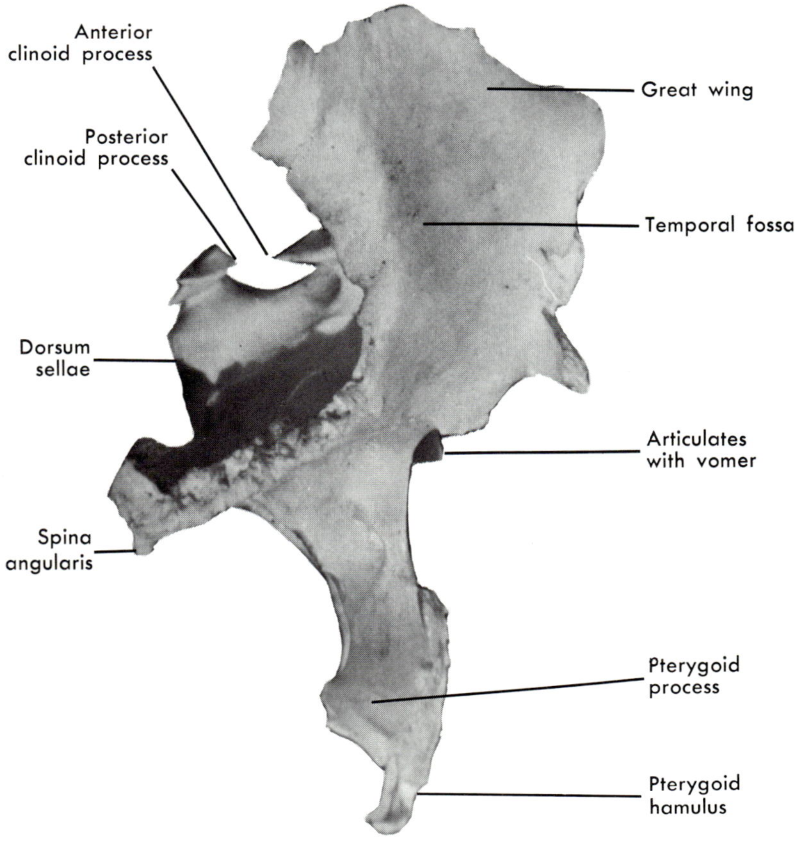

Fig. 10-4. Sphenoid, lateral surface.

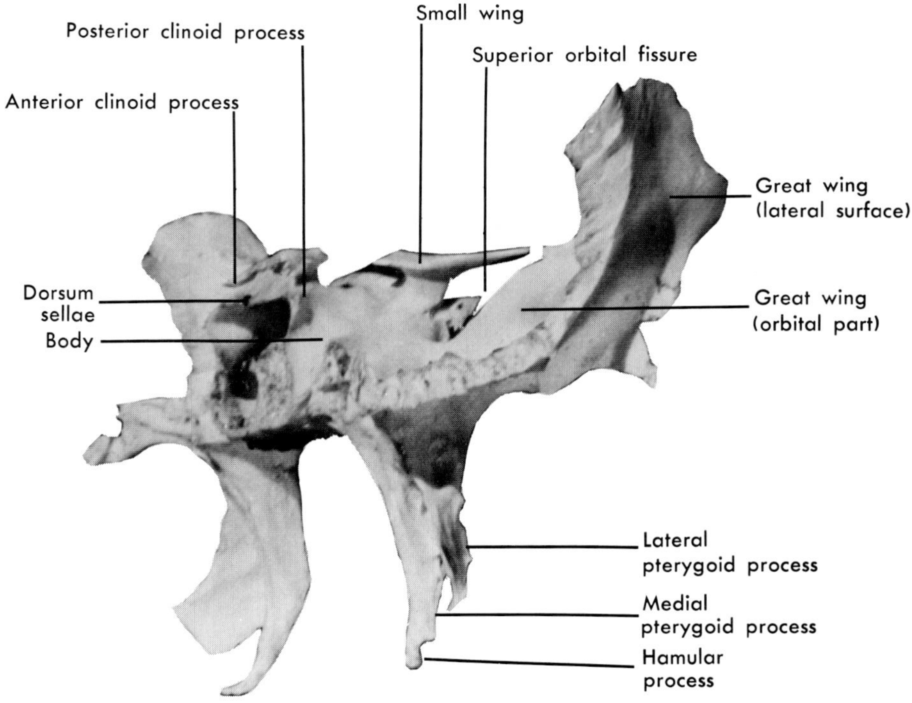

Fig. 10-5. Sphenoid, latero-oblique aspect.

tion adjacent to both the squamosal and petrous portions of the temporal bone. The *pterion* is a point at the junction of the frontal, parietal, and temporal bones and great wing of the sphenoid bone, about 3 cm posterior to the external angular process of the orbit. Frequently, a point is formed by the junction of the parietal, temporal, and sphenoid bones; however, in many skulls this part of the sphenoid bone is broad and separates the frontal bone from the temporal bone. The smaller wings are superior to the body and extend bilaterally. They contain the *optic foramina* and form the anterior clinoid processes. The pterygoid processes are paired. They are inferior to the junction of the body and the greater wings. There are two sphenoidal conchae between the nasal cavity and the sphenoidal sinus, which permit the passage of air between the nasal cavity and the sinus. The sphenoid bone is demonstrated radiographically by the use of the open-mouth sphenoid and lateral sinus views. The anterior (P-A) view demonstrates the optic foramen. The sphenoid bone articulates with the parietal bones, zygomatic bones, palatine bones, temporal bones, vomer, ethmoid bone, frontal bone, and occipital bone. The maxillary tuberosities occasionally articulate with the sphenoid bone.

Occipital bone

The occipital bone forms parts of the posterior and inferior, or basal, portions of the cranium. It consists of three parts: the *basilar,* which articulates anteriorly with the basilar part of the sphenoid bone; the *lateral,* which are situated bilateral to the *foramen magnum;* and the *squamous,* which lies posterior, superior, and anterior to the foramen magnum and contributes to the formation of the lambdoidal suture. The *occipital condyles* are located on the inferior surfaces of the lateral parts and articulate with the superior articular facets of the atlas. The squama of the occipital bone, like the squama of the frontal bone, curves toward its perimeter. Its cranial surface faces the posterior part of the brain. The spinal cord passes through the foramen magnum to connect with the brain. The occiput is demonstrated radiographically by the use of the occipital view. The occipital bone articulates with both temporal bones, both parietal bones, the atlas, and the sphenoid bone.

Parietal bone

The paired parietal bones articulate with each other in the midsagittal plane, forming the sagittal suture. Each bone articulates inferiorly with the temporal bone, posteriorly with the occipital bone, and anteriorly with the frontal bone. Near the sagittal and lambdoidal sutures, each parietal bone contains a small foramen called the *parietal foramen.* These foramina are not always visualized. The junction of the sagittal and coronal sutures is named the *anterior fontanelle* (bregma), and the junction of the lambdoidal and sagittal sutures is named the *posterior fontanelle* (lambda). The parietal bone is demonstrated radiographically by the use of the lateral skull position. Each parietal bone articulates with the temporal bone, sphenoid bone, frontal bone, occipital bone, and opposite parietal bone.

Temporal bone

Obtaining radiographs that demonstrate well the numerous parts of the temporal bones requires both anatomic knowledge and radiographic skill. Careful study of the anatomy of the temporal bone is essential. Although not demonstrable radiographically, the *auditory ossicles* are in the cavity of the tympanum. These bones are the *malleus, incus,* and *stapes.*

The temporal bones are inferior to the parietal bones between the occipital bone and great wing of the sphenoid bone. (See Figs. 10-6 and 10-7.) The *squama* of the temporal bone is surrounded by the sphenoid bone and parietal bone. The *zygomatic process* extends anteriorly from the inferior portion of the squama and articulates anteriorly with the zygomatic bone. The *mastoid portion* is posterior and inferior to the squama. The mastoid process contains the *mas-*

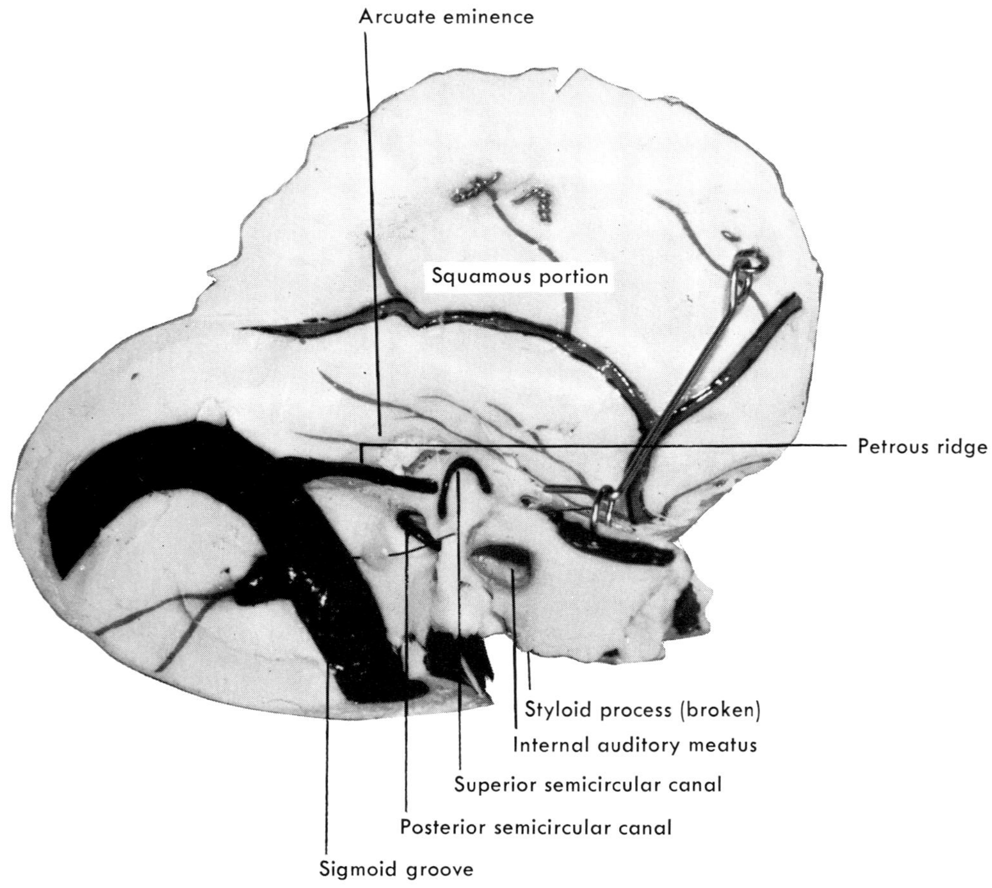

Fig. 10-6. Left temporal, internal surface. (Courtesy Clay-Adams, Inc.)

toid cells and extends posteriorly and inferiorly below the *external auditory meatus.* The *tympanic antrum* is medial to the cells and lateral and posterior to the *epitympanic recess.* Most of the important auditory organs, among which are the *semicircular canals* and *membranous labyrinth,* are in the petrous portion, which separates the occipital bone and sphenoid bone. The *styloid process* is directed inferiorly and anteriorly from beneath the tympanic part. The external auditory meatus is located in the petrous portion. The temporal bone is demonstrated radiographically by the use of the lateral skull view; the petrous ridges, by the use of the posterior (A-P) axial view, anterior (P-A) axial view, and the occipital view; and the mastoids, by the use of the lateral view. The temporal bone articulates with the parietal bone, occipital bone, sphenoid bone, zygomatic bone, and mandible.

Points of importance

1. The floor of the cranium is formed by the ethmoid bone, sphenoid bone, both temporal bones, frontal bone, and occipital bone.
2. The flat bones of the skullcap are composed of three layers: *outer table, diploë,* and *inner table.* The diploë contains the major supply of the nerves and blood vessels of the skullcap. It is the nutrient layer for the entire outer table and for part of the inner table.
3. The foramen magnum in the occipital bone is surrounded by the lateral parts, basilar part, and squamous part.
4. The basilar part of the occipital bone articulates anteriorly with the basilar portion of the sphenoid bone.
5. The basilar portion of the sphenoid bone articulates anteriorly and inferiorly with the vomer.
6. The following bones and parts contribute to the formation of the nasal septum: nasal crests and frontal spine, perpendicular plate of the ethmoid, sphenoidal rostrum and vomer, and maxillary crests.
7. The sagittal suture is formed by the junction of the parietal bones.
8. The coronal suture is formed by the junction of the frontal bone with the parietal bones.
9. The anterior fontanelle (bregma) is at the junction of the sagittal and coronal sutures.
10. The posterior fontanelle (lambda) is at the junction of the sagittal and lambdoidal sutures.
11. The lambdoidal suture is situated between the occipital bone and the parietal bones.
12. The squamous sutures are between the temporal bones and parietal bones.
13. The pterion is located at the junction of the coronal and squamosal sutures.
14. The *asterion* is located at the junction of the lambdoidal and squamosal sutures.

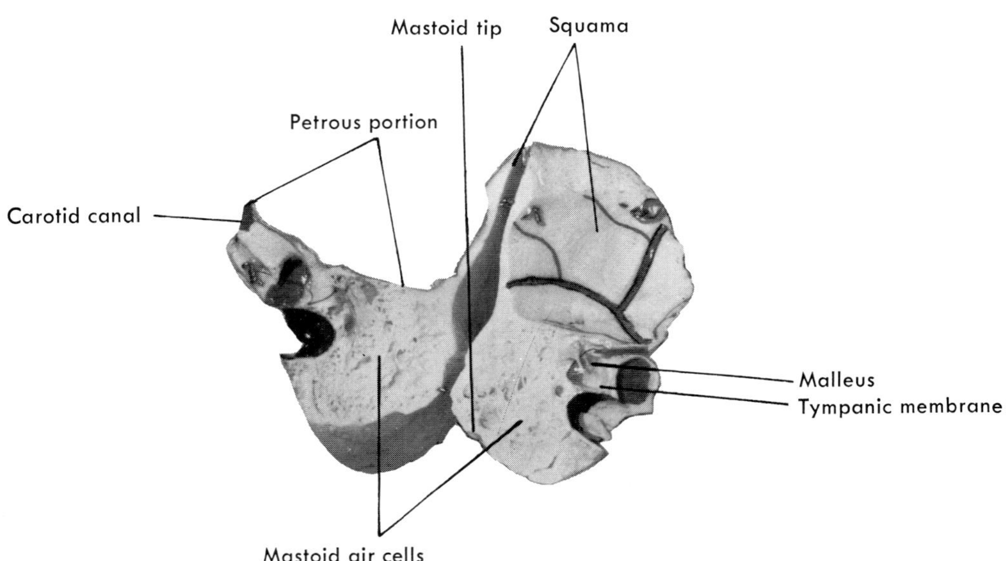

Fig. 10-7. Left temporal, oblique section through mastoid and petrous portions. (Courtesy Clay-Adams, Inc.)

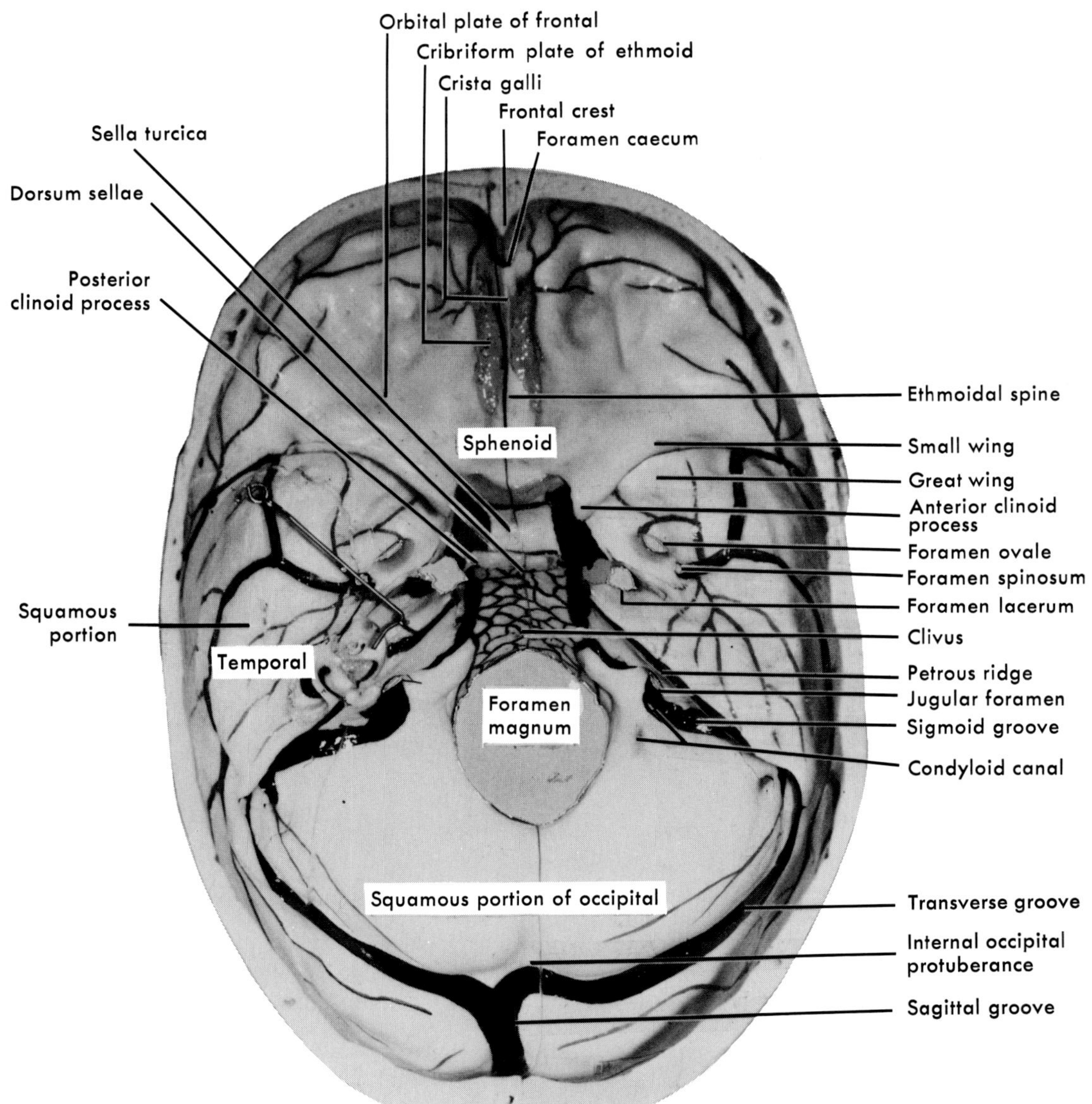

Fig. 10-8. Cranial floor, superior aspect. (Courtesy Clay-Adams, Inc.)

15. The *obelion* is located at the junction of a line drawn between the parietal foramina with the sagittal suture.

16. The *inion* is the midpoint of the external occipital protuberance.

For a better understanding of the relation of the bones forming the base of the cranium, see Fig. 10-8. The verticosubmental view is frequently used to demonstrate the cranial floor.

FACIAL BONES

Including the mandible, there are fourteen facial bones: two nasal, two zygomatic, two lacrimal, two maxillae, two palatine, two inferior nasal turbinates, mandible, and vomer. They are generally responsible for the shape and appearance of the face.

Nasal bones

The nasal bones are quite small and articulate with each other in the midsagittal plane. Each articulates with the corresponding frontal process of the maxilla. The lateral cartilage of the nose is inferior to each nasal bone. The vertical crest articulates with the frontal spine and the perpendicular plate of the ethmoid bone and extends below the sagittal border. The nasal bones are demonstrated radiographically by the use of the axial, anterior (P-A) (Waters) sinus views, and lateral nasal bone view. The nasal bone articulates with the frontal bone, ethmoid bone, maxilla, and opposite nasal bone.

Lacrimal bone

The smallest facial bone is the lacrimal bone. It occupies the space surrounded by the lamina papyracea of the ethmoid bone, two parts of the maxilla, frontal orbital plate, and inferior nasal turbinate and forms a part of the medial orbital wall. The lacrimal bones are not well demonstrated radiographically. The anterior (P-A) view is used.

Zygomatic (malar) bone

The zygomatic bone occupies the space bordering on the temporal bone, frontal bone, maxilla, and sphenoid bone and has processes that articulate with these bones. It is situated inferior and lateral to the outer canthus of the eye and is commonly called the cheek bone. It is concerned with the formation of the lateral border of the eye orbit in its articulation with the frontal bone and also with the formation of the zygomatic arch in its articulation with the zygomatic process of the temporal bone. The zygomatic bone is demonstrated radiographically by the use of the zygomatic arch, tangential view.

Maxillae

The second largest bones of the facial group are the maxillae, which form the upper jaw. The maxilla articulates with, and occupies the space bordering on, the nasal bone, lacrimal bone, zygomatic bone, inferior nasal turbinate bone, vomer, palatine bone, ethmoid bone, frontal bone, and opposite maxilla. It contains one of the *maxillary sinuses (nasal antra)* lateral to the median plane and superior to the bicuspid, when demonstrated in an anterior projection. It borders on the buccal, nasal, and orbital cavities. Each maxilla forms one half of the anterior nasal spine. The *frontal process* extends superiorly between the nasal and lacrimal bones and articulates with the frontal bone. The *zygomatic process* faces and articulates posteriorly with the zygomatic bone. The strong *palatine process* is horizontal. It articulates in the midsagittal plane with the palatine process of the opposite maxilla. Posteriorly each palatine process articulates with the horizontal portion of the palatine bone. The palatine processes of the maxillae with the horizontal parts of the palatine bones separate the nasal and oral cavities and form the *hard palate*. The *alveolar process* is the ridge from which the teeth of the upper jaw erupt. The *alveolar arch* is composed of the two alveolar processes. The maxillary sinus is described on pp. 308 and 310. The maxilla is demonstrated radiographically by the use of the oblique maxilla and anterior (P-A) (Waters) views. The antra are demonstrated by the use of the erect anterior (P-A) (Waters) view, whereas the maxillae, inferior (superoinferior) view demonstrates the hard palate and palatine processes.

Palatine bone

The palatine bone, above the roof of the mouth, occupies the space bordering on the palatine process of the maxilla, the opposite palatine bone, ethmoid bone, vomer, and inferior nasal turbinate bone and articulates with these bones. The palatine borders on the nasal and oral cavities and the orbit of the eye. It is comprised of five distinct parts: three processes (pyramidal, orbital, and sphenoidal) and a horizontal part and a vertical part. The *horizontal part* articulates with the corresponding part of the other palatine bone in the midsagittal plane. This articulation is described under the palatine processes of the maxillae. It is inferiorly placed on the palatine bone and extends medially from the main structure. The *vertical part* extends above the horizontal part and includes the orbital, sphenoidal, and pyramidal processes. The palatine bone is demonstrated radiographically by the use of the maxillae, inferior (superoinferior) view for the hard palate. The horizontal part of the palatine bones is always included in radiographs of the hard palate.

Inferior nasal turbinate bone (concha)

The inferior nasal turbinate bone resembles a conch shell and is truly osseous, while the middle and superior turbinate bones are chiefly cartilaginous. The middle and superior nasal turbinates are parts of the ethmoid. The inferior nasal turbinate bones are lateral and inferior in the nasal cavity, one turbinate bone being located on each lateral wall. This bone is best demonstrated radiographically in the anterior (P-A) skull view, although it may be visualized in the anterior (P-A) (Waters) sinus view. The inferior nasal turbinate bone articulates with the ethmoid bone, maxilla, lacrimal bone, and palatine bone.

Vomer

The vomer occupies the space surrounded by the ethmoid bone, sphenoid bone, both maxillae, and both palatine bones and articulates with these bones. It is near the center of the base of the skull. A lateral projection bears a fair resemblance to a blunt arrowhead, with the blunted end directed toward the *alveolar point*. The *choanae* (posterior nares) are separated by the posterior margin of the vomer. The vomer contributes to the formation of the nasal septum and is the most posterior part of the nasal septum. Although difficult to visualize, the vomer is demonstrated radiographically by the use of the lateral skull, submentovertex, and verticosubmental views.

Mandible

The largest bone of the facial section of the skull is the mandible. Ossification begins in two different centers in intrauterine life, and the mandibular body is in two parts at birth. In the first few months of extrauterine life, the two parts of the body are fused anteriorly in the midsagittal plane *(symphysis mandibulus)*. Superiorly on each side of the body is the *alveolar ridge (process)*, from which the teeth of the lower jaw erupt. From the posterior ends of the body the bone turns upward, forming the *ramus* on each side. This turn is called the *angle* of the mandible. The *condylar process* extends posteriorly and superiorly from the ramus to support the *head (condyle)*, which articulates in the mandibular fossa of the temporal bone, forming the *temporomandibular joint*. There is one head for each ramus. The *coronoid process* extends anteriorly and superiorly from the ramus. It has no articulation. There is one coronoid process for each ramus. The mandible is demonstrated radiographically by the use of the lateral and oblique mandible views, and the symphysis and rami are demonstrated by the use of the anterior (P-A) view. Frequently, it is inconvenient to obtain satisfactory views in the routine positioning. The use of dental films intraorally and extraorally is of extreme value in certain cases.

Hyoid bone

Although the hyoid bone is not one of the bones of the skull, it is usually discussed immediately following them. It is U shaped, has no osseous articulations, and is attached by ligaments to the styloid processes of the temporal bones. It is superior to the thyroid cartilage and anterior to the base of the tongue. The hyoid bone is demonstrated radiographically by the use of the lateral cervical spine view.

SINUSES

The *paranasal sinuses (frontal, two ethmoid, sphenoid,* and *two maxillary* or *nasal antra)* form a border of air spaces around the nasal cavity. Each sinus has openings into the nasal cavity. The sinuses are frequently examined radiographically. The major positions for examinations were mentioned briefly in conjunction with the description of their respective bones. In addition to these sinuses, a discussion of the *nasal cavity* is pertinent in this section. (See Figs. 10-9 and 10-10.)

Frontal sinus

The frontal sinus is located in the frontal bone posterior to the glabella and medially between the supraorbital ridges in the diploë.

Ethmoid sinuses

The two ethmoid sinuses are anterior and posterior to each other. They are located in the ethmoid bone superior and bilateral to the nasal septum and anterior and superior to the sphenoid sinus.

Sphenoid sinus

The sphenoid sinus is located in the sphenoid bone, anterior and inferior to the sella turcica.

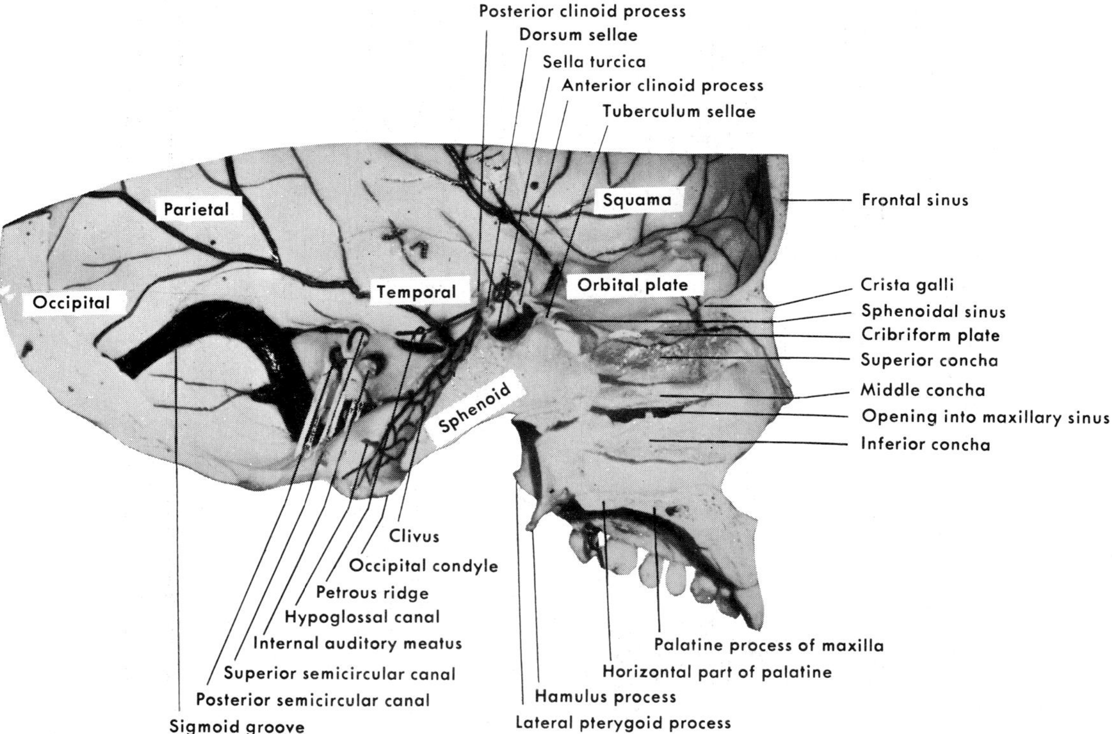

Fig. 10-9. Skull, midsagittal section, showing relationship of paranasal sinuses to other structures. (Courtesy Clay-Adams, Inc.)

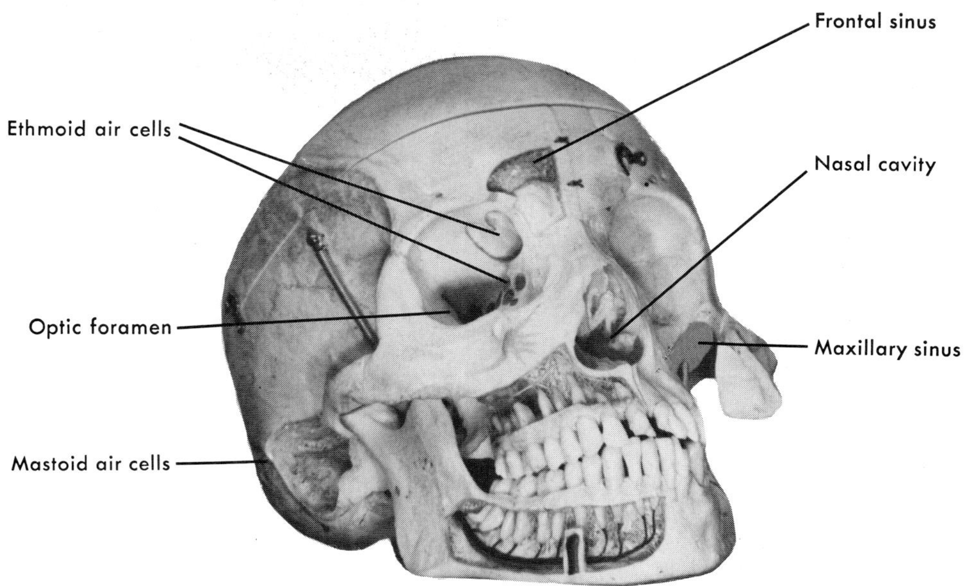

Fig. 10-10. Skull, antero-oblique aspect.

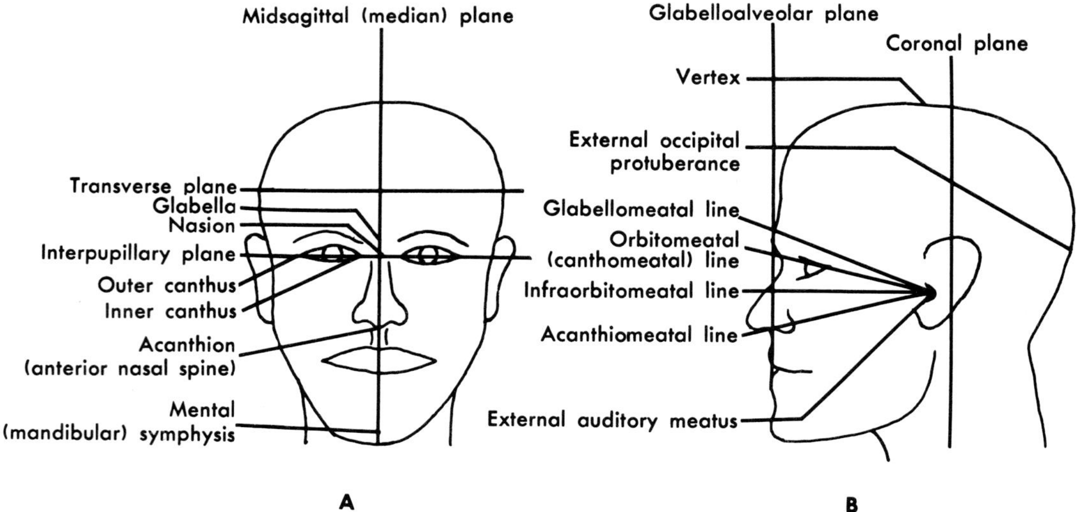

Fig. 10-11. A, Guidelines. **B,** Skull landmarks.

Nasal antra

The nasal antra are located in the maxillae, bilateral to the nasal cavity and inferior to the orbital floors of the eye cavities.

Nasal cavity

The nasal septum divides the nasal cavity into two parts. It is situated between the oral cavity and the cranial floor. The nasal bone, frontal spine, cribriform plate of the ethmoid bone, body of the sphenoid bone, sphenoidal conchae, alae of the vomer, and the palatine sphenoidal processes form the roof of the nasal cavity. The palatine processes of the maxillae and half of the horizontal parts of the palatine bones form the floor of the nasal cavity. The medial wall is the nasal septum and is described in item 6 under Points of Importance. The frontal process of the maxilla, lacrimal bone, ethmoid bone, body of the maxilla, inferior nasal turbinate bone, vertical plate of the palatine bone, and the medial pterygoid plate of the sphenoid bone form the lateral wall. The nasal cavity opens to the outside through the *anterior nares* (bony parts of the nose) and into the pharynx through the choanae (posterior nares). It is demonstrated radiographically by the use of the routine sinus views. See Fig. 10-11 for some of the landmarks and guidelines used in skull and sinus radiography.

REFERENCES

Anthony, C. P., and Kolthoff, N. J.: Textbook of anatomy and physiology, ed. 9, St. Louis, 1975, The C. V. Mosby Co.

Goss, Charles M.: Gray's anatomy, ed. 28, Philadelphia, 1966, Lea & Febiger.

Jacobi, C. A.: Textbook of anatomy and physiology in radiologic technology, ed. 2, St. Louis, 1975, The C. V. Mosby Co.

Meschan, Isadore: Atlas of anatomy basic to radiology, Philadelphia, 1975, W. B. Saunders Co.

QUESTIONS

1. Name the bones that compose the cranial vault.
2. Name the bones that compose the cranium.
3. Name the bones that make up the facial section of the skull.
4. What bones form the eye orbit?
5. What important gland is situated within the sella turcica?
6. What parts of what bones comprise the zygomatic arches?
7. In what bone(s) are found the optic foramina?
8. The petrous processes are important parts of what bones?
9. What lesser bones are contained within each tympanic part?
10. In what bone is the foramen magnum? What important structure passes through it?
11. Describe and locate the following: coronal and sagittal sutures and anterior fontanelle.
12. Describe and locate the following: lambdoidal and squamosal sutures and posterior fontanelle.
13. Describe the processes of the maxilla.
14. Describe in detail the mandible.
15. What bone of the head and neck region has no osseous articulation?
16. Describe the paranasal sinuses.
17. What other, than paranasal, sinuses are found in the skull? Where?
18. What are the movable articulations of the skull?
19. Of what bone(s) is the cribriform plate a part?
20. What passes through the cribriform plate? How?

11 · POSITIONING FOR THE SKULL

Skull—anterior (P-A) view (Figs. 11-1 and 11-2)

Film size—10″ × 12″
Cassette
Lengthwise
Bucky
Collimate to cover

Technique

Factors	Screen film cassette (par)
mA	100
Time	0.6
mAs	60
Thickness in cm	18
kVp	78
Distance	40

Patient preparation

Remove all metallic and plastic articles from the head and neck region.

Palpation point

Vertex.

Procedure

Place the patient in the prone position with the median plane of the skull and body over the center line of the table. Place the hands in a comfortable position at the sides of the head. Place the forehead and nose on the table so that both the midsagittal plane and the canthomeatal line are perpendicular to the tabletop. Align the top of the cassette 1½ inches above the vertex of the skull.

Central ray

Direct the central ray perpendicular through the nasion to the film holder. Collimate to film holder.

Immobilization

Place large sponges on each side of the skull and hold them in place with sandbags or the patient's hands. Employ suspended expiration.

Right-left markers

Place the *R* marker on the right side, center border of the film holder.

Technical tips

For thin patients, place a pillow or positioning sponges under the anterior thorax.

Structures demonstrated

Anterior (P-A) view of the anterior wall of the cranium, the frontal sinuses, the ethmoid sinuses, and the crista galli. The petrous ridges should fill the lower two thirds of the eye orbits.

Note: To demonstrate a larger area of the petrous portion within the bony eye orbits, make an anteroposterior view, reversing the above procedure.

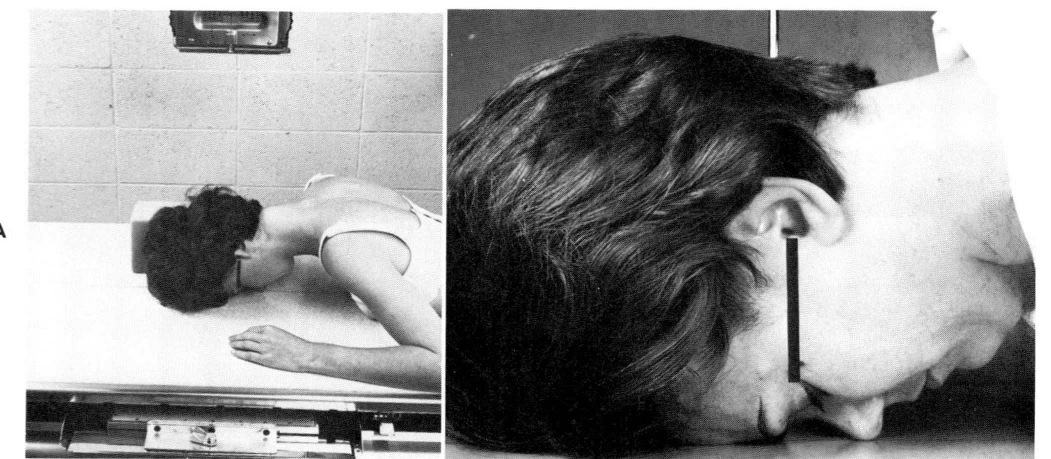

Fig. 11-1. Skull. **A** and **B,** Anterior (P-A) positions.

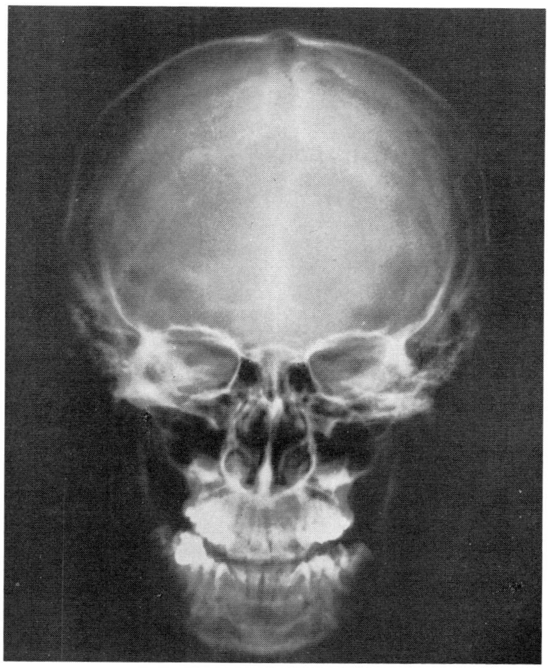

Fig. 11-2. Skull—anterior (P-A) view. (Courtesy Dr. E. I. L. Cilley, Dr. T. W. Crowell, Dr. R. E. Waud, and Dr. G. H. Hoffman.)

Skull—lateral view (Figs. 11-3 and 11-4)

Film size—10″ × 12″
Cassette
Crosswise
Bucky
Collimate to cover

Technique

Factors	Screen film cassette (par)
mA	100
Time	0.5
mAs	50
Thickness in cm	15
kVp	68
Distance	40

Patient preparation

Remove all metallic and plastic articles from the head and neck region.

Palpation point

Vertex.

Procedure

Place the patient in the prone position with the side of the skull being examined on the table. Elevate the opposite side of the body; flex this knee and elbow for support. The midsagittal plane of the skull is parallel with the tabletop. Flex the neck so that the canthomeatal line is perpendicular to the side of the table. Support the chin with a sponge or the patient's fist. On the canthomeatal line, center a point ¾ inch anterior and ¾ inch superior to the external auditory meatus over the center line of the table. Align the top of the cassette 1½ inches above the vertex of the skull.

Central ray

Direct the central ray perpendicular through the selected point to the film holder. Collimate to film holder.

Immobilization

Place large sponges against the top and back of the skull; hold them in place with sandbags. Employ suspended expiration.

Right-left markers

Place the correct marker on the anterior center border of the film holder.

Technical tips

Make bilateral views on patients with traumatic injuries.

Structures demonstrated

Lateral view visualizing the anterior and posterior clinoid processes, sella turcica, dorsum sellae, and superimposed parietal bones.

Note: For stereographic views, make two separate views, shifting the tube 2 inches inferior from the centering point and then 2 inches superior from the centering point. The patient *must retain the same position* for both radiographic exposures.

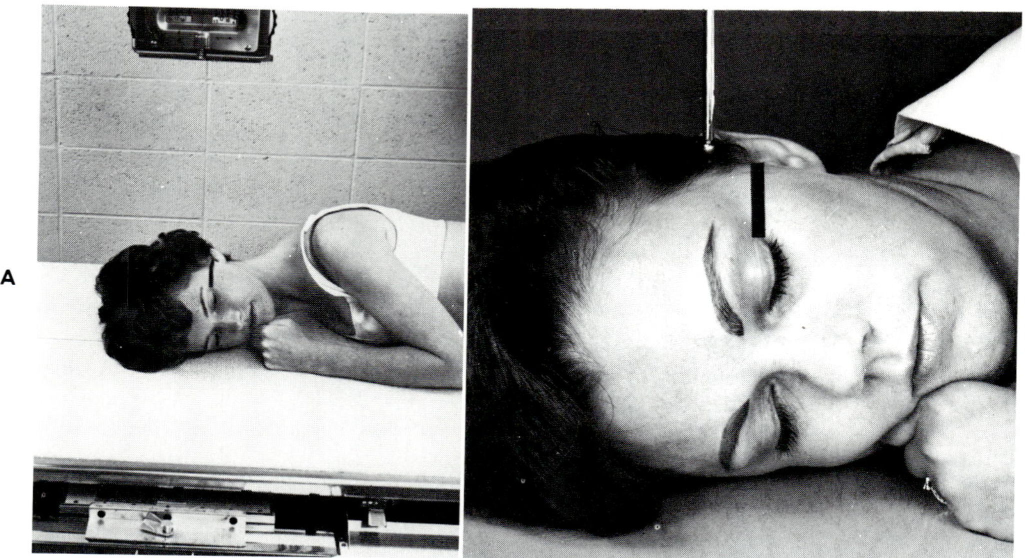

Fig. 11-3. Skull. **A** and **B,** Lateral positions.

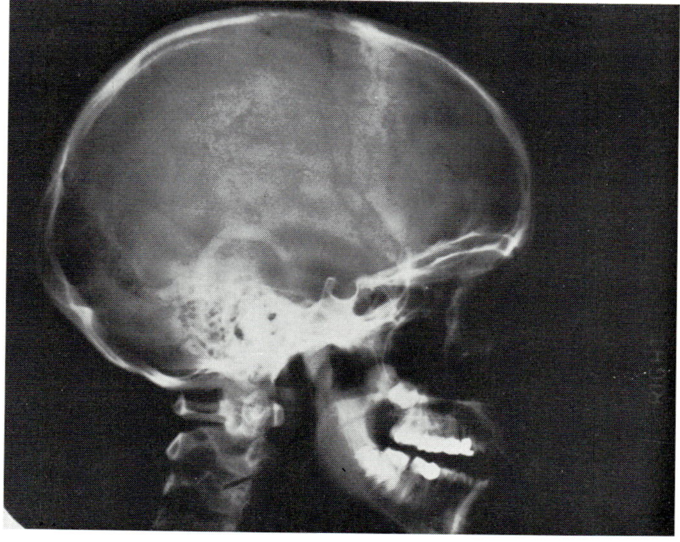

Fig. 11-4. Skull—lateral view. (Courtesy Dr. E. I. L. Cilley, Dr. T. W. Crowell, Dr. R. E. Waud, and Dr. G. H. Hoffman.)

Skull—occipital (Towne) view (Figs. 11-5 and 11-6)

Film size—10″ × 12″
Cassette
Lengthwise
Bucky
Collimate to cover

Technique

Factors	Screen film cassette (par)
mA	100
Time	0.7
mAs	70
Thickness in cm	23
kVp	80
Distance	40

Patient preparation

Remove all metallic and plastic articles from the head and neck region.

Palpation point

Vertex.

Procedure

Place the patient in the supine position with the median plane of the skull and body over the center line of the table. The midsagittal plane is perpendicular to the tabletop. Flex the chin so that the canthomeatal line is perpendicular to the tabletop. Align the top of the cassette with the vertex of the skull.

Central ray

Direct the central ray 35 degrees caudad through a point in line with the external auditory meatus to the film holder. Collimate to film holder.

Immobilization

Place a sandbag on top of the chin and chest and instruct the patient to hold the sandbag in place. Employ suspended expiration.

Right-left markers

Place the *R* marker on the right lateral center border of the film holder.

Technical tips

The posterior clinoid processes and the dorsum sellae will be demonstrated within the foramen magnum when the view is exact.

Structures demonstrated

Posterior (A-P) view of the occipital region visualizing the bilateral petrous pyramids, foramen magnum, dorsum sellae, occipital squama, and the posterior portions of both parietal bones.

Note: For prone patients, place the forehead on the tabletop and reverse the central ray angulation described above.

A

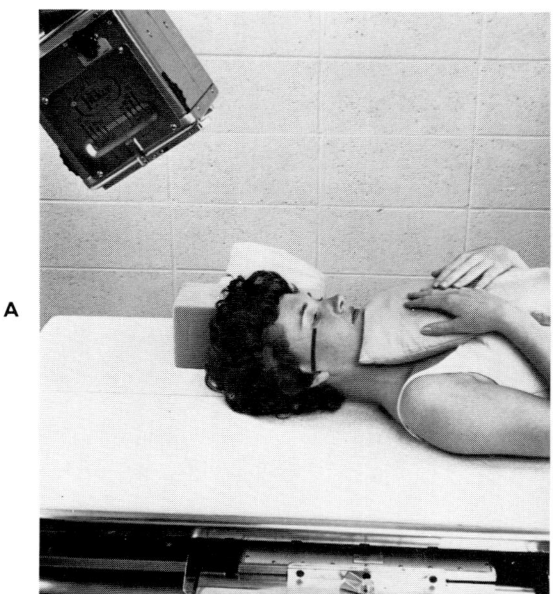

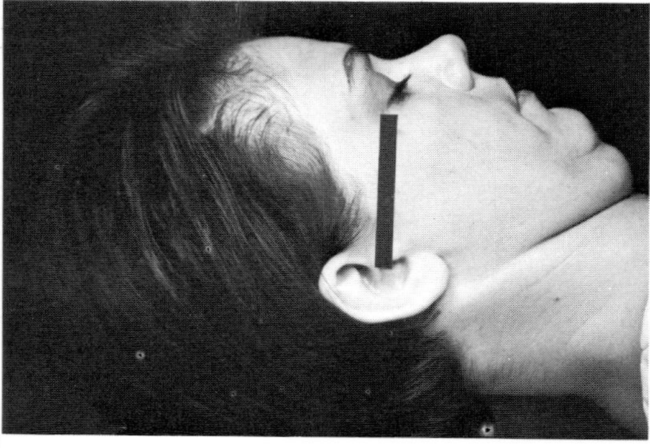

B

Fig. 11-5. Skull. **A** and **B,** Occipital (Towne) positions.

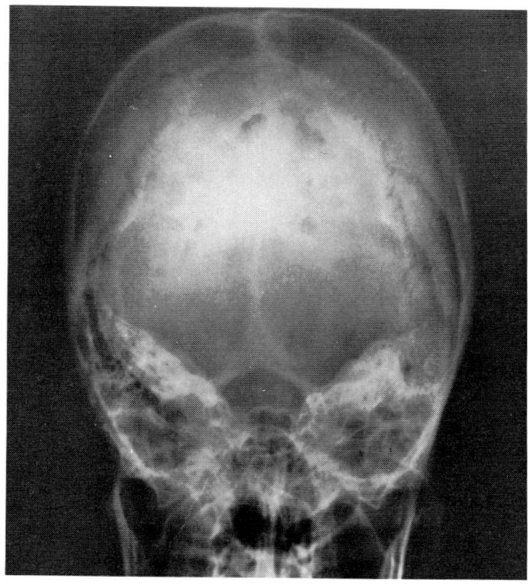

Fig. 11-6. Skull—occipital (Towne) view. (Courtesy Dr. E. I. L. Cilley, Dr. T. W. Crowell, Dr. R. E. Waud, and Dr. G. H. Hoffman.)

Skull—basilar (submentovertex) view (Figs. 11-7 and 11-8)

Film size—10″ × 12″
Cassette
Lengthwise
Bucky
Collimate to cover

Technique

Factors	Screen film cassette (par)
mA	100
Time	0.8
mAs	80
Thickness in cm	23
kVp	80
Distance	40

Patient preparation

Remove all metallic and plastic articles from the head and neck region.

Palpation points

Vertex; mandibular angles.

Procedure

Place the patient in the supine position on a large cushion or pillow with the median plane of the skull and body over the center line of the table. Extend the head backward so that the vertex of the skull rests on the tabletop. The midsagittal plane is perpendicular to the tabletop.

Central ray

Direct the central ray perpendicular to the infraorbitomeatal line, to enter a point midway between the angles of the mandible, and to the center of the film holder. Collimate to film holder.

Immobilization

Place sponges supported by sandbags against the forehead. Flex both knees and place both feet on the table to relieve neck strain. Employ suspended expiration.

Right-left markers

Place the *R* marker on the right lateral center border of the film holder.

Technical tips

For a better demonstration of the jugular foramen, decrease the cervical extension 20 degrees.

Structures demonstrated

Axial view of the basilar region visualizing the bilateral petrous ridges, mastoid processes, atlas, sphenoidal sinuses, maxillary sinuses, mandible, and the bilateral zygomatic arches.

Note: For elderly or wheelchair patients, use an erect table or a film holder with the patient seated.

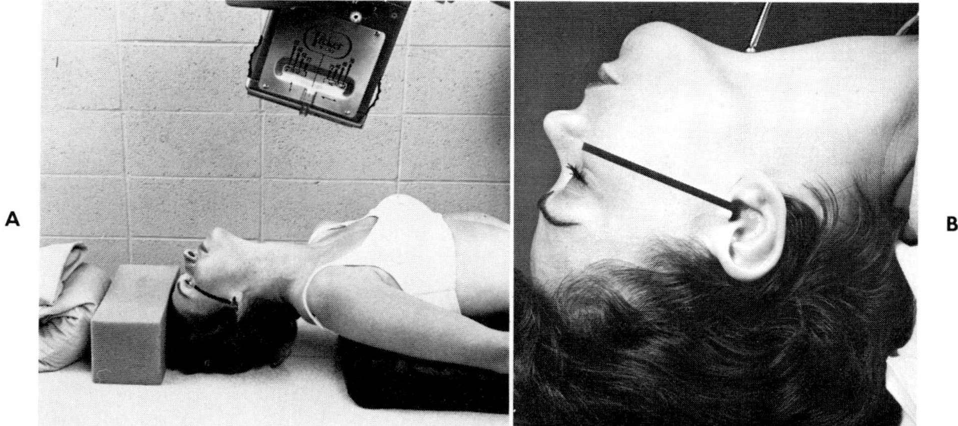

Fig. 11-7. Skull. **A** and **B**, Basilar (submentovertex) positions.

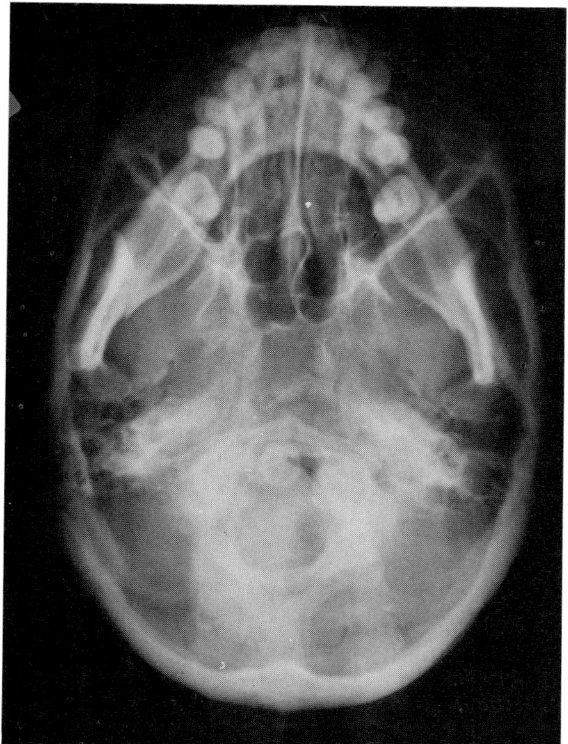

Fig. 11-8. Skull—basilar (submentovertex) view. (Courtesy Dr. Frank S. Cavallaro and Valley Hospital, Las Vegas, Nevada.)

Skull—verticosubmental view (Figs. 11-9 and 11-10)

Film size—10″ × 12″
Cassette
Lengthwise

Bucky
Collimate to cover

Technique

Factors	Screen film cassette (par)
mA	100
Time	0.8
mAs	80
Thickness in cm	23
kVp	80
Distance	40

Patient preparation

Remove all metallic and plastic articles from the head and neck region.

Palpation points

Vertex; mandibular condyles.

Procedure

Place the patient in the prone position with the median plane of the skull and body over the center line of the table. Place the hands on the table at the sides of the head. Extend the chin as far as possible and rest it on the center line of the table. The midsagittal plane of the skull is perpendicular to the tabletop.

Central ray

Direct the central ray perpendicular to the infraorbitomeatal line, through a point in line with the condyles of the mandible, and to the center of the film holder. Collimate to film holder.

Immobilization

Place large sponges against the sides of the skull, and sandbags against the sponges; instruct the patient to hold the sandbags in place with his hands. Employ suspended expiration.

Right-left markers

Place the *R* marker on the right lateral center border of the film holder.

Technical tips

Use of a grid cassette or portable Bucky will reduce both magnification and distortion of the image.

Structures demonstrated

Axial view of the base of the skull visualizing the sphenoidal sinuses and anterior cranial base.

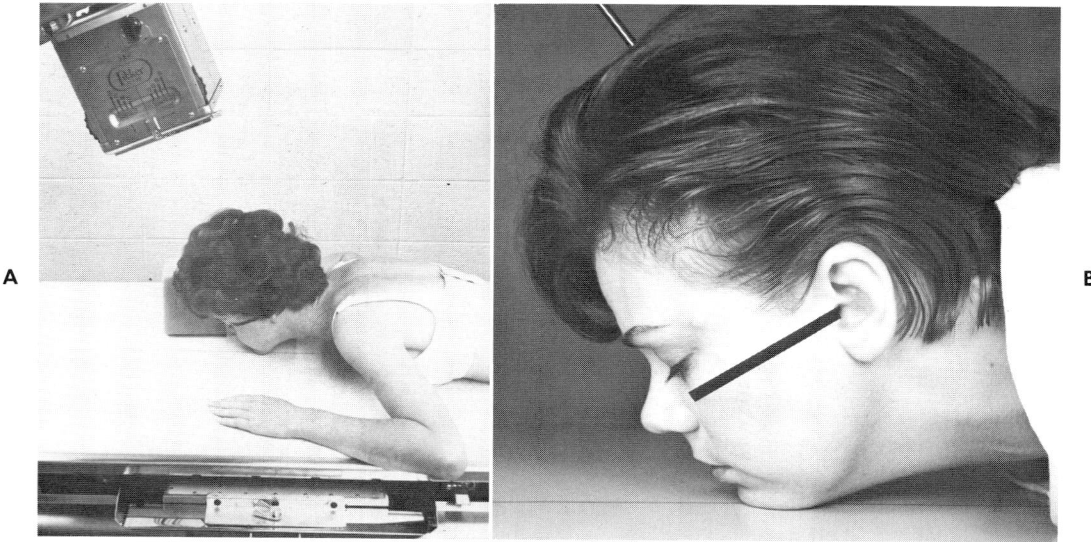

Fig. 11-9. Skull. **A** and **B**, Verticosubmental positions.

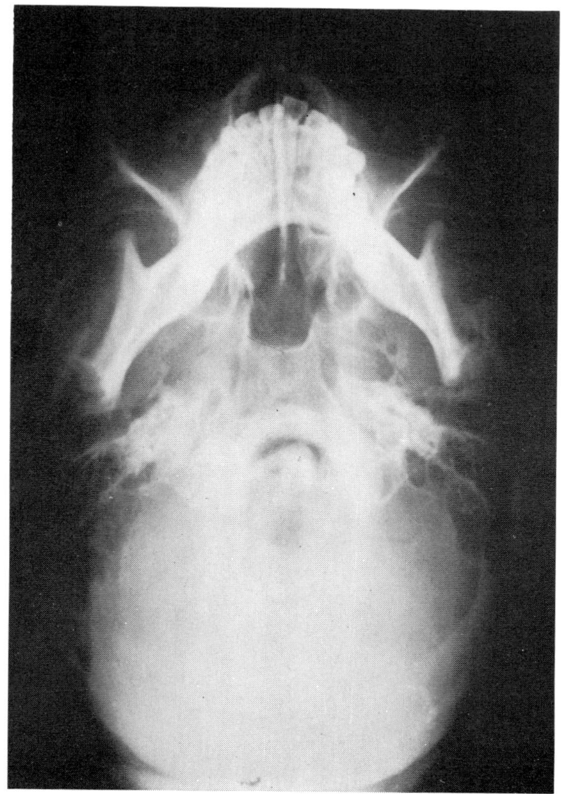

Fig. 11-10. Skull—verticosubmental view.

Sinuses—maxillary (Water) view (Figs. 11-11 to 11-13)

Film size—8″ × 10″ | *Erect Bucky*
Cassette | *Extension cone*
Lengthwise

Technique

Factors	Screen film cassette (par) Bucky	Screen film cassette (par) tabletop
mA	100	100
Time	0.5	0.25
mAs	50	25
Thickness in cm	21	21
kVp	78	78
Distance	30	30

Patient preparation

Remove all metallic and plastic articles from the head and neck region.

Palpation point

Acanthion.

Procedure

Seat the patient facing the erect Bucky with the median plane of the skull over the center line of the erect Bucky. Extend the chin both upward and forward to rest against the center line of the erect Bucky. The canthomeatal line forms a 37-degree angle with the erect Bucky, and the midsagittal plane of the skull is perpendicular to it.

Central ray

Direct the central ray perpendicular through the anterior nasal spine to the center of the film holder.

Immobilization

Instruct the patient to grasp each side of the table with his hands. Place the extension cone against the back of the skull. Employ suspended expiration.

Right-left markers

Burn the erect and *L* markers in the upper left border of the film holder above the cone field after the exposure is made.

Technical tips

Increase the cervical extension to decrease the amount of petrous portion demonstrated.

Structures demonstrated

Anterior (P-A) views of the maxillary antra to demonstrate possible fluid levels, the nasal septum, and the posterior walls of the eye orbits.

Note: Prone positioning will allow for better immobilization but will not demonstrate fluid level.

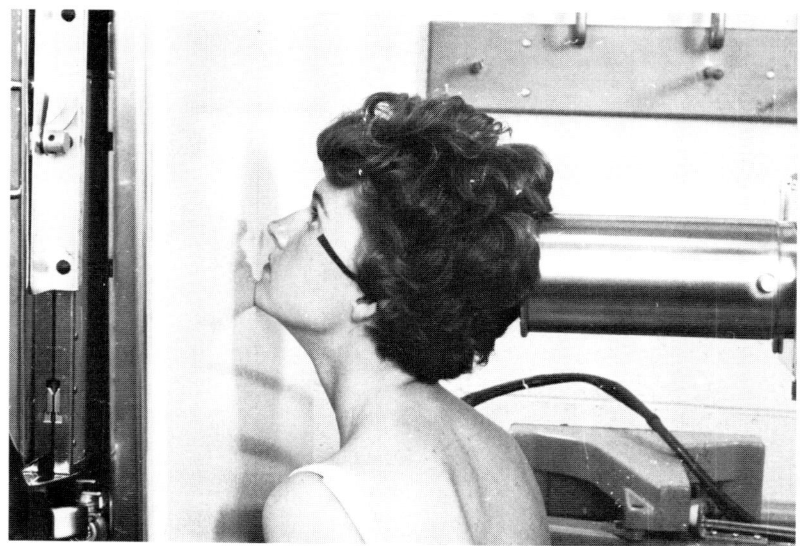

Fig. 11-11. Sinuses—maxillary (Water) erect position.

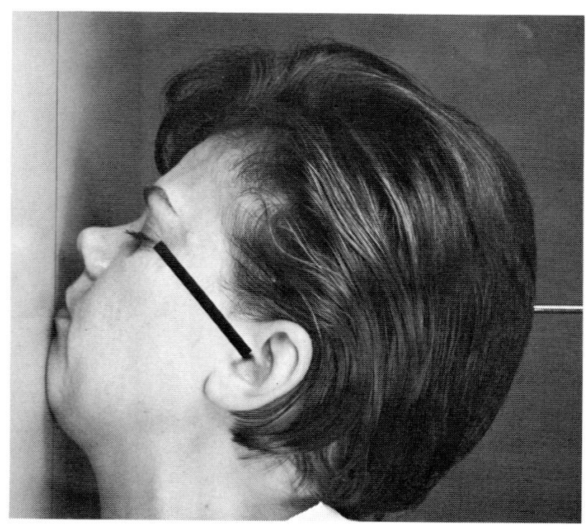

Fig. 11-12. Sinuses—maxillary (Water) erect position.

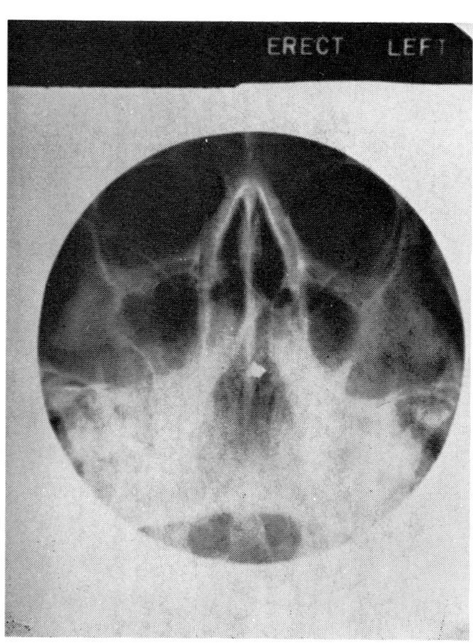

Fig. 11-13. Sinuses—maxillary (Water) erect view. (Courtesy Dr. E. I. L. Cilley, Dr. T. W. Crowell, Dr. R. E. Waud, and Dr. G. H. Hoffman.)

Sinuses—frontal-ethmoidal (modified Caldwell) view (Figs. 11-14 and 11-15)

Film size—8″ × 10″
Cassette
Lengthwise
Bucky
Extension cone

Technique

Factors	Screen film cassette (par) Bucky	Screen film cassette (par) tabletop
mA	100	100
Time	0.5	0.25
mAs	50	25
Thickness in cm	19	19
kVp	74	74
Distance	30	30

Patient preparation

Remove all metallic and plastic articles from the head and neck region.

Palpation points

Glabella; nasal bones.

Procedure

Place the patient in the prone position with the median plane of the skull and body over the center line of the table. Place the hands at the sides of the head. Place the forehead and nose on the center line of the table. Both the canthomeatal line and the midsagittal plane are perpendicular to the tabletop.

Central ray

Direct the central ray 15 degrees caudad through the nasion to the center of the film holder.

Immobilization

Place large sponges against the sides of the skull; instruct the patient to hold them in place with his hands, or hold them in place with sandbags. Employ suspended expiration.

Right-left markers

Burn the *L* marker in the upper left border of the film holder above the cone field after the exposure is made.

Technical tips

For thin patients, place a pillow or positioning sponges under the anterior thorax.

Structures demonstrated

Anterior (P-A) view of the frontal sinuses, anterior ethmoid cells, and the superior optic fissures.

Note: For a true Caldwell view, angle the central ray 23 degrees caudad through the glabella to the center of the film holder.

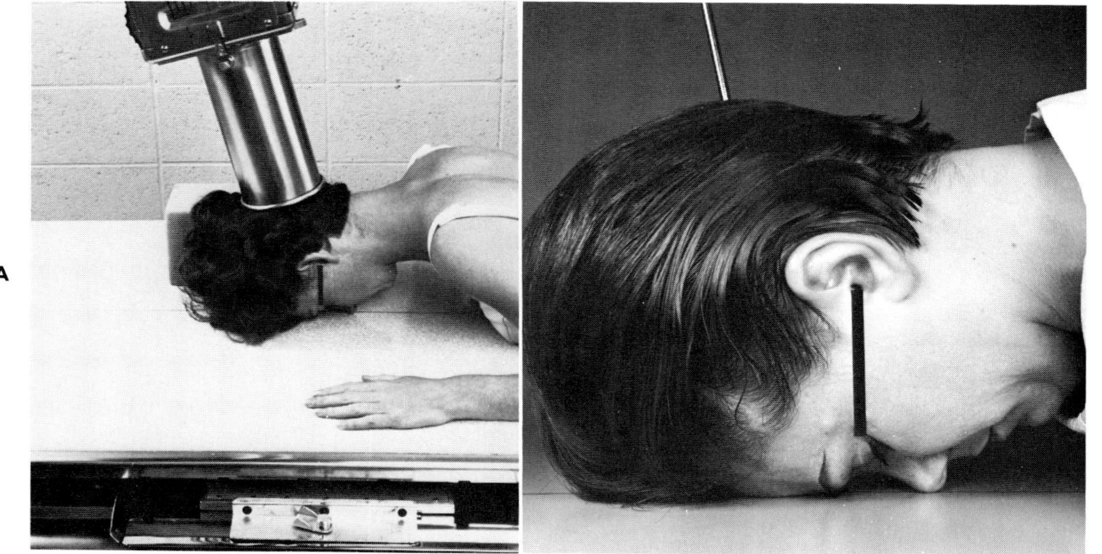

Fig. 11-14. Sinuses. **A** and **B,** Frontal-ethmoidal (modified Caldwell) positions.

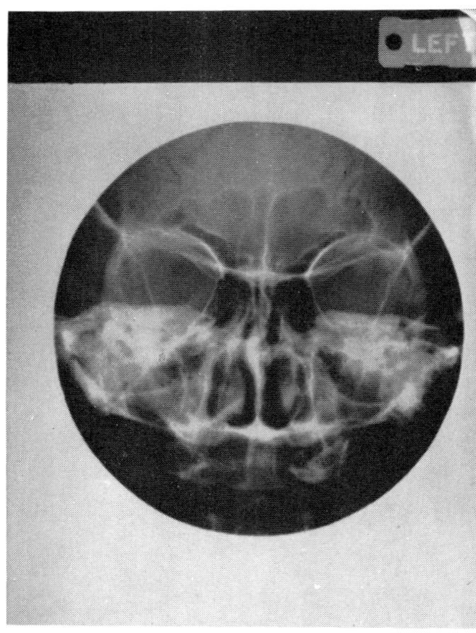

Fig. 11-15. Sinuses—frontal-ethmoidal (modified Caldwell) view. (Courtesy Dr. E. I. L. Cilley, Dr. T. W. Crowell, Dr. R. E. Waud, and Dr. G. H. Hoffman.)

Sinuses—lateral view (Figs. 11-16 and 11-17)

Film size—8″ × 10″ | *Bucky*
Cassette | *Extension cone*
Lengthwise

Technique

Factors	Screen film cassette (par) Bucky	Screen film cassette (par) tabletop
mA	100	100
Time	0.2	0.1
mAs	20	10
Thickness in cm	15	15
kVp	62	62
Distance	30	30

Patient preparation

Remove all metallic and plastic articles from the head and neck region.

Palpation point

Lateral margin of bony orbit.

Procedure

Place the patient in the prone position with the side of the head being examined on the table. Elevate the opposite side of the body and flex this knee and elbow for support. The midsagittal plane of the head is parallel with the tabletop. Flex the neck so that the canthomeatal line is perpendicular to the side of the table. Support the chin with a sponge or the patient's fist. Center a point ½ inch posterior to the outer canthus of the eye over the center line of the table.

Central ray

Direct the central ray perpendicular through the selected point to the center of the film holder.

Immobilization

Place large sponges against the top and back of the head and hold them in place with sandbags. Employ suspended expiration.

Right-left markers

Burn the correct marker in the upper center border of the film holder above the cone field after the exposure is made.

Technical tips

The rim of the extension cone should just clear the anterior border of the external auditory meatus.

Structures demonstrated

Lateral view of the paranasal sinuses and sella turcica.

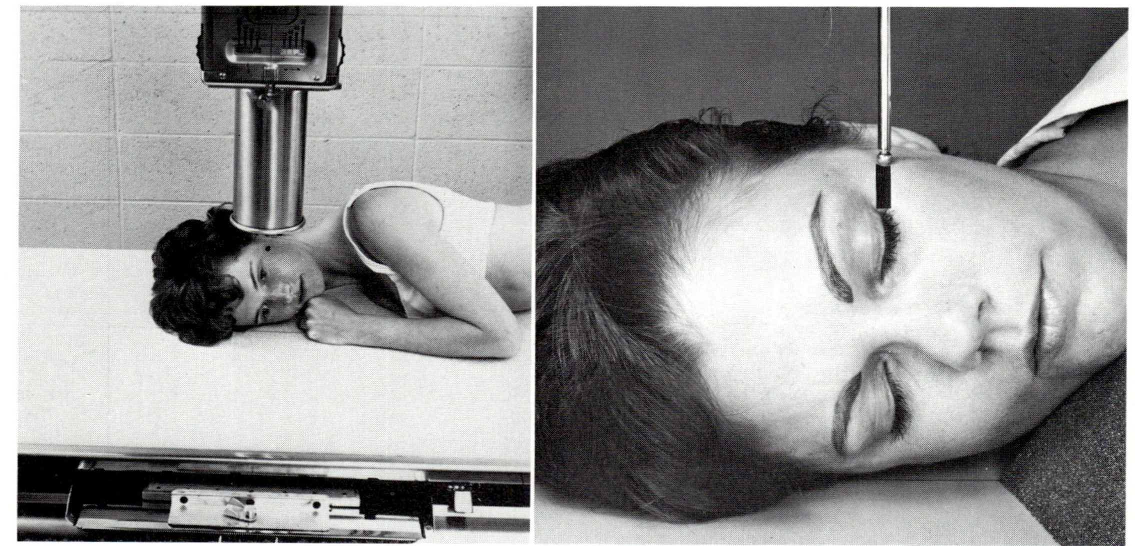

Fig. 11-16. Sinuses. **A** and **B,** Lateral positions.

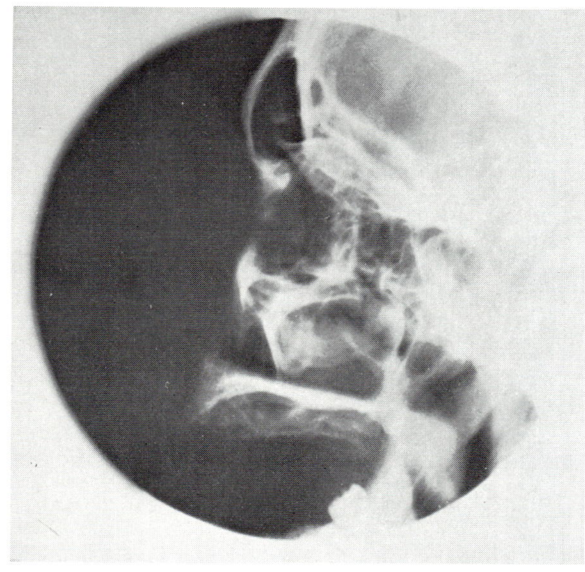

Fig. 11-17. Sinuses—lateral view. (Courtesy Dr. E. I. L. Cilley, Dr. T. W. Crowell, Dr. R. E. Waud, and Dr. G. H. Hoffman.)

Sinuses—open-mouth, sphenoid view (Figs. 11-18 and 11-19)

Film size—8″ × 10″
Cassette
Lengthwise
Bucky
Extension cone

Technique

Factors	Screen film cassette (par) Bucky	Screen film cassette (par) tabletop
mA	100	100
Time	0.5	0.25
mAs	50	25
Thickness in cm	21	21
kVp	76	76
Distance	30	30

Patient preparation

Remove all metallic and plastic articles from the head and neck region.

Palpation point

Temporal bone.

Procedure

Place the patient in the prone position with the median plane of the head and body over the center line of the table. Place the hands at the sides of the head. Have the patient open the mouth as far as possible and place it on the center line of the table. The midsagittal plane is perpendicular to the tabletop.

Central ray

Direct the central ray 23 degrees caudad through the sella turcica and the center of the open mouth to the center of the film holder.

Immobilization

Place large sponges against the sides of the head, and instruct the patient to hold them in place with his hands, or use sandbags. Employ suspended expiration.

Right-left markers

Burn the *L* marker in the upper left border of the film holder above the cone field after the exposure is made.

Technical tips

Decreased central-ray angulation may be necessary to align the sella turcica with the center of the open mouth.

Structures demonstrated

Anterior (P-A) view of the sphenoidal sinuses projected through the open mouth.

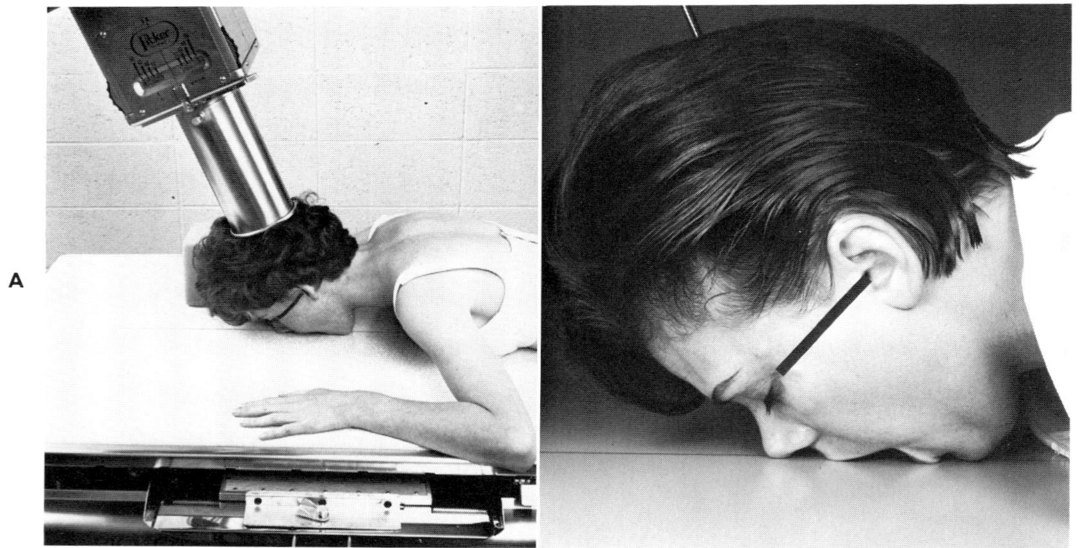

Fig. 11-18. Sinuses. **A** and **B**, Sphenoid (open-mouth) positions.

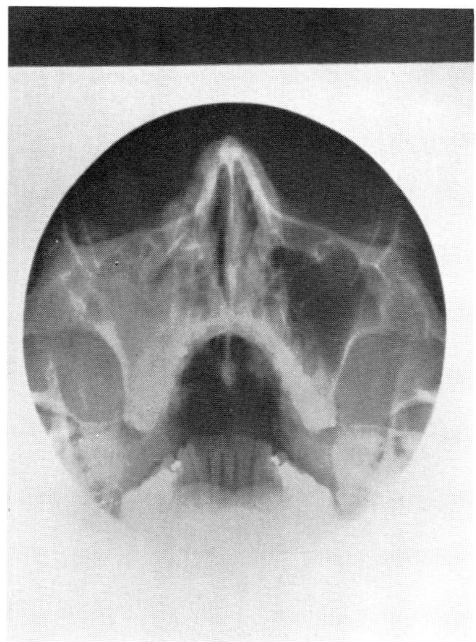

Fig. 11-19. Sinuses—sphenoid (open-mouth) view. (Courtesy Dr. E. I. L. Cilley, Dr. T. W. Crowell, Dr. R. E. Waud, and Dr. G. H. Hoffman.)

Mastoids—lateral (15°-15° Law) view (Figs. 11-20 and 11-21)

Film size—8″ × 10″
Cassette
Lengthwise
Bucky
Extension cone

Technique

Factors	Screen film cassette (par) Bucky	Screen film cassette (par) tabletop
mA	100	100
Time	0.4	0.2
mAs	40	20
Thickness in cm	18	18
kVp	70	64
Distance	30	30

Patient preparation

Remove all metallic and plastic articles from the head and neck region.

Palpation points

Mastoid processes.

Procedure

Tape the auricle of each ear forward. With a wax pencil make a mark 1 inch posterior to the external auditory meatus on each side of the head in line with the infraorbitomeatal line. Place the patient in the prone position with the side of the head being examined on the table. Elevate the opposite side of the body, and flex this knee and elbow for support. The midsagittal plane is parallel with the tabletop. Rotate the face 15 degrees toward the side being examined. The infraorbitomeatal line is perpendicular to the long axis of the table. Center the lower pencil mark over the center line of the table.

Central ray

Direct the central ray 15 degrees caudad through the lower pencil mark to the center of the film holder.

Immobilization

Support the patient's chin with a sponge. Employ suspended expiration.

Right-left markers

Burn the correct marker in the upper center border of the film holder above the cone field after the exposure is made.

Technical tips

To improve centering accuracy, precenter the central ray to a point on the table and down to the film center. Position the selected mark on the patient over the point on the table.

Structures demonstrated

Lateral view of the mastoid air cells, and of the superimposed internal and external auditory meatuses.

Note: Make bilateral views for comparison.

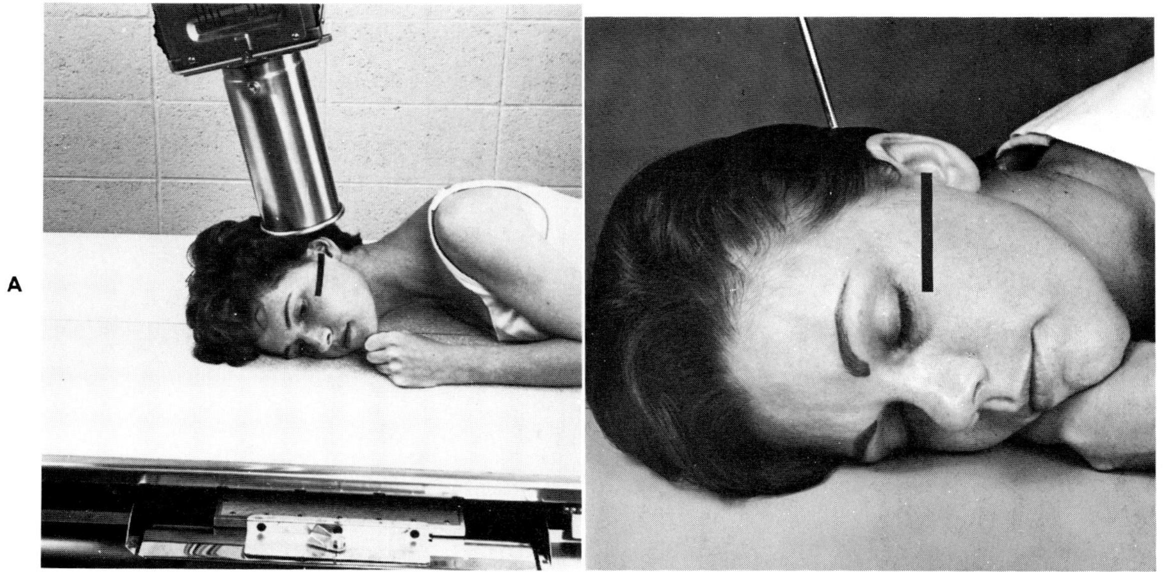

Fig. 11-20. Mastoids. A and B, Lateral (15°-15° Law) positions.

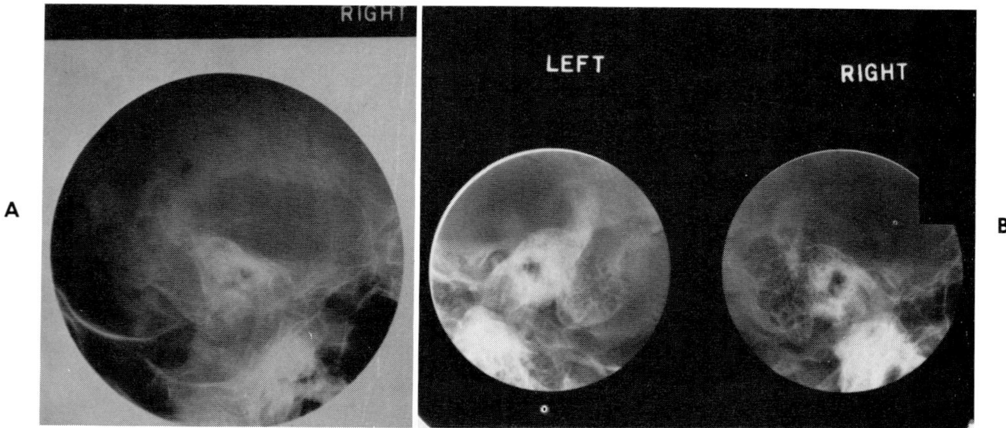

Fig. 11-21. Mastoids. A, Lateral (15°-15° Law) view—Bucky technique. B, Lateral (15°-15° Law) view—angle-board technique. (Courtesy Dr. E. I. L. Cilley, Dr. T. W. Crowell, Dr. R. E. Waud, and Dr. G. H. Hoffman.)

Pars petrosa, petrous portion—posterior (A-P) oblique (Arcelin) view
(Figs. 11-22 and 11-23)

Film size—8″ × 10″
Cassette
Lengthwise

Bucky
Extension cone

Technique

Factors	Screen film cassette (par) Bucky	Screen film cassette (par) tabletop
mA	100	100
Time	0.4	0.3
mAs	40	30
Thickness in cm	16	16
kVp	70	56
Distance	30	30

Patient preparation

Remove all metallic and plastic articles from the head and neck region.

Palpation points

Mastoid processes.

Procedure

With a wax pencil make a mark 1 inch anterior and superior to the external auditory meatus on the canthomeatal line on each side of the head. Place the patient in the supine position. Rotate the face 45 degrees away from the side being examined. The infraorbitomeatal line is perpendicular to the long axis of the table. Center the pencil mark on the upper side of the skull over the center line of the table.

Central ray

Direct the central ray 15 degrees caudad through the upper pencil mark to the center of the film holder.

Immobilization

Place a wedge sponge under the face; hold the sponge in place with a sandbag. A compression band may be placed across the head. Employ suspended expiration.

Right-left markers

Burn the correct marker in the upper center border of the film holder above the cone field after the exposure is made.

Technical tips

To improve centering accuracy, precenter the central ray to a point on the table and down to the film center. Position the patient so that the central ray is in line through the selected mark on the upper side of the skull to the film center.

Structures demonstrated

Posterior (A-P) view of the petrous pyramid, apex, internal acoustic canal, antral and labyrinthal areas, and mastoid air cells.

Note: Make bilateral views for comparison.

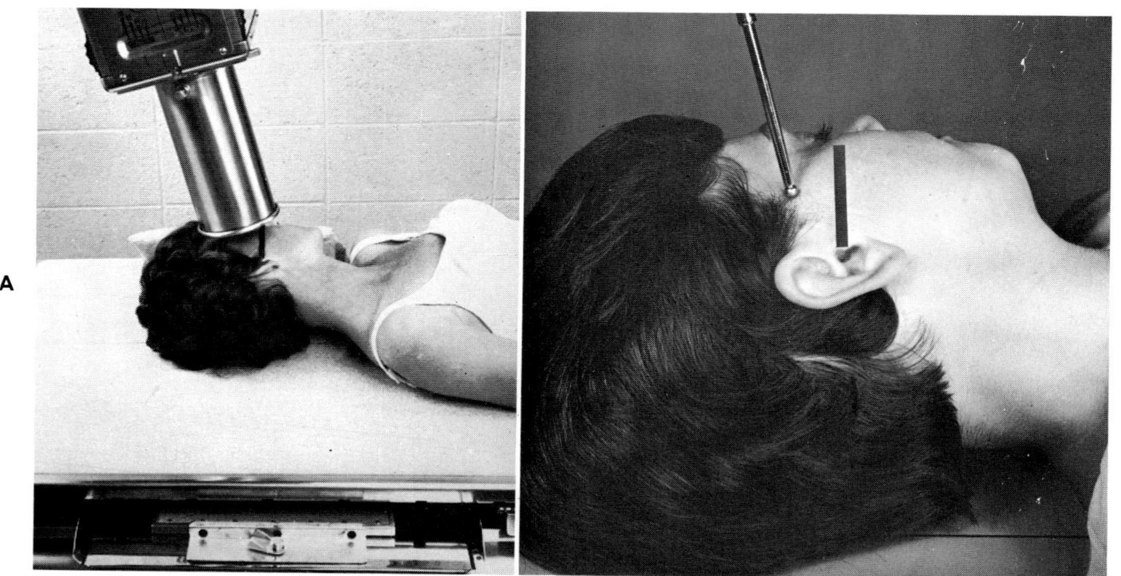

Fig. 11-22. Pars petrosa. **A** and **B,** Posterior (A-P) oblique (Arcelin) positions.

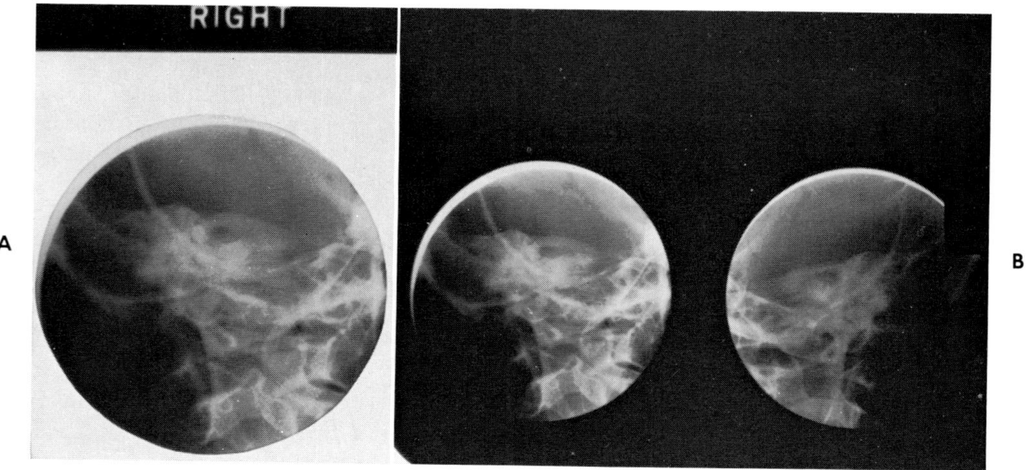

Fig. 11-23. Pars petrosa. **A,** Posterior (A-P) oblique (Arcelin) view—Bucky technique. **B,** Posterior (A-P) oblique (Arcelin) view—angle-board technique. (Courtesy Dr. E. I. L. Cilley, Dr. T. W. Crowell, Dr. R. E. Waud, and Dr. G. H. Hoffman.)

Petrous portion—anterior (P-A) oblique (Stenver) view (Figs. 11-24 and 11-25)

Film size—8″ × 10″ *Bucky*
Cassette *Extension cone*
Lengthwise

Technique

Factors	Screen film cassette (par) Bucky	Screen film cassette (par) tabletop
mA	100	100
Time	0.4	0.3
mAs	40	30
Thickness in cm	16	16
kVp	70	56
Distance	30	30

Patient preparation

Remove all metallic and plastic articles from the head and neck region.

Palpation points

Mastoid processes.

Procedure

With a wax pencil make a mark 1 inch anterior to the external auditory meatus on the infraorbitomeatal line on each side of the head. Place the patient in the prone position with the forehead and nose on the tabletop. Place the hands at the sides of the head. Rotate the face 45 degrees away from the side being examined. The infraorbitomeatal line is perpendicular to the long axis of the table. Center the lower pencil mark over the center line of the table.

Central ray

Direct the central ray 12 degrees cephalad through the lower pencil mark to the center of the film holder.

Immobilization

Place a wedge sponge under the posterior portion of the head and instruct the patient to hold the sponge in place with his hand, or use a sandbag. Employ suspended expiration.

Right-left markers

Burn the correct marker in the upper center border of the film holder above the cone field after the exposure is made.

Technical tips

The superior and horizontal semicircular canals should be clearly defined when positioning accuracy is achieved.

Structures demonstrated

Anterior (P-A) view of the petrous pyramid, apex, internal acoustic canal, antral and labyrinthal areas, and mastoid air cells.

Note: Make bilateral views for comparison.

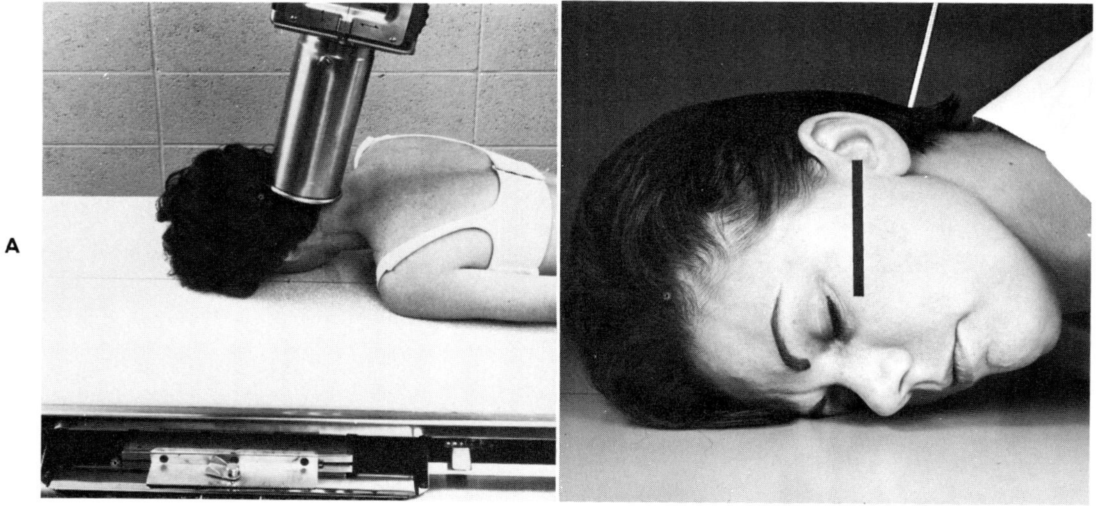

Fig. 11-24. Pars petrosa. **A** and **B,** Anterior (P-A) oblique (Stenver) positions.

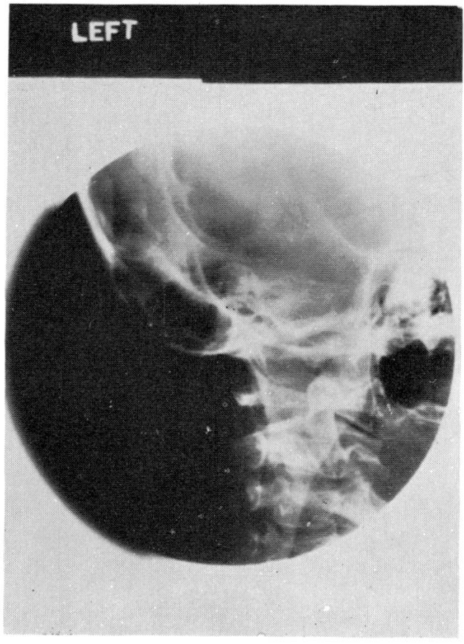

Fig. 11-25. Pars petrosa–anterior (P-A) oblique (Stenver) view. (Courtesy Dr. E. I. L. Cilley, Dr. T. W. Crowell, Dr. R. E. Waud, and Dr. G. H. Hoffman.)

Petrous portion—axial (Mayer) view (Figs. 11-26 and 11-27)

Film size—8″ × 10″
Cassette
Lengthwise
Bucky
Extension cone

Technique

Factors	Screen film cassette (par) Bucky	Screen film cassette (par) tabletop
mA	100	100
Time	0.6	0.3
mAs	60	30
Thickness in cm	22	22
kVp	78	60
Distance	30	30

Patient preparation

Remove all metallic and plastic articles from the head and neck region.

Palpation points

Mastoid processes.

Procedure

Tape the auricle of each ear forward. With a wax pencil make a mark behind each ear on the posterior border of the external auditory meatus. Place the patient in the supine position with the median plane of the body over the center line of the table. Rotate the face 45 degrees toward the side being examined. The infraorbitomeatal line is perpendicular to the tabletop. Place the lower pencil mark over the center line of the table.

Central ray

Direct the central ray 45 degrees caudad through the lower pencil mark to the center of the film holder.

Immobilization

Place a wedge sponge under the face and hold the sponge in place with sandbags. Employ suspended expiration.

Right-left markers

Burn the correct marker in the upper center border of the film holder above the cone field after the exposure is made.

Technical tips

For stocky patients with short necks, use an angle board on the tabletop to minimize distortion.

Structures demonstrated

Axial views of the internal and external auditory canals, the labyrinthal area, the mastoid cells, and the carotid canal.

Note: Make bilateral views for comparison.

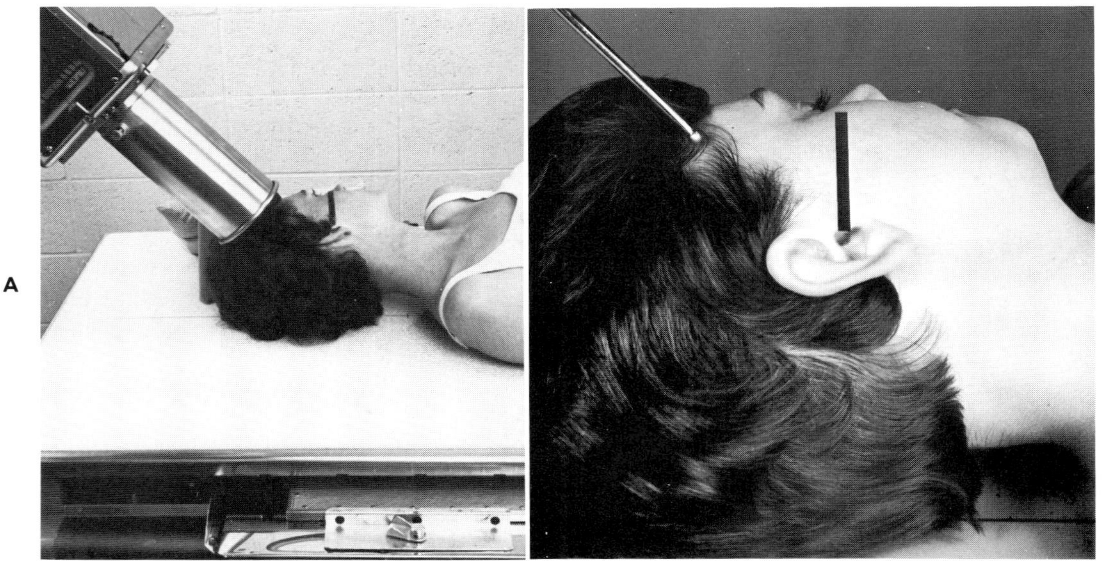

Fig. 11-26. Pars petrosa. **A** and **B,** Axial (Mayer) positions.

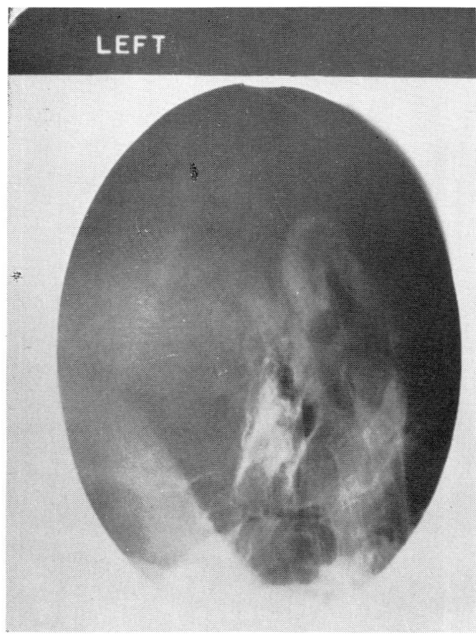

Fig. 11-27. Pars petrosa–axial (Mayer) view. (Courtesy Dr. E. I. L. Cilley, Dr. T. W. Crowell, Dr. R. E. Waud, and Dr. G. H. Hoffman.)

Temporomandibular joints—lateral (T.M.J.) view (mouth open and mouth closed) (Figs. 11-28 and 11-29)

Film size—8″ × 10″
Cassette
Lengthwise
Bucky
Extension cone

Technique

Factors	Screen film cassette (par) Bucky	Screen film cassette (par) tabletop
mA	100	100
Time	0.5	.15
mAs	50	15
Thickness in cm	18	18
kVp	68	66
Distance	30	30

Patient preparation

Remove all metallic and plastic articles from the head and neck region.

Palpation points

Lateral mandibular condyles.

Procedure

Closed—With a wax pencil make a mark ¾ inch anterior to the external auditory meatus on the acanthiomeatal line on each side of the head. Place the patient in the prone position. Place the side of the head being examined on the table. Elevate the opposite side of the body and flex this knee and elbow for support. Place the lower pencil mark over the center line of the table. The midsagittal plane is parallel with the tabletop. The acanthiomeatal line is perpendicular to the long axis of the table. The jaw must be closed.

Open—Open the mouth and insert a sterile cork. Recheck the acanthiomeatal line for position.

Central ray

Direct the central ray 15 degrees caudad through the lower pencil mark to the center of the film holder.

Immobilization

Place a fist or sponge under the chin. Employ suspended expiration.

Right-left markers

Burn the correct marker in the upper center border of the film holder above the cone field.

Technical tips

To improve centering accuracy, precenter the central ray to a point on the table and down to the film center. Position the selected mark on the patient over the point on the table.

Structures demonstrated

Lateral views of the condyle in relationship to the mandibular fossa.

Note: Make bilateral views for comparison.

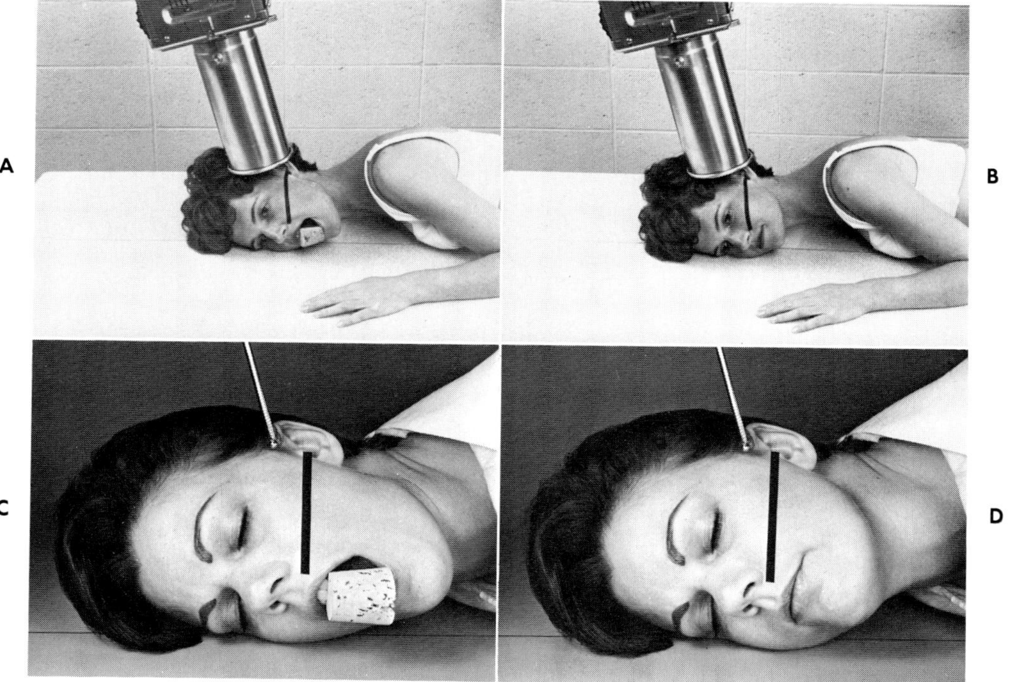

Fig. 11-28. Temporomandibular joint positions. **A** and **C**, Lateral (T.M.J.) positions, mouth open. **B** and **D**, Lateral (T.M.J.) positions, mouth closed.

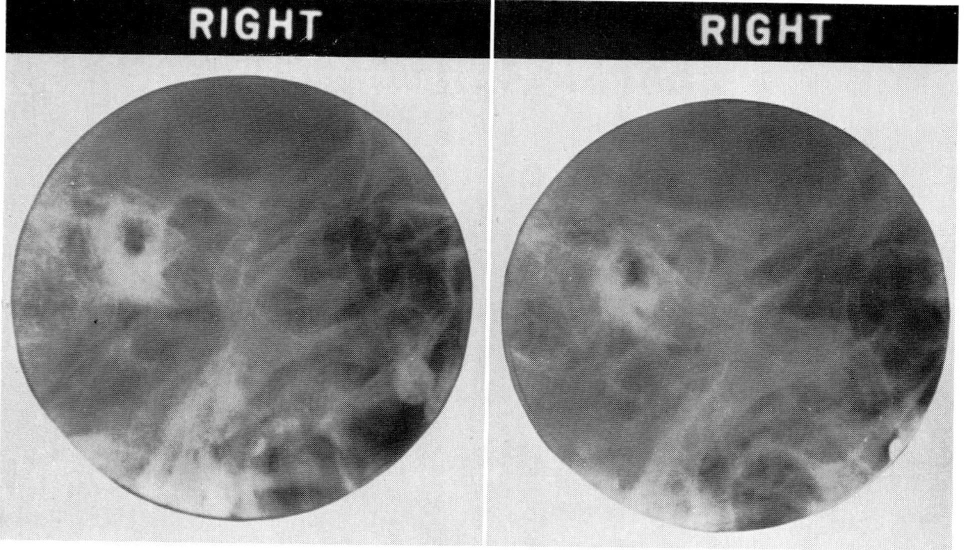

Fig. 11-29. Temporomandibular joint views. Lateral (T.M.J.) views, mouth open and mouth closed. (Courtesy Dr. E. I. L. Cilley, Dr. T. W. Crowell, Dr. R. E. Waud, and Dr. G. H. Hoffman.)

Facial bones—zygomatic arch, tangential view (Figs. 11-30 and 11-31)

Film size—8″ × 10″
Cassette
Lengthwise
Tabletop
Extension cone

Technique

Factors	Screen film cassette (par)
mA	100
Time	0.2
mAs	20
Thickness in cm	20
kVp	54
Distance	30

Patient preparation

Remove all metallic and plastic articles from the head and neck region.

Palpation points

Lateral wall of the cranial vault; zygomatic arch; angle and body of the mandible.

Procedure

Place the patient in the prone position with the chest supported by a folded pillow. Extend the chin as far as possible and place it on the cassette face. The center of the zygomatic arch being examined is over the center line of the cassette. Shift the mandible to the opposite side; instruct the patient to bite down to hold the mandible in place. Tilt the head toward the opposite side so that a tangent from the side of the skull to the side of the mandible is perpendicular to the face of the cassette.

Central ray

Direct the central ray perpendicular to the infraorbitomeatal line, through the zygomatic arch, and to the center of the film holder.

Immobilization

Place the patient's thumbs on the anterior corners of the cassette to hold it in place. Extend the cone to contact the head. Employ suspended expiration.

Right-left markers

Burn the correct marker in the upper center border of the film holder above the cone field after the exposure is made.

Technical tips

For better demonstration of the zygomatic bone, angle the central ray 20 degrees toward the anterior (face).

Structures demonstrated

Tangential view of the zygomatic arch.

Note: Make bilateral views for comparison.

For supine patients, make a submentovertex skull view on 10 ″ × 12″ film with tabletop technique. See p. 317.

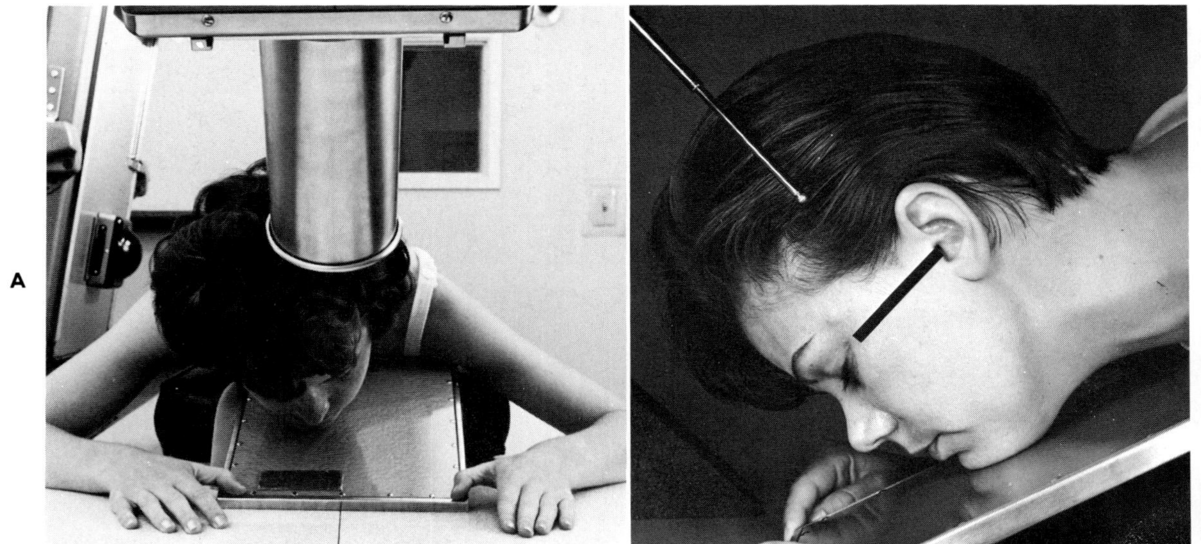

Fig. 11-30. Facial bones. **A** and **B,** Zygomatic arch—tangential positions.

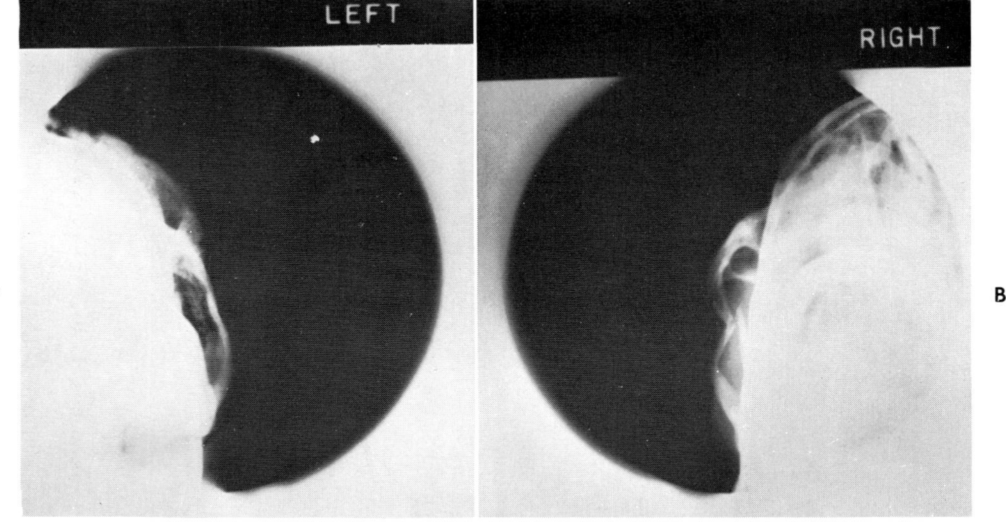

Fig. 11-31. Facial bones: zygomatic arch—tangential view. **A,** Normal. **B,** With fracture. (Courtesy Dr. E. I. L. Cilley, Dr. T. W. Crowell, Dr. R. E. Waud, and Dr. G. H. Hoffman.)

Facial bones—orbital ridges, anterior (P-A) view (Figs. 11-32 and 11-33)

Film size—8″ × 10″
Cassette
Lengthwise
Bucky
Collimate to cover

Technique

Factors	Screen film cassette (par)
mA	100
Time	0.5
mAs	50
Thickness in cm	20
kVp	76
Distance	30

Patient preparation

Remove all metallic and plastic articles from the head and neck region.

Palpation point

Acanthion.

Procedure

Place the patient in a prone position with the median plane of the head and body over the center line of the table. Extend the chin both upward and forward to rest on the center line of the table. The canthomeatal line forms a 37-degree angle with the tabletop, and the midsagittal plane of the head is perpendicular to it.

Central ray

Direct the central ray perpendicular through the anterior nasal spine to the center of the film holder. Collimate to film holder.

Immobilization

Place sponges on each side of the head. Instruct the patient to hold them in place with his hands, or use sandbags. Employ suspended expiration.

Right-left markers

Place the *R* marker on the right lateral center border of the film holder.

Technical tips

For a variation of this view, angle the central ray 10 degrees caudad.

Structures demonstrated

Anterior (P-A) view of the orbits, nasal bones, nasal septum, zygomas, and maxillary antra.

Note: This view may be used as a survey radiograph for a foreign body in the eye.

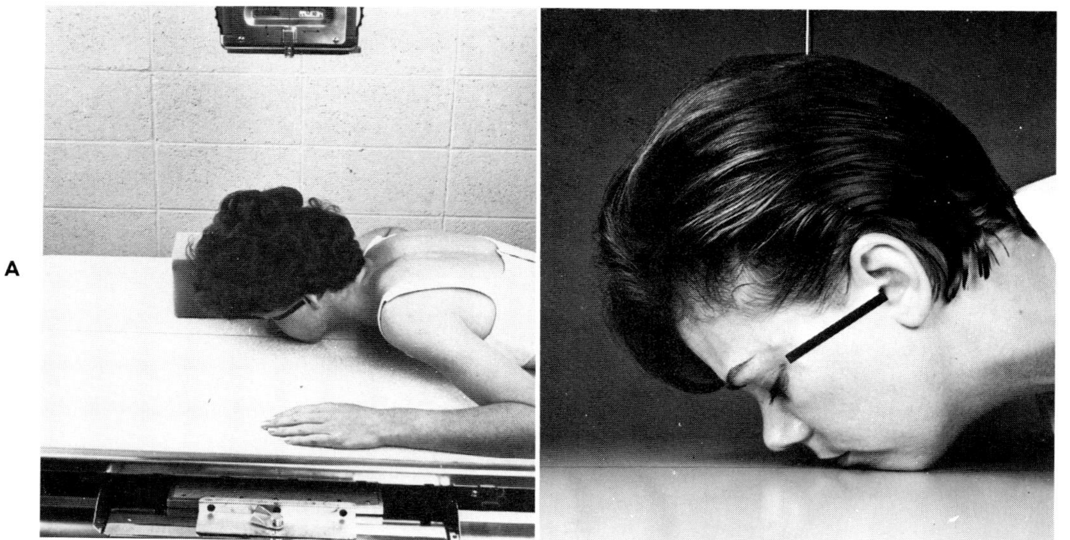

Fig. 11-32. Facial bones. A and B, Orbital ridges—anterior (P-A) positions.

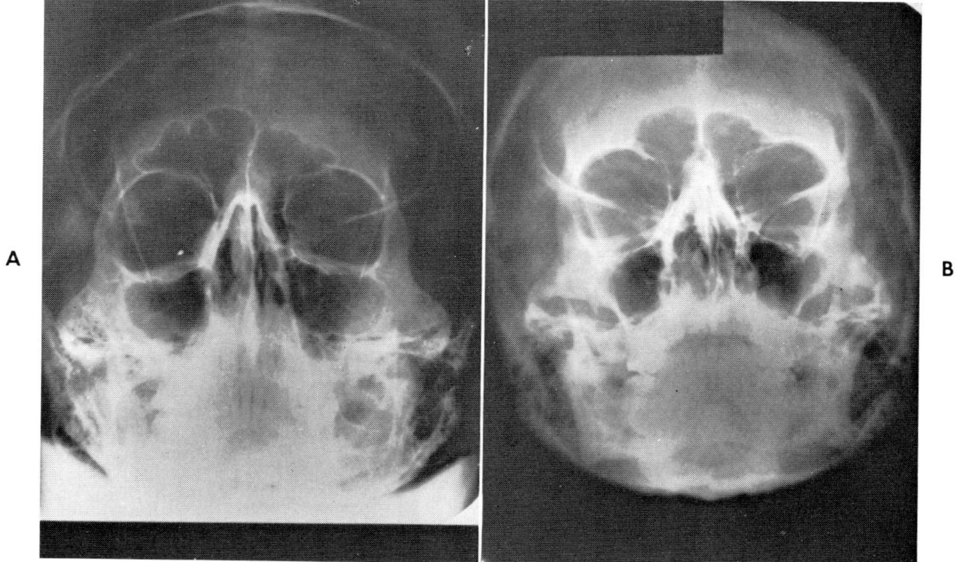

Fig. 11-33. Facial bones: orbital ridges—anterior (P-A) view. A, With 90-degree (perpendicular) angle. B, With 10-degree caudad angle. (Courtesy Dr. E. I. L. Cilley, Dr. T. W. Crowell, Dr. R. E. Waud, and Dr. G. H. Hoffman.)

Facial bones—lateral view (Figs. 11-34 and 11-35)

Film size—8″ × 10″
Cassette
Lengthwise
Bucky
Collimate to cover

Technique

Factors	Screen film cassette (par)
mA	100
Time	0.2
mAs	20
Thickness in cm	15
kVp	62
Distance	30

Patient preparation

Remove all metallic and plastic articles from the head and neck region.

Palpation point

Lateral ridge of the eye orbit.

Procedure

Place the patient in the prone position with the side of the head being examined on the table. Elevate the opposite side of the body and flex this knee and elbow for support. The midsagittal plane of the head is parallel with the tabletop. The canthomeatal line is perpendicular to the long axis of the table. Center a point ½ inch posterior to the outer canthus over the center line of the table.

Central ray

Direct the central ray perpendicular through the selected point to the center of the film holder. Collimate to film holder.

Immobilization

Instruct the patient to brace the tip of the chin with his fist, or use a sponge. Place large sponges on the top of and behind the skull, and hold them in place with sandbags. Employ suspended expiration.

Right-left markers

Place the correct marker on the anterior center border of the film holder.

Technical tips

For better visualization of soft tissue structures, use a no-screen film holder on the tabletop.

Structures demonstrated

Lateral view of the bones of the face with the right and left sides superimposed.

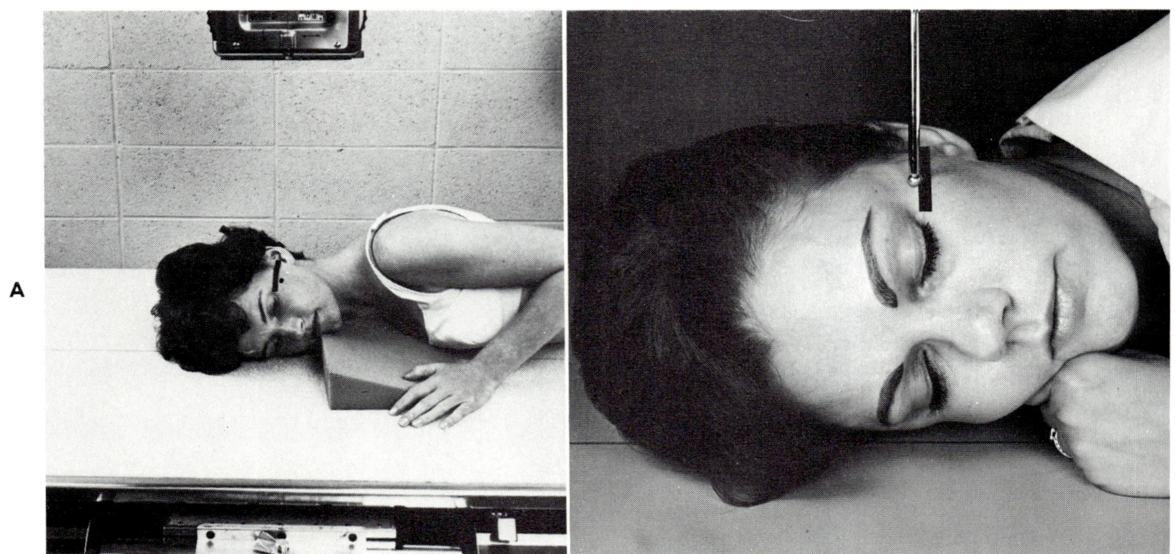

Fig. 11-34. Facial bones. **A** and **B,** Lateral positions.

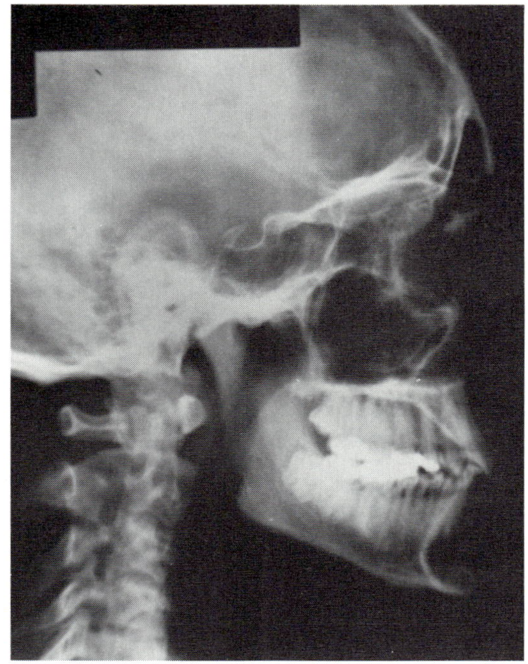

Fig. 11-35. Facial bones—lateral view. (Courtesy Dr. E. I. L. Cilley, Dr. T. W. Crowell, Dr. R. E. Waud, and Dr. G. H. Hoffman.)

Facial bones—nasal bones, axial view (Figs. 11-36 to 11-38)

Film size—occlusal
Dental type
Lengthwise
Intraoral
Extension cone

Technique

Factors	No-screen film occlusal (fast)
mA	100
Time	0.2
mAs	20
Thickness in cm	—
kVp	64
Distance	30

Patient preparation

Remove all metallic and plastic articles from the face region.

Palpation points

Glabella; nasion; acanthion.

Procedure

Seat the patient at the end of the table. Place both elbows on the table with the forearms in the vertical plane and the fists together. Place the lower part of the chin on the fists, and insert half of the length of the occlusal film between the teeth.

Central ray

Direct the central ray perpendicular along the glabelloalveolar line to the film holder.

Immobilization

Place the extension cone in contact with the forehead. Employ suspended expiration.

Right-left markers

Place a *small letter r* in the right anterior corner of the film holder.

Technical tips

For a film substitute, use a regular dental film, or the corner of a no-screen film holder and the finger technique.

Structures demonstrated

Axial view of the nasal bones that extend beyond the glabelloalveolar line.

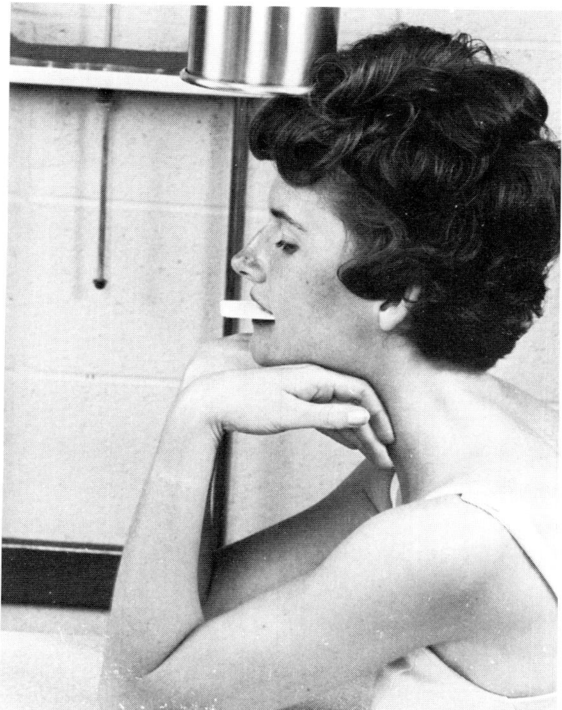

Fig. 11-36. Facial bones: nasal bones—axial position.

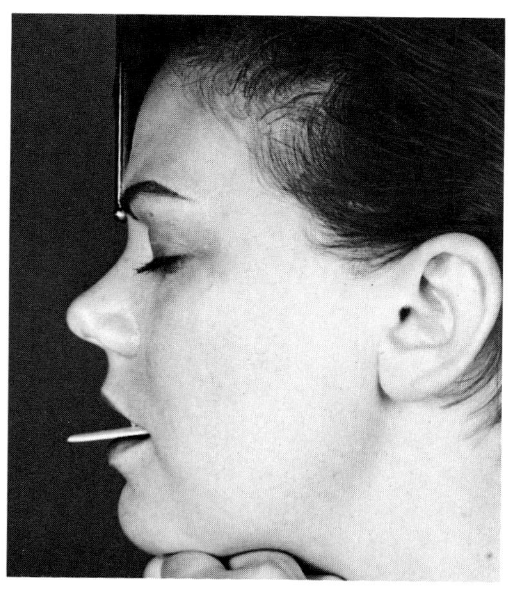

Fig. 11-37. Facial bones: nasal bones—axial position.

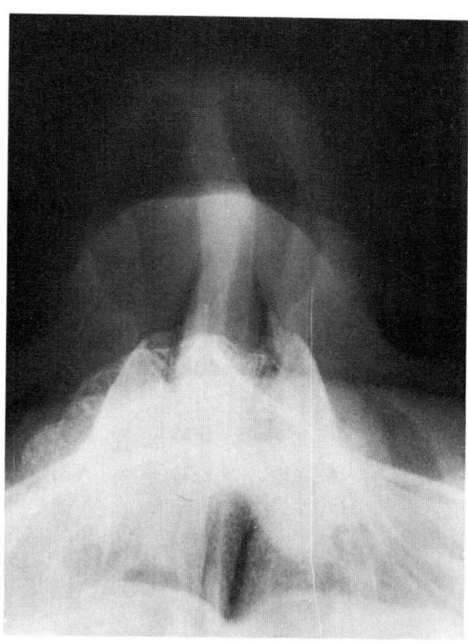

Fig. 11-38. Facial bones: nasal bones—axial view. (Courtesy Dr. E. I. L. Cilley, Dr. T. W. Crowell, Dr. R. E. Waud, and Dr. G. H. Hoffman.)

Facial bones—nasal bones, lateral view (Figs. 11-39 and 11-40)

Film size—8″ × 10″ *Tabletop*
Cardboard *Extension cone*
Lengthwise

Technique

Factors	Screen film cardboard	No-screen film occlusal (fast)
mA	100	100
Time	0.7	0.2
mAs	70	20
Thickness in cm	3	3
kVp	56	60
Distance	30	30

Patient preparation

Remove all metallic and plastic articles from the face region.

Palpation point

Nasion.

Procedure

Place the patient in the prone position with the side of the face being examined on the table. Elevate the opposite side of the body and flex this knee and elbow for support. The midsagittal plane of the head is parallel with the tabletop. The canthomeatal line is perpendicular to the long axis of the table. Center the nasion over the center of the no-screen film holder.

Central ray

Direct the central ray perpendicular through the nasion to the center of the film holder.

Immobilization

Brace the tip of the chin with the patient's fist, or use a sponge. Employ suspended expiration.

Right-left markers

Burn the correct marker in the upper center border of the film holder above the cone field after the exposure is made.

Technical tips

For a film substitute, use a dental or occlusal film, inserting the corner of the film gently into the inner canthus of the eye.

Structures demonstrated

Lateral view of the nasal bones and of the soft tissue structures of the nose.

Note: Some routines call for bilateral views on one radiograph.

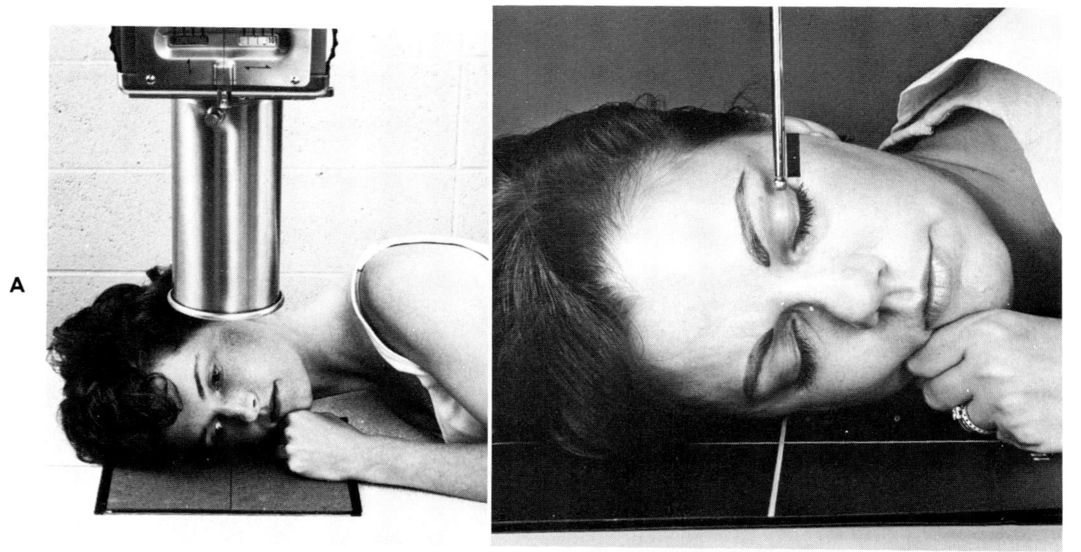

Fig. 11-39. Facial bones. **A** and **B**, Nasal bones—lateral positions.

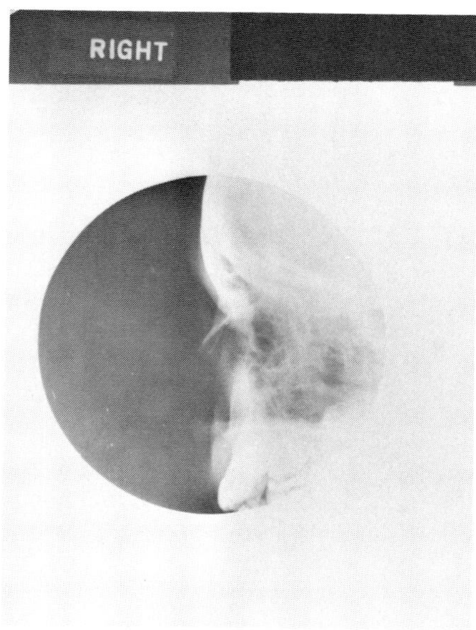

Fig. 11-40. Facial bones: nasal bones—lateral view. (Courtesy Dr. E. I. L. Cilley, Dr. T. W. Crowell, Dr. R. E. Waud, and Dr. G. H. Hoffman.)

Facial bones—optic foramen, anterior (P-A) view (Figs. 11-41 and 11-42)

Film size—8″ × 10″
Cassette
Lengthwise
Bucky
Extension cone

Technique

Factors	Screen film cassette (par) Bucky	Screen film cassette (par) tabletop
mA	100	100
Time	0.4	0.2
mAs	40	20
Thickness in cm	18	18
kVp	70	64
Distance	30	30

Patient preparation

Remove all metallic and plastic articles from the head region.

Palpation point

Lateral ridge of the eye orbit.

Procedure

Place the patient in the prone position with the median plane of the head and body over the center line of the table. Place the hands at the sides of the head. Rotate the face 40 degrees away from the side being examined, resting the selected eye orbit on the table. The acanthiomeatal line is perpendicular to the long axis of the table. Center a point ¼ inch medial to the outer canthus of the eye being examined over the center line of the table.

Central ray

Direct the central ray perpendicular through the selected point to the center of the film holder.

Immobilization

Place a wedge sponge under the lower side of the head, and instruct the patient to hold this in place with his hand, or use sandbags. Place the extension cone in contact with the head. Employ suspended expiration.

Right-left markers

Burn the correct marker in the upper center border of the film holder above the cone field after the exposure is made.

Technical tips

To project the optic foramen lower in the orbit, increase the cervical extension; to project the optic foramen lateral in the orbit, increase the head rotation.

Structures demonstrated

Anterior (P-A) view of the optic foramen projected in the lower lateral area of the orbit.

Note: Make bilateral views for comparison.

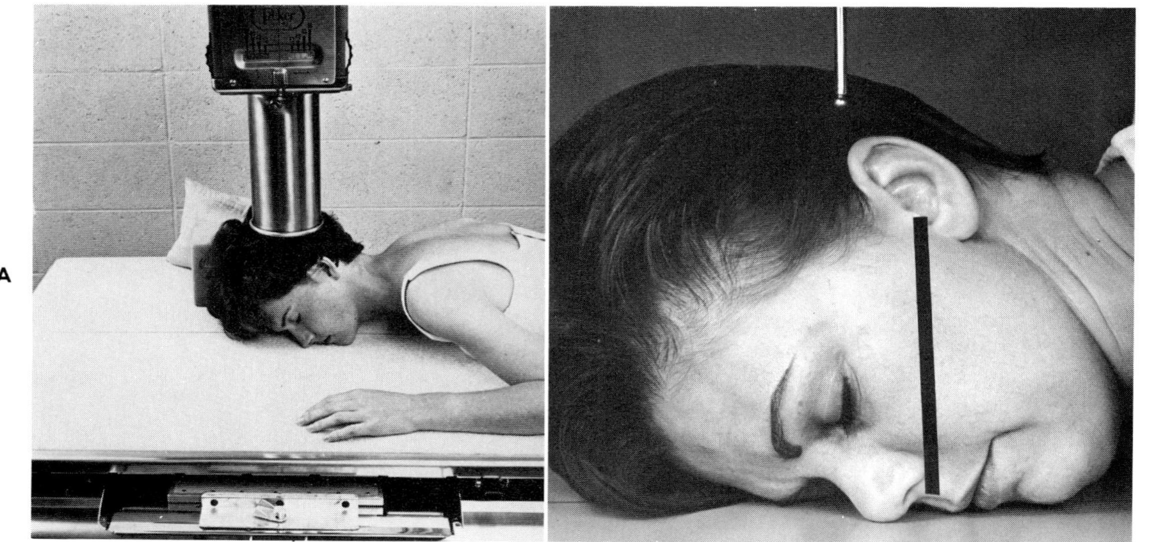

Fig. 11-41. Facial bones. **A** and **B,** Optic foramen—anterior (P-A) positions.

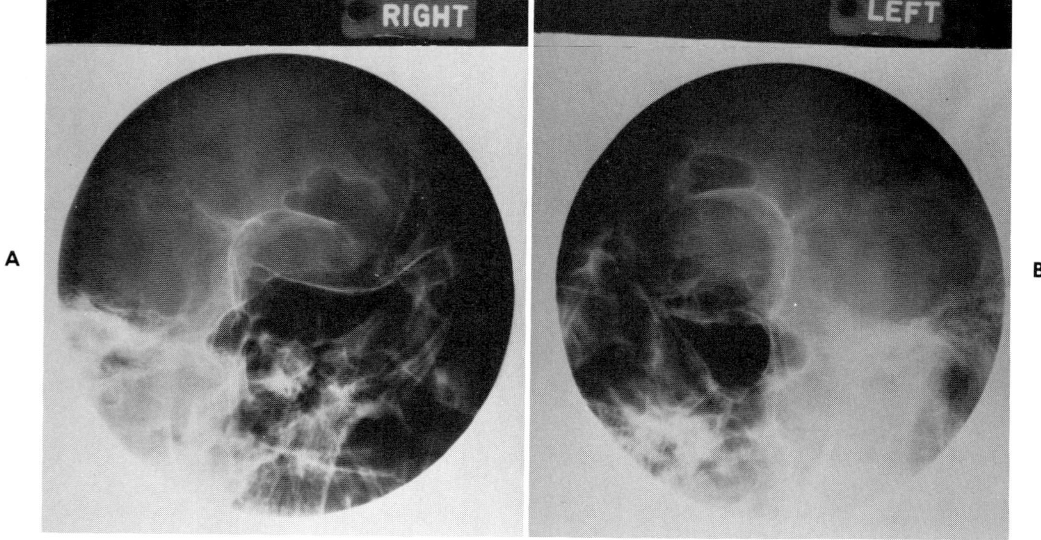

Fig. 11-42. Facial bones: optic foramen—anterior (P-A) view. **A,** Right optic foramen. **B,** Left optic foramen. (Courtesy Dr. E. I. L. Cilley, Dr. T. W. Crowell, Dr. R. E. Waud, and Dr. G. H. Hoffman.)

Facial bones—maxilla, oblique view (Figs. 11-43 to 11-45)

Film size—occlusal
Dental type
Lengthwise

Intraoral
Extension cone

Technique

Factors	No-screen film occlusal (fast)
mA	100
Time	0.2
mAs	20
Thickness in cm	—
kVp	70
Distance	30

Patient preparation

Remove all metallic and plastic articles from the face region.

Palpation point

Maxillary bone.

Procedure

Seat the patient at the end of the table. Place both elbows on the table with the forearms in a vertical plane and the fists together. Place the lower part of the chin on fists, and insert the occlusal film between the teeth of the side being examined.

Central ray

Direct the central ray 45 degrees from vertical toward the face and 45 degrees from anterior toward the median plane through the maxilla being examined to the film holder.

Immobilization

Employ suspended expiration.

Right-left markers

Place the correct marker in the anterior lateral corner of the film holder.

Technical tips

To better demonstrate the posterior portion of the maxilla, direct the central ray 60 degrees from the anterior toward the median plane.

Structures demonstrated

Oblique views of the alveolar process and hard palate, and of the bicuspids and molars of the side of the maxilla being examined.

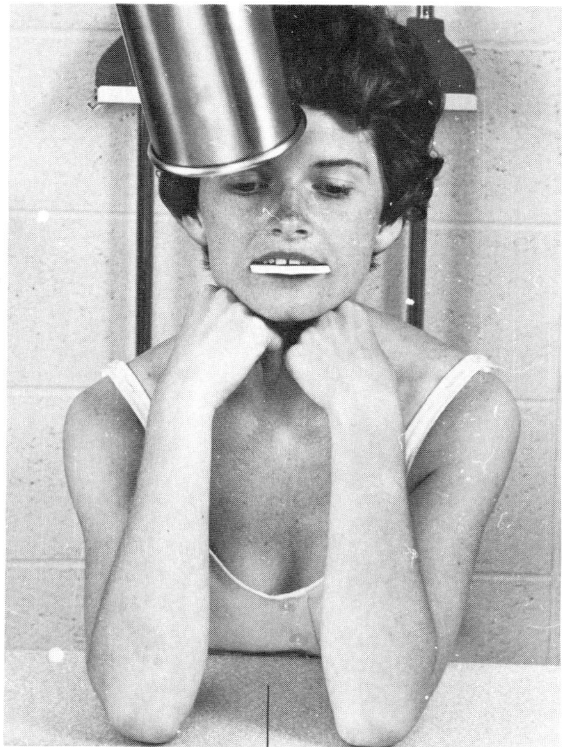

Fig. 11-43. Facial bones: maxilla–oblique position.

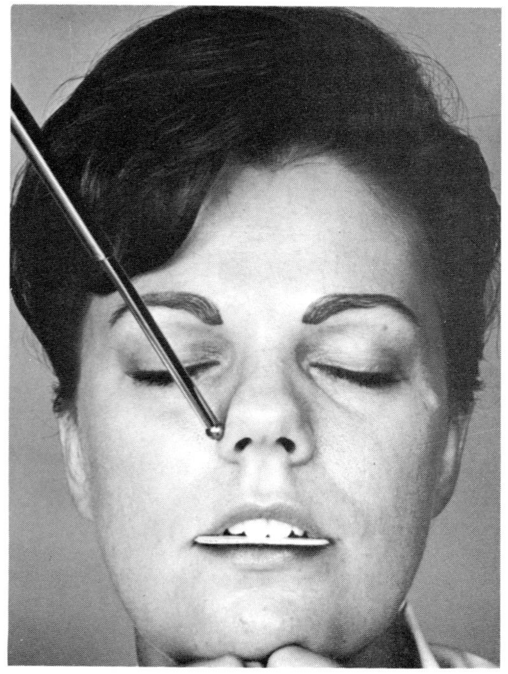

Fig. 11-44. Facial bones: maxilla–oblique position.

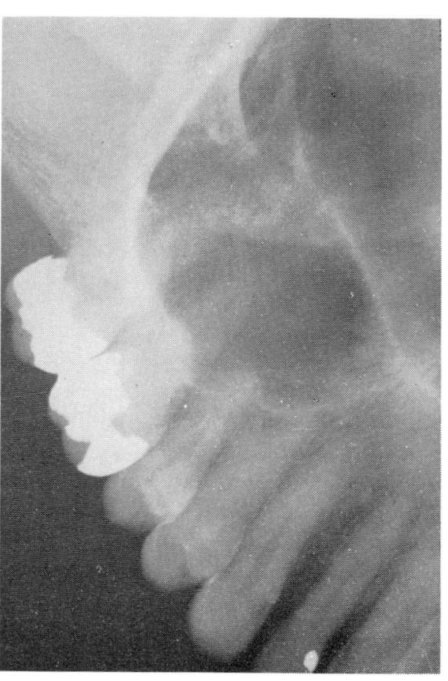

Fig. 11-45. Facial bones: maxilla–oblique view. (Courtesy Dr. E. I. L. Cilley, Dr. T. W. Crowell, Dr. R. E. Waud, and Dr. G. H. Hoffman.)

Facial bones—maxillae, inferior (superoinferior) view (Figs. 11-46 to 11-48)

Film size—occlusal
Dental type
Lengthwise
Intraoral
Extension cone

Technique

Factors	No-screen film occlusal (fast)
mA	100
Time	0.2
mAs	20
Thickness in cm	—
kVp	70
Distance	30

Patient preparation

Remove all plastic and metallic articles from the face region.

Palpation point

Maxillary bone.

Procedure

Seat the patient at the end of the table. Place both elbows on the table with the forearms in a vertical plane and the fists together. Place the lower part of the chin on the fists, and insert the occlusal film as far as possible between the teeth.

Central ray

Direct the central ray 45 degrees from vertical toward the face through the anterior nasal spine to the film holder.

Immobilization

Employ suspended expiration.

Right-left markers

Place a *small letter r* in the right anterior corner of the film holder.

Technical tips

For a film substitute, use a regular dental film or the corner of a no-screen film holder.

Structures demonstrated

Inferior (superoinferior) view of the upper incisors, the alveolar processes, and the hard palate.

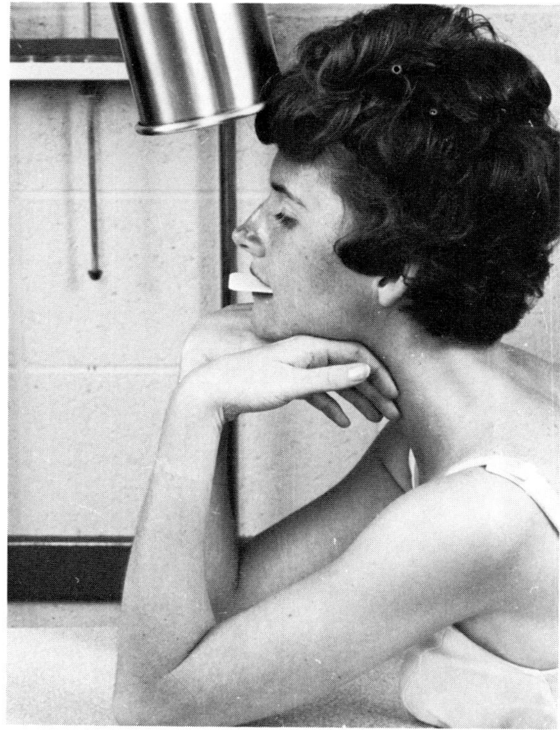

Fig. 11-46. Facial bones: maxillae—inferior (superoinferior) position.

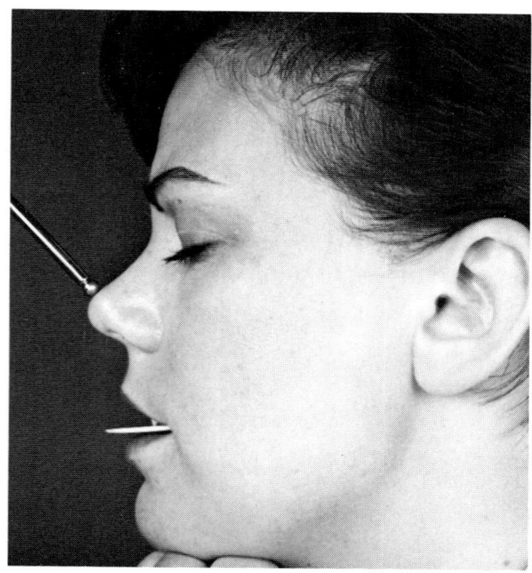

Fig. 11-47. Facial bones: maxillae—inferior (superoinferior) position.

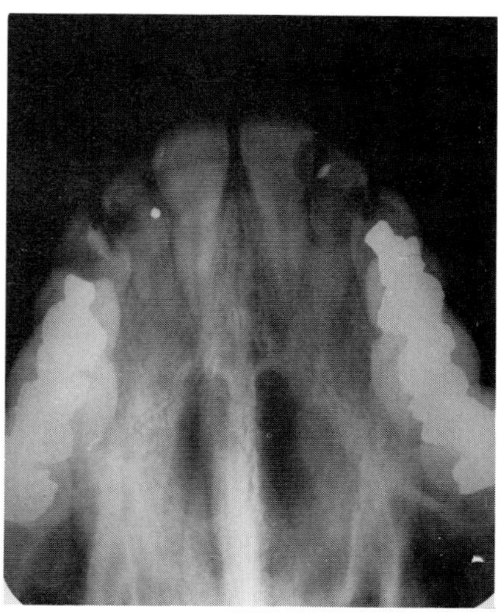

Fig. 11-48. Facial bones: maxillae—inferior (superoinferior) view. (Courtesy Dr. E. I. L. Cilley, Dr. T. W. Crowell, Dr. R. E. Waud, and Dr. G. H. Hoffman.)

Facial bones—mandible (rami), anterior (P-A) view (Figs. 11-49 and 11-50)

Film size—8″ × 10″
Cassette
Lengthwise

Bucky
Collimate to cover

Technique

Factors	Screen film cassette (par) Bucky	Screen film cassette (par) tabletop
mA	100	100
Time	0.5	0.4
mAs	50	40
Thickness in cm	16	16
kVp	66	56
Distance	40	40

Patient preparation

Remove all metallic and plastic articles from the head and neck region.

Palpation points

Mandibular rami and angles; spinous processes of the cervical vertebrae.

Procedure

Place the patient in the prone position with the median plane of the head and body over the center line of the table. Place the hands at the sides of the head. Place the forehead and nose on the center line of the table. The canthomeatal line is perpendicular to the tabletop, and the midsagittal plane is perpendicular to the tabletop.

Central ray

Direct the central ray perpendicularly in line with the angles of the mandible, to the center of the film holder. Collimate to film holder.

Immobilization

Place large sponges on each side of the head, and instruct the patient to hold them in place with his hands, or use sandbags. Employ suspended expiration.

Right-left markers

Place the *R* marker on the right lower later side of the film holder.

Technical tips

For thin patients, elevate the thorax with a pillow or sponges.

Structures demonstrated

Anterior (P-A) view of the mandibular body and rami. The mental area is demonstrated superimposed on the cervical vertebrae.

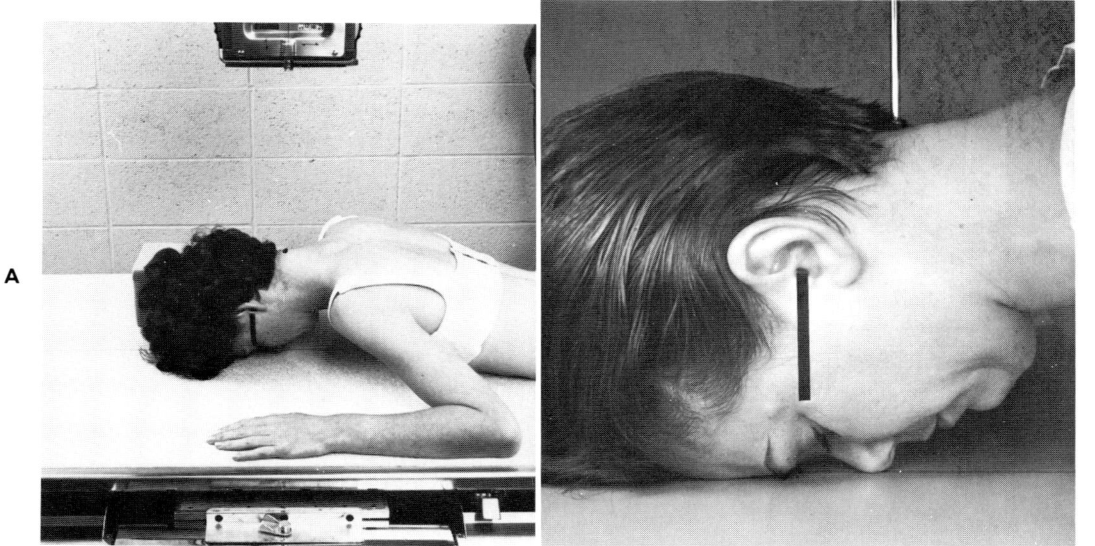

Fig. 11-49. Facial bones. A and B, Mandible (rami)—anterior (P-A) positions.

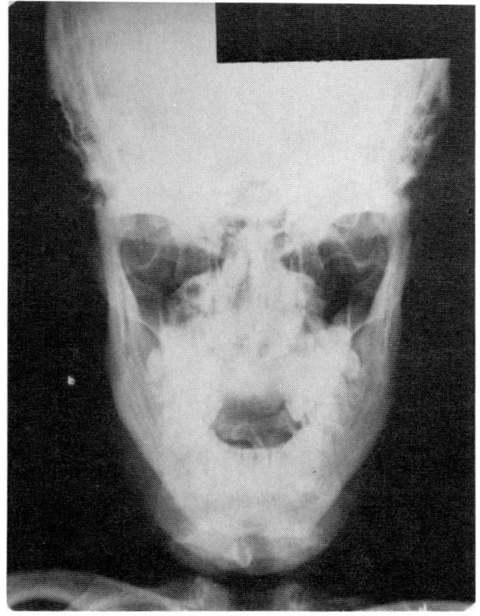

Fig. 11-50. Facial bones: mandible (rami)—anterior (P-A) view. (Courtesy Dr. E. I. L. Cilley, Dr. T. W. Crowell, Dr. R. E. Waud, and Dr. G. H. Hoffman.)

Facial bones—mandible (condyles), anterior (P-A) view (Figs. 11-51 and 11-52)

Film size—8″ × 10″
Cassette
Lengthwise
Bucky
Collimate to cover

Technique

Factors	Screen film cassette (par) Bucky	Screen film cassette (par) tabletop
mA	100	100
Time	0.5	0.4
mAs	50	40
Thickness in cm	16	16
kVp	66	56
Distance	40	40

Patient preparation

Remove all metallic and plastic articles from the head and neck region.

Palpation points

Mandibular rami and angles; spinous processes of the cervical vertebrae.

Procedure

Place the patient in the prone position with the median plane of the head and body over the center line of the table. Place the hands at the sides of the head. Place the forehead and nose on the center line of the table. The canthomeatal line is perpendicular to the tabletop, and the midsagittal plane is perpendicular to the tabletop. Open the patient's mouth as far as possible and insert a sterile cork between the teeth.

Central ray

Direct the central ray 12 degrees cephalad through the nasion to the center of the film holder. Collimate to film holder.

Immobilization

Place large sponges on each side of the head and instruct the patient to hold them in place with his hands, or use sandbags. Employ suspended expiration.

Right-left markers

Place the *R* marker on the right lower lateral side of the film holder.

Technical tips

If the base of the occiput is superimposed over the condyles, increase cervical flexion 5 degrees.

Structures demonstrated

Anterior (P-A) view of the mandibular body, rami, and condyles.

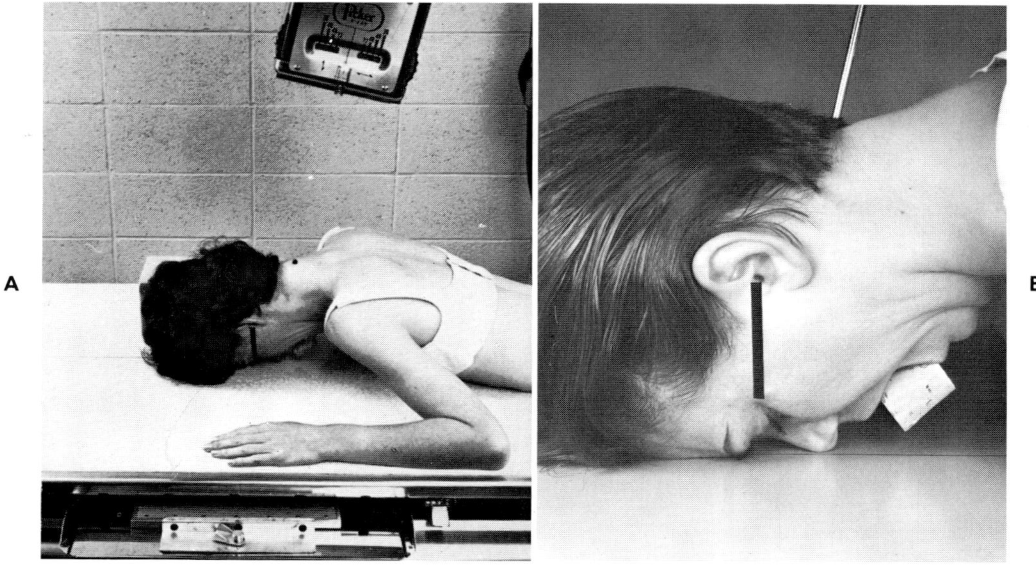

Fig. 11-51. Facial bones. **A** and **B,** Mandible (condyles)—anterior (P-A) positions.

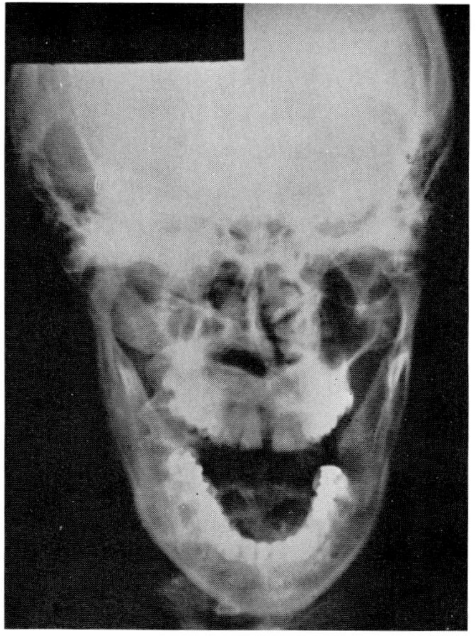

Fig. 11-52. Facial bones: mandible (condyles)—anterior (P-A) view. (Courtesy Dr. E. I. L. Cilley, Dr. T. W. Crowell, Dr. R. E. Waud, and Dr. G. H. Hoffman.)

Facial bones—mandible, lateral view (Figs. 11-53 to 11-55)

Film size—8″ × 10″
Cassette
Lengthwise

Erect film holder
Collimate to cover

Technique

Factors	Screen film cassette (par)
mA	100
Time	0.3
mAs	30
Thickness in cm	8
kVp	64
Distance	72

Patient preparation

Remove all metallic and plastic articles from the head and neck region.

Palpation points

Mandibular rami, angles, and bodies.

Procedure

Place the patient in the erect position, either sitting or standing, with the side of the face being examined against the center of the erect film holder. Place a sandbag in each hand of the patient and instruct him to extend each arm down the side of the body. Extend the chin upward and inward so that the long axis of the mandibular body being examined is parallel with both the erect film holder and the floor. Tilt the head 25 degrees, and rest the parietal region against the erect film holder.

Central ray

Direct a horizontal central ray perpendicular through the center of the mandibular body to the center of the film holder. Collimate to film holder.

Immobilization

A compression band may be used across the patient's head. Employ suspended expiration.

Right-left markers

Place the correct marker on the anterior center border of the film holder.

Technical tips

To eliminate superimposition of mandibular bodies, increase the tilt of the head.

Structures demonstrated

Mediolateral (lateral) view of the mandibular body. The symphysis and ramus may be demonstrated with a variation in head rotation.

Note: Make bilateral views for comparison.

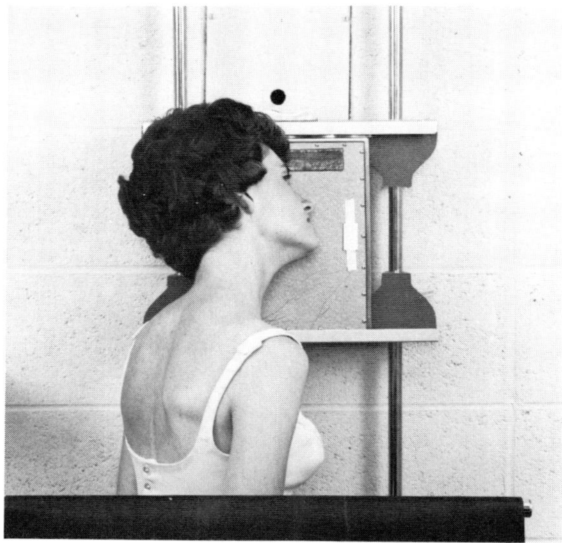

Fig. 11-53. Facial bones: mandible–lateral position.

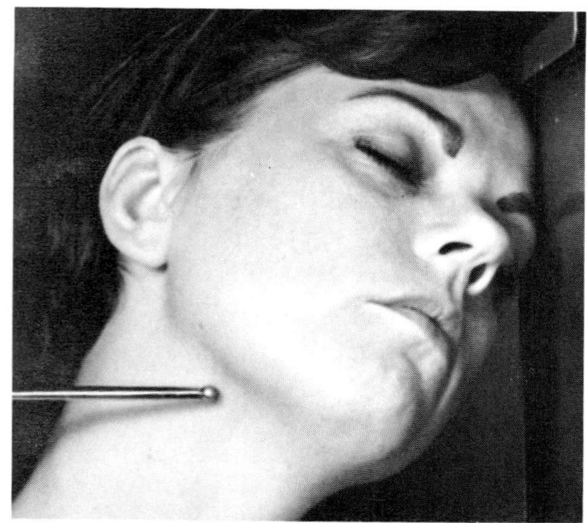

Fig. 11-54. Facial bones: mandible–lateral position.

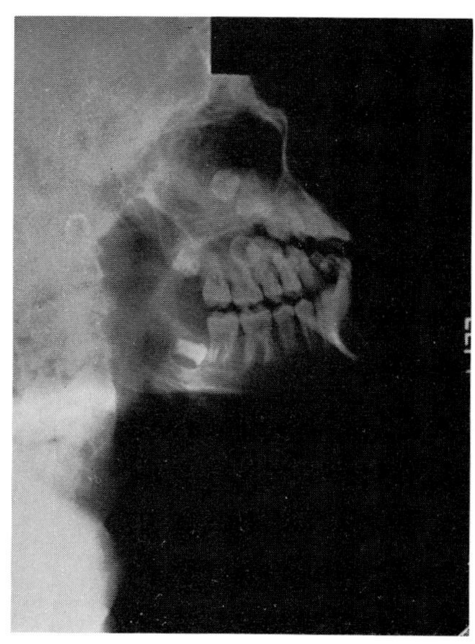

Fig. 11-55. Facial bones: mandible–lateral view. (Courtesy Dr. E. I. L. Cilley, Dr. T. W. Crowell, Dr. R. E. Waud, and Dr. G. H. Hoffman.)

Facial bones—mandible (symphysis), submentovertical view (Figs. 11-56 to 11-58)

Film size—occlusal
Dental type
Lengthwise
Intraoral
Extension cone

Technique

Factors	No-screen film occlusal (fast)
mA	100
Time	0.2
mAs	20
Thickness in cm	5
kVp	66
Distance	30

Patient preparation

Remove all metallic and plastic articles from the face and neck region.

Palpation point

Mandibular symphysis.

Procedure

Place the patient in a supine position on a large cushion or folded pillows, with the vertex of the head against the table. Insert half the length of the occlusal film between the teeth.

Central ray

Direct the central ray perpendicular through the mandibular symphysis to the film holder.

Immobilization

Place a sandbag against the forehead. Employ suspended expiration.

Right-left markers

Place a *small letter r* on the right anterior corner of the film holder.

Technical tips

For a film substitute, use a regular dental film, or the corner of a no-screen film holder and the finger technique.

Structures demonstrated

Submentovertical view of the mandibular symphysis.

Note: For a variation of this view, place an occlusal film beneath the chin and direct the central ray superoinferior, 45 degrees from perpendicular, through the symphysis to the center of the film holder.

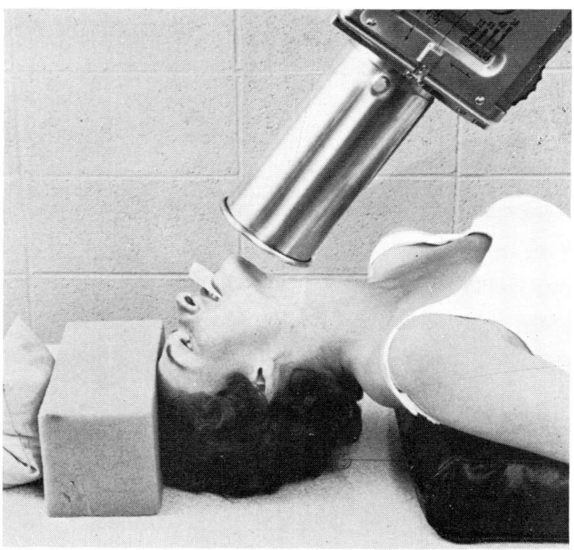

Fig. 11-56. Facial bones: mandible (symphysis)—submentovertical position.

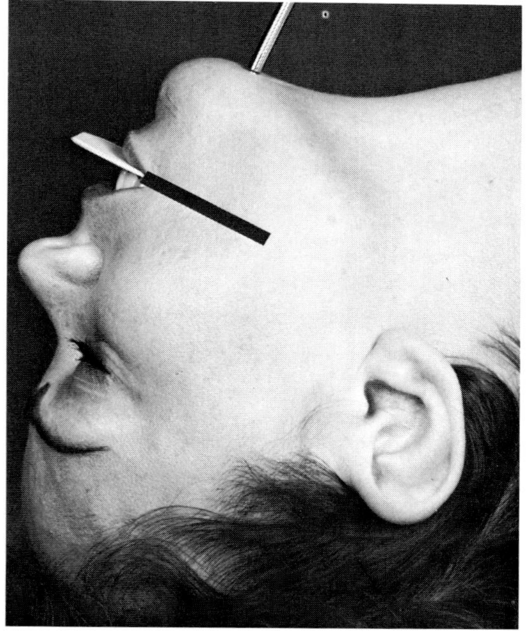

Fig. 11-57. Facial bones: mandible (symphysis)—submentovertical position.

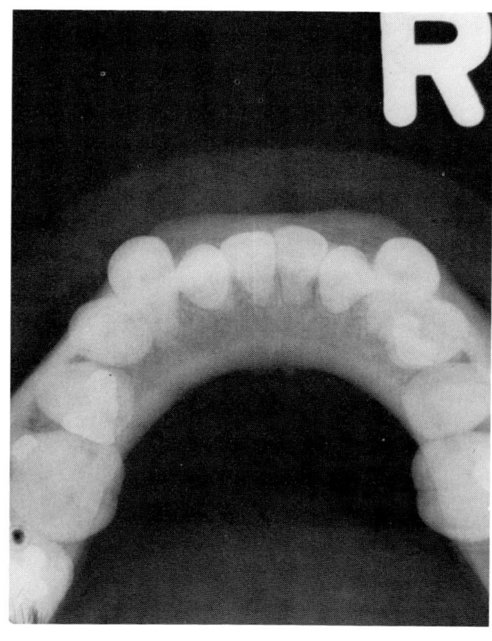

Fig. 11-58. Facial bones: mandible (symphysis)—submentovertical view. (Courtesy Dr. E. I. L. Cilley, Dr. T. W. Crowell, Dr. R. E. Waud, and Dr. G. H. Hoffman.)

QUESTIONS

1. Describe the radiographic procedure for a posteroanterior view of the skull.
2. What method is used to locate the centering point for a lateral skull?
3. Name four major structures demonstrated in the occipital (Towne) view of the skull.
4. Describe the radiographic procedure for the basilar (submental vertex) view of the skull.
5. In the verticosubmental view of the skull, what major guideline is used to determine central ray angulation?
6. What four radiographic views are considered routine in the sinus series?
7. In the maxillary Water's sinus view, why is it necessary for the canthomeatal line to form a 37-degree angle with the film holder?
8. What is the degree of central ray angulation in the true Caldwell projection of the sinuses?
9. Describe the radiographic procedure for demonstrating fluid level in the maxillary sinuses.
10. Describe the reason for the 23-degree caudad central ray angulation in the open-mouth sphenoid view.
11. What is the degree of central ray angulation in the lateral Law's mastoid view?
12. What major guideline is used in the lateral Law's mastoid view?
13. Name the major palpation points used in Arcelin's view of the pars petrosa.
14. Name four major structures demonstrated in Arcelin's anteroposterior oblique view of the pars petrosa.
15. When positioning accuracy is achieved in Stenver's view of the pars petrosa, what important structure will be clearly defined?
16. State the degree of central ray angulation in Mayer's view of pars petrosa.
17. Describe the radiographic procedure for the open- and closed-mouth temporal mandibular joints.
18. Describe two different methods for demonstrating the zygomatic arches.
19. What radiographic view may be used as an adequate survey radiograph for a foreign body in the eye?
20. Describe three different radiographic views for demonstrating fractures of the nasal bones.
21. Give one synonym for the anterior nasal spine.
22. State the degree of head rotation used in the optic foramen radiographic procedure.
23. In a radiographic view of an optic foramen, describe the head manipulations that are necessary to correctly relocate an optic foramen that is found in the center of the eye orbit.
24. Describe the radiographic procedure for a superoinferior view of the maxilla.
25. What major guideline is used to position the posteroanterior view of the mandibular rami?
26. In the posteroanterior projection of the mandible, state the degree and angle of the central ray.
27. In the posteroanterior projection of the mandible, what method is employed to demonstrate the condyle?
28. State the average degree of head tilt used in the lateral view of the mandible.
29. In a lateral view of the mandible, describe the head manipulation that is necessary to better demonstrate the mandibular symphysis.
30. Describe the radiographic procedure for demonstrating a submentovertical view of the mandibular symphysis.

12 • ANATOMIC PHYSIOLOGY

DIGESTIVE SYSTEM

The major parts of the digestive system form a canal that is open at both ends. The tract passes through the thoracic and abdominal cavities. Beginning with the mouth and terminating with the anus, this canal, commonly known as the *gastrointestinal tract,* is 840 to 1,020 cm* (28 to 34 feet) in length. The chief organs of digestion are the mouth, pharynx, esophagus, stomach, and small and large intestines. (See Fig. 12-1.) The accessory organs, which are contained within, or open into, the gastrointestinal tract, include the teeth, tongue, salivary glands, pancreas, liver, gallbladder, and appendix. The digestive system receives and prepares food for absorption and use by all the body cells. In the mouth the food is masticated and mixed with saliva into a *bolus,* which, through the act of *deglutition,* passes into the stomach. *Peristaltic motion* then conducts the *bolus* through the stomach into the duodenum, jejunum, ileum, and finally the large intestine, from which it is eliminated as waste. After the bolus has undergone gastric digestion, it is called *chyme.* After undergoing intestinal digestion, the *chyle,* a milky fluid taken from the food during digestion, is absorbed by the lacteals, intestinal lymphatics. Chyle consists of lymph and emulsified fat and passes from the lacteals via the thoracic duct to empty into the blood at the formation of the left brachiocephalic vein.

Oral cavity

The oral cavity (mouth) is bounded laterally by the cheeks, anteriorly by the lips, superiorly by the hard and soft palates, inferiorly by the tongue and associated muscles, and posteriorly by the pharynx and uvula. The oral cavity proper (cavitum oris proprium) is inside the teeth, whereas the buccal cavity (cavitum oris externum) is the vestibule of the oral cavity and is outside the teeth. It contains the teeth, which masticate the food; the tongue, which aids in mastication and deglutition; and the salivary glands, which manufacture and excrete saliva through their openings into this cavity. The salivary excretion contains *salivary amylase,* an enzyme that attacks starch and hydrolyzes it into maltose, and *mucin,* a very sticky substance that mixes with the food to form the bolus. There are three pairs of salivary glands: the *parotids,* which are inferior and anterior to the ears and are emptied by the *parotid (Stensen's) ducts,* which drain into the buccal cavity through small orifices in the cheeks (the orifices are near the upper second molars); the *submandibulars* (submaxillaries), which are on the posterior portions of the floor of the mouth near the angles of the mandibles and are emptied by the *submandibular (Wharton's) ducts,* which drain into the anterior part of the buccal cavity inferior to the tongue; and the *sublinguals,* which are in the floor of the mouth inferior to the free end of the tongue and empty into this cavity through several small ducts and direct openings. Special radiographic studies of the salivary glands are discussed in Chapter 13.

*Use 1 foot as being equal to 30 cm.

Teeth

The normal adult mouth contains thirty-two teeth, sixteen in each jaw. These teeth are called the *permanent teeth,* whereas those of the child, which are shed at various ages, are called *deciduous teeth.* The name of each tooth and the number per jaw are given in Table 12-1.

The teeth are contained in the alveolar processes of the mandible and maxillae. The plane of

Table 12-1. Dentition*

Name of tooth	Number per jaw	
	deciduous set	**permanent set**
Central incisors	2	2
Lateral incisors	2	2
Cuspids (canines)	2	2
Premolars (bicuspids)	0	4
Molars (tricuspids)	4	6
Total per jaw	10	16
Total per set	20	32

*From Anthony, C. P., and Kolthoff, N. J.: Textbook of anatomy and physiology, ed. 9, St. Louis, 1975, The C. V. Mosby Co.

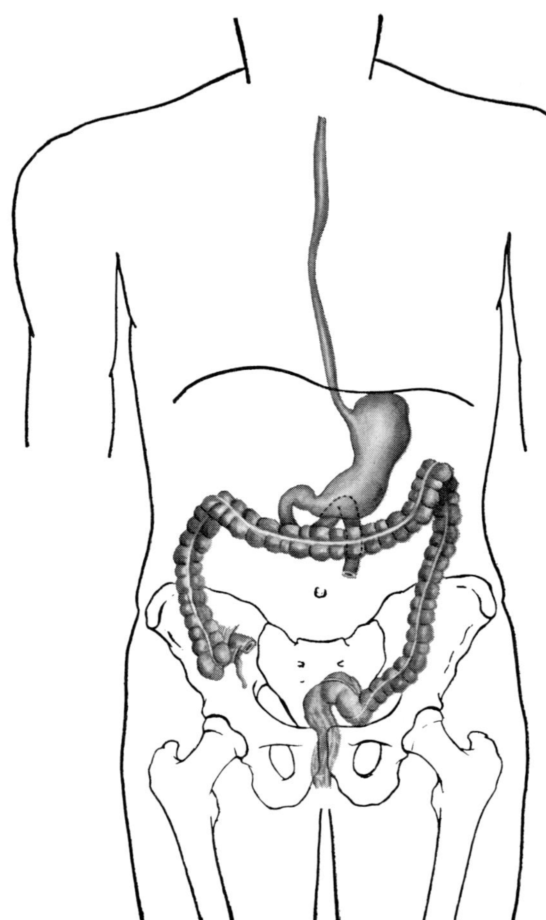

Fig. 12-1. Normal position of some of the digestive organs. (From Francis, Carl C: Introduction to human anatomy, ed. 5, St. Louis, 1968, The C. V. Mosby Co.)

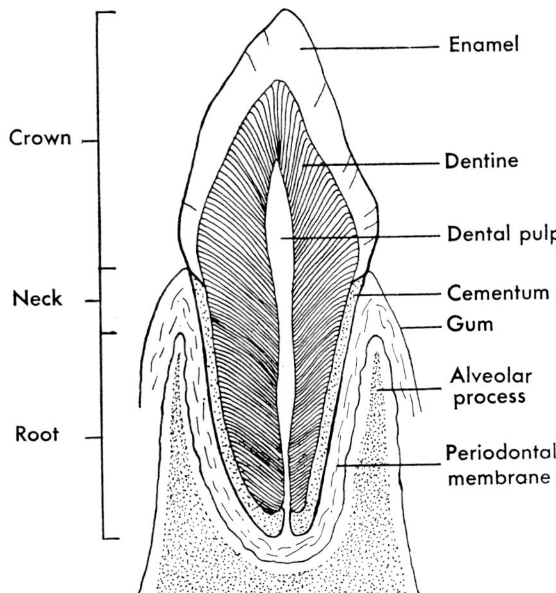

Fig. 12-2. Incisor, longitudinal section. (From Francis, Carl C: Introduction to human anatomy, ed. 5, St. Louis, 1968, The C. V. Mosby Co.)

closing the teeth is called the *occlusal plane.* In dental radiography, emphasis is placed on the periodontal membrane, roots, and neck. There is less radiographic interest in the crown. It is extremely important to prevent elongation or foreshortening of the roots. The construction and placement of a tooth in its alveolar socket is shown in Fig. 12-2.

Pharynx

The pharynx (throat) is a muscular structure common to both the digestive and respiratory systems and aids in the act of deglutition. It is about 12.5 cm long and lies between the cranial floor and the esophagus anterior to the cervical spine. Each auditory tube opens into the sides of the nasopharynx; the choanae open into the anterior part of the nasopharynx; the oral cavity opens into the anterior part of the *oropharynx;* and the pharynx opens posteroinferiorly into the larynx *(laryngopharynx)* and anteroinferiorly into the esophagus. The opening from the mouth is called the *fauces.* (See Fig. 12-3.) The pharynx is demonstrated radiographically by use of the lateral projection for the esophagus.

Esophagus

The esophagus is a muscular tube located chiefly in the thoracic cavity and partially in the abdominal cavity. It serves as the connection between the pharynx and the stomach and is approximately 22.5 to 27.5 cm in length. It passes through the *diaphragm* in the *esophageal hiatus* and is located posterior to the trachea and heart. True peristalsis does not begin in the esophagus, although a peristaltic-like action begins below the upper third of the esophagus and conveys the bolus into the stomach. Lateral and oblique positions (sometimes erect) are used to demonstrate the esophagus radiographically.

Stomach

The stomach is inferior to the diaphragm on the left side of the median line in the abdominal

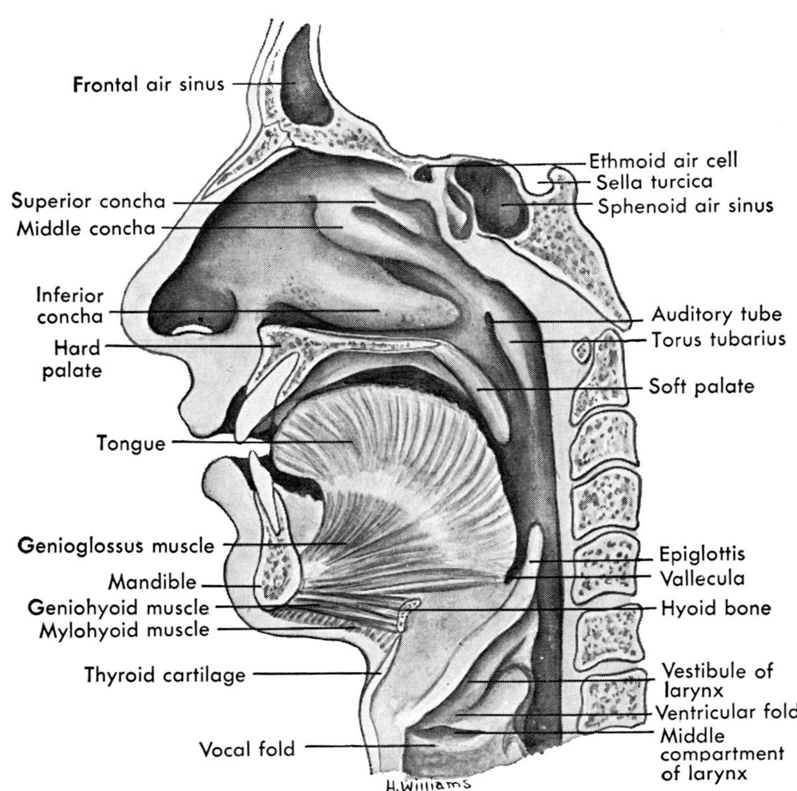

Fig. 12-3. Face and neck, sagittal section. (From Francis, Carl C: Introduction to human anatomy, ed. 5, St. Louis, 1968, The C. V. Mosby Co.)

cavity. Its capacity varies from 500 to 1,000 ml. It is located chiefly in the epigastrium, but small parts are in the left hypochondrium and umbilical regions. The superior opening, called the *cardiac orifice,* is the junction of the esophagus with the stomach and is near the level of the eleventh thoracic vertebra. The inferior opening (outlet), the *pylorus,* opens into the first part of the duodenum. The stomach has three divisions: the *cardiac third (fundus),* which is that part superior to a horizontal plane passing through the cardiac orifice; the *pyloric third,* which is the distal portion; and the *body,* which is the portion between the cardiac and pyloric thirds. The shorter margin of the stomach between the cardiac and pyloric orifies is called the *lesser curvature,* whereas the opposite, longer margin is called the *greater curvature.* Throughout the stomach are heavy folds of mucosa called *rugae,* the majority of which extend the length of the stomach. The circular muscle in the cardiac orifice is called the cardiac sphincter. A similar muscle in the pylorus is called the pyloric sphincter. Numerous glands located throughout the entire gastric mucosa excrete the gastric juices. The principal excretions of the stomach are *hydrochloric acid,* which acidifies the gastric juice and aids in proteolytic hydrolysis; pepsinogen, a precursor to *pepsin,* which hydrolyzes proteins to proteoses and peptones; *lipase,* which hydrolyzes some of the emulsified fats to fatty acids and glycerol; and *rennin* in infants, which acts upon caseinogen to form paracasein. (See Fig. 12-4.)

Small intestine

Duodenum. The duodenum is the first part of the small intestine and is approximately 22.5 cm long. The major percentage of true digestion, or absorption, occurs in the *villi* of its walls. It is divided into four parts: *bulb (cap), descending, transverse,* and *ascending.* The bulb is attached to the pylorus, and the ascending portion attaches to the jejunum. The duodenum is located primarily in the epigastrium to the right of the stomach and is the only part of the small intestine not completely attached to the mesentery. Approximately 7.5 cm inferior to the pylorus and on the posteromedial surface is the *hepatopancreatic ampulla,* through which the bile and pancreatic juice enter the duodenum. The principal intestinal juices are *peptidase,* which hydrolyzes peptones and peptides to amino acids; *lactase,* which hydrolyzes lactose to glucose and galactose; *maltase,* which hydrolyzes maltose to glucose; and *sucrase,* which hydrolyzes sucrose to glucose and fructose. The head of the pancreas is enveloped by the loop of the duodenum. The duodenum joins the jejunum in the *duodenojejunal flexure* approximately on the level of the second lumber vertebra and slightly left of the aorta. Radiographic examination of the esophagus, stomach, and duodenum comprises an upper gastroin-

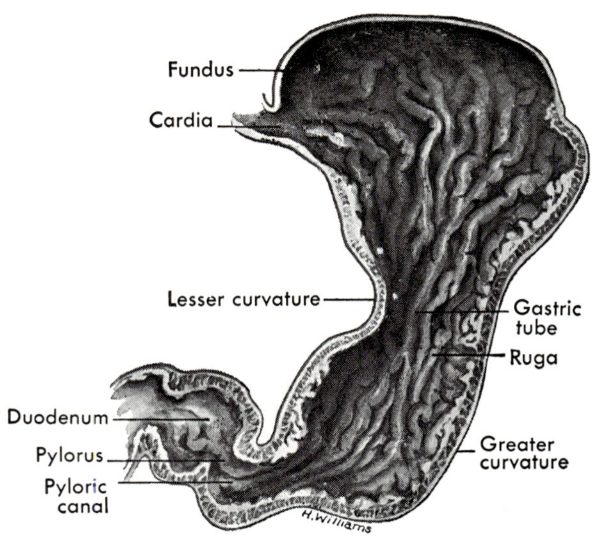

Fig. 12-4. Stomach, frontal section. (From Francis, Carl C: Introduction to human anatomy, ed. 5, St. Louis, 1968, The C. V. Mosby Co.)

testinal tract study, often called an E.S.D. or U.G.I.

Jejunum. The jejunum is about 270 cm long and lies in the umbilical, left lumbar, and left iliac regions. It joins distally with the ileum. The villi become progressively smaller at this junction. Some digestion occurs in the ileum and jejunum. (See Fig. 12-5.)

Ileum. The ileum is the distal part of the small intestine. It is approximately 390 cm long and begins with the jejunum and terminates in its junction with the cecum. It is located primarily in the pelvic cavity. The junction with the cecum contains the *ileocecal valve,* which prevents regurgitation of the feces into the ileum. When this valve is *patent,* it has lost its function, and feces may enter the ileum. *Meckel's diverticulum* extends from the ileum in a very small percentage of persons. It is located about 90 cm above the ileocecal valve. The jejunum and ileum are examined radiographically following the procedures for E.S.D. studies.

Bile ducts and gallbladder

This system of ducts and glands plays an important part in radiography. The gallbladder is located beneath the right lobe of the liver. It has three divisions: the *fundus,* which is inferior, the *body,* and the *neck,* both of which extend above the fundus. The gallbladder is drained by the *cystic duct,* which is very short. It stores and concentrates the bile and is stimulated to contract and excrete the bile by a hormone *(cholecystokinin)* secreted in the intestinal mucosa. The *hepatic duct* from the liver originates from two branches, one each from the right and left lobes. The short hepatic duct joins the cystic duct to form the *common bile duct.* The latter is about as long as the combined lengths of the cystic and hepatic ducts. The common bile duct joins with the *pancreatic duct (duct of Wirsung)* to form the *hepatopancreatic ampulla* (of Vater), which is extremely short. The *choledochal sphincter (of Oddi)* is in the terminus of the common bile duct. The hepatopancreatic ampulla opens into the duodenum through the *major duodenal papilla.* The *accessory pancreatic duct (duct of Santorini)* opens into the duodenum slightly above the ampulla through the *lesser duodenal papilla.* (See Fig. 12-6.) The bile ducts and gallbladder are demonstrated radiographically by cholangiography and cholecystography.

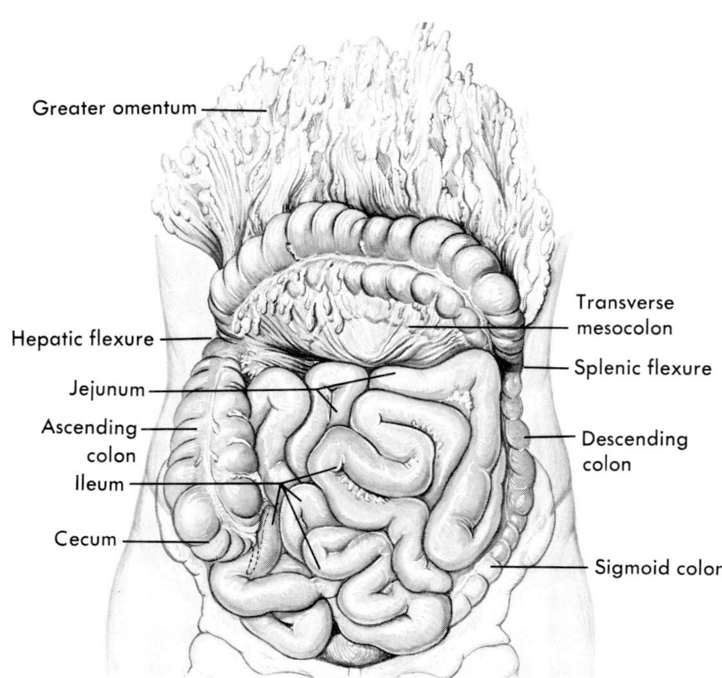

Fig. 12-5. Abdominal viscera. (From Anthony, C. P., and Kolthoff, N. J.: Textbook of anatomy and physiology, ed. 9, St. Louis, 1975, The C. V. Mosby Co.)

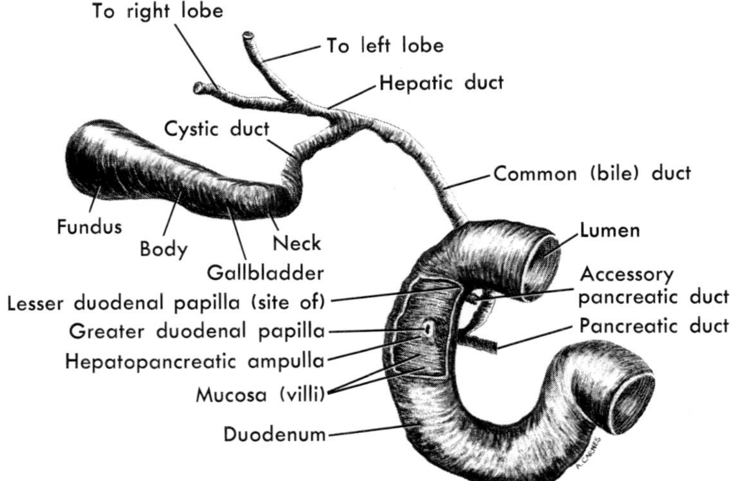

Fig. 12-6. Biliary tract and associated structures.

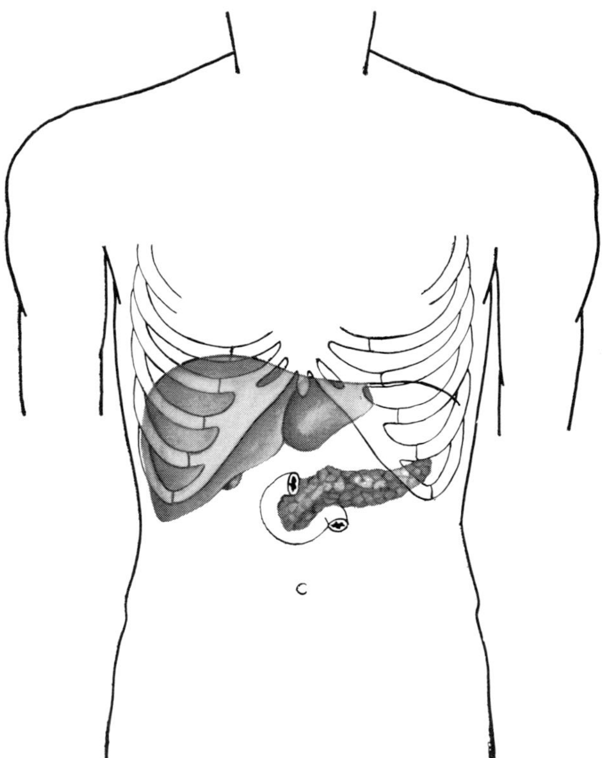

Fig. 12-7. Normal position of liver and pancreas. (From Francis, Carl C: Introduction to human anatomy, ed. 5, St. Louis, 1968, The C. V. Mosby Co.)

Pancreas

The pancreas excretes juices into the duodenum via the pancreatic duct (of Wirsung). Included with these juices are the enzymes *trypsin, amylase,* and *lipase.* In addition, the pancreas contains several groups of specialized cells, called the *islands of Langerhans,* which secrete a hormone, *insulin.* The pancreas lies posteriorly in the epigastric and left hypochondriac regions in a transverse position. (See Fig. 12-7.) Its head lies within the curve of the duodenum, with the tail extending to the left.

Large intestine

The large intestine, which begins with the cecum and terminates in the anus, is between 150 and 180 cm in length. It consists of the *cecum, colon (ascending, transverse, descending, iliac,* and *sigmoid* portions), *rectum,* and *anal canal.*

The cecum is located in the right iliac region and has about the same capacity as the stomach. The ileum enters the large intestine at the junction of the cecum with the colon. The fundus of the cecum is directed inferiorly. The appendix projects distally from the cecum and is infrequently demonstrated radiographically during the course of examination with barium enemas. (See Fig. 12-8.) The ascending colon extends from the cecum to the right lobe of the liver. At this point the colon bends, forming the *hepatic flexure.* Then it passes across the abdomen (transverse portion), approximately in line with the division between the epigastric and umbilical regions, making another bend in the left hypochondrium (the *splenic flexure*). The splenic flexure is usually higher than the hepatic flexure and is attached to the diaphragm on a level between the tenth and eleventh ribs. From the splenic flexure, the colon extends down through the left hypochondrium and left lumbar regions as the descending colon. Below the left kidney the descending colon extends medially toward the crest of the left ilium. At this point it becomes the iliac colon (frequently included as a part of the descending colon by various authors). The short iliac colon becomes the sigmoid colon as it enters into the lesser pelvis. The sigmoid colon is usually entirely in the pelvis. It is S shaped and terminates in the rectum. The rectum projects down and back to terminate in the anal canal. The anal canal is very short and terminates with the anus. The large intestine is demonstrated radiographically by the use of radiopaque and radiolucent contrast media. The media of choice are barium sulfate and air.

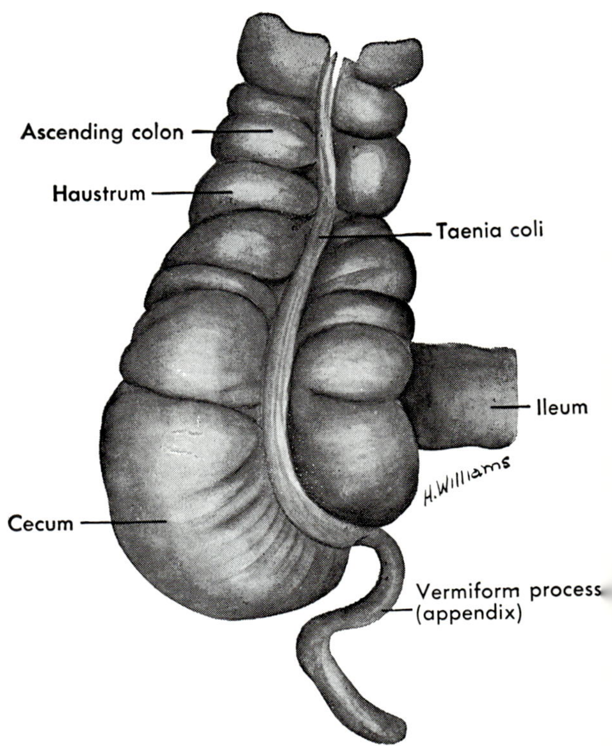

Fig. 12-8. Cecum and appendix. (From Francis, Carl C: Introduction to human anatomy, ed. 5, St. Louis, 1968, The C. V. Mosby Co.)

For descriptive purposes the abdominal cavity may be divided in two ways: *four quadrants* or *nine regions.* Both divisions include all or most of the pelvic cavity. Sagittal and transverse lines at right angles to each other and through the *umbilicus* (navel) outline the four quadrants. The nine regions are as follows: right hypochondrium, epigastrium, left hypochondrium, right lumbar, umbilical, left lumbar, right iliac, hypogastrium, and left iliac. In Table 12-2 are listed the more important parts of the viscera according to the regions shown in Fig. 12-9. There are many other portions of the abdominal viscera that are not mentioned in relation to each of these regions, since they are of little importance to radiologic technologists.

GENITOURINARY SYSTEM

The genital and urinary systems are considered together because both systems share a common outlet in both sexes. Also, the procedure of radiographic examination is similar in both sexes and in both systems.

Table 12-2. Major viscera of the nine regions of the abdomen

Right hypochondrium	Epigastrium	Left hypochondrium
Most of right lobe of liver Hepatic flexure of colon Part of right renal body	Most of left lobe and remainder of right lobe of liver Gallbladder Most of stomach, duodenum, and pancreas Part of spleen Suprarenals Parts of renals	Greater curvature of stomach Remainder of spleen Tail of pancreas Splenic flexure of colon Part of left renal body
Right lumbar	**Umbilical**	**Left lumbar**
Ascending colon Most of right renal body	Most of transverse colon Parts of duodenum, jejunum, and ileum Parts of renal bodies Most of ureters	Descending colon Part of jejunum Most of left renal body
Right iliac	**Hypogastrium**	**Left iliac**
Cecum Appendix Terminal end of ileum Ileocecal valve	Ileum Flexure of sigmoid colon	Sigmoid colon Jejunum Ileum Iliac colon

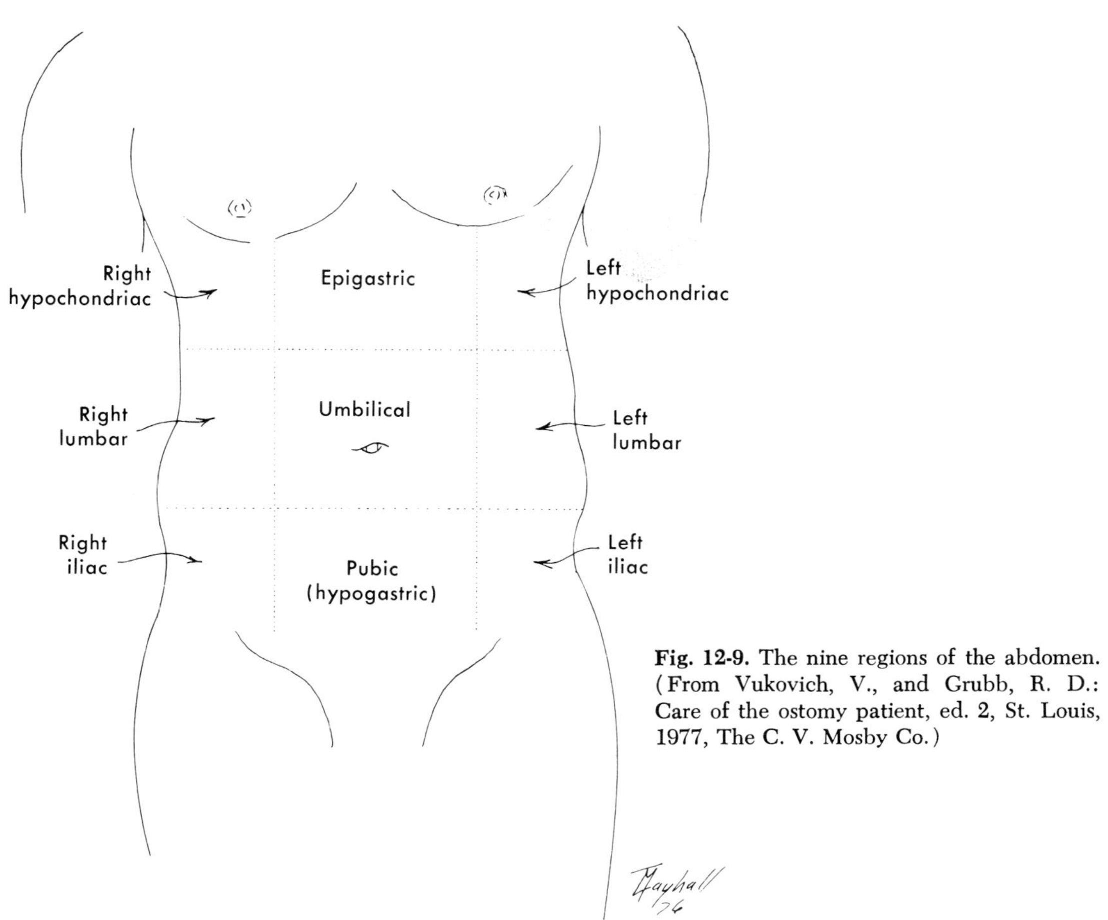

Fig. 12-9. The nine regions of the abdomen. (From Vukovich, V., and Grubb, R. D.: Care of the ostomy patient, ed. 2, St. Louis, 1977, The C. V. Mosby Co.)

Urinary system

The urinary system is a rather complex excretory system and has two distinct functions: filtration of the urine from the blood and elimination of the urine from the body. It is vitally concerned with the maintenance of *homeostasis* and includes two kidneys, two ureters, the urinary bladder, and the urethra. (See Fig. 12-10.)

Kidneys. The paired kidneys are located bilateral to the midsagittal plane behind the parietal peritoneum of the abdomen in the area of the twelfth thoracic to the third lumbar vertebra. The right kidney is slightly lower and smaller than the left. The kidney is a bean-shaped organ approximately 10 cm in total length. Its concave surface faces the midsagittal plane. In the center of this concavity is located the *hilar space,* through which the nerves, blood vessels, and ureters pass. The waste products of the kidneys may either be liquid or be suspended in liquid. The functional unit of the kidneys is called the *nephron.*

Frequently, requests are made for erect radiographs of the kidneys and ureters for the demonstration of any possible ptosis of either of the kidneys or ureters. The kidneys are sometimes demonstrated radiographically without opacification but are always opacified for study. Opacification is obtained by either of two methods: by intravenous injection of a radiopaque medium and utilization of the normal function of blood filtration, called *intravenous pyelography,* or by the injection of a radiopaque substance into the kidneys directly through catheters placed in the kidneys, called *retrograde pyelography.* After opacification the *calyces* and the *renal pelves* are

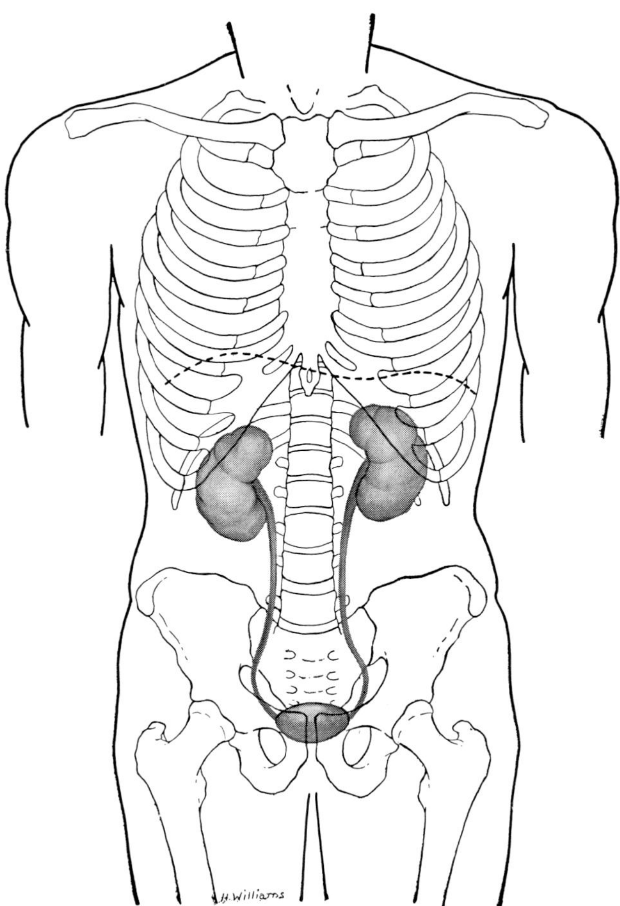

Fig. 12-10. Normal position of urinary organs. (From Francis, Carl C: Introduction to human anatomy, ed. 5, St. Louis, 1968, The C. V. Mosby Co.)

visualized radiographically. The *renal pelvis* narrows inferiorly to form the *ureter,* which drains the kidney. (See Fig. 12-11.)

Ureters. The ureters are about 27.5 cm in length and are quite small in diameter. Their walls are muscular. They are located bilateral to the midsagittal plane, are extraperitoneal, and connect the hilar spaces of the kidneys to the posterior surface of the bladder. (See Fig. 12-12.) The urine is moved through the ureters into the bladder by peristalsis. The ureteral orifices are located laterally and posteriorly in the bladder. These, together with the urethral orifice (anteriorly), form the *trigone.*

Bladder. The urinary bladder receives urine from the ureters. Its capacity has been stated to be from 400 to 600 ml. The total quantity of urine eliminated in a 24-hour period has been stated to be from 1 to 2 liters. The urinary bladder has a *vertex,* which is ventral and slightly superior, and a *fundus,* which is dorsal and slightly inferior. In the male the bladder is superior to the prostate. In the female it is inferior to the uterus and anterior to the vagina. (See Figs. 12-13 and 12-14.) Radiographic examinations of the bladder are called *cystograms,* and the visual examination is called *cystoscopy.* The procedure of radiographic examination may be either intravenous or retrograde.

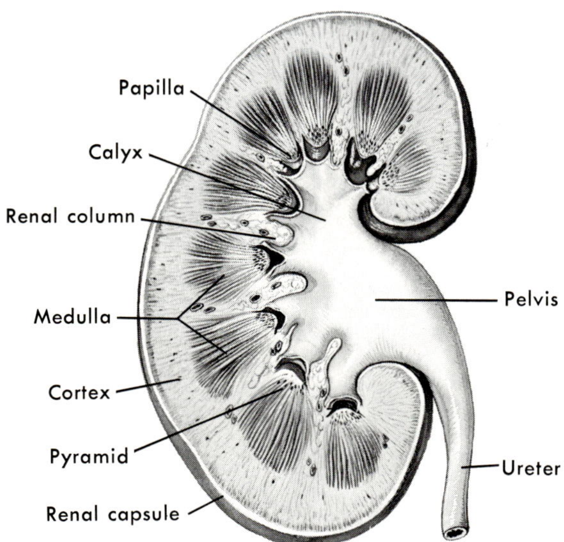

Fig. 12-11. Kidney, coronal section. (From Anthony, C. P., and Kolthoff, N. J.: Textbook of anatomy and physiology, ed. 9, St. Louis, 1975, The C. V. Mosby Co.)

Urethra. In both sexes the bladder is drained by the urethra, which extends between the urinary bladder and the external urethral orifice. In the male the external orifice *(meatus)* is in the distal end of the penis, while in the female, it is between the labia minora and posterior to the glans clitoris. (See Figs. 12-13 and 12-14.) In the male the urethra is approximately 18 cm long, whereas in the female it is approximately 4 cm long. The urethra is the excretory canal of the bladder for the urine. In the male it also serves

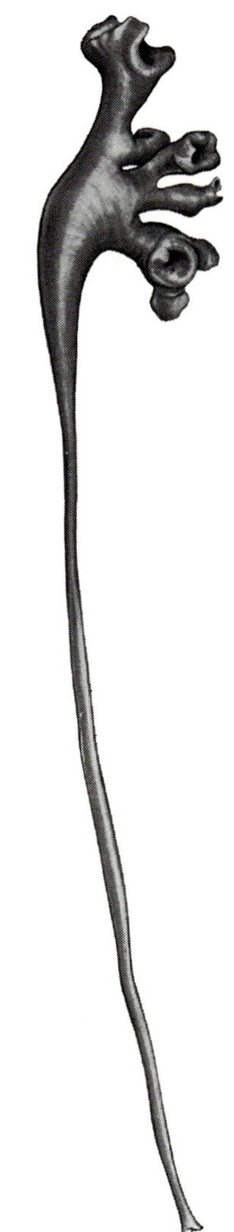

Fig. 12-12. Left ureter, renal pelvis, and calyces, anterior view. (From Francis, Carl C: Introduction to human anatomy, ed. 5, St. Louis, 1968, The C. V. Mosby Co.)

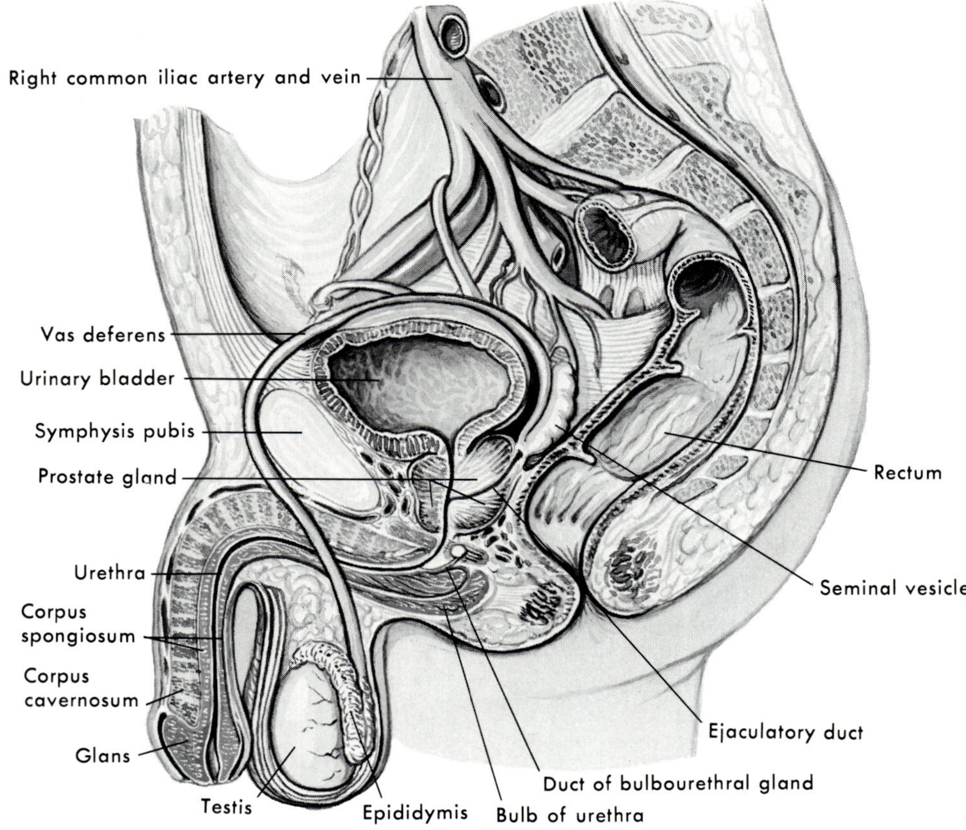

Fig. 12-13. Male pelvis, sagittal section. (From Anthony, C. P., and Kolthoff, N. J.: Textbook of anatomy and physiology, ed. 9, St. Louis, 1975, The C. V. Mosby Co.)

as the excretory duct for the semen. The male urethra passes directly from the urinary bladder through the prostate gland, where it receives the excretions from the ejaculatory ducts, vas deferens, and testes. Radiographic examination, *urethrography,* of the urethra in the female is seldom requested; however, this procedure is not infrequent in the male. Urethrography is also a method of examination of the *prostate* in certain cases.

Reproductive system

Male. The male reproductive system consists of the testes, ductus deferens, seminal vesicles, ejaculatory ducts, and penis and includes the accessory prostate and bulbourethral (Cowper's) glands. (See Fig. 12-13.) There are no radiographic procedures (other than urethrography) that are peculiar to the male reproductive system.

Female. The female reproductive system consists of the ovaries, uterine tubes (salpinges, fallopian tubes), uterus, vagina, clitoris, and vulva, along with the associated accessory glands. (See Fig. 12-14.) From the radiographic viewpoint, interest lies in the technique of *uterosalpingography* (hysterosalpingography), which is radiography of the uterus and salpinges after opacification with an iodized oil or other contrast media. The uterine walls are thick and muscular. The *uterus* separates the rectum and urinary bladder and opens into the vagina through the *cervix.* The fundus is anterior and superior to the body of the uterus. The *salpinges* join the uterus superiorly and bilaterally in the cornu. They are not directly attached to the ovaries but have a funnellike terminus called the *fimbria,* which catches the ova from the ovaries. The salpinges (less than 13 cm long) extend bilaterally from the uterus in the broad ligament.

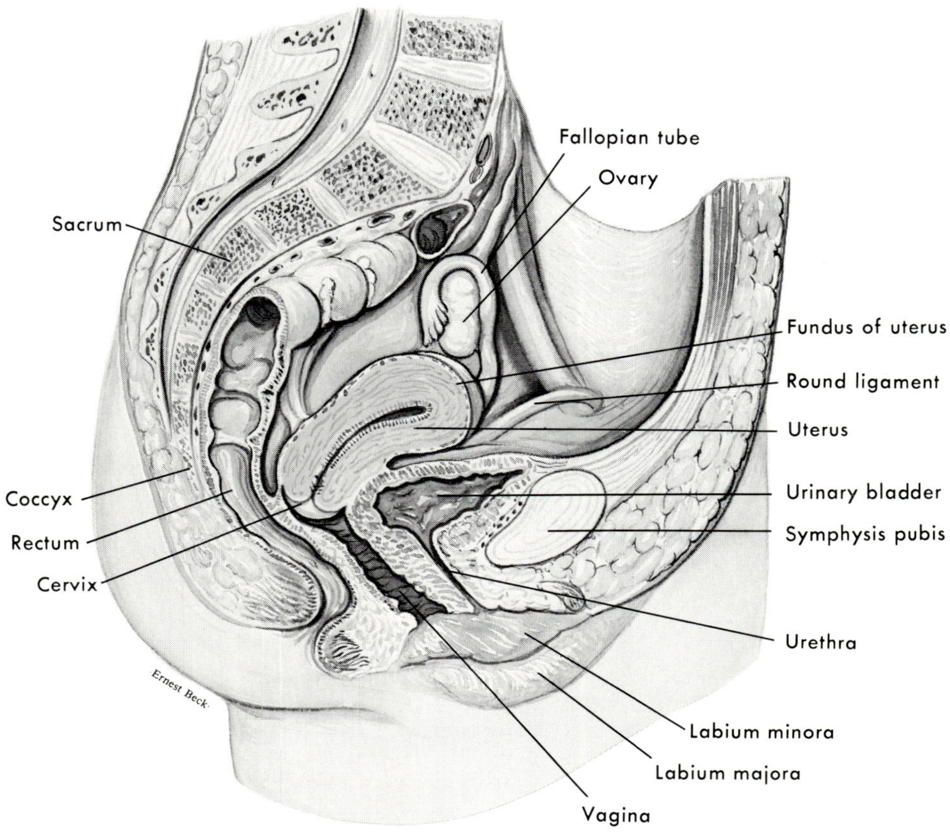

Fig. 12-14. Female pelvis, sagittal section. (From Anthony, C. P., and Kolthoff, N. J.: Textbook of anatomy and physiology, ed. 9, St. Louis, 1975, The C. V. Mosby Co.)

CIRCULATORY SYSTEM

In recent years the circulatory system has presented many interesting radiographic studies, among which are angiograms, venograms, arteriograms, and angiocardiograms. In addition to the lymphatic system, which will be discussed in the following section, the circulatory system consists of four distinct, closely interrelated systems: the *pulmonary circulation,* which is the flow of blood from the heart to the lungs and back to the heart for the purpose of gaseous exchange; the *portal circulation,* which is the flow of blood from the digestive viscera to the liver, allowing the blood to absorb the nutrients that feed the body cells; the *systemic circulation,* which is the flow of blood to the remainder of the body cells to deliver nutrition and oxygen and to return waste materials and carbon dioxide; and the *coronary circulation,* which is the flow of blood from the origin of the aorta, in the left ventricle, to the myocardium and return to the right atrium. The organs of the circulatory system include the heart, arteries, veins, capillaries, and lymphatic vessels.

Pulmonary circulation

The right atrium receives blood from the superior and inferior vena cavas during the same period that the left atrium is receiving blood from the pulmonary veins. These chambers are in *diastole* during the filling period. The atria begin to contract, or begin the *systole,* and force the blood into the corresponding ventricles, which are now in diastole. When the atria are completely contracted, they begin to relax, and the ventricles begin the systole, which forces the blood from the right ventricle into the pulmonary artery and from the left ventricle into the aorta. The blood in the pulmonary artery is forced into the lungs, where the carbon dioxide is exchanged for oxygen. From the lungs the blood flows via the pulmonary veins into the left atrium. The blood in the aorta flows into the systemic and portal systems to all of the body cells.

Portal circulation

The blood from the systemic circulation enters the spleen, pancreas, stomach, small intestine, and greater part of the large intestine but does not directly return to the right atrium. It flows via the portal vein to the liver and into the liver sinusoids and from the liver via the hepatic vein to the inferior vena cava. This portal system is a vital part of the digestive and nutritive processes. The portal system commences with the superior mesenteric and splenic veins. The inferior mesenteric vein conveys water from the large intestine (chiefly) to the splenic vein that joins the superior mesenteric vein to form the portal vein that empties into the liver. The portal system, per se, terminates in the liver.

Systemic circulation

The systemic circulation is that which leaves the left ventricle, circulates through the body, and returns to the right atrium. It is this system that receives the various radiopaque media injected for radiographic studies.

Coronary circulation

The coronary circulation conveys blood to the myocardium via the right and left coronary arteries. Blood flows from the myocardium via the

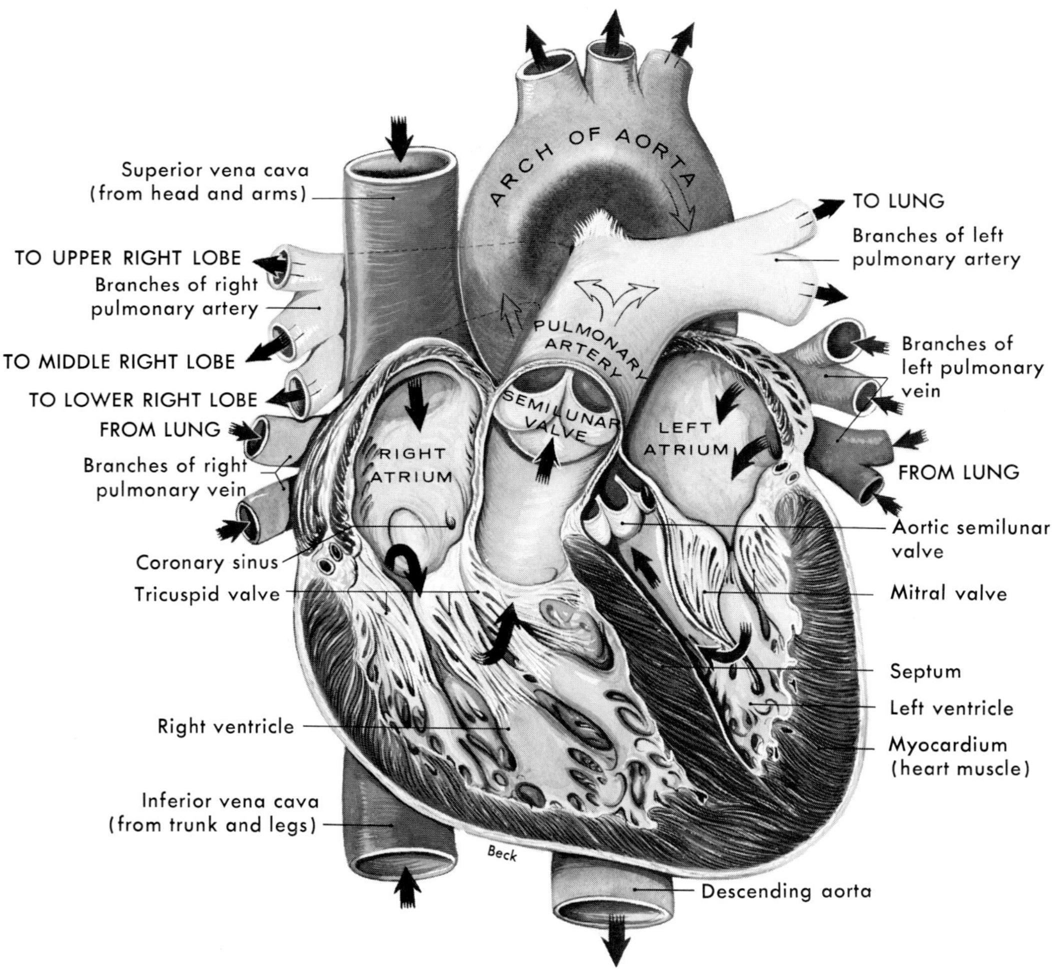

Fig. 12-15. Heart, frontal section. (From Anthony, C. P., and Kolthoff, N. J.: Textbook of anatomy and physiology, ed. 9, St. Louis, 1975, The C. V. Mosby Co.)

right and left coronary veins and the coronary sinus to the right atrium.

Heart

The heart is a very muscular organ located in the thoracic cavity in the mediastinum and enveloped by the pericardium. It resembles an inverted cone and lies posterior to the sternum, with about twice as much to the left of the midsagittal plane as to the right. The *apex* is inferior to and slightly to the right of the left nipple. The heart is divided into four chambers: right and left *atria* (or auricles) and right and left *ventricles.* Blood from the vena cavas enters the right atrium, passes to the right ventricle through the *tricuspid valve,* and then passes from the right ventricle to the lungs via the pulmonary arteries. From the lungs via the pulmonary veins it enters the left atrium, passes into the left ventricle through the *bicuspid valve,* and then passes from the left ventricle via the aorta. Semilunar valves are located in the inferior vena cava, pulmonary vein, pulmonary artery, and aortic orifices. (See Fig. 12-15.) The heart is demonstrated radiographically without opacification in the routine chest exposures. However, it is always opacified by the injection of suitable radiopaque media for certain studies. These studies usually precede surgery.

Major arteries

The aorta arises from the left ventricle and makes an arch to the left of the median line. Posteriorly and inferiorly from the arch the descending aorta commences. Two coronary arteries for the heart muscles rise from sinuses in the ascending portion origin. There are three major arteries arising from the arch: brachiocephalic (innominate), which branches into the right common carotid and right subclavian arteries; left common carotid; and left subclavian. The carotid arteries supply the head and neck along with the vertebral arteries, and the subclavian arteries supply the upper extremities. After the aorta begins its descent, it is called the descending or thoracic aorta in the thorax and the abdominal aorta in the abdomen. A little below the umbilicus the aorta branches into the two common iliac arteries, which are the major arteries supplying the lower extremities. The subclavian arteries, abdominal artery, and iliac arteries all branch into many smaller arteries, which supply various organs and parts. (See Fig. 12-16.)

The femur, tibia, and other long bones contain small nutrient foramina, located usually near the center of the shaft. One of the arterial branches, the nutrient artery, enters a foramen to supply the marrow of the bone. The tibial nutrient artery is one of the larger of these.

Major veins

The arteries all terminate in minute vessels known as capillaries, which join with the venules that join with each other to form veins. The veins receive other veins and become progressively larger as they approach the heart. The veins of major importance in radiography are those into which the contrast media are injected. In the lower extremity the anterior and posterior tibial veins join to form the popliteal vein, which receives the lesser saphenous vein superior to the knee on the posterior surface. The popliteal vein receives the greater saphenous vein just inferior to the inguinal region and becomes the femoral vein, which later becomes the external iliac vein. The external iliac vein receives the hypogastric vein and becomes the common iliac vein; the two common iliac veins join to form the inferior vena cava. The inferior vena cava receives numerous other veins as it approaches the right atrium. In the upper extremities the radial and ulnar veins join just superior to the elbow to form the brachial vein. The brachial vein receives the basilic vein to form the axillary vein. Just above this vein it receives the cephalic vein to form the subclavian vein. The subclavian vein receives the corresponding internal jugular vein from the head and neck to form the brachiocephalic (innominate) vein; the two brachiocephalic veins join to form the superior vena cava. (See Fig. 12-17.) As the veins pass through the anterior surface of the elbow, they are easily palpated. It is in this area, called the *antecubital space,* that intravenous injections are usually administered. The veins and arteries are usually named after the particular region of the body in which they are located or after a bone or organ in that particular region.

LYMPHATIC SYSTEM

The lymphatic system is actually a part of the circulatory system, but the lymph flows only toward the heart: from the extremities and head to the subclavian veins. The thoracic duct drains all of the left side of head, neck, thorax, the left upper extremity, and all of the remainder of the body into the left subclavian vein at its junction with the left internal jugular vein. The lymphatic duct drains the right side of the head, neck, thorax, and the upper right extremity into the right

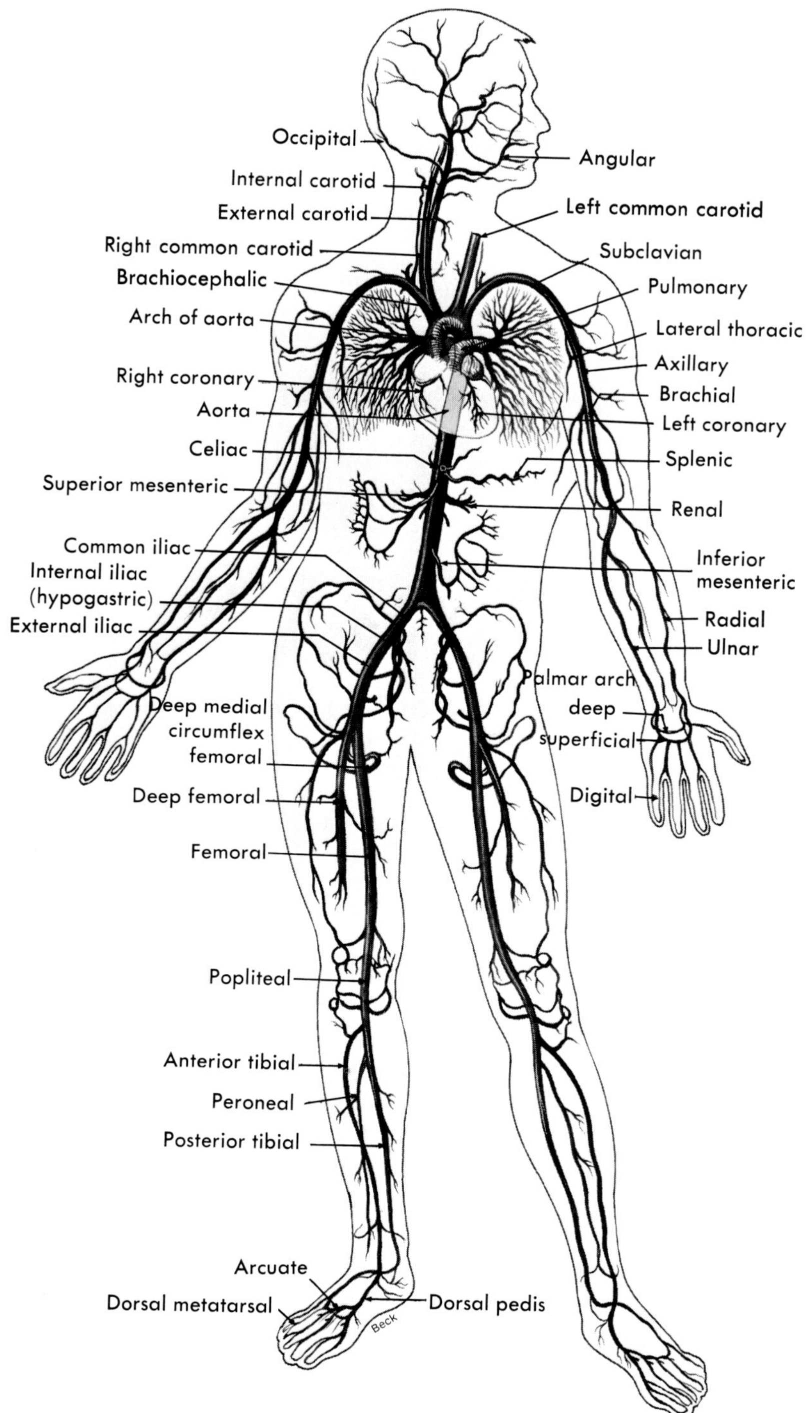

Fig. 12-16. Chief arteries. (Modified from Anthony, C. P., and Kolthoff, N. J.: Textbook of anatomy and physiology, ed. 9, St. Louis, 1975, The C. V. Mosby Co.)

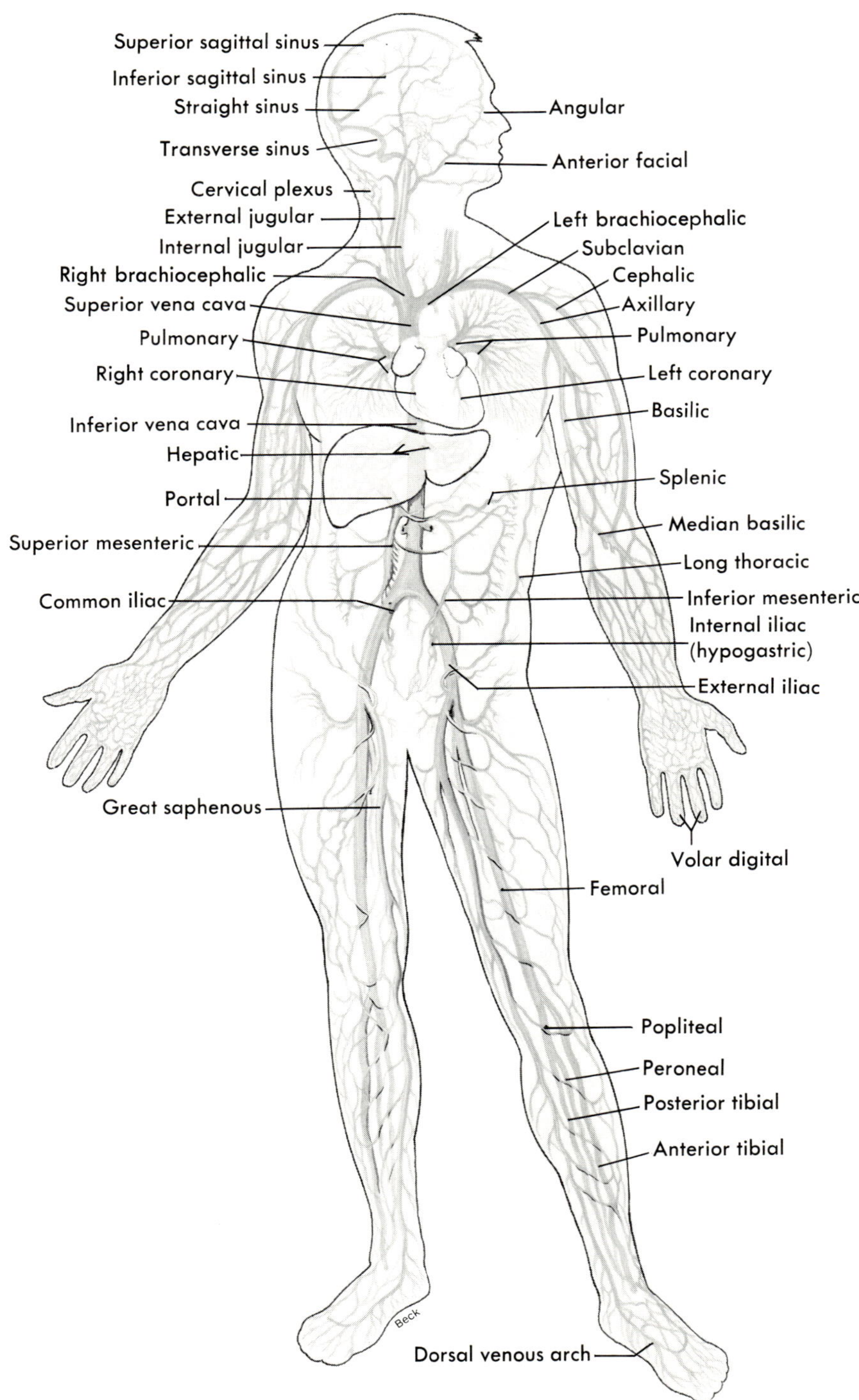

Fig. 12-17. Chief veins. (Modified from Anthony, C. P., and Kolthoff, N. J.: Textbook of anatomy and physiology, ed. 9, St. Louis, 1975, The C. V. Mosby Co.)

subclavian vein at its junction with the right internal jugular vein. There are major concentrations of lymph nodes in the inguinal, mediastinal, axillary, subclavicular, supraclavicular and cervical regions.

RESPIRATORY SYSTEM

The respiratory system includes the nose, pharynx, larynx, trachea, bronchi, and lungs. (See Fig. 12-18.) All of the organs of respiration are contained in the thorax, head, and neck, with the external openings (anterior nares) in the nose.

Nose

The nose opens into the nasal cavity, which opens directly into the pharynx through the choanae. The nasal septum was discussed elsewhere (p. 305). Air passes between the nasal cavities

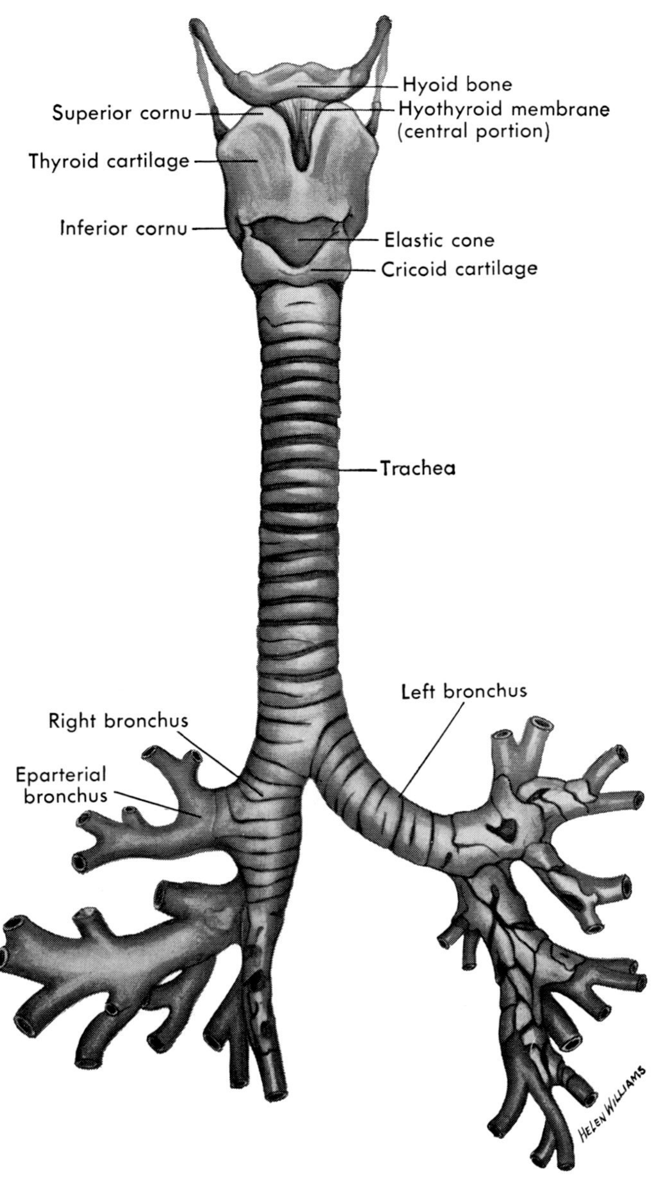

Fig. 12-18. Larynx and bronchial tree, anterior view. (From Francis, Carl C: Introduction to human anatomy, ed. 5, St. Louis, 1968, The C. V. Mosby Co.)

and the frontal, maxillary, ethmoid, and sphenoid sinuses. The formation of the nasal cavity was discussed on p. 310, as was the radiography of this cavity.

Pharynx

The pharynx was described on p. 366.

Larynx

The larynx enables us to speak. It is located between the trachea and the tongue in the neck in the area between the fourth and sixth cervical vertebrae. The larynx connects the pharynx with the trachea. Its walls are comprised of nine pieces of cartilage that contain the vocal cords within the cavity so formed. Among these cartilaginous parts are the *thyroid cartilage* (Adam's apple), *epiglottis* (lid) of the larynx, and the *cricoid cartilage*. The thyroid cartilage is very prominent in many males because of its more acute angle. The epiglottis prevents food from entering the trachea during deglutition. The cricoid cartilage forms the inferior surface of the larynx. The *glottis* is a space separating the true vocal cords. The vocal cords are fibers that expand and contract to control the frequency (pitch) of the voice. (See Fig. 12-3.)

Trachea

The *tracheal* walls contain incomplete circular cartilaginous rings that lend support to the walls and keep the lumen of the trachea open at all times. The trachea is usually less than 12.5 cm long and occupies the area between the sixth cervical and fifth thoracic vertebrae. It bifurcates inferiorly, usually near the fifth thoracic vertebra, and the two major bronchi are formed at this bifurcation. The bronchi are of the same general construction as the trachea.

Bronchi

The *bronchi* enter the lungs through the *hila*. The right hilum is approximately opposite the fifth thoracic vertebra, and the left hilum is approximately opposite the sixth. The right bronchus extends almost directly into the right hilum, while the superior border of the left bronchus makes a more acute angle with the lateral margin of the trachea. In the lungs the bronchi branch into progressively smaller subdivisions, which are finally called *alveolar ducts*. The ducts are comprised of *alveolar sacs*, which consist of many very small structures known as *alveoli*. The *gaseous exchange* takes place between the capillaries and the alveoli.

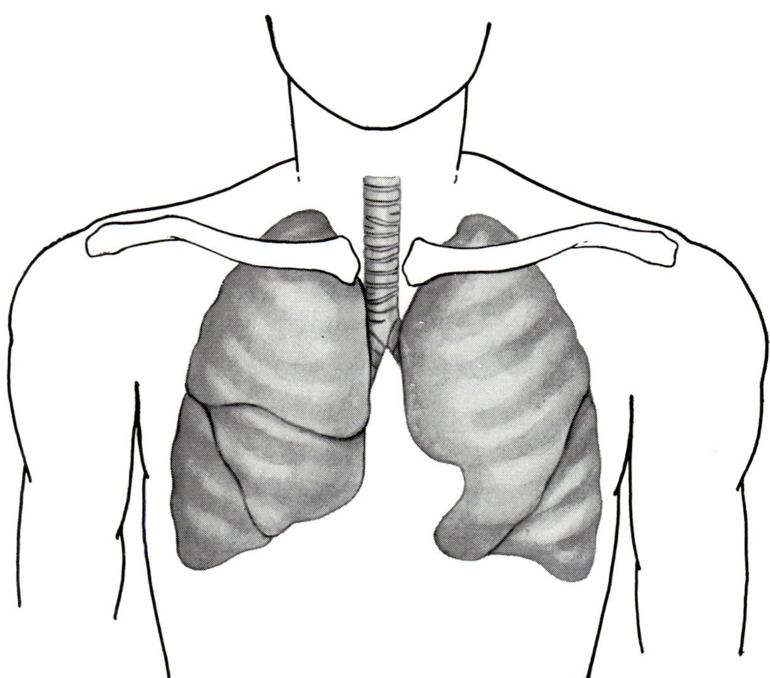

Fig. 12-19. Normal position of lungs and trachea. (From Francis, Carl C: Introduction to human anatomy, ed. 5, St. Louis, 1968, The C. V. Mosby Co.)

Lungs

The major respiratory organs, the *lungs,* are separated by the mediastinal viscera. The right lung is somewhat larger than the left and is divided into three lobes, whereas the left lung is divided into two lobes. Both lungs resemble cones. The *apex* of the lung is directed superiorly and is demonstrated radiographically by the use of the *apical lordotic position.* The base of each lung rests on the diaphragm. The medial surfaces of the lungs are concave and contain the hila. It is through the hila that all of the nerves and blood vessels as well as the bronchi enter the lungs. (See Fig. 12-19.) The major portion of the respiratory system is located in the thoracic cavity.

Thoracic cavity

The ribs and thoracic vertebrae form the posterior wall of the thoracic cavity, the ribs and related muscles form the lateral walls, and the ribs and sternum form the anterior wall. The superior border is narrowed and is bounded by the manubrium, the first ribs, and the first thoracic vertebra. The diaphragm forms the inferior border and separates the thoracic cavity from the abdominal cavity. The diaphragm is very important in respiration. It has three major openings through it and several lesser openings that actually are posterior to it. The *aortic hiatus* is slightly to the left of the center and near the spine. The *esophageal hiatus* is slightly to the left of the midsagittal plane and nearly in the center. The *vena cavic foramen* is slightly anterior to the esophageal hiatus and to the right of the midsagittal plane. (See Fig. 12-20.) The diaphragm is a frequent object for radiographic study when a *diaphragmatic hernia* is suspected. Such herniations are demonstrable during gastrointestinal studies employing contrast media.

The thoracic cavity consists of three divisions: *pleural,* which contains the lungs; *mediastinal,* which contains the ascending aorta, descending aorta, aortic arch, inferior vena cava, thoracic duct, lymphatic duct, esophagus, bronchi, and azygos veins; and the *pericardial,* which contains the heart. These divisions are separated from each other by pleural partitions.

NERVOUS SYSTEM

The nervous system contains the *central* and *peripheral* divisions. The central nervous system includes the brain and spinal cord, whereas the peripheral system includes all the nerves of the body tissues and their connections to the central nervous system. Since nerves are radiolucent, they are difficult to radiograph. Opacification of surrounding tissues and insufflation of air surrounding the nerve tissue under consideration are the methods used in such radiographic techniques as *myelography* to examine the spinal cord, *encephalography* to examine the brain, and *ventriculography* to examine the ventricles of the brain. The spinal cord passes through the vertebral foramina of the vertebral column, the formation of which is discussed in Chapter 8.

The adult human brain includes the cerebrum, diencephalon, midbrain, pons, medulla oblongata, cerebellum, and ventricles.

The cerebrum includes the two cerebral hemispheres. The cerebral hemispheres are connected in several places by the commissures, bands of nerve tissue; the principal commissure is the corpus callosum, situated in the bottom of the longitudinal fissure. Each hemisphere consists of the following four lobes: frontal, parietal, temporal, and occipital.

The following five pairs of cranial nerves arise from the two cerebral hemispheres: olfactory

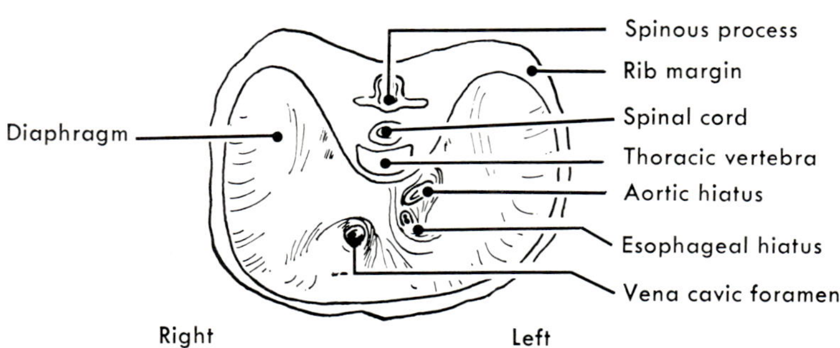

Fig. 12-20. Major openings of diaphragm.

(first), optic (second), oculomotor (third), trochlear (fourth), and abducens (sixth).

The diencephalon is situated between the cerebrum and the midbrain and consists of the thalamus and hypothalamus.

The cerebral peduncles* form the midbrain and are two in number. These function to attach the cerebellum to the brainstem.

The pons, a large round structure connecting the cerebellar hemispheres, lies inferior to and connects with the midbrain. The trigeminal (fifth), facial (seventh), and acoustic (eighth) cranial nerve pairs attach to the pons.

The medulla oblongata is inferior to and connects with the pons superiorly and is continuous with the spinal cord at the level of the foramen magnum. The glossopharyngeal (ninth), vagus

*A peduncle is a supporting part, or stem.

Table 12-3. Glands having endocrine function

	Location
Gland	
Pituitary	Sella turcica in sphenoid
Thyroid	Anteriorly in neck, inferior to larynx
Parathyroids	Posterior surfaces of lobes of thyroid
Adrenals	Proximal poles of each kidney
Ovaries	Female pelvic cavity
Testes	Scrotum in male
Islands of Langerhans	Throughout pancreas
Indefinite glands	
Thymus	Posteriorly in neck from about C-6 to T-4
Pineal	Midbrain, superior and posterior to pituitary

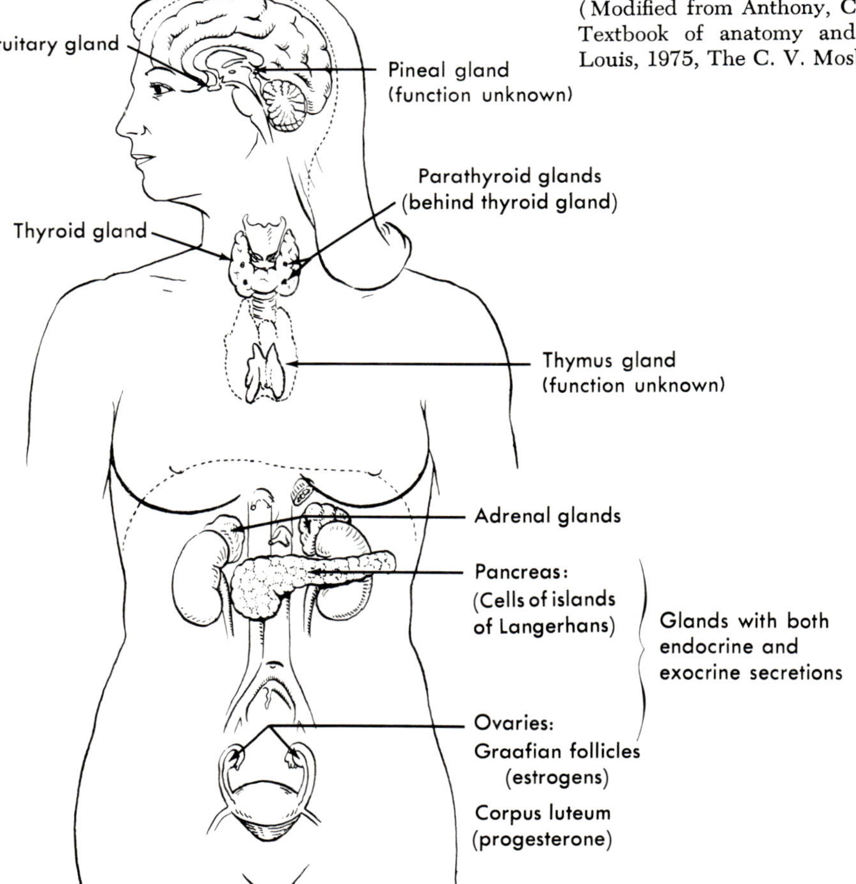

Fig. 12-21. Location of some of the endocrine glands. (Modified from Anthony, C. P., and Kolthoff, N. J.: Textbook of anatomy and physiology, ed. 9, St. Louis, 1975, The C. V. Mosby Co.)

(tenth), spinal accessory (eleventh), and hypoglossal (twelfth) cranial nerve pairs attach to the medulla oblongata.

The cerebellum is situated inferior to the occipital lobes of the cerebrum and posterior to the brainstem.

Cerebrospinal fluid is manufactured in the four brain ventricles. Two of the ventricles are paired and lie to the right and left of the midline, the lateral ventricles; one is in each cerebral hemisphere. These are each connected to the third ventricle, posteriorly and inferiorly, via one of two interventricular foramina. The third ventricle is contained within the diencephalon and is continuous with the cerebral aqueduct, which is continuous inferiorly with the fourth ventricle.

Cerebrospinal fluid circulates through the ventricles from laterals to third to fourth and through the length of the spinal cord in the central canal and between the meninges, coverings of the spinal cord. The meninges, from inside to outside, are the pia mater, arachnoid membrane, and dura mater.

The spinal cord tapers in the conus medularis and terminates near the level of the first lumbar vertebra to the second lumbar vertebra. The filum terminale interna continues below this level to terminate with the dura mater at the level of the first sacral vertebra. The filum terminale externa continues below the first sacral vertebra to terminate usually even with the first coccygeal segment.

ENDOCRINE SYSTEM

The endocrine system of ductless glands includes all structures of the body that secrete hormones. Hormones are discrete chemical substances, each one of which exhibits a specific effect on the activities of other organs. Since these glands and specialized tissues in other glands are ductless and quite small, radiologic examination of them is an uncommon procedure. The true endocrine glands include the pituitary, thyroids, parathyroids, and adrenals. The ovaries, testes, and pancreas are compound glands having specific endocrine function. Several hormones are secreted in the walls of the small intestines. The true endocrine glands and principal glands known to secrete hormones are listed in Table 12-3; some of these are shown in Fig. 12-21.

REFERENCES

Anthony, Catherine Parker, and Kolthoff, N. J.: Textbook of anatomy and physiology, ed. 9, St. Louis, 1975, The C. V. Mosby Co.

Goss, Charles M.: Gray's anatomy, ed. 28, Philadelphia, 1966, Lea & Febiger.

Meschan, Isadore: An atlas of anatomy basic to radiology, Philadelphia, 1975, W. B. Saunders Co.

QUESTIONS

1. List in order the structures that compose the digestive tube.
2. Differentiate between the buccal and oral cavities.
3. Name the ducts that drain the upper salivary glands.
4. Name the ducts that drain the lower salivary glands.
5. From what bony processes do the teeth erupt?
6. Describe the shape and openings of the pharynx.
7. What is the common name for the pharynx?
8. Through what normal opening in the diaphragm does the esophagus pass?
9. Differentiate between false and true peristalsis.
10. What is the name of the longitudinal folds of the stomach?
11. Name the parts of the small intestine.
12. Name the parts of the first section of the small intestine.
13. What is the name of the stomach outlet? Inlet?
14. Describe in detail the biliary system.
15. What are the proteolytic enzymes of the stomach, intestinal tract, and pancreas?
16. Name the lipolytic enzyme(s).
17. What part does bile play in the digestive process?
18. Explain the function of the ileocecal valve.
19. The functional unit of the kidney is called what?
20. Differentiate between intravenous and retrograde pyelography.
21. What two structures does each ureter connect?
22. In its passage from the urinary bladder, the male urethra passes through what structure not passed through by the female urethra?
23. What is the name of the rather common radiographic examination of the female reproductive system?
24. Name the four divisions of the circulatory system.
25. Describe each of the systems mentioned in 24.
26. Describe the flow of blood through the heart naming each compartment and valve.
27. In its flow through the heart, does the blood at any time leave the heart before entering the aorta?
28. Name in order the principal arteries of the head and neck.
29. Name in order the principal arteries of the upper extremity.
30. Name in order the principal arteries of the lower extremity.
31. Name in order the principal veins of the lower extremity.

32. Name in order the principal veins of the upper extremity.
33. What veins drain blood into the heart?
34. Where does the lymph drain into the blood stream?
35. What and where are the antecubital spaces?
36. In order of decreasing size name the structures of the respiratory system contained completely within the lungs.
37. Through what natural opening in the diaphragm passes the aorta?
38. Name the cranial nerves arising from the cerebral hemispheres.
39. List in order from anterior to posterior the pairs of cranial nerves.
40. Where is the site of manufacture of the cerebrospinal fluid?
41. From outside to inside name the meninges.
42. Name the true endocrine glands.
43. Differentiate endocrine from simple glands.
44. What are compound glands?
45. What are hormones?
46. Differentiate hormones from enzymes.
47. Locate specifically the site of the pituitary gland.
48. Locate specifically the sites of the adrenal glands.
49. Name and locate the four ventricles of the brain.
50. Name the arteries supplying blood to the adrenal glands.

13 • POSITIONING FOR CONTRAST STUDIES

CONTRAST MEDIA

A contrast medium is a substance or material that makes it possible to examine by means of radiography specific organ systems and areas of the body that would otherwise have to be examined by actual observation or by relying on interpretation of the patient's symptoms.

There are many advantages to the use of contrast media:

1. They make the examination easier and faster in many cases and the diagnosis faster, more exact, and more complete.
2. In many cases the use of contrast media eliminates the necessity of resorting to surgery to study an organ or an area.
3. It can eliminate searching and probing on the part of the doctor; he can go directly to the area he wants to study and carry out his examination quickly and easily.
4. Completing a study using a contrast medium will in many cases give the patient peace of mind by reassuring him that there is no injury or disease to "worry about."

Normally, bone radiography presents no problem, since the bone structures are sufficiently dense to present a good diagnostic demonstration on the x-ray film or the fluoroscopic screen. Since most internal organs and structures are composed of soft tissue, the demonstration of the organ or area is difficult unless it is filled with a medium that is either radiolucent or opaque to x rays. For example, all the organs in the abdominal cavity are of about the same density, and it is difficult to distinguish one from the other on a routine radiograph. However, by filling the gallbladder with a radiopaque contrast medium, the gallbladder stands out in sharp contrast to the other organs in the abdominal cavity. This concentration of radiopaque chemicals in a certain area makes that area opaque to x ray and so demonstrates the area on x-ray film.

Air or gas can be used as a contrast medium in certain areas, such as the brain ventricles, sinuses, and lungs. Air or gas makes the area of interest less opaque to x rays than the surrounding areas; the presence of air causes the area to offer less resistance to the passage of x rays than would be offered if the area were filled with fluid or with folds of tissue. On the film, the area is seen as having increased radiographic density (darker).

There are different forms of contrast media specific to examination of various areas and organs. Most forms—liquid, powder, pill forms—are opaque; air or gas, however, is used as a radiolucent (nonradiopaque) contrast medium. The methods of introducing contrast media include intravenous injections, drinking in the form of liquids, ingesting orally in pill or granular form, injecting rectally in the form of an enema, and injecting the contrast medium directly into the space or area to be examined.

Characteristics of diagnostic opaques

Regardless of chemical composition, the contrast media (except, of course, air and gas) all contain some material or chemical that is opaque to x rays. The type of diagnostic opaque to be used is selected with the foreknowledge that its radiopaque chemicals will concentrate in the area under consideration.

The radiopaque chemical in many contrast media is a form of iodine, usually in organic chemical combination. One disadvantage of this is that some persons are overly sensitive to the iodine, so the contrast media should only be given following specific sensitivity tests.

Barium sulfate is a radiopaque mineral powder that is mixed with water and administered into the digestive system: it may be swallowed as a liquid, swallowed as a paste, or given in enema form to fill the colon; it is completely nonabsorbable through the intestinal walls.

Examples of contrast media and their uses are set out in Table 13-1.

Table 13-1. Contrast media*

Viscera or structures	Examination name	Media
Cranial blood vessels	Cerebral angiography	Diodrast solution, Hypaque sodium, Urokon sodium, Conray 60
Paranasal sinuses	None	Iodochlorol, Lipiodol, Sinografin
Salivary ducts	Sialography	Diodrast solution, Lipiodol, Iodochlorol, Mulsopaque, Neo-Iopax, Sinografin
Esophagus, laryngopharynx	ESD, UGI, esophagus	Barium sulfate, Baropaque A, B, or C, Microtrast, Rugar, Baridol, Basolac, Barosperse, Esophatrast, Gastrografin
Articulations	Arthrograms	Diodrast solution, Lipiodol, Iodochlorol, Hypaque sodium
	Pneumoarthrograms	Oxygen or air
Heart and great vessels	Angiocardiography	Diodrast concentrate, Urokon sodium, Conray 400, Renografin 60
Arteries and veins	Arteriography, aortography, venography	Diodrast 70%, Diodrast solution, Hypaque sodium, Urokon sodium, Conray 60
Lymph vessels	Lymphangiography	Ethiodol
Lungs	Routine chest	Air
Bronchioles	Bronchography	Dionosil, Lipiodol, Iodochlorol
Breasts	Mammography	Diodrast solution, Lipiodol, Iodochlorol, Mulsopaque, Neo-Iopax
Stomach and small intestine	Gastrolntestinal (GI) study	Barium sulfate, Baropaque A, B, or C, Micropaque, Baridol, Baroloid, Barotrast, Basolac, Gelobarin, Barosperse, Gastrografin
Stomach mucosa	GI study	Micropaque, Rugar, Umbrathor, Gastrografin
Spleen	Splenography	Air and Ethiodol
Gallbladder	Cholecystography	Telepaque, Cholografin sodium, Cholografin methylglucamine, GBD tablets, Oragrafin, Cholebrine
Bile ducts	Cholangiography	Cholografin sodium, Cholografin methylglucamine, Diodrast solution, Iodochlorol, Lipiodol, Medopaque H, Mulsopaque, Neo-Iopax, Hypaque sodium

*Note: Not all the media are listed in this table, nor are all the media listed used routinely. The table simply presents ready reference material. The physician always orders a specific medium. Several preparations have been developed to aid the completion of certain studies. Among these preparations are Pitressin and Stamyl to aid in gas elimination and Cholex, Neo-Cholex, safflower oil, and Bilevac to substitute for the fatty meal following *filled* gallbladder radiographs.

Continued.

Table 13-1. Contrast media—cont'd

Viscera or structures	Examination name	Media
Intestinal mucosa	ESD, UGI, GI study, colon, barium enema (BE)	Micropaque, Rugar, barium sulfate, Umbrathor, Barosperse, Gastrografin
Colon	Barium enema (BE), colon	Barium sulfate, barium sulfate compound, Baropaque A and B, Barotrast, Micropaque, Baridol, Baroloid, Gastriolid, Umbrathor
Spinal canal	Myelography	Lipiodol, Pantopaque
Intervertebral discs	Discography	Pantopaque, Hypaque
Kidneys, ureters	IVP, retrograde pyelogram	Diodrast solution, Hypaque sodium solution, Renografin, Diodrast compound, Miokon sodium, Neo-Iopax, Conray 400, Urokon sodium
Urinary bladder, urethra	Cystogram, urethrogram	Diodrast solution, Hypaque sodium, Renografin, Diodrast compound, Miokon sodium, Neo-Iopax
Bladder mucosa	Bladder mucosa	Umbrathor, Urokon sodium
Seminal vesicles	Seminal vesicles	Diodrast solution, Lipiodol, Iodochlorol, Sinografin
Uterus and salpinges	Hysterosalpinography, uterosalpinography, uterography, salpinography	Diodrast solution, Ethiodol, Lipiodol, Salpix, Iodochlorol, Medopaque H
Draining sinuses, fistulae	None	Diodrast solution, Ethiodol, Lipiodol, Iodochlorol, Mulsopaque, Neo-Iopax, Sinografin

CONTRAST STUDIES

Contrast studies are increasing both in number and in the percentage of total studies performed as knowledge of assimilation and excretion of newer contrast media increases. One of the most common contrast studies, air contrast for lung detail, presents more practical application to Chapter 9 than to this chapter. Many contrast studies fall into the classification of special techniques. This chapter includes the more common contrast studies of the digestive, urinary, reproductive, respiratory, and nervous systems. The digestive system begins with the mouth, and the first contrast study is of the salivary glands and ducts.

SIALOGRAPHY

ROUTINE RADIOGRAPHIC POSITIONS

Salivary glands—submaxillary (submandibular) and sublingual, submentovertical view (Figs. 13-1 and 13-2)

Film size—occlusal
Dental type
Lengthwise

Intraoral
Extension cone

Technique

Factors	No-screen film occlusal (fast)
mA	100
Time	0.2
mAs	20
Thickness in cm	5
kVp	64
Distance	30

Patient preparation

Remove all metallic and plastic articles from the head and neck region.

Contrast medium

Fill a sterile syringe with 1 ml of warmed iodized oil (Lipiodol).

Palpation points

Mandibular angles.

Procedure

Place the patient in the supine position, with shoulders elevated on a folded pillow. Extend the chin so that the vertex of the head rests on the table. Place the film lengthwise as far into the mouth as possible. The rough surface of the film packet must face the tube.

Central ray

Direct the central ray cephalad and perpendicular through a point just anterior to the mandibular angles to the center of the film holder.

Immobilization

Place a sandbag against the patient's forehead. Employ suspended respiration.

Right-left markers

Tape an *L* or *R* on the corresponding corner of the film holder

Examination

The doctor introduces a fine gold, chrome, or silver cannula into the duct orifice and injects the contrast medium until the patient experiences some discomfort. The radiographs must be made as quickly as possible in order to visualize the ducts before the oil diffuses into the alveoli.

Structures demonstrated

Submentovertical projection of the sublingual area to demonstrate pathology of the salivary ducts and alveoli.

Note: This view is used in many routine series as a survey film for demonstrating calculi without the use of contrast media.

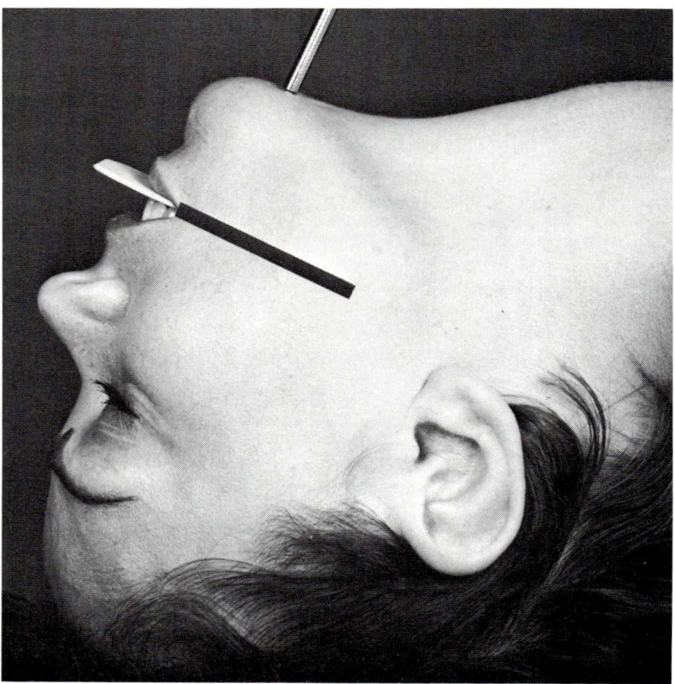

Fig. 13-1. Sialogram (salivary glands): submaxillary (submandibular) and sublingual glands—submentovertical position.

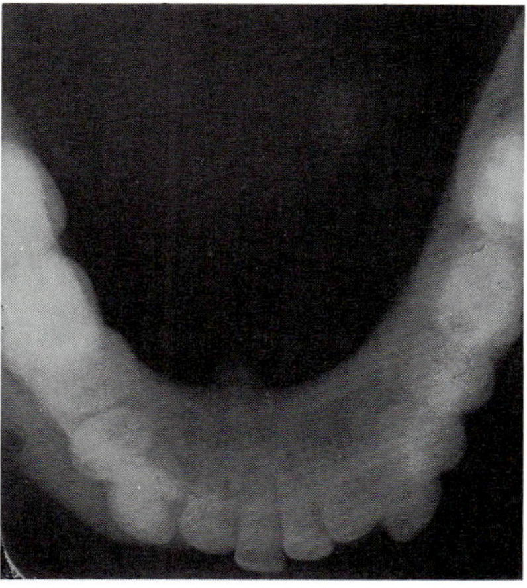

Fig. 13-2. Sialogram (salivary glands): submaxillary (submandibular) and sublingual glands—submentovertical view. (Courtesy Dr. James M. Hilton.)

Salivary glands—parotid gland, anterior (P-A) view (Figs. 13-3 to 13-5)

Film size—8″ × 10″
Cassette
Lengthwise
Erect film holder
Collimate to cover

Technique

Factors	Screen film cassette (par)
mA	100
Time	0.3
mAs	30
Thickness in cm	10
kVp	62
Distance	72

Patient preparation

Remove all metallic and plastic articles from the head and neck region.

Contrast medium

Fill a sterile syringe with 1 ml of warmed iodized oil (Lipiodol).

Palpation points

Mandibular angles.

Procedure

Place the patient in the prone or erect anterior (P-A) position. Rotate the head so that the long axis of the mandibular body of the side being examined is perpendicular to the film surface. Center that mandibular angle to the center of the film holder; the chin and nose are in contact with the film holder.

Central ray

Direct the central ray perpendicular to the center of the film holder. Collimate to film holder.

Immobilization

Place a positioning sponge against the opposite side of the face in contact with the film holder. Have the patient hold the sponge in place. Employ suspended respiration.

Right-left markers

Place a right or left marker on the corresponding lateral center border of the film holder.

Examination

The doctor introduces a fine gold, chrome, or silver cannula into the duct orifice and injects the contrast medium until the patient experiences some discomfort. The radiographs must be made as quickly as possible in order to visualize the ducts before the oil diffuses into the alveoli.

Structures demonstrated

Anterior (P-A) projection of the parotid area to demonstrate pathology of the salivary ducts and alveoli.

Note: This view is used in many routine series as a survey film for demonstrating calculi without the use of contrast media.

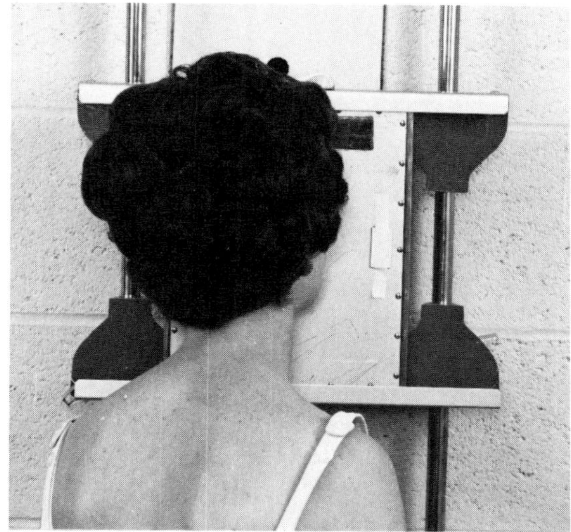

Fig. 13-3. Sialography: parotid gland—anterior (P-A) position.

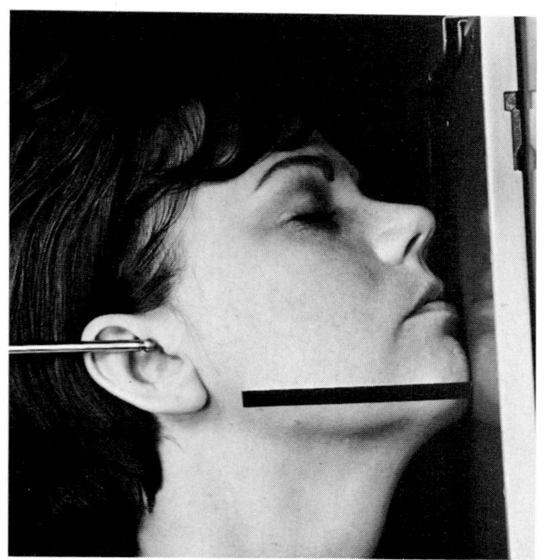

Fig. 13-4. Sialography: parotid gland—anterior (P-A) position.

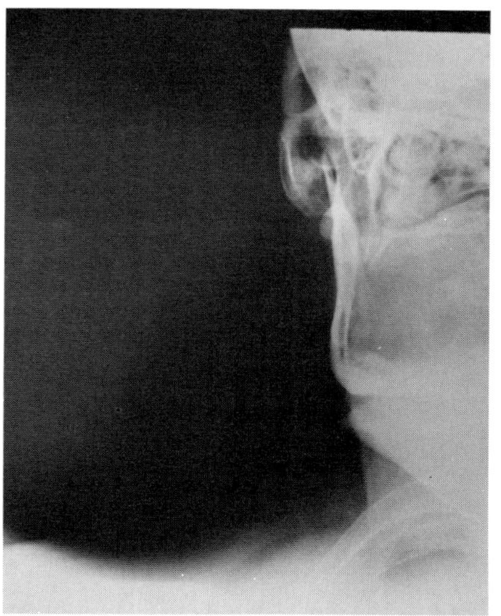

Fig. 13-5. Sialogram: parotid gland—anterior (P-A) view. (Courtesy Dr. E. I. L. Cilley, Dr. T. W. Crowell, Dr. R. E. Waud, and Dr. G. H. Hoffman.)

Salivary glands—parotid gland, posterior (A-P) view (Figs. 13-6 to 13-8)

Film size—8″ × 10″
Cassette
Lengthwise
Tabletop
Extension cone

Technique

Factors	Screen film cassette (par)
mA	100
Time	0.2
mAs	20
Thickness in cm	10
kVp	58
Distance	30

Patient preparation

Remove all metallic and plastic articles from the head and neck region.

Contrast medium

Fill a syringe with 1 ml of warmed iodized oil (Lipiodol).

Palpation points

Mandibular bodies and angles.

Procedure

Place the patient in the supine or erect posterior (A-P) position. Rotate the head so that the long axis of the mandibular body of the side being examined is perpendicular to the film holder. Center that mandibular angle to the center of the film holder; the canthomeatal line is perpendicular to the film holder.

Central ray

Direct the central ray perpendicular to the film holder.

Immobilization

Place a positioning sponge against the opposite side of the head. Have the patient hold the sponge in place. Employ suspended respiration.

Right-left markers

Burn a right or left marker over the superior center border of the film holder.

Examination

The doctor introduces a fine gold, chrome, or silver cannula into the duct orifice and injects the contrast medium until the patient experiences some discomfort. The radiographs must be made as quickly as possible in order to visualize the ducts before the oil diffuses into the alveoli.

Structures demonstrated

Posterior (A-P) projection of the parotid area to demonstrate pathology of the parotid ducts and alveoli.

Note: This view is used in many routine series as a survey film for demonstrating calculi wthout the use of contrast media.

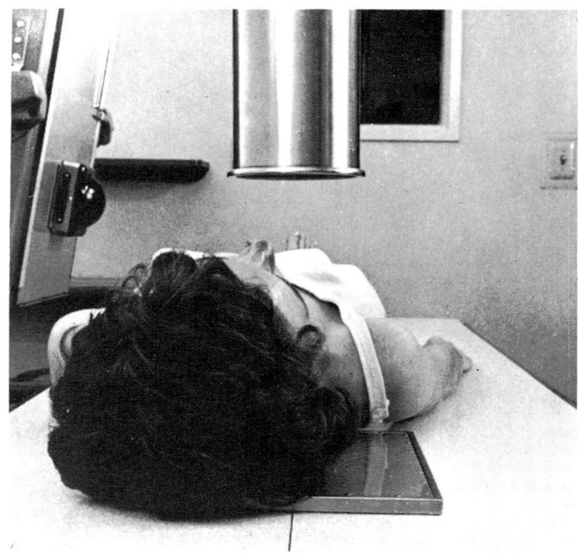

Fig. 13-6. Sialography: parotid gland–posterior (A-P) position.

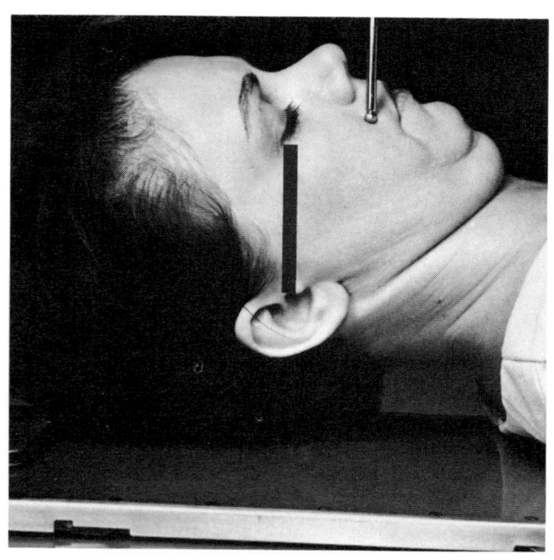

Fig. 13-7. Sialogram: parotid gland–posterior (A-P) position.

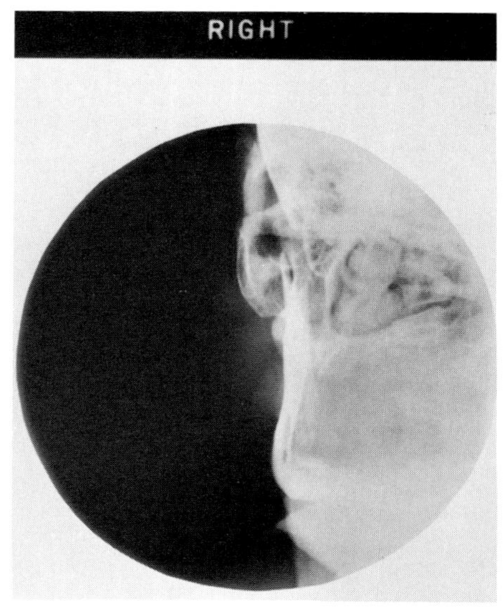

Fig. 13-8. Sialogram: parotid gland–posterior (A-P) view. (Courtesy Dr. E. I. L. Cilley, Dr. T. W. Crowell, Dr. R. E. Waud, and Dr. G. H. Hoffman.)

Salivary glands—parotid and submaxillary glands, lateral view (Figs. 13-9 and 13-10)

Film size—8″ × 10″
Cassette
Lengthwise
Erect film holder
Collimate to cover

Technique

Factors	Screen film cassette (par)
mA	200
Time	0.1
mAs	20
Thickness in cm	11
kVp	66
Distance	72

Patient preparation

Remove all metallic and plastic articles from the head and neck region.

Contrast medium

Fill a syringe with 1 ml of warmed iodized oil (Lipiodol).

Palpation points

Mandibular rami and bodies.

Procedure

Place the patient in the lateral erect position with the shoulder of the side being examined against the film holder. Extend the arms down the sides. The midsagittal plane of the head and body is parallel with the film holder. Elevate the chin so that the long axis of the mandibular body is parallel with the floor. Center a point 1 inch anterior to the external auditory meatus over the center of the film holder.

Central ray

Direct the central ray perpendicular through the selected point to the center of the film holder. Collimate to film holder.

Immobilization

Place a rectangular sponge between the patient's head and the erect film holder. A compression band may be used around the head. Employ suspended respiration.

Right-left markers

Place a right or left marker over the anterior center border of the film holder.

Examination

The doctor introduces a fine gold, chrome, or silver cannula into the duct orifice and injects the contrast medium until the patient experiences some discomfort. The radiographs must be made as quickly as possible in order to visualize the duct before the oil diffuses into the alveoli.

Structures demonstrated

Lateral projection of the salivary glands to demonstrate pathology of the parotid and submandibular glands, ducts, and alveoli.

Note: This view is used in many routine series as a survey radiograph for demonstrating calculi without the use of contrast media.

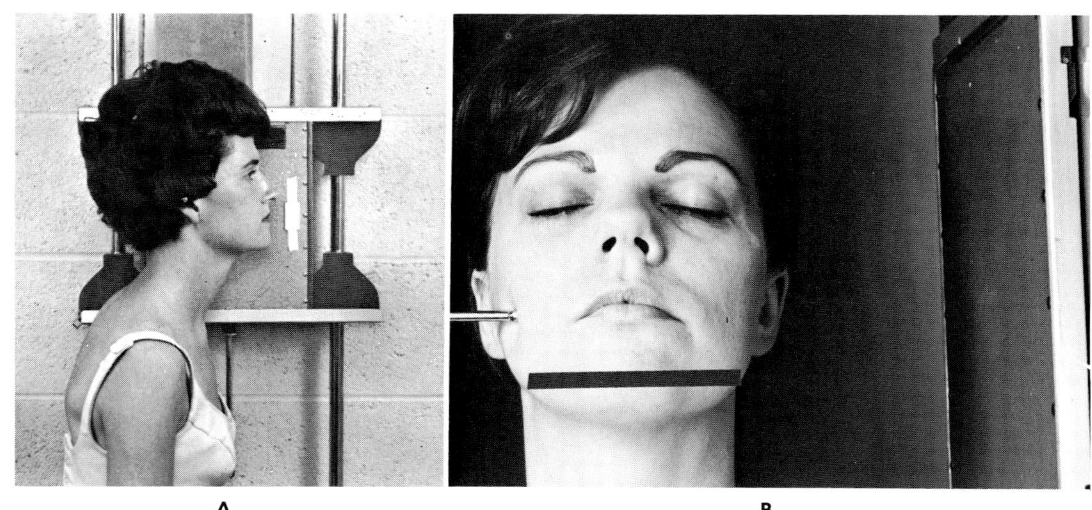

Fig. 13-9. Sialography. **A** and **B**, Parotid and submaxillary (submandibular) glands—lateral positions.

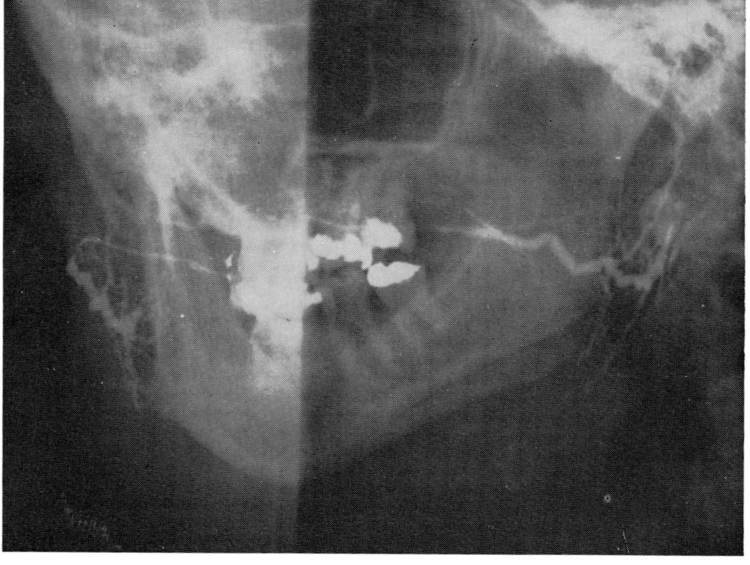

Fig. 13-10. Sialogram: parotid and submaxillary (submandibular) glands—tangential and lateral views. (Courtesy Dr. Earl L. Lawson.)

GASTROINTESTINAL STUDIES

Department routine

The first part of the morning is usually reserved for gallbladder, stomach, and colon studies. Each of these examinations requires previous appointments. After opening the department for the day, note the number of gallbladder and gastrointestinal studies scheduled and then prepare the barium for the day's examinations. Valuable time can be saved and department routine can be smoother when the barium mixtures are prepared correctly. The opacity of a given suspension of barium sulfate in water is in direct relation to the quantity of barium used. Use of a hydrometer especially designed to measure the specific gravity of barium sulfate suspensions assures consistent results from day to day.

Next, check the temperatures of the darkroom solutions, adjust if necessary, add replenishers, and completely mix and stir the solutions. After this, prepare the previous day's unread films for interpretation. By this time one of the patients scheduled for gallbladder study should have arrived for radiography. If there is an interval of time between the completion of his radiographic examination and the arrival of the next patient, who is probably scheduled for gastrointestinal examination, file the previous day's films. To avoid confusion, accomplish filing between other duties and as often as possible. We do not intend to recommend departmental operation but to emphasize the need for a routine and to demonstrate or suggest how a routine enables one person to accomplish a large volume of work easily and thus aid his employer in maintaining a smooth, efficiently operating department.

Radiography of the viscera, or soft tissue radiography, requires considerably different combinations of factors than does bone radiography. Usually, higher peak voltage and proportionally lower milliampere-seconds are required; however, the milliamperage is often quite high near the maximum capacity of the tube on the large focal spot. If the maximum milliamperage of the tube is 200, then 100 milliampere-seconds are usually used.

Various conditions limit or control the specific starting factors for visceral radiography; first, the radiologist must determine what combination of factors on any given machine will deliver the maximum tissue differentiation; second, the tube capacity and output of the transformer place limitations on the selected factors; third, the physiologic variability of the patients modifies many parts of the routine and selected factors.

FLUOROSCOPIC EXAMINATION

Esophagus

Patient preparation

No special preparation of the patient is necessary. Remove all garments down to the waist. Provide a gown for female patients.

Contrast media

Prepare approximately 4 ounces of regular barium sulfate mixture (two parts barium to one part water) with added flavoring if desired, or use flavored commercial preparations per instructions.

Equipment preparation

1. Lock a footstand on the fluoroscopy table.
2. Stand the fluoroscopy table erect and lock the Bucky diaphragm at the lower end of the table.
3. Unlock and position the fluoroscopy tower.
4. Insert a cassette into the spot-film device on the fluoroscopy tower and set the selector switch.
5. Place the foot switch to the left or right of the erect table, and position the radiologist's fluoroscopy stool in front of the table.
6. Close the line switch on the control panel and select the fluoroscopy technique (usually 3 to 5 mA).
7. Provide the mixed contrast medium, a tablespoon, an emesis basin, towels, a marking pencil, etc.
8. Darken the fluoroscopy room and energize the safelights.
9. Notify the radiologist that you are prepared and assist him with lead gloves and lead apron.

Note: If an *image intensifier* is used, attach the *intensifier* to the fluoroscopy tower according to instructions.

Examination

1. Introduce the radiologist to the patient.
2. Instruct the patient to stand on the footstand with his back against the table.
3. A cursory screening of the area under consideration may be performed by the doctor.
4. The technologist places a spoonful of the thick contrast medium mixture in the patient's mouth and cautions the patient to turn his face to the left and follow the doctor's instructions.
5. In most cases the doctor will make various *spot films* and require additional loaded cassettes.
6. Fluoroscopy may be conducted with the patient in the horizontal or Trendelenburg* position with additional contrast medium mixture.
7. The doctor will instruct the technologist as to the number and kind of radiographic views desired.

---

*The head is lower than the feet.

ROUTINE RADIOGRAPHIC POSITION

Esophagus—right anterior oblique (R.A.O.) view (Figs. 13-11 and 13-12)

Film size—14″ × 17″ (two)
Cassette
Lengthwise
Bucky
Collimate to cover

Technique

Factors	Screen film cassette (par)
mA	300
Time	0.1
mAs	30
Thickness in cm	30
kVp	80
Distance	40

Palpation points

Spinous processes of the thoracic vertebrae.

Procedure

Place the patient in the prone position. Flex the left elbow and knee, rotating the patient into a 35-degree right anterior oblique position. Center a point midway between the spinous processes and the vertebral border of the scapula on the elevated side over the midline of the table. Place the top of the film holder in line with the external auditory meatus.

Central ray

Direct the central ray perpendicular to the center of the film holder. Collimate to film holder.

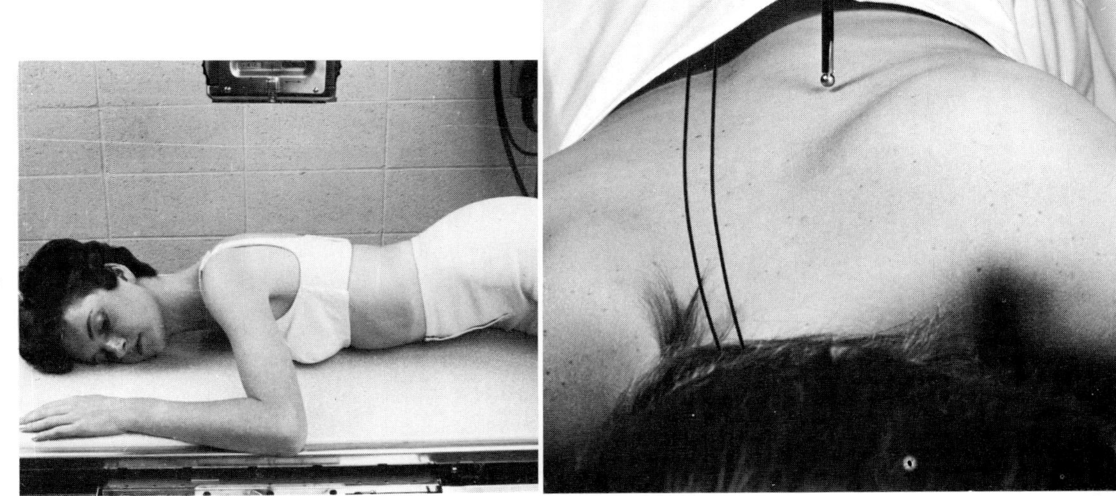

Fig. 13-11. Esophagus. **A** and **B**, Right anterior oblique (R.A.O.) positions.

Immobilization

Employ suspended inspiration.

Right-left markers

Place an R.A.O. marker on the right lateral center border of the film holder.

Examination

1. Have the patient swallow 1 tablespoonful of thick contrast medium mixture.
2. Place a second tablespoonful of this mixture in the patient's mouth and caution him to swallow when instructed to by the doctor.
3. Energize the cathode and instruct the patient to suspend breathing on deep inspiration; then to swallow.
4. After the patient swallows, count one, two, and then make the exposure.
5. Inform the patient that a 1-ounce saline purgative and a copious amount of water may be necessary to eliminate the contrast medium.

Structures demonstrated

R.A.O. view of the entire esophagus and cardiac orifice filled with contrast medium.

Note: For examination of the upper lateral esophagus, position the patient for a lateral cervical spine view (p. 215), using rapid exposure and thick contrast medium mixture.

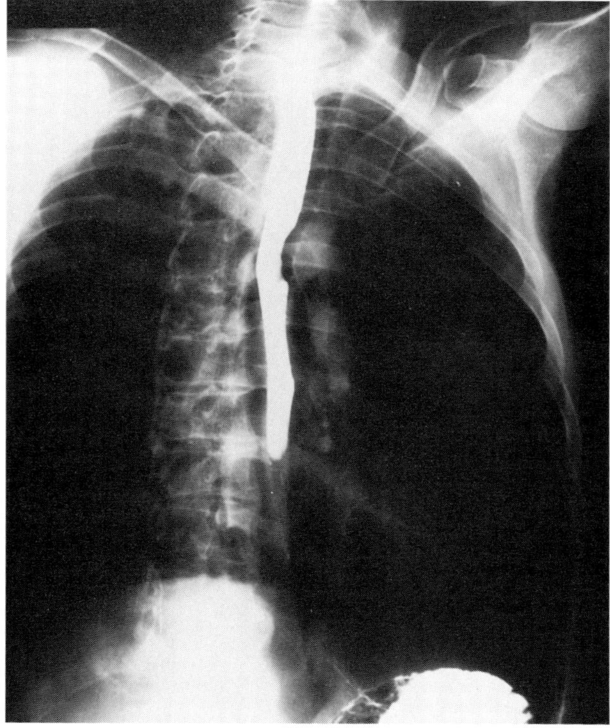

Fig. 13-12. Esophagus–right anterior oblique (R.A.O.) view. (Courtesy Dr. E. I. L. Cilley, Dr. T. W. Crowell, Dr. R. E. Waud, and Dr. G. H. Hoffman.)

FLUOROSCOPIC EXAMINATION

Stomach and duodenum—upper G.I., barium meal, E.S.D.

Patient preparation

The patient is to have nothing by mouth after 10 P.M. the night prior to the examination. On the morning of the examination, remove all garments except shoes and socks. Provide a gown and instruct the patient to tie the open ends together in the back.

Make a 14″ × 17″ posterior (A-P) abdominal scout (survey) radiograph of the patient, centering at the iliac crest. (See p. 430.)

Contrast media

Prepare approximately 8 ounces of regular barium sulfate mixture (one part barium to one part water) with added flavoring as desired, or use flavored commercial preparations per instructions.

Equipment preparation

1. Lock a footstand on the fluoroscopy table.
2. Stand the fluoroscopy table erect and lock the Bucky diaphragm at the lower end of the table.
3. Unlock and position the fluoroscopy tower.
4. Insert a loaded cassette into the spot-film device on fluoroscopy tower and set the selector switch.
5. Place the foot switch to the left or right of the erect table and position the radiologist's fluoroscopy stool in front of the table.
6. Close the line switch on the control panel and select the fluoroscopy technique (usually 3 to 5 mA).
7. Provide the mixed contrast medium, a drinking tube, an emesis basin, towels, a marking pencil, etc.
8. Darken the fluoroscopy room and energize the safelights.
9. Notify the radiologist that you are prepared and assist him with lead gloves and lead apron.

Note: If an *image intensifier* is used, leave the table horizontal and attach the *intensifier* to the fluoroscopy tower.

Examination

1. Introduce the radiologist to the patient.
2. Instruct the patient to stand on the footstand with his back against the table.
3. Instruct the patient to hold the glass of barium sulfate mixture in his left hand and to rest the hand against his left shoulder, turn his face to the left, and follow the doctor's instructions.
4. A cursory screening of the area under consideration may be performed by the doctor.
5. In most cases the doctor will make various *spot films* and will require additional loaded cassettes.
6. Fluoroscopy may be conducted with the patient in the horizontal or Trendelenburg position with the use of additional contrast medium and drinking tube.
7. The doctor will mark the region of interest and instruct the technologist as to the number and kind of radiographic views desired.

ROUTINE RADIOGRAPHIC POSITIONS

Stomach—anterior (P-A) view (Figs. 13-13 and 13-14)

Film size—10″ × 12″
Cassette
Crosswise

Bucky
Collimate to cover

Technique

Factors	Screen film, cassette (par) Regular kVp—12:1 grid	Screen film, cassette (par) High kVp—16:1 grid
mA	300	200
Time	0.2	0.1
mAs	60	20
Thickness in cm	20	20
kVp	78	120
Distance	40	40

Palpation points

Spinous processes of the thoracic vertebrae.

Procedure

Place the patient in the prone position with the arms relaxed at the sides. Center a point 2½ inches to the left of the eleventh thoracic spinous process or xiphoid process over the center line of the table.

Central ray

Direct the central ray perpendicular through the selected point to the center of the film holder. Collimate to film holder.

Immobilization

Employ suspended expiration.

Right-left markers

Markers are not necessary on this view.

Technical tips

For the hypersthenic (large, obese) patient, position the film holder crosswise and 2 or more inches higher than normal. For the asthenic (thin, slender) patient, position the film holder lengthwise and 2 or more inches lower than normal.

Structures demonstrated

Anterior (P-A) view of the entire stomach, including the terminal end of the esophagus and the duodenal cap (bulb) with the proximal duodenum.

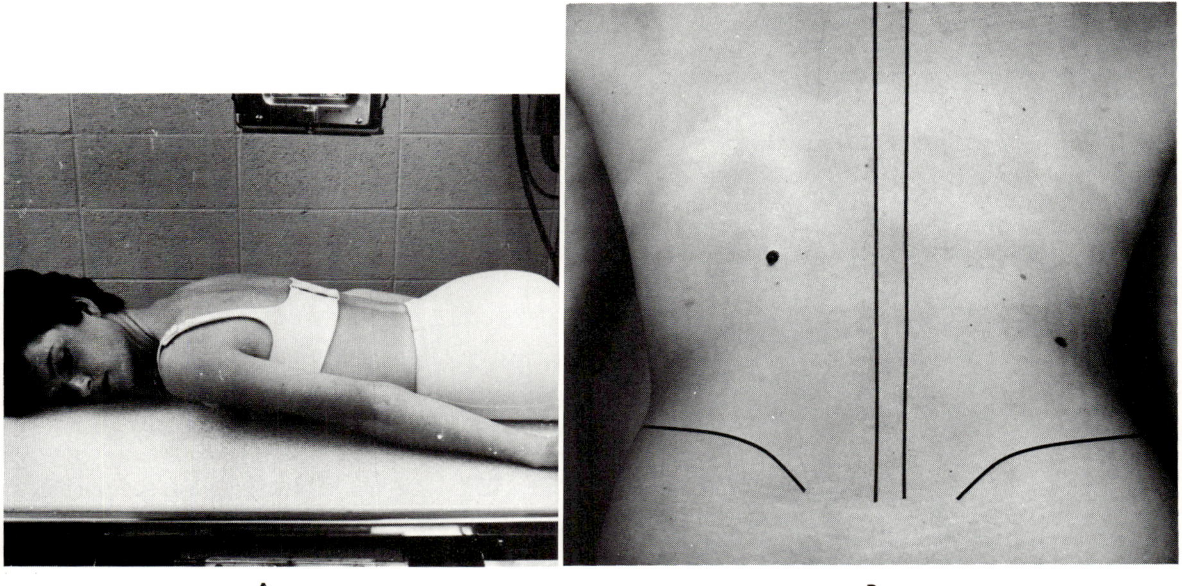

A B

Fig. 13-13. Stomach. **A** and **B,** Anterior (P-A) positions.

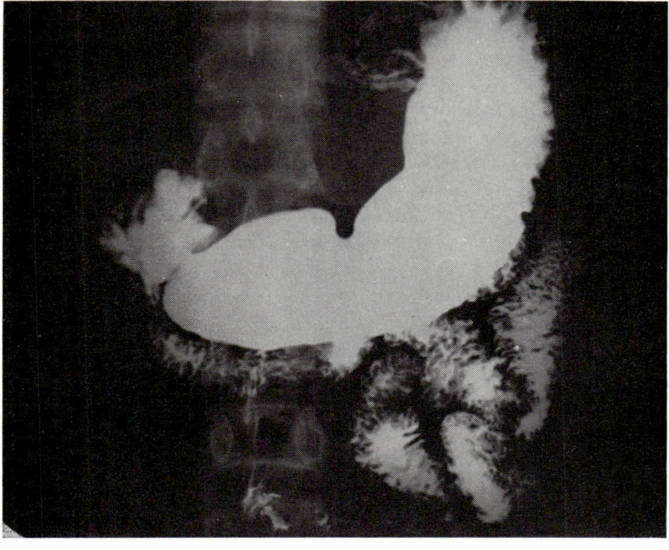

Fig. 13-14. Stomach—anterior (P-A) view. (Courtesy Dr. E. I. L. Cilley, Dr. T. W. Crowell, Dr. R. E. Waud, and Dr. G. H. Hoffman.)

Stomach—right anterior oblique (R.A.O.) view (Figs. 13-15 to 13-17)

Film size—10″ × 12″
Cassette
Lengthwise
Bucky
Collimate to cover

Technique

Factors	Screen film cassette (par) Regular kVp—12:1 grid	Screen film cassette (par) High kVp—16:1 grid
mA	300	400
Time	0.3	0.1
mAs	90	40
Thickness in cm	25	25
kVp	78	120
Distance	40	40

Palpation points

Spinous processes of lumbar vertebrae; lateral ribs.

Procedure

Place the patient in the prone position. Flex the left elbow and knee, rotating the patient into a 45-degree right anterior oblique position. Center the area marked by the radiologist (during fluoroscopy) over the center line of the table. If no marks are present, center a point in line with the first lumbar vertebra and midway between the spinous processes and the lateral ribs on the elevated side over the center line of the table.

Central ray

Direct the central ray perpendicular to the center of the film holder. Collimate to film holder.

Immobilization

Employ suspended expiration.

Right-left markers

Markers are not necessary on this view.

Technical tips

For the hypersthenic (large, obese) patient, position the film holder crosswise and 2 or more inches higher than normal. For the asthenic (thin, slender) patient, position the film holder lengthwise and 2 or more inches lower than normal.

Structures demonstrated

R.A.O. view of the entire stomach, including the terminal end of the esophagus and the duodenal cap (bulb) with the proximal duodenum.

Note: Some routine series call for more than one radiograph in this position, at 2- or 3-minute time intervals and on inspiration as well as expiration. Also, many radiologists request that the patient return for a 2- or 3-hour *stasis* film; the patient is usually requested to abstain from anything to eat or drink during this period.

Upon completion of the entire radiographic procedure, inform the patient that a 1-ounce saline purgative and copious amounts of water may be necessary to eliminate the contrast medium.

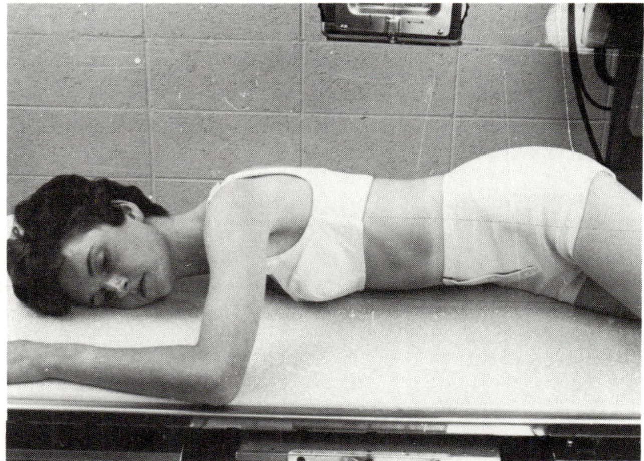

Fig. 13-15. Stomach—right anterior oblique (R.A.O.) position.

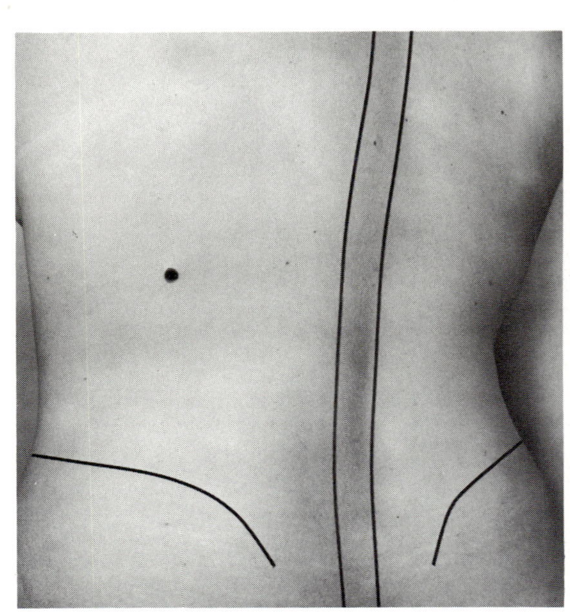

Fig. 13-16

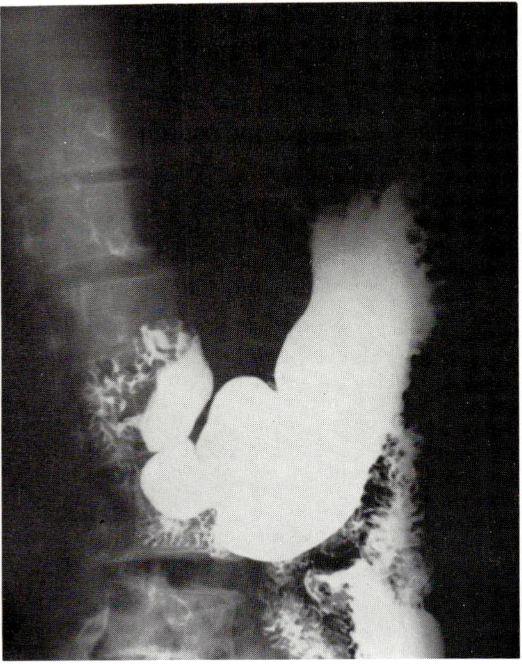

Fig. 13-17

Fig. 13-16. Stomach—right anterior oblique (R.A.O.) position.
Fig. 13-17. Stomach—right anterior oblique (R.A.O.) view. (Courtesy Dr. E. I. L. Cilley, Dr. T. W. Crowell, Dr. R. E. Waud, and Dr. G. H. Hoffman.)

FLUOROSCOPIC EXAMINATION

Small intestine beyond duodenum—stasis

Patient preparation

The patient is to have nothing by mouth after 10 P.M. the night prior to the examination. On the morning of the examination, remove all garments except shoes and socks. Provide a gown and instruct the patient to tie the open ends together in the back. Make a 14″ × 17″ posterior (A-P) abdominal scout (survey) radiograph of the patient, centering at the iliac crest. (See p. 430.)

Contrast media

Prepare approximately 4 ounces of regular barium sulfate mixture (one part barium sulfate to one part water) with added flavoring as desired, or use flavored commercial preparations per instructions.

Equipment preparation

1. Lock a footstand on the fluoroscopy table.
2. Stand the fluoroscopy table erect and lock the Bucky diaphragm at the lower end of the table.
3. Unlock and position the fluoroscopy tower.
4. Insert a loaded cassette into the spot-film device on the fluoroscopy tower and set the selector switch.
5. Place the foot switch to the left or right of the erect table and position the radiologist's fluoroscopy stool in front of the table.
6. Close the line switch on the panel and select the fluoroscopy technique (usually 3 to 5 mA).
7. Provide the mixed contrast medium, an emesis basin, towels, a marking pencil, etc.
8. Darken the fluoroscopy room and energize the safelights.
9. Notify the radiologist that you are prepared and assist him with lead gloves and lead apron.

Note: If an *image intensifier* is used, leave the table horizontal and attach the *intensifier* to the fluoroscopy tower.

Examination

1. Introduce the radiologist to the patient.
2. Instruct the patient to stand on the footstand with his back against the table.
3. Instruct the patient to hold the glass of barium sulfate mixture in his left hand and to rest the hand against his left shoulder, turn his face to the left, and follow the doctor's instructions.
4. A cursory screening of the area under consideration may be performed by the doctor.
5. In most cases the doctor will instruct the patient to drink all of the contrast medium. (The technologist should note the approximate time required for Step 5.)
6. In most cases the doctor will make various *spot films* and require additional loaded cassettes.
7. Fluoroscopy may be conducted with the patient in the horizontal or Trendelenburg position.
8. The doctor will instruct the technologist as to the number and kind of radiographs desired.

Note: Many routines specify that the patient be given 2 ounces of cold isotonic saline solution or carbonated water after the initial fluoroscopic examination to accelerate the travel of the contrast medium through the small intestine.

ROUTINE RADIOGRAPHIC POSITION
Small intestine—posterior (A-P) view (Figs. 13-18 and 13-19)

Film size—14″ × 17″ | *Bucky*
Cassette | *Collimate to cover*
Lengthwise

Technique

Factors	Screen film cassette (par) Regular kVp—12:1 grid	Screen film cassette (par) High kVp—16:1 grid
mA	300	200
Time	0.2	0.1
mAs	60	20
Thickness in cm	20	20
kVp	78	120
Distance	40	40

Palpation points

Iliac crests.

Procedure

Place the patient in the supine position with the median line of the body over the center line of the table. Elevate the knees with sponges or sandbags to aid in patient comfort. Center the film holder to the crest of the ilium.

Central ray

Direct the central ray perpendicular to the center of the film holder. Collimate to film holder.

Immobilization

Employ suspended expiration.

Right-left markers

Place a right marker on the right lateral center border of the film holder.

Examination

The radiologist may request a progress film of this type every 30 to 60 minutes after the contrast medium has been ingested and until it reaches the cecum. Also, it may be routine for the radiologist to check the patient fluoroscopically prior to each progress film.

Structures demonstrated

Posterior (A-P) view of the abdomen demonstrating contrast meduim at various stages of progression from the stomach through the small intestine.

Note: Each progress film must have the time interval identified on it during exposure.

Upon completion of the entire radiographic procedure, inform the patient that a 1-ounce saline purgative and copious amounts of water may be necessary to eliminate the contrast medium.

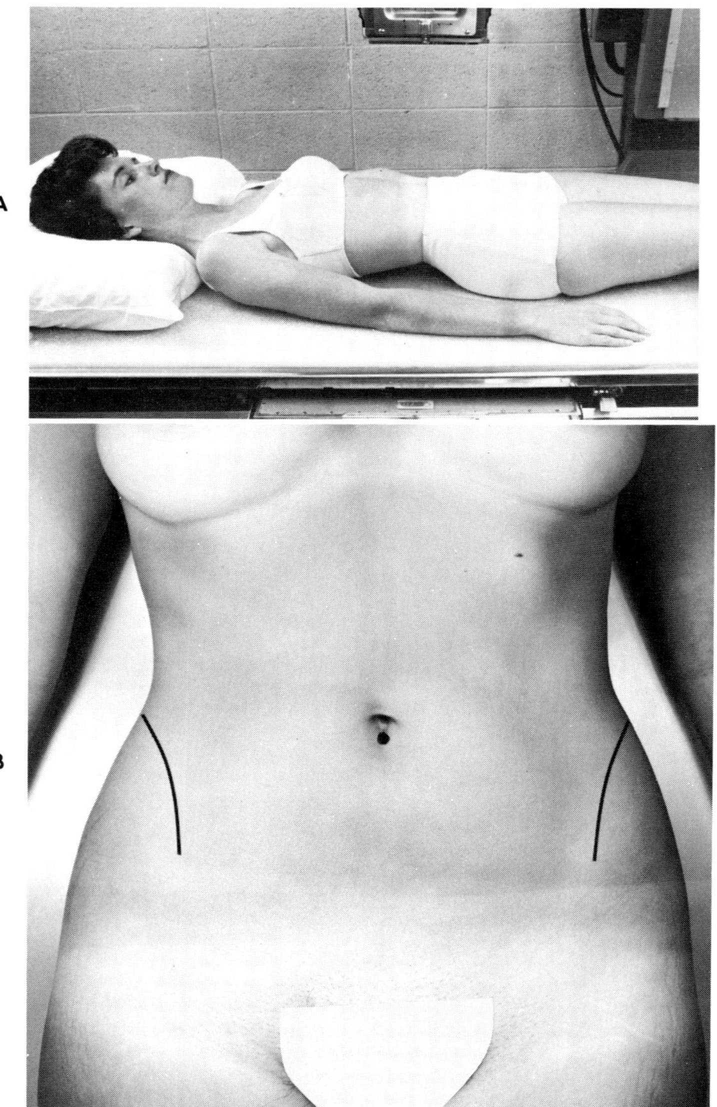

Fig. 13-18. Small intestine. **A** and **B,** Posterior (A-P) positions.

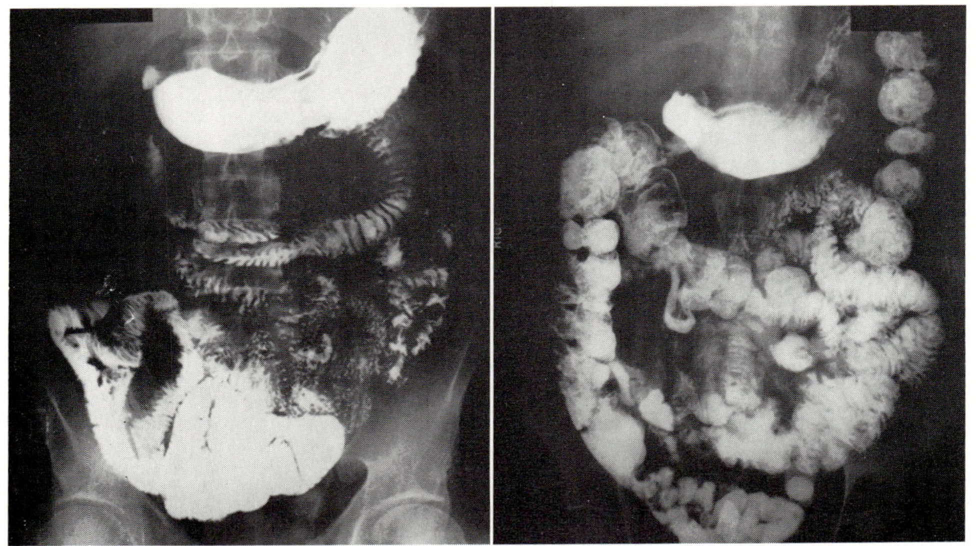

Fig. 13-19. Small intestine—posterior (A-P) view. **A,** One hour after barium meal. **B,** Two hours after barium meal. (Courtesy Dr. E. I. L. Cilley, Dr. T. W. Crowell, Dr. R. E. Waud, and Dr. G. H. Hoffman.)

FLUOROSCOPIC EXAMINATION

Large intestine—barium enema

Patient preparation

1. On the day prior to the examination, the patient should avoid eating roughage and dairy products. A liquid diet is desirable.
2. Between 3 and 5 P.M. on the day prior to the examination, the patient must take 2 ounces of castor oil. *This may be disguised with root beer or orange juice.*
3. He must take an enema consisting of 1½ to 2 pints of warm soapsuds at bedtime of the day prior to the examination.
4. On the morning of the examination he must take an enema consisting of 1 pint of warm water, repeated until a clear return is obtained.
5. He must omit breakfast except for a cup of black coffee or clear tea. (Omit this if a complete gastrointestinal study is to be made.)
6. When the patient is admitted, remove all garments except shoes and socks. Provide a gown and instruct the patient to tie the open ends together in the back.
7. Make a 14″ × 17″ posterior (A-P) abdominal scout (survey) radiograph of the patient, centering at the iliac crest. (See p. 430.)

Note: Ascertain from the patient whether he is able to retain an enema.

Contrast media

Prepare approximately 1 quart of regular barium sulfate mixture (one part barium sulfate to two parts water), or use commercial preparations per instructions. Solution must be *tepid* (100° F.) and mixed thoroughly.

Attach the enema tip to the tube. Pour the mixture into the enema container and allow it to run through the tube and tip before clamping off the tube. For commercial disposable containers, follow directions as indicated. (A hemostat makes an excellent clamp.)

Equipment preparation

1. Position and lock the Bucky diaphragm at the foot end of the horizontal table.
2. Unlock and position the fluoroscopy tower.
3. Insert loaded cassette into the spot-film device on the fluoroscopy tower and set the selector switch.
4. Place the foot switch to the center of the working side of the table.
5. Close the line switch on the control panel and select the fluoroscopy technique (usually 3 to 5 mA).
6. Provide the following:
   a. Enema container with tepid contrast medium
   b. Ceiling hook or I.V. stand for enema container
   c. Lubricant for enema tip (water-soluble preferred)
   d. Bedpan
   e. Paper towels
   f. A Bardex catheter with two hemostats in place of the regular enema tip if patient has difficulty in retaining an enema
7. Darken the fluoroscopy room and energize the safelights.
8. Notify the radiologist that you are prepared and assist him with lead gloves and lead apron.

Note: If an *image intensifier* is used, attach the *intensifier* to the fluoroscopy tower.

Examination

1. Introduce the radiologist to the patient.
2. Place the patient on the table on his left side with knees flexed.
3. Separate the gluteal folds and insert the well-lubricated enema tip (or Bardex catheter) into the rectum.
4. Instruct the patient to lie in the supine position. Recheck the enema tube to eliminate any twisting or kinking.
5. Explain the procedure to the patient and inform him that he may experience some cramping.
6. The technologist will stand to the right of the doctor and manipulate the barium sulfate mixture flow as directed.
7. A cursory screening of the area under consideration may be performed by the doctor.
8. In most cases the doctor will make various *spot films* during the barium sulfate mixture injection and will require additional loaded cassettes.
9. The fluoroscopy procedure is usually concluded when the contrast medium reaches the ileocecal valve.
10. The doctor will instruct the technologist as to the number and kind of radiographs desired.
11. After preevacuation radiographs have been made, the technologist will escort the patient to the lavatory to eliminate the enema mixture.

Note: If a disposable enema container is used, the contrast medium is returned to the container, thus eliminating Step 11 in some examinations.

ROUTINE RADIOGRAPHIC POSITION

Large intestine (colon)—anterior (P-A) views, preevacuation and postevacuation (Figs. 13-20 to 13-22)

Film size—14″ × 17″
Cassette
Lengthwise

Bucky
Collimate to cover

Technique

Factors	Screen film cassette (par) Regular kVp—12:1 grid	Screen film cassette (par) High kVp—16:1 grid
mA	300	200
Time	0.2	0.1
mAs	60	20
Thickness in cm	20	20
kVp	78	120
Distance	40	40

Palpation points

Iliac crests.

Procedure

Place the patient in the prone position with the median line of the body over the center line of the table. Center the film holder to the crest of the ilium.

Central ray

Direct the central ray perpendicular to the center of the film holder. Collimate to film holder.

Immobilization

Employ suspended expiration.

Right-left markers

Place a right marker on the right lateral border of the film holder.

Technical tips

When the patient must eliminate the contrast medium in the lavatory, speed as well as accuracy is essential in radiographic procedures. Allow a sufficient amount of time for the elimination of the contrast medium before making the postevacuation exposures.

Structures demonstrated

Anterior (P-A) view of the large intestine demonstrating contrast meduim between the rectum and the ileocecal junction.

Note: For anterior (P-A) erect views, lower the film holder position 2 inches and increase the technique factors approximately 10 kVp or the equivalent. Upon completion of the entire radiographic procedure, inform the patient that a 1-ounce saline purgative and copious amounts of water may be necessary to eliminate the contrast medium.

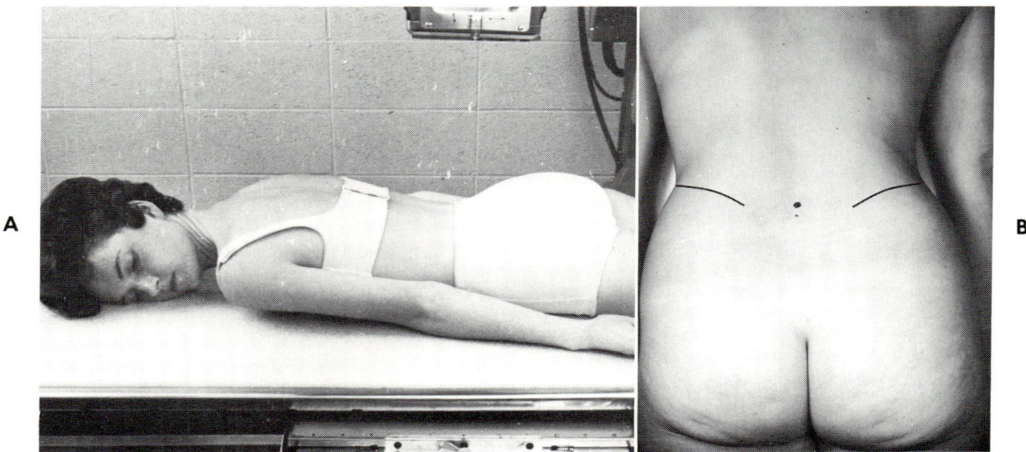

Fig. 13-20. Large intestine (colon). **A** and **B**, Anterior (P-A) positions.

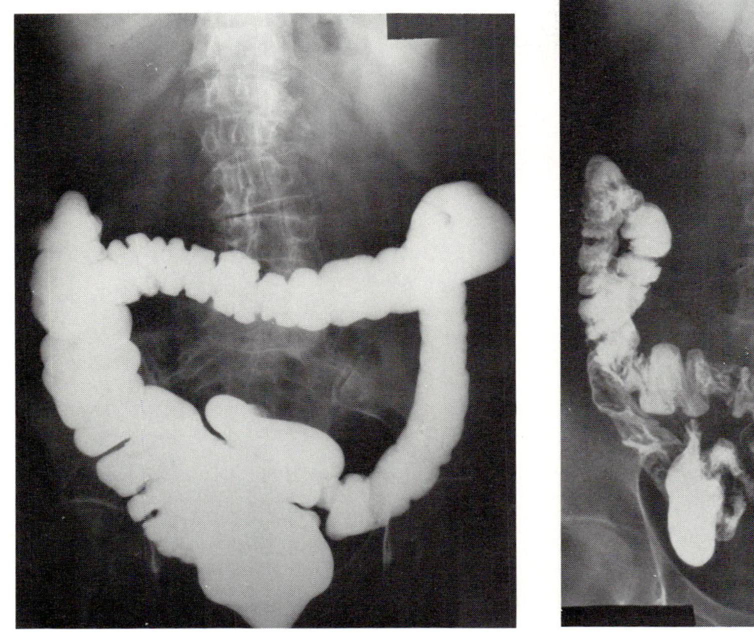

Fig. 13-21

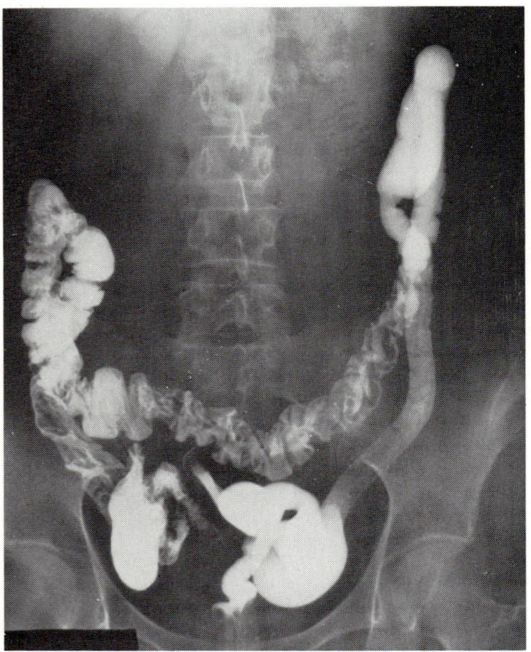

Fig. 13-22

Fig. 13-21. Large intestine (colon)—anterior (P-A) view, preevacuation. (Courtesy Dr. E. I. L. Cilley, Dr. T. W. Crowell, Dr. R. E. Waud, and Dr. G. H. Hoffman.)
Fig. 13-22. Large intestine (colon)—anterior (P-A) view, postevacuation. (Courtesy Dr. E. I. L. Cilley, Dr. T. W. Crowell, Dr. R. E. Waud, and Dr. G. H. Hoffman.)

FLUOROSCOPIC EXAMINATION

Large intestine—double contrast (D.C. colon) (Fig. 13-23)

Patient preparation

The patient is given the barium enema with the same procedure described in the preceding section (p. 410), except that after the scout (survey) film has been completed, instruct patient to ingest approximately 16 ounces of water in order to retard *flaking* (caused by dehydration) of the contrast medium in the colon.

Contrast medium

The contrast medium is the same as that used for the barium enema (p. 410).

Equipment preparation

The equipment needed is the same as that required for the barium enema (p. 410), except for the addition of a Bardex catheter with air insufflator.

Examination

The examination proceeds in the same manner as the barium enema study (p. 411), except that after the patient has eliminated approximately 50% of the barium sulfate mixture, air is injected by means of an air insufflator attached to the Bardex catheter. Fluoroscopy procedures are resumed, and appropriate preevacuation radiographs are made.

Note: Modern disposable barium enema containers will eliminate the need for the patient to evacuate intestinal contents in the lavatory.

Cholecystography

Cholecystography is a functional radiographic examination of the gallbladder by means of an orally ingested contrast medium.

Patient preparation

1. The patient's noon meal on the day before the examination should include two pats of butter or a fried egg.
2. The evening meal should be light and free of fatty foods, as directed on the package of contrast medium tablets.
3. The patient must take the contrast medium tablets with plenty of water approximately *12* hours prior to the examination:
   a. Sthenic (average build) patients require six tablets (ex.: Telepaque).
   b. Asthenic (thin, slender) patients require four tablets.
   c. Hypersthenic (large, obese) patients require eight to ten tablets.
4. On the morning of the examination, the patient must omit breakfast except for water, black coffee, or clear tea.
5. He must take an enema consisting of warm tap water, using an amount sufficient to produce a clear return.
6. When the patient is admitted, remove all garments except shoes and socks; provide a gown and instruct patient to tie open ends together in back.

Note: Recent commercial preparations that are prescribed by some departments and that are taken orally 15 to 18 hours prior to the examination eliminate the necessity for Step 5 (warm water enema).

Contrast media

Various commercial preparations (Telepaque, Oragrafin, or the like) may be purchased from local pharmacies by the patient or provided by the radiology department. (See Step 3 above.)

Note: Inform the patient that varying degrees of diarrhea may result from the ingestion of this type of contrast media, so that it may become necessary for him to control this reaction with some type of paregoric elixir.

Complications

Gas shadows may exist in the intestinal tract; they may be overcome by one of the following:

1. Breathing technique; inspiration or expiration
2. Rotation of the patient
3. Angulation (direction) of the central ray
4. Erect positions; gallbladder will drop approximately 2½ inches in the average-sized patient
5. Trendelenburg position (anterior, P-A); gallbladder will move slightly cephalad; gas shadows will rise caudad
6. Right lateral decubitus position; gallbladder will drop toward the right midaxillary region; gas shadows will rise toward medial plane
7. Use of Pitressin, carminative (a medium to relieve flatulence, gas) (Use 0.5 ml intradermal injection. **Caution: Permission must** be obtained from the referring physician.)

Contrast medium may be absent in the gallbladder; this may be caused by one on the following:

1. Functional disturbance of the patient
2. Gallbladder previously removed
3. Patient vomited contrast medium or had diarrhea
4. Contrast medium ingested too late
5. Improper patient preparation

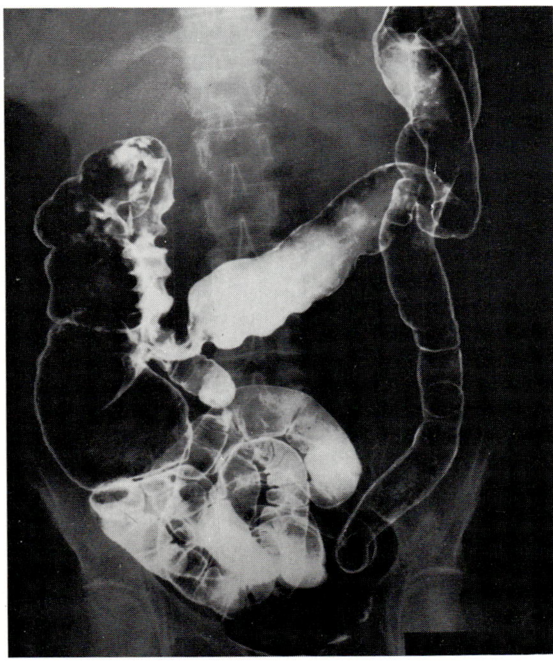

Fig. 13-23. Large intestine (colon)—anterior (P-A) view, air contrast, postevacuation. (Courtesy Dr. E. I. L. Cilley, Dr. T. W. Crowell, Dr. R. E. Waud, and Dr. G. H. Hoffman.)

ROUTINE RADIOGRAPHIC POSITIONS

Cholecystography (oral)—anterior (P-A) scout (survey) view (Figs. 13-24 and 13-25)

Functional examination
Film size (scout)–14″ × 17″
(regular)–8″ × 10″
Cassette
Lengthwise
Bucky (or grid)
Collimate to cover

Technique

Factors	Screen film cassette (par)	Screen film cassette (par) High kVp—16:1 grid
mA	300	200
Time	0.3	0.1
mAs	90	20
Thickness in cm	20	20
kVp	68	120
Distance	40	40

Palpation points

Spinous processes; lateral ribs.

Procedure

Place the patient in the prone position with the median plane of the body over the center line of the table. Rotate the patient's head toward the righ side. Extend the arms down the sides. Palpate the second lumbar spinous process and mark this point with a skin pencil. Center the cassette, with right marker, to the selected point.

Central ray

Direct the central ray perpendicular through a point 2 to 3 inches to the right of "L-2" to the center of the film holder. Collimate to film holder.

Immobilization

Employ suspended expiration. A compression band should be used to compress the viscera in obese patients.

Right-left markers

Place a right marker on the right lateral center border of the film holder.

Technical tips

For large or obese patients, center 2 to 3 inches higher than normal. For slender patients, center 2 to 3 inches lower than normal.

Structures demonstrated

Anterior (P-A) scout (survey) view of the abdomen demonstrating the degree of function and the location of the gallbladder by means of an orally ingested contrast medium.

Note: Locate the gallbladder on the radiograph by measuring from the center of the film holder, which is in line with the right marker and skin pencil mark on the patient.

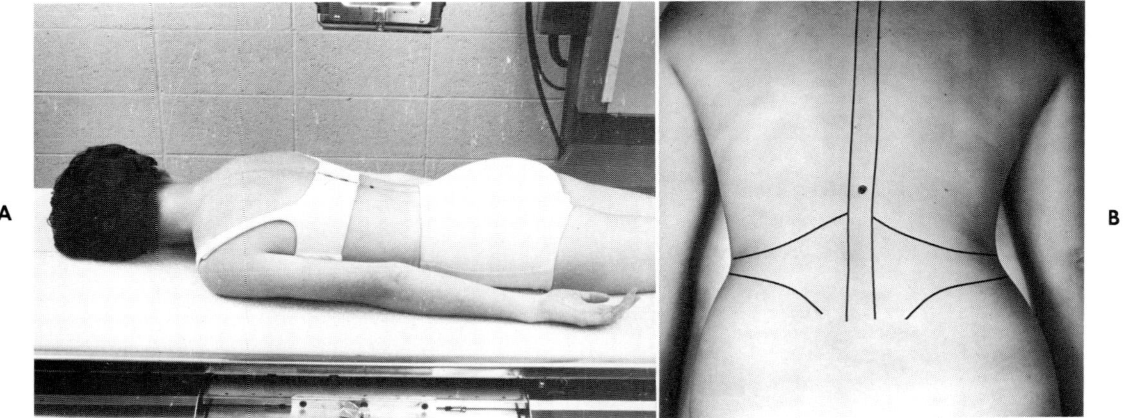

Fig. 13-24. Gallbladder. **A** and **B,** Anterior (P-A) scout positions.

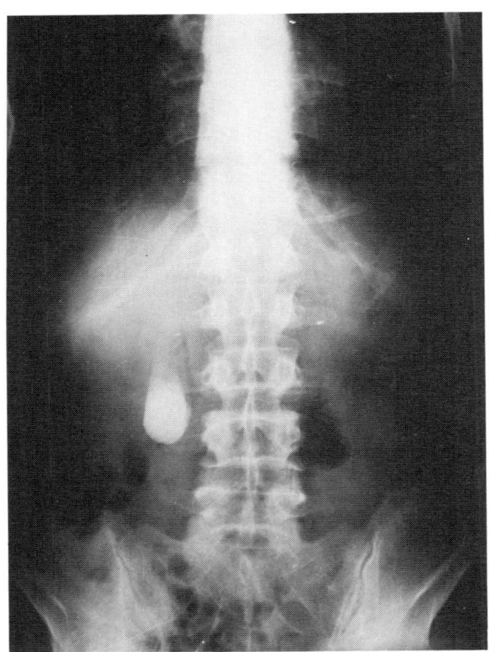

Fig. 13-25. Gallbladder–anterior (P-A) scout view. (Courtesy Dr. E. I. L. Cilley, Dr. T. W. Crowell, Dr. R. E. Waud, and Dr. G. H. Hoffman.)

Cholecystography (oral)—left anterior oblique (L.A.O.) view (Figs. 13-26 and 13-27)

Functional examination
Film size—8″ × 10″
Cassette
Lengthwise
Bucky (or grid)
Collimate to cover

Technique

Factors	Screen film cassette (par)	Screen film cassette (par) High kVp—16:1 grid
mA	300	300
Time	0.3	0.1
mAs	90	30
Thickness in cm	23	23
kVp	74	120
Distance	40	40

Palpation points

Spinous processes; lateral ribs.

Procedure

Place the patient in the prone position. Flex the right elbow and knee, rotating the patient into a 20- to 30-degree L.A.O. position. Center a point (transversely) halfway between the spinous processes and the right lateral rib margin over the center line of the table. Center the cassette (longitudinally) in line with the gallbladder (located from the scout film).

Central ray

Direct the central ray perpendicular to the center of the film holder. (See preceding note.) Collimate to film holder.

Immobilization

Employ suspended expiration.

Right-left markers

Markers are not necessary on this view.

Technical tips

1. Deep suspended *inspiration* may be used to move the gallbladder lower.
2. In large or obese patients, the gallbladder will usually move to the outer third of the lateral abdomen.
3. In slender patients, the gallbladder will usually remain close to the original anterior (P-A) location.
4. High kVp technique may be used to better visualize radiopaque stones.

Structures demonstrated

Left anterior oblique (L.A.O.) view of the abdomen demonstrating the degree of function and the location of the gallbladder (free from superimposed gas shadows) by means of an orally ingested contrast medium.

Note: For a variation of this view, direct the central ray 15 degrees caudad through the level of the gallbladder to the center of the film holder. When satisfactory preevacuation radiographs (free of superimposed gas shadows) have been completed, provide the patient with a commercial *fatty meal* (Neo-Cholex) preparation per instructions and repeat the radiograph film series (postevacuation) in 20 to 30 minutes.

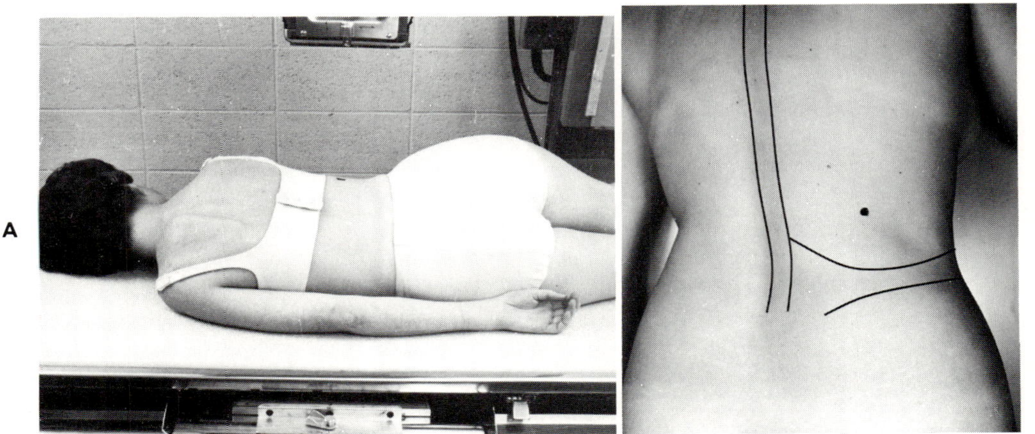

Fig. 13-26. Gallbladder. **A** and **B,** Left anterior oblique (L.A.O.) positions.

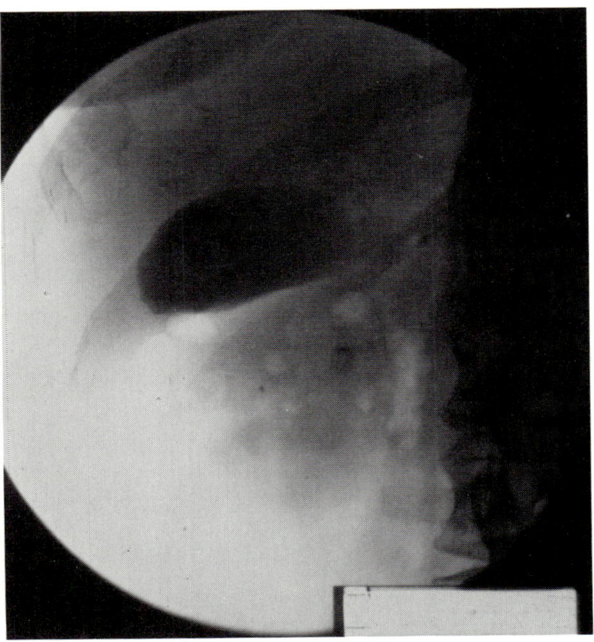

Fig. 13-27. Gallbladder—left anterior oblique (L.A.O.) view. (Scottsdale Memorial Hospital, Scottsdale, Arizona.)

Cholecystography (oral)—right lateral decubitus view (Figs. 13-28 and 13-29)

Functional examination
Film size—8″ × 10″
Grid cassette
Lengthwise

Bucky (or grid)
Collimate to cover

Technique

Factors	Screen film cassette (par)	Screen film cassette (par) High kVp—16:1 grid
mA	300	300
Time	0.3	0.1
mAs	90	30
Thickness in cm	23	23
kVp	74	120
Distance	40	40

Palpation points

Spinous processes; lateral ribs.

Procedure

Place the patient with his right side on the table. Place a fine-line grid-cassette on edge and against the abdomen with the film center in line with the gallbladder (located from scout film). The gallbladder tends to drop near the midaxillary line in this position, so consider this condition when centering.

Central ray

Direct the central ray perpendicular to the center of the film holder. Collimate to film holder.

Immobilization

Employ suspended expiration for one view and suspended inspiration for the second view.

Right-left markers

Place a *decubitus* marker on upper center border of film holder. *R* and *L* markers are not necessary on this view.

Technical tips

In large or obese patients, the gallbladder will usually move slightly superior. In slender patients, the gallbladder will move very close to the midaxillary line and slightly inferior.

Structures demonstrated

Right lateral decubitus (anterior, P-A) view of the right lateral abdomen, demonstrating the degree of function and the layering or stratification of small stones that may concentrate in the fundus of the gallbladder.

Note: When satisfactory preevacuation radiographs (free of superimposed gas shadows) have been completed, give the patient a *fatty meal* (commercial) preparation per instructions and repeat the film series (postevacuation) in 20 minutes.

The cystic duct may be demonstrated on some patients 5 to 10 minutes after the *fatty meal* (commercial) preparation has been ingested.

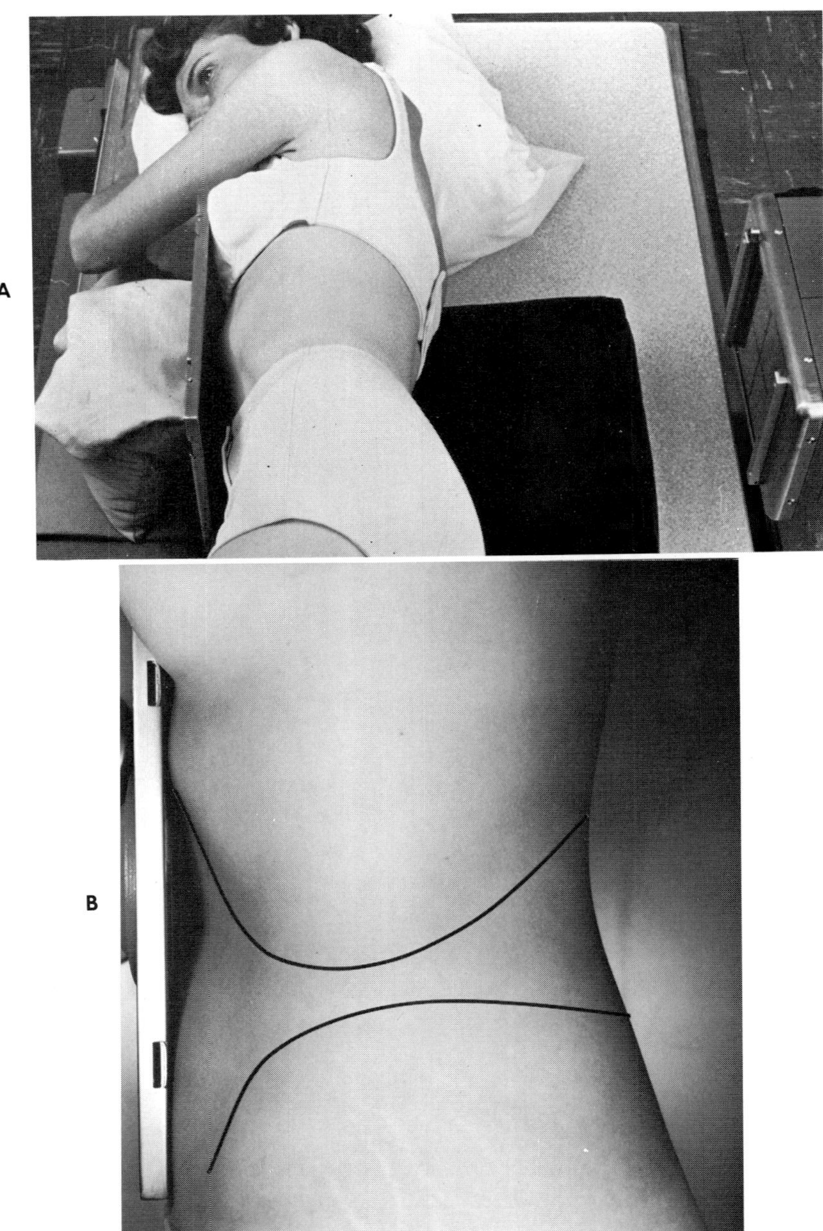

Fig. 13-28. Gallbladder. **A** and **B,** Right lateral decubitus positions.

Cholangiography

Cholangiography is the term used to describe the radiographic examination of the biliary tract. This examination is obtained by three methods: surgical cholangiography, postoperative cholangiography (T tube), and intravenous cholangiography. The purpose of the examination is to detect the presence of small stones or calculi in the bile ducts and, indirectly, to determine the patency of the cystic and common ducts and the condition of the choledochal sphincter.

Surgical cholangiography

Surgical cholangiography is a nonfunctional radiographic examination of the biliary ducts performed in surgery by means of a contrast medium injected directly into these ducts.

Patient preparation

Routine surgical preparation of the patient is performed by surgical personnel.

Contrast media

A sterile 20 cc syringe filled with Diodrast, Renografin, or another selected water-soluble urographic medium is prepared and provided by the surgical department.

Equipment preparation

Provide a mobile radiographic unit, extension cords, and a minimum of two 10″ × 12″ cassettes.

Examination

The cassette is positioned in the surgical table and the radiographic equipment is prepared before the patient arrives in surgery. The patient is positioned on the table in a posterior (A-P) or slight right posterior oblique (R.P.O) position under aseptic conditions by surgical personnel. After surgically exposing the biliary system, the surgeon aspirates existing bile and probes the biliary ducts for existing stones. The contrast medium is then injected and the sterile field is covered.

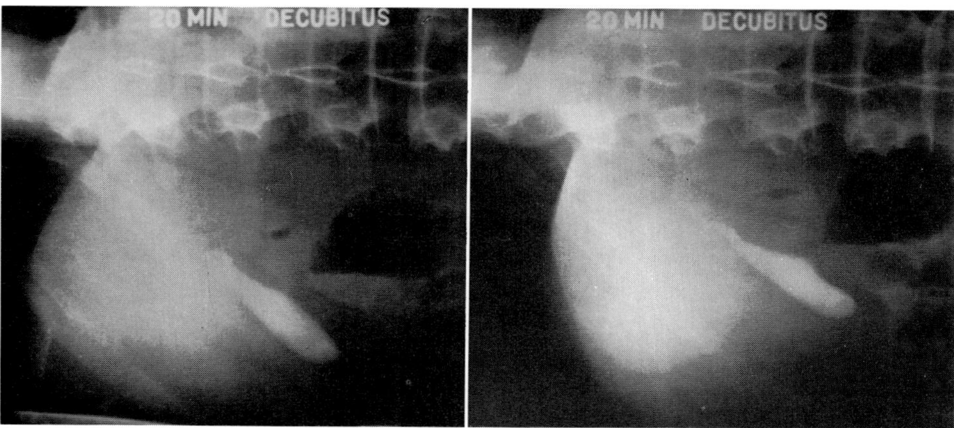

Fig. 13-29. Gallbladder—right lateral decubitus view with expiration and right lateral decubitus view with inspiration. (Courtesy Dr. E. I. L. Cilley, Dr. T. W. Crowell, Dr. R. E. Waud, and Dr. G. H. Hoffman.)

ROUTINE RADIOGRAPHIC POSITION

Surgical cholangiography—right posterior oblique (R.P.O.) view (Fig. 13-30)

Nonfunctional examination
Film size—10″ × 12″
Grid-cassette
Lengthwise
Bucky or film tunnel
Collimate to cover
Mobile radiographic unit

Technique

Factors	Screen film cassette (par)	Screen film cassette (par) High kVp—16:1 grid
mA	300	300
Time	0.3	0.1
mAs	90	30
Thickness in cm	23	23
kVp	74	120
Distance	40	40

Palpation point

The center of the biliary system is located by the surgeon.

Procedure

Move the preset mobile raidographic unit into position and make the exposure during the injection.

Central ray

Direct the central ray perpendicular to the center of the film holder. Collimate to film holder.

Immobilization

Employ suspended expiration if the patient is under spinal anesthesia; otherwise, a rapid exposure time is required.

Right-left markers

Preevacuation or postevacuation markers are placed on the right lateral center border of the film holder.

Structures demonstrated

Right posterior oblique (R.P.O.) view of the right abdominal cavity with the use of a contrast medium to detect the presence of small stones or calculi in the bile ducts, and, indirectly, to determine the patency of the cystic and common ducts, and the condition of the choledochal sphincter.

Note: Additional postevacuation radiographs may be required.

Postoperative cholangiography (choledochogram, T tube)

A nonfunctional, postoperative (10 days) radiographic examination of the bile ducts by means of a contrast medium injected, through a surgically implanted T tube, directly into the biliary system.

Patient preparation

1. The patient is usually instructed to follow a special regimen prescribed by the referring physician.
2. The evening meal should be light and free of fatty foods.
3. On the morning of the examination, the patient must omit breakfast except for water, black coffee, or clear tea.
4. On the morning of the examination he must take an enema consisting of warm tap water, using an amount sufficient to produec a clear return.
5. When the patient is admitted, remove all garments except shoes and socks. Provide a gown and instruct the patient to tie the open ends together in the front.
6. Make a 14″ × 17″ posterior (A-P) abdominal scout (survey) radiograph of the patient, centering at the iliac crest. (See p. 430.)

Contrast media

Fill a sterile 20 cc syringe with Diodrast or other selected contrast medium. (See Table 13-1.)

Equipment preparation

Place a radiolucent sponge mat on the tabletop for the patient's comfort. Provide the following items:

1. Sterile 20 cc syringe with contrast medium (see above)
2. Cannula (tapered)
3. Hemostat (clamp)
4. Emesis basin
5. Cotton sponges

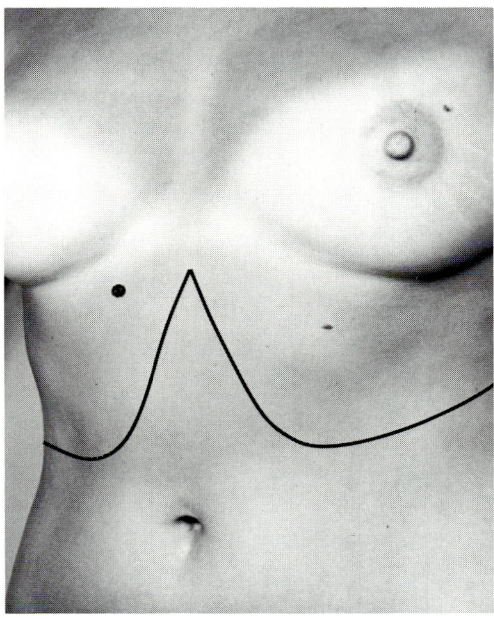

Fig. 13-30. Cholangiogram—posterior (R.P.O.) position.

Examination

1. After the scout (survey) radiograph has been completed, the following steps must be carried out:
   a. Expose the T tube (remove the tube tip from the bile receptacle) and insert the cannula into the opening of the T tube.
   b. Allow the bile to drain into the emesis basin. (Repeated deep respiration will aid in this.)
   c. Remove air bubbles from the tube by directing the tube in the vertical position; then clamp the tube with a hemostat.
   d. Insert the 20 cc syringe with contrast medium into the cannula orifice.
2. Inform the radiologist that you are prepared, and introduce the radiologist to the patient.
3. Assist the radiologist with lead gloves and lead apron.
4. The radiologist will release the clamp and inject the contrast medium (usually 10 ml).
5. The hemostat is applied and the first exposure is made as rapidly as possible.

Note: Additional injections and exposures may be necessary.

ROUTINE RADIOGRAPHIC POSITION

Postoperative cholangiography (choledochogram, T tube)—right posterior oblique (R.P.O.) view (Figs. 13-31 and 13-32)

Nonfunctional examination
Film size—10″ × 12″ (two)
Cassette
Lengthwise
Bucky
Collimate to cover

Technique

Factors	Screen film cassette (par) Regular kVp—12:1 grid	Screen film cassette (par) High kVp—16:1 grid
mA	300	300
Time	0.3	0.1
mAs	90	30
Thickness in cm	23	23
kVp	74	120
Distance	40	40

Palpation point

Xiphoid process of sternum.

Procedure

Place the patient in the supine position with the left side elevated approximately 35 degrees. Center a point midway between the xiphoid process and the right lateral ribs over the center line of the table. Center the cassette to a point in line with the tip of the xiphoid process.

Central ray

Direct the central ray perpendicular to the center of the film holder. Collimate to film holder.

Immobilization

Place a wedge-shaped positioning sponge (or sponges) beneath the elevated side. Employ suspended expiration for one exposure and suspended inspiration for the second exposure.

Right-left markers

Place numerical sequence markers on the right lateral center border of the film holder.

Structures demonstrated

Right posterior oblique (R.P.O.) view of the right abdominal cavity with the use of a contrast medium to detect the presence of small stones or calculi in the bile ducts (usually 10 days to 2 weeks after surgical removal of the gallbladder).

Note: A subsequent radiograph (postevacuation) is made after the contrast medium has been aspirated into the syringe by the radiologist.

Intravenous cholangiography

Intravenous cholangiography is a functional radiographic examination of the gallbladder by means of an intravenously injected contrast medium.

Patient preparation

1. The patient's noon meal on the day prior to the examination should include two pats of butter or a fried egg.
2. Between 3 and 5 P.M. on the day prior to the examination, the patient must take 2 ounces of castor oil or other prescribed laxative. *This may be disguised with root beer or orange juice.*

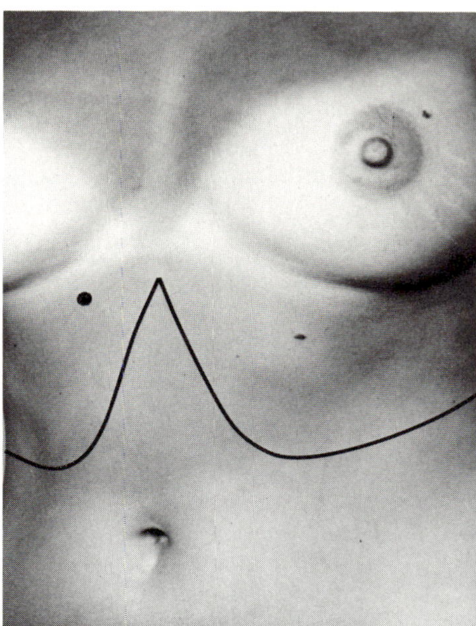

Fig. 13-31. Cholangiogram—posterior (R.P.O.) position.

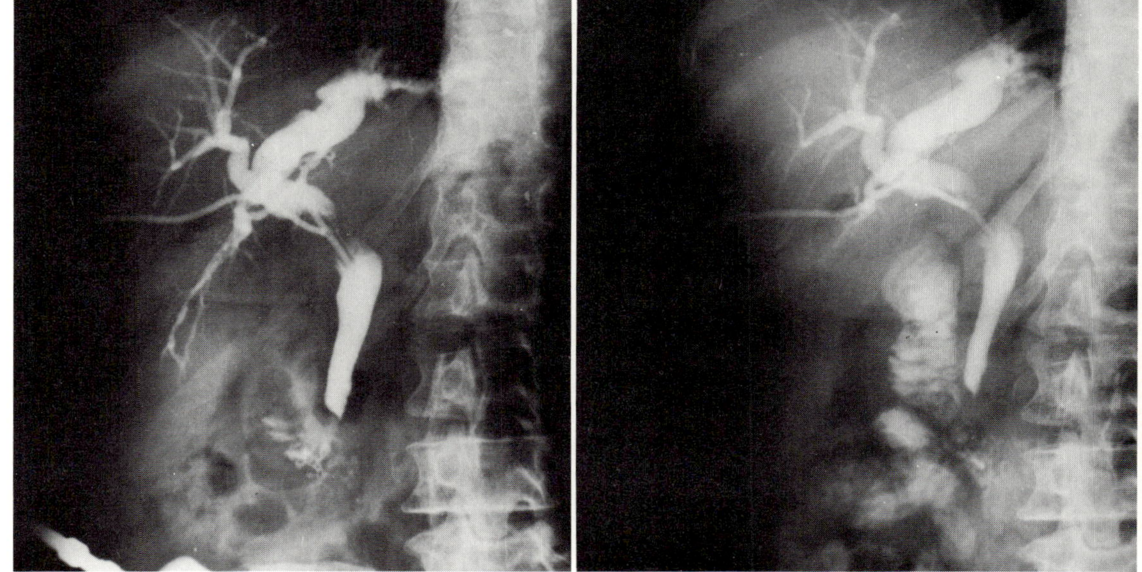

Fig. 13-32. Cholangiogram. **A** and **B,** Postoperative posterior (A-P) views. (Courtesy Dr. E. I. L. Cilley, Dr. T. W. Crowell, Dr. R. E. Waud, and Dr. G. H. Hoffman.)

3. The patient must have only clear liquids for the evening meal.
4. On the morning of the examination the patient must take an enema consisting of 1½ to 2 pints of warm soapsuds, followed by a warm water enema until the return is clear.
5. The patient must omit breakfast and all liquids on the morning of the examination.
6. When the patient is admitted, remove all garments except shoes and socks. Provide a short-sleeved gown, and instruct the patient to tie the open ends together in the back.
7. Make a 14″ × 17″ posterior (A-P) abdominal scout (survey) radiograph of the patient, centering at the iliac crest. (See p. 430.)

Contrast media

Fill a sterile 20 cc syringe with Cholografin sodium or another selected contrast medium. Fill a sterile 2 cc syringe with 1 ml of Cholografin sodium (test dose) or another selected contrast medium. (See Table 13-1.)

Equipment preparation

Place a radiolucent sponge mat on the tabletop for the patient's comfort. Provide the following items:

1. A sterile 20 cc syringe with contrast medium
2. A sterile 2 cc syringe with contrast medium *(test dose)*
3. A sterile 21-gauge × 1½-inch needle
4. A sterile 25-gauge × 1-inch needle
5. A sterile towel
6. A tourniquet and sandbag or sponge for support of the arm
7. Alcohol sponges
8. An emesis basin
9. An emergency kit *consisting in part of oxygen,* Adrenalin* [injectable], and Chlor-trimeton [injectable])

Examination

1. After the scout (survey) radiograph has been completed and checked, make the following preparations:
   a. Place a tourniquet around the upper right arm.
   b. Place a sandbag or sponge under the right extended elbow for support.
   c. Place an alcohol-dampened sponge on the antecubital space (anterior elbow surface).
   d. Place the 25-gauge needle on the sterile 2 cc syringe.
2. Inform the radiologist that you are prepared, and introduce the radiologist to the patient.
3. The radiologist will inject the test dose (1 ml); then approximately 10 minutes later he will inject the full dose from the loaded 20 cc syringe.

   Note: Contrast medium instructions caution that injection of the full dose should be made very slowly, over a 10-minute period. Rapid injection will produce nausea or vomiting or both.
4. For visualization of the ducts, serial 10-minute radiographs should be started 10 minutes after the injection.
5. Gallbladder studies may be started 2 hours after the injection.

---

*There are some objections to having Adrenalin on an emergency tray.

ROUTINE RADIOGRAPHIC POSITION

Intravenous cholangiography—posterior (A-P) view (Fig. 13-33)

Film size—10″ × 12″ (two)
Cassette
Lengthwise
Bucky
Collimate to cover

Technique

Factors	Screen film cassette (par) Regular kVp—12:1 grid	Screen film cassette (par) High kVp—16:1 grid
mA	300	300
Time	0.3	0.1
mAs	90	30
Thickness in cm	23	23
kVp	74	120
Distance	40	40

Palpation point

Xiphoid process of the sternum.

Procedure

Place the patient in the supine position with the left side elevated approximately 35 degrees. Center a point midway between the xiphoid process and the right lateral ribs over the center line of the table. Center the cassette to a point in line with the tip of the xiphoid process.

Central ray

Direct the central ray perpendicular to the center of the film holder. Collimate to film holder.

Immobilization

Place wedge-shaped positioning sponges beneath the elevated side. Employ suspended expiration.

Right-left markers

Place time-sequence markers on the right lateral center border of the film holder.

Structures demonstrated

Right posterior oblique (R.P.O.) view of the right abdominal cavity with the use of a contrast medium to detect the presence of small stones or calculi or other pathology or both in the bile ducts or gallbladder.

Note: For a variation of this view, direct the central ray 20 degrees cephalad through the level of the gallbladder to the center of the film holder.

If the patient has a nonfunctioning gallbladder, this method of administration of the contrast medium will not demonstrate the gallbladder or any defect causing the nonfunction.

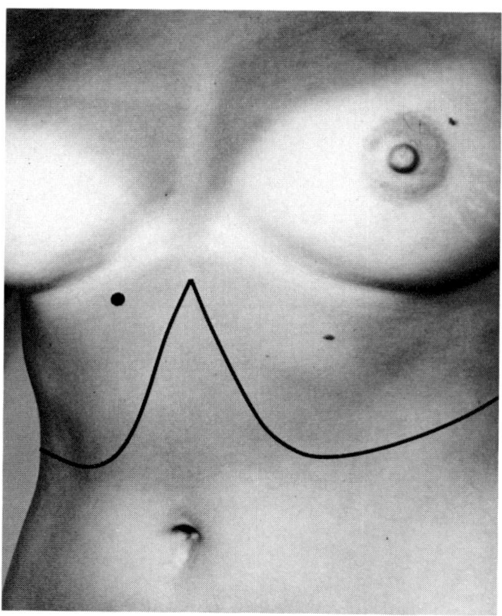

Fig. 13-33. Cholangiogram—posterior (R.P.O.) position.

ABDOMEN

The abdomen radiograph is a view of abdominal viscera that includes the gastrointestinal tract, pancreas, spleen, aorta, suprarenal glands, liver, and diaphragm. The abdomen radiographic exposure may be made with the patient in the horizontal, erect, or decubitus positions as a scout (survey) film for numerous radiographic series, acute abdominal conditions, or foreign bodies.

Abdomen—flat—posterior (A-P) or anterior (P-A) view (Fig. 13-34)

Film size—14″ × 17″
Cassette
Lengthwise

Bucky
Collimate to cover

Technique

Factors	Screen film cassette (par)	Screen film cassette (par) High kVp—16:1 grid
mA	300	200
Time	0.3	0.1
mAs	90	20
Thickness in cm	20	20
kVp	68	120
Distance	40	40

Patient preparation

Remove all garments except shoes and socks. Provide a gown and instruct the patient to tie the open ends together in the back.

Palpation point

Crest of the ilium.

Procedure

Place the patient in either the supine or prone position, with the median line of the body over the center line of the table. Center the film holder to the crest of the ilium.

Central ray

Direct the central ray perpendicular to the center of the film holder. Collimate to film holder.

Immobilization

For the supine position, elevate the knees with sponges for comfort. For the prone position, elevate the ankles with sponges for comfort. Use a compression band for obese patients. Employ suspended expiration.

Right-left markers

Place a right marker on the right lateral center border of the film holder.

Technical tips

Excellence in longitudinal positioning exists when the symphysis pubis is demonstrated as being transversely bisected by the lower film border.

Structures demonstrated

A posterior (A-P) or anterior (P-A) view of the abdominal viscera demonstrating conformation, size, and shape of the pancreas, spleen, aorta, suprarenal glands, liver, and diaphragm. It serves as an excellent scout (survey) view for intestinal obstructions, numerous tumor masses, calcifications, and foreign bodies.

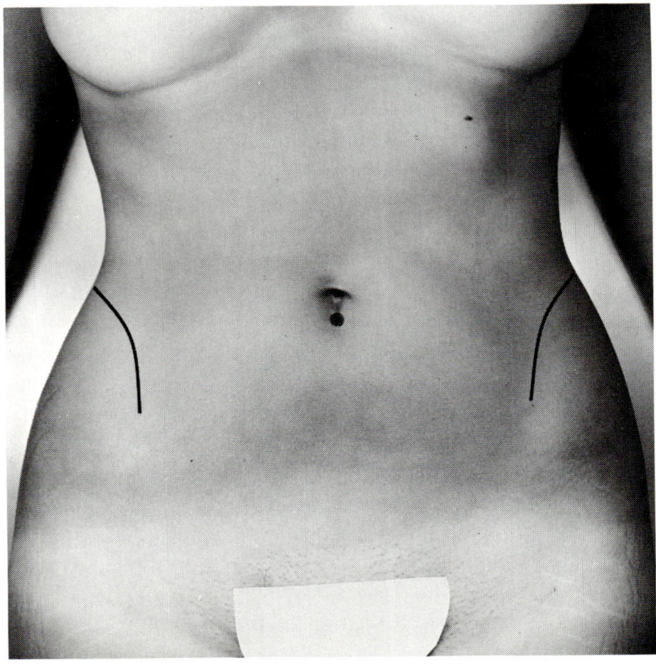

Fig. 13-34. Abdomen—flat—posterior (A-P) position.

Abdomen—erect—anterior (P-A) view (Fig. 13-35)

Film size—14" × 17"
Cassette
Lengthwise

Erect Bucky
Collimate to cover

Technique

Factors	Screen film cassette (par)	Screen film cassette (par) High kVp—16:1 grid
mA	300	300
Time	0.3	0.1
mAs	90	30
Thickness in cm	23	23
kVp	74	120
Distance	40	40

Patient preparation

Remove all garments except shoes and socks. Provide a gown and instruct the patient to tie the open ends together in the back.

Palpation point

Crest of the ilium.

Procedure

Place the table in the erect (vertical) position and instruct the patient to stand facing the table with the median line of the body over the center line of the table. Extend the arms along the sides with the hands grasping the edge of the table. Center the film holder 1 inch above the crest of the ilium.

Central ray

Direct the central ray horizontal and perpendicular to the center of the film holder. Collimate to film holder.

Immobilization

Use a compression band. Employ suspended expiration.

Right-left markers

Place a right-erect marker on the right lateral center border of the film holder.

Technical tips

It is necessary to include the *diaphragm* in the radiograph, since the free air will rise to and be under it, so adjust the film holder centering to accommodate the size of the patient.

Structures demonstrated

Anterior (P-A) erect view of the abdominal viscera to include the diaphragm for the demonstration of free air under the diaphragm, and for visualization of fluid levels.

Note: Many routines call for both the erect (upright) and the horizontal flatplate abdomen radiographs.

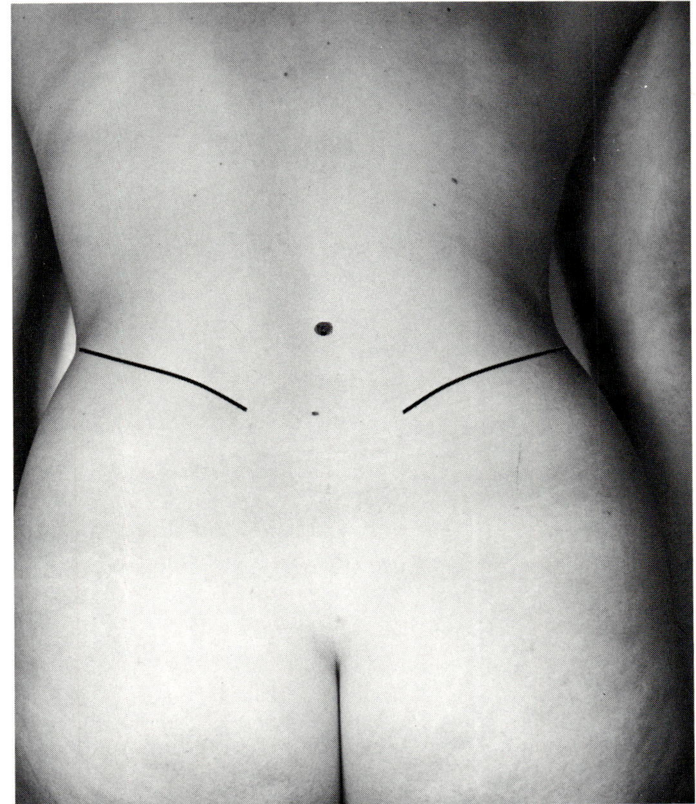

Fig. 13-35. Abdomen—erect—anterior (P-A) position.

Abdomen—lateral decubitus—right or left view

A decubitus position refers to a situation wherein the skin of a given surface of the body is in contact with the tabletop. The patient is horizontal and the central ray is horizontal. Thus a left anterior decubitus position has the left side down and the anterior surface of the body next to the film; the central ray passes from dorsal to ventral (posterior to anterior) to the film.

Film size—14″ × 17″
Cassette
Lengthwise
Erect Bucky
Collimate to cover

Technique

Factors	Screen film cassette (par)	Screen film cassette (par) High kVp—16:1 grid
mA	300	200
Time	0.3	0.1
mAs	90	20
Thickness in cm	20	20
kVp	68	120
Distance	40	40

Patient preparation

Remove all garments except shoes and socks. Provide a gown and instruct the patient to tie the open ends together in the back.

Palpation point

Crest the ilium.

Procedure

Place the table in an erect (vertical) position. Place the patient in the desired lateral position on a stretcher or gurney, which may be rolled to the table. Flex lower elbow beneath pillow. Position the stretcher or gurney so that the crest of the ilium is aligned over the center line of the table, then secure the wheel locks.

Central ray

Direct the central ray horizontal and perpendicular through the median line of the body to the center of the film holder. Collimate to film holder.

Immobilization

Instruct the patient to grasp the edge of the table with his upper hand. Employ suspended expiration.

Right-left markers

Place the correct decubitus marker on the upper lateral center border of the film holder.

Structures demonstrated

Anterior (P-A) or posterior (A-P) lateral decubitus view of the abdominal viscera for demonstration of free air and for visualization of fluid levels.

URINARY EXCRETORY SYSTEM

Radiographic examinations of the urinary excretory system include views of the kidneys, ureters, urinary bladder, and urethra. The examinations are the K.U.B., intravenous pyelogram, retrograde pyelogram, and retrograde urethrogram.

K.U.B.

A K.U.B. is a two-film radiographic scout (survey) examination of the kidneys, ureters, and urinary bladder without the use of contrast media.

ROUTINE RADIOGRAPHIC POSITION

K.U.B.—posterior (A-P) view (Figs. 13-36 and 13-37)

Film size—14″ × 17″ (two)
Cassette
Lengthwise
Bucky
Collimate to cover

Technique

Factors	Screen film cassette (par)	Screen film cassette (par) High kVp—16:1 grid
mA	300	200
Time	0.3	0.1
mAs	90	20
Thickness in cm	20	20
kVp	68	120
Distance	40	40

Patient preparation

Remove all garments except shoes and socks. Provide a gown and instruct the patient to tie the open ends together in the back.

Note: If the examination is prescheduled, instruct patient to follow *Patient preparation instructions* per intravenous pyelography (p. 438).

Palpation point

Crest of the ilium.

Procedure

Place the patient in the supine position with the median line of the body over the center line of the table. For the first view, center the first film holder to the crest of the ilium. For the second view, center the second film holder 3 inches above the crest of the ilium.

Central ray

Direct the central ray perpendicular to the center of the film holder for each view. Collimate to film holder.

Immobilization

Elevate the knees with sponges for patient comfort. A compression band may be used across large or obese patients. Employ suspended expiration for each view.

Right-left markers

Place a right marker on the right lateral center border of the film holder.

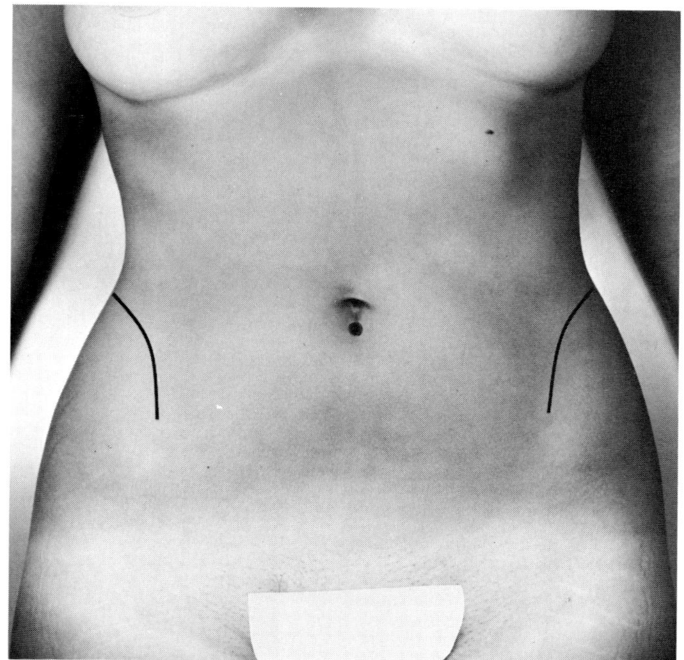

Fig. 13-36. K.U.B.—posterior (A-P) lower abdomen position.

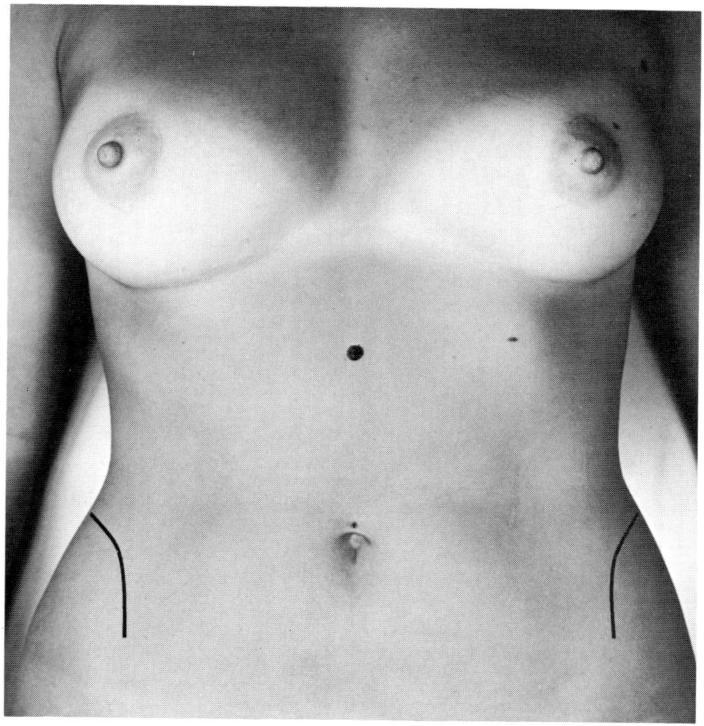

Fig. 13-37. K.U.B.—posterior (A-P) upper abdomen position.

Structures demonstrated

A posterior (A-P) view (two-film scout-survey series) of the abdomen demonstrating stones, calcifications, and certain tumor masses associated with kidneys, ureters, and urinary bladder without the aid of a contrast medium.

Intravenous pyelography (I.V.P.)

Intravenous pyelography is a functional radiographic examination of the kidneys, ureters, and urinary bladder with the use of an intravenously injected contrast medium.

Patient preparation

1. Between 3 and 5 P.M. on the afternoon before the examination the patient must take 2 ounces of castor oil or other prescribed laxative. *This may be disguised with root beer or orange juice.*
2. He may have clear liquids only for the evening meal preceding the day of the examination.
3. On the morning of the examination the patient must take an enema consisting of 1½ to 2 pints of warm soapsuds, followed by a warm water enema until the return is clear.
4. On the morning of the examination, the patient must restrict breakfast to a slice of toast and a half-cup of liquid. He may *not* drink any other liquids that morning.
5. When the patient is admitted, remove all garments except shoes and socks. Provide a short-sleeved gown and instruct the patient to tie the open ends together in the back.
6. Make a 14″ × 17″ posterior (A-P) abdominal scout (survey) radiograph of the patient, centering at the iliac crest. (See p. 430.)

Contrast media

Fill a sterile 2 cc syringe with 1 ml (test dose) of Renografin, Hypaque sodium, or another selected water soluble urographic medium. (See Table 13-1.) Fill a sterile 20 or 30 cc syringe with the identical type of contrast medium as used for the test dose.

Equipment preparation

Place a radiolucent sponge mat on the table top for the patient's comfort. Provide the following items:

1. A sterile 2 cc syringe with contrast medium (test dose)
2. A sterile 20 or 30 cc syringe with contrast medium
3. A sterile 25-gauge × 1-inch needle (test dose)
4. A sterile 21-gauge × 1½-inch needle (main dose)
5. A sterile 18-gauge × 1½-inch needle (filler)
6. A sterile towel
7. A tourniquet and sandbag or sponge for support of the arm
8. Alcohol sponges
9. An emesis basin
10. A compression band and I.V.P. block
11. An emergency kit (*consisting in part of* oxygen, Adrenalin [injectable], and Chlor-trimeton [injectable])

Examination

1. After scout (survey) radiograph has been completed and checked, make the following preparations:
   a. Place a tourniquet around the upper right arm.
   b. Place sandbags or sponges under the right extended elbow for support.

   c. Place alcohol-dampened sponge on antecubital space (anterior elbow surface).
   d. Position the I.V.P. compression block between the anterior superior iliac spines and hold in place with compression band. *Do not tighten compression band.*
   e. Place a 25-gauge needle on the sterile 2 cc syringe and the 21-gauge needle on the sterile 20 or 30 cc syringe.
2. Inform the radiologist that you are prepared, and introduce the radiologist to the patient.
3. The radiologist will inject the test dose (1 ml), then approximately 10 minutes later he will inject the full dose from the loaded 20 or 30 cc syringe.
4. Immediately after the main injection, apply firm pressure to the I.V.P. block with the compression band and position the table 10 degrees Trendelenburg.

   Note: Some radiologists prefer not to use compression or Trendelenburg positioning.
5. An acceptable radiographic routine series is as follows:
   a. 5 minutes after injection (with pressure)
   b. 15 minutes after injection (with pressure)
   c. 25 minutes after injection (with pressure released)
   d. 35 minutes after injection (erect postvoiding without pressure)

   Note: For hypertensive patients, the radiographic routine series should be 1, 2, and 3 minutes. Also, a 90 cc bolus injection may be preferred by the radiologist.

ROUTINE RADIOGRAPHIC POSITION

Intravenous pyelography (I.V.P.)—posterior (A-P) view (Figs. 13-38 to 13-40)

Film size—14″ × 17″
Cassette
Lengthwise

Bucky
Collimate to cover

Technique

Factors	Screen film cassette (par)	Screen film cassette (par) High kVp—16:1 grid
mA	300	200
Time	0.3	0.1
mAs	90	20
Thickness in cm	20	20
kVp	68	120
Distance	40	40

Palpation point

Crest of the ilium.

Procedure

With the patient remaining in the supine position and with the median line of the body over the center line of the table, center the film holder to the crest of the ilium.

Central ray

Direct the central ray perpendicular to the center of the film holder. Collimate to film holder.

Immobilization

With the compression band and I.V.P. block in place and firm pressure applied to the abdomen, employ suspended expiration.

Right-left markers

Place the right and correct time-interval markers on the right lateral center border of the film holder.

Structures demonstrated

Posterior (A-P) view (5-film routine series) of the posterior abdomen with the use of an injectable contrast medium to *functionally* demonstrate stones, calcifications tumor masses, and other pathology associated with the kidneys, ureters, and urinary bladder.

Note: For female patients within the childbearing age, cover the pelvis with lead protection and use a 10″ × 12″ film holder *crosswise,* aligning the bottom edge of the film holder with the crest of the ilium for the 5- and 15-minute views.

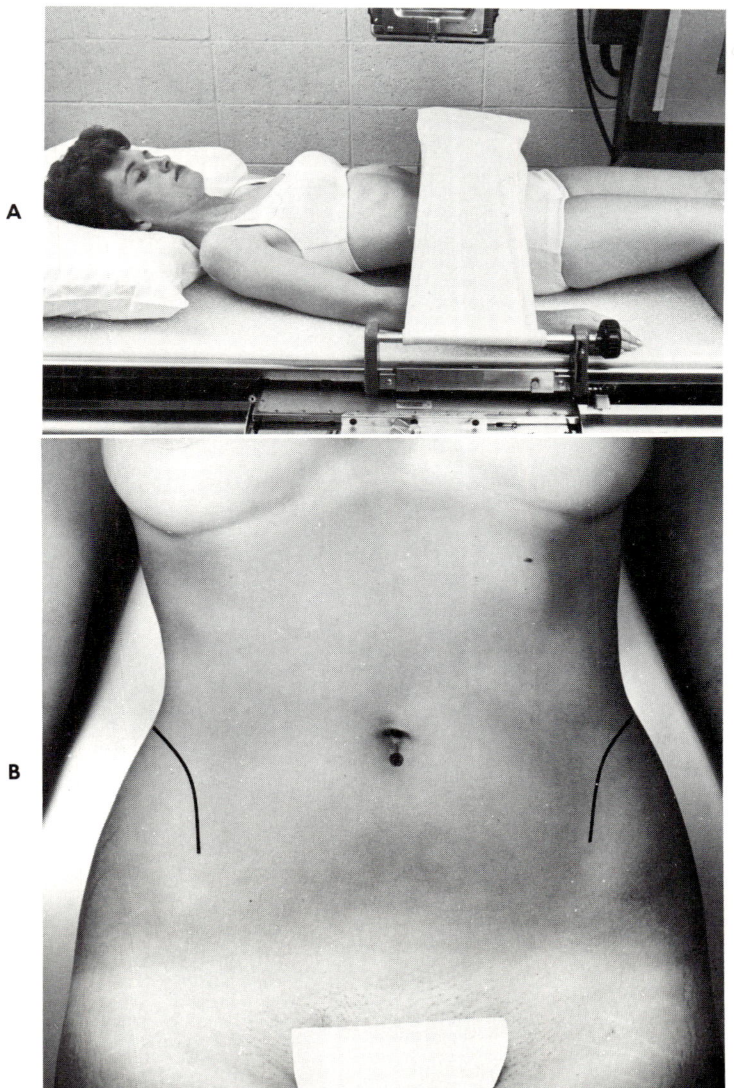

Fig. 13-38. Intravenous pyelography. **A** and **B,** Posterior (A-P) positions.

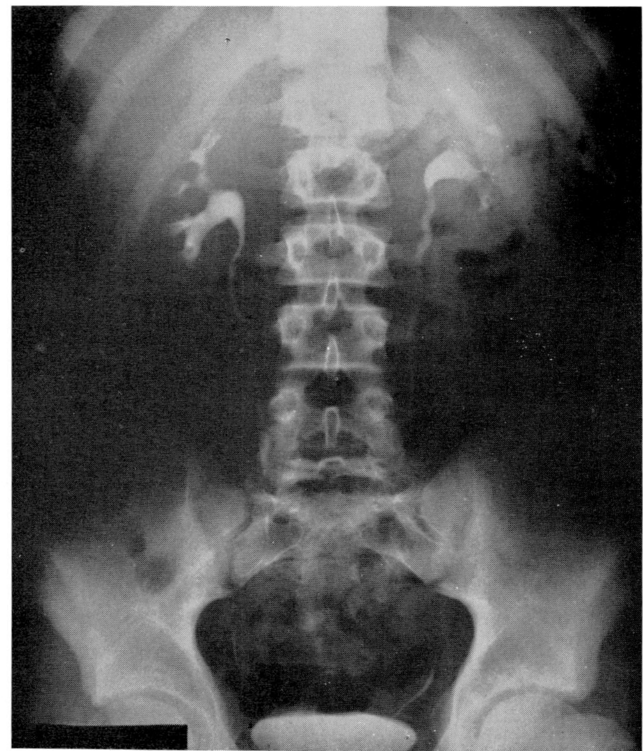

Fig. 13-39. Intravenous pyelogram—posterior (A-P) view. (Courtesy Dr. E. I. L. Cilley, Dr. T. W. Crowell, Dr. R. E. Waud, and Dr. G. H. Hoffman.)

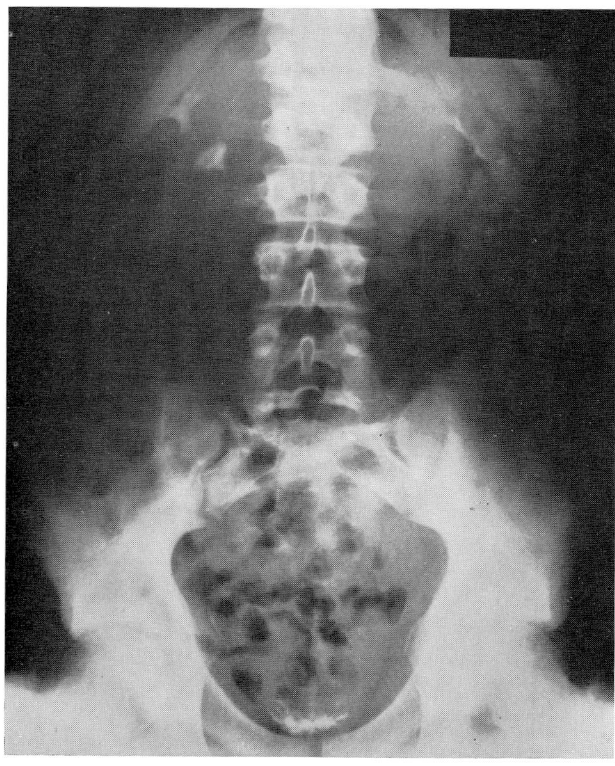

Fig. 13-40. Intravenous pyelogram—erect posterior (A-P) view, postevacuation. (Courtesy Dr. E. I. L. Cilley, Dr. T. W. Crowell, Dr. R. E. Waud, and Dr. G. H. Hoffman.)

Retrograde pyelography—renal pelves and ureters

Retrograde pyelography is a nonfunctional radiographic examination of the kidneys, ureters, urinary bladder, and urethra with the use of a contrast medium injected through ureteral catheters.

Patient preparation

1. Between 3 and 5 P.M. on the afternoon before the examination the patient must take 2 ounces of castor oil or other prescribed laxative. *This may be disguised with root beer or orange juice.*
2. He may have clear liquids only for the evening meal.
3. On the morning of the examination the patient must take an enema consisting of 1½ to 2 pints of soapsuds, followed by a warm water enema until the return is clear.
4. The patient must be instructed to omit breakfast and to drink copious amounts of water a few hours prior to the examination (for urine specimens).
5. Routine surgical preparation of the genitourinary region is performed by surgical personnel.
6. Make a 14″ × 17″ posterior (A-P) abdominal scout (survey) radiograph of the patient, centering at the iliac crest. (See p. 430.)

Contrast media

Diodrast, Renografin, or another selected water-soluble urographic medium along with a sterilized urographic-retrograde instrument kit is provided by the surgical department.

Equipment preparation

Provide a cystoscopic-radiographic unit or suitable table with leg stirrups, and a minimum of four loaded 14″ × 17″ cassettes.

Examination

The patient is placed in a posterior (A-P) position on the cystoscopy table with the thighs abducted, knees flexed and resting in leg stirrups. A sterile field is prepared around the genitourinary region by the doctor or assistants. A urethral catheter is inserted and a urine specimen collected. A cystoscopic examination is performed, and ureteral catheters are inserted, usually as far as the ureteropelvic junction. A scout radiograph is made to demonstrate catheter placement. The contrast medium is then injected. An acceptable radiographic routine series is as follows:

1. A scout (survey) radiograph of the abdomen
2. A radiograph demonstrating the catheters in position
3. A radiograph demonstrating the ureters
4. A radiograph after the contrast medium has been injected and the catheters removed

ROUTINE RADIOGRAPHIC POSITION

Retrograde pyelography—renal pelves and ureters, posterior (A-P) view
(Figs. 13-41 and 13-42)

Film size—14″ × 17″
Cassette
Lengthwise
Bucky
Collimate to cover

Technique

Factors	Screen film cassette (par)	Screen film cassette (par) High kVp—16:1 grid
mA	300	200
Time	0.3	0.1
mAs	90	20
Thickness in cm	20	20
kVp	68	120
Distance	40	40

Palpation point

Crest of the ilium.

Procedure

The patient remains in the supine position with the median line of the body over the center line of the table. The crest of the ilium is precentered over the center line of the fixed Bucky.

Central ray

The central ray is automatically precentered to the fixed Bucky. Collimate to film holder.

Immobilization

Knees are secured in the leg stirrups. Use a compression band if necessary. Employ suspended expiration.

Right-left markers

Place the right marker on the right lateral center border of the film holder.

Structures demonstrated

Posterior (A-P) views (four-film routine series) of the posterior abdomen with the use of a contrast medium injected through ureteral catheters to demonstrate stones, calcifications, tumor masses, and other pathology associated with the kidneys, ureters, urinary bladder, and urethra.

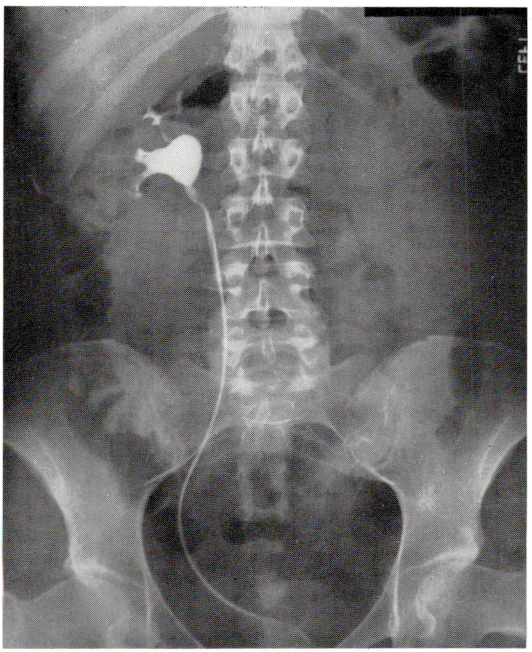

Fig. 13-41. Retrograde pyelogram—posterior (A-P) view. (Courtesy Dr. E. I. L. Cilley, Dr. T. W. Crowell, Dr. R. E. Waud, and Dr. G. H. Hoffman.)

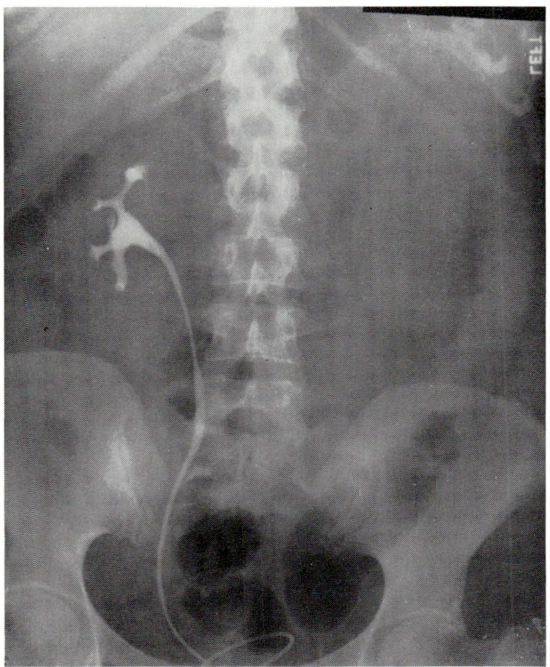

Fig. 13-42. Retrograde pyelogram—posterior (A-P) view. (Courtesy Dr. E. I. L. Cilley, Dr. T. W. Crowell, Dr. R. E. Waud, and Dr. G. H. Hoffman.)

Retrograde urography—urinary bladder (cystogram)

A retrograde cystogram is a nonfunctional radiographic examination of the urinary bladder with the use of a contrast medium injected through a urethral catheter. This examination may be performed on any regular radiographic table.

Patient preparation

1. In some cases the preparation may be as extensive as that for the intravenous pyelogram (p. 438); in most cases, however, a routine warm water enema prior to the examination is sufficient.
2. When the patient is admitted, remove all garments except shoes and socks. Provide a gown and instruct the patient to tie the open ends together in the front.
3. Instruct the patient that the bladder must be voided prior to the examination.
4. Make a 10″ × 12″ posterior (A-P) pelvic scout (survey) radiograph, centering the film holder (lengthwise), with the central ray 1 inch above the greater trochanter.

Contrast media

Dilute approximately 75 ml of Renografin, Hypaque sodium, or another selected water-soluble urographic medium (Table 13-1) with an equal volume of sterile water.

Equipment preparation

Provide the following items:

1. A sterile 50 cc syringe
2. A sterile urethral catheter
3. A sterile two-way stopcock
4. A hemostat (clamp)
5. A sterile kidney basin
6. Adhesive tape
7. Bandage shears

Examination

After the scout (survey) radiograph has been completed and checked, the doctor will introduce a urethral catheter. The bladder will be drained and then irrigated. The contrast medium will be injected through the catheter until the bladder capacity has been reached. The catheter will be clamped and taped to the thigh (usually the left one).

ROUTINE RADIOGRAPHIC POSITIONS

Posterior (A-P), right oblique, and left oblique are the usual routine positions.

Retrograde urography—urinary bladder (cystogram), posterior (A-P) view (Figs. 13-43 and 13-44)

Film size—10″ × 12″
Cassette
Lengthwise

Bucky
Collimate to cover

Technique

Factors	Screen film cassette (par)	Screen film cassette (par) High kVp—16:1 grid
mA	300	200
Time	0.3	0.1
mAs	90	20
Thickness in cm	20	20
kVp	68	120
Distance	40	40

Palpation point

Greater trochanter of the femur.

Procedure

The patient remains in the supine position with the median line of the body over the center line of the table. Center the film holder 1 inch above the greater trochanter.

Central ray

Direct the central ray 15 degrees caudad to the center of the film holder. Collimate to film holder.

Immobilization

Employ suspended expiration.

Right-left markers

Place the right marker on the right lateral center border of the film holder.

Structures demonstrated

Posterior (A-P) view of the pelvic region with the use of a catheter-injected contrast medium to demonstrate stones, calcifications, tumor masses, and other pathology associated with the urinary bladder.

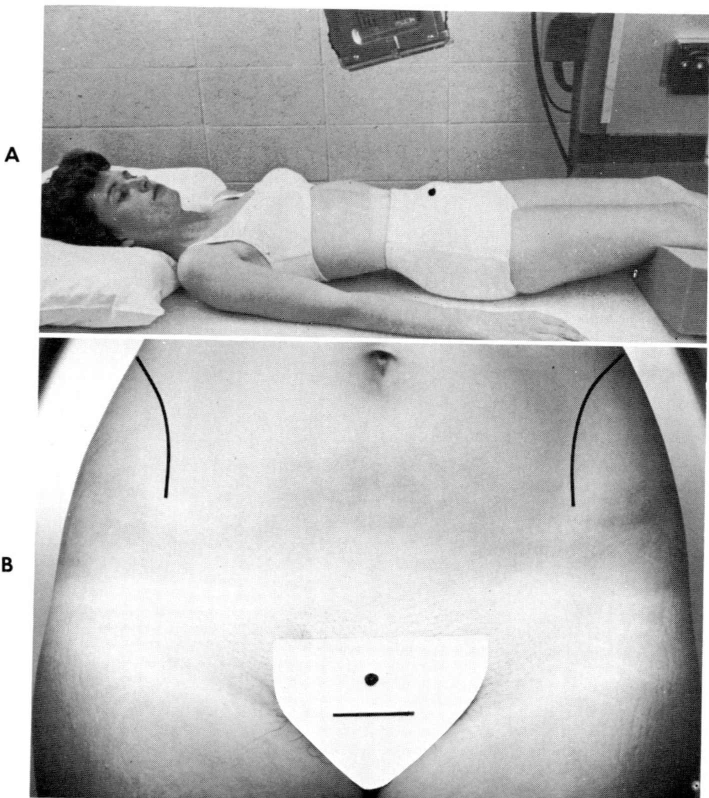

Fig. 13-43. Cystography. **A** and **B**, Posterior (A-P) positions.

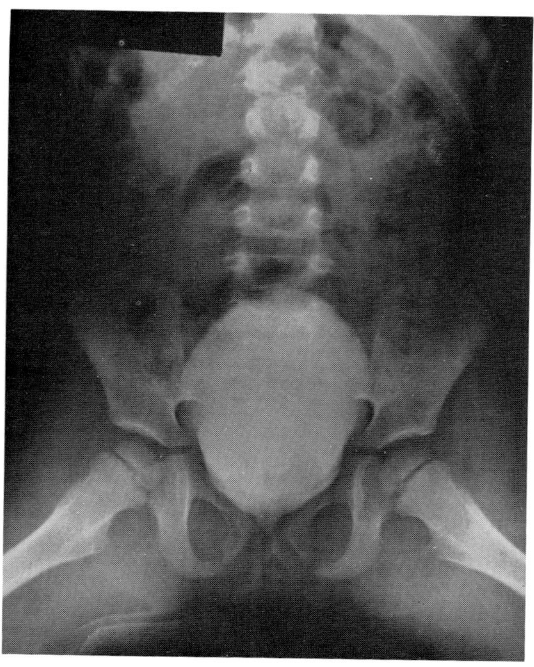

Fig. 13-44. Cystogram—posterior (A-P) view. (Courtesy Dr. E. I. L. Cilley, Dr. T. W. Crowell, Dr. R. E. Waud, and Dr. G. H. Hoffman.)

Retrograde urography—urinary bladder (cystograms), right posterior oblique (R.P.O.) view (Figs. 13-45 and 13-46)

Film size—10″ × 12″
Cassette
Lengthwise
Bucky
Collimate to cover

Technique

Factors	Screen film cassette (par)	Screen film cassette (par) High kVp—16:1 grid
mA	300	300
Time	0.3	0.1
mAs	90	30
Thickness in cm	23	23
kVp	74	120
Distance	40	40

Palpation points

Greater trochanter of the femur; anterior superior iliac spines.

Procedure

From the supine position, elevate the left side of the body 45 degrees. Flex the right knee, placing the right ankle under the opposite leg. Have the patient grasp the right side of the table with the left hand. Center a point midway between the anterior superior iliac spines over the center line of the table. Center the film holder 1 inch superior to the greater trochanter.

Central ray

Direct the central ray perpendicular to the center of the film holder. Collimate to film holder.

Immobilization

Place wedge-shaped positioning sponges beneath the elevated side. Employ suspended expiration.

Right-left markers

Place an R.P.O. marker on the right lateral center border of the film holder.

Structures demonstrated

Right posterior oblique (R.P.O.) view of the pelvic region with the use of a catheter-injected contrast medium to demonstrate stones, calcifications, tumor masses, and other pathology associated with or contained within the urinary bladder. The prostate gland and urethra may also be demonstrated.

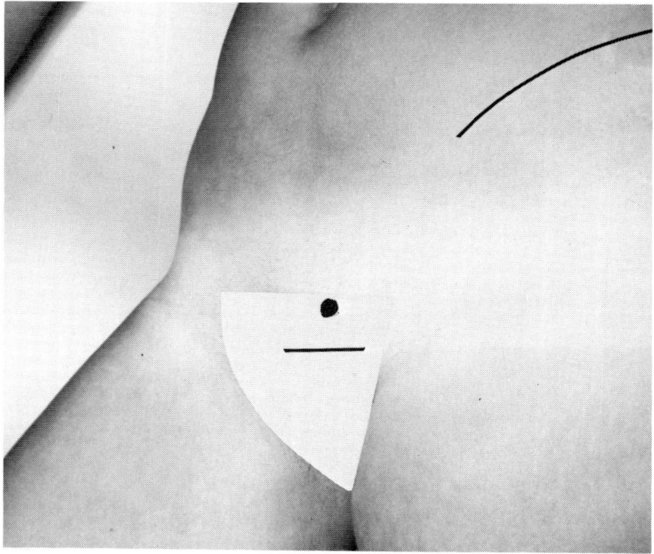

Fig. 13-45. Retrograde urogram—urinary bladder (cystogram), right posterior oblique (R.P.O.) position.

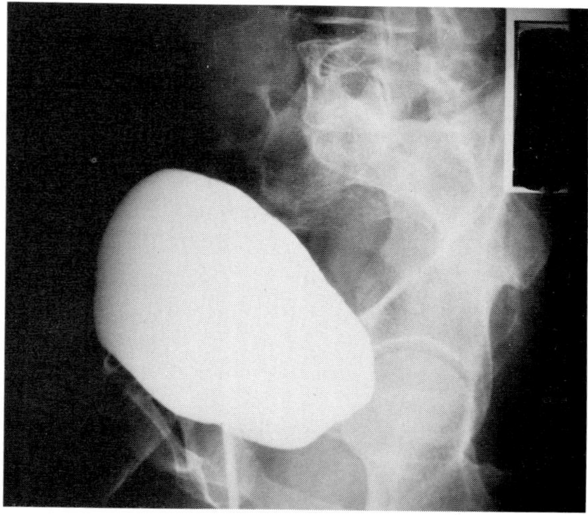

Fig. 13-46. Retrograde urogram—urinary bladder (cystogram), right posterior oblique (R.P.O.) view. (Courtesy Scottsdale Memorial Hospital, Scottsdale, Arizona.)

Retrograde urography—urinary bladder (cystogram), left posterior oblique (L.P.O.) view

This view is the reverse of the preceding view.

Retrograde urography—urethra and prostate (urethrography)

A retrograde urethrogram is a nonfunctional radiographic examination of the urethra with the use of a contrast medium injected through a urethral catheter. This examination may be performed on any regular radiographic table.

Patient preparation

1. When the patient is admitted, remove all garments except shoes and socks. Provide a gown and instruct the patient to tie the open ends together in the front.
2. Instruct the patient that the bladder must be voided prior to the examination.
3. Make a 10″ × 12″ posterior (A-P) pelvic scout (survey) radiograph, centering the film holder (lengthwise), with the central ray in line with the greater trochanter.

Contrast media

Dilute approximately 25 ml of Renografin, Hypaque sodium, or another selected water-soluble urographic medium (Table 13-1) with an equal volume of sterile water.

Equipment preparation

Provide the following items:

1. A sterile 30 or 50 cc syringe
2. A sterile urethral catheter
3. A sterile two-way stopcock
4. A hemostat (clamp)
5. A sterile kidney basin
6. Adhesive tape
7. Bandage shears

Examination

After the scout (survey) radiograph has been completed and checked, the doctor will introduce a urethral catheter. The bladder will be drained and then irrigated. (Radiographic positioning and procedure must now be readied; see the following position.) The doctor next inserts a urethral syringe into the orifice of the urethra and prepares to inject the contrast medium.

ROUTINE RADIOGRAPHIC POSITION

Retrograde urography—urethra and prostate, bicycle view (Fig. 13-47)

Film size—10″ × 12″
Cassette
Crosswise
Bucky
Collimate to cover

Technique

Factors	Screen film cassette (par)	Screen film cassette (par) High kVp—16:1 grid
mA	300	200
Time	0.15	0.05
mAs	45	10
Thickness in cm	16	16
kVp	64	120
Distance	40	40

Palpation points

Greater trochanter of the femur; symphysis pubis.

Procedure

From the supine position, elevate the left side of the body approximately 35 degrees. Flex the right knee, placing the right ankle under the opposite leg. Have the patient grasp the right side of the table with the left hand. Center the symphysis pubis over the center line of the table. Center the film holder to the greater trochanter.

Central ray

Direct the central ray perpendicular to the center of the film holder. Collimate to film holder.

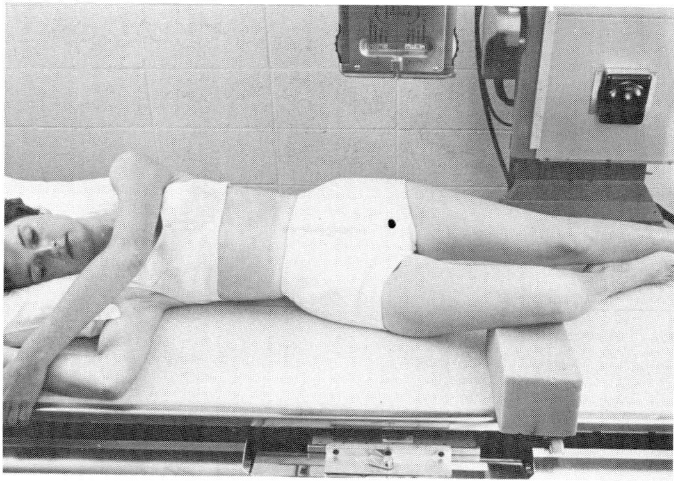

Fig. 13-47. Urethrography—bicycle position.

Immobilization

Place wedge-shaped positioning sponges beneath the elevated side. Employ suspended expiration.

Right-left markers

Place an R.P.O. marker on the right lateral center border of the film holder.

Examination

Extend the penis along the upper thigh. The doctor will inject the contrast medium, and as soon as the urethra distends *fully*, the doctor will signal the technologist. The exposure is then made.

Structures demonstrated

Right posterior oblique (R.P.O.) view of the lower pelvic region with the use of a catheter-injected contrast medium to demonstrate stones or other pathology associated with or contained within the urethra. The prostate gland may also be demonstrated.

Note: For a variation of this examination, the following is recommended: with the patient in a semisitting position (the arms extended backward for support), abduct the legs and direct the central ray 10 degrees cephalad through the symphysis pubis to the center of the film holder.

REPRODUCTIVE SYSTEM

Hysterosalpingography

Hysterosalpingography is a nonfunctional radiographic examination of the uterus, uterine tubes (oviducts), and ovaries with the use of a heavy contrast medium injected through a special uterine catheter.

Patient preparation

1. The patient should be scheduled 7 to 8 days following cessation of menstruation.
2. Instruct the patient to take a warm-water enema (1½ pints) and a cleansing douche prior to the examination.
3. When the patient is admitted, remove all garments except shoes and socks. Provide a gown and instruct the patient to tie the open ends together in the front.
4. Instruct the patient that the bladder must be voided prior to the examination.
5. Make a 10″ × 12″ posterior (A-P) pelvic scout (survey) radiograph of the patient, centering the film holder (lengthwise), with the central ray 2 inches above the greater trochanter.

Contrast media

Fill a sterile 20 cc syringe with warm Sinografin, Salpix, or another selected contrast medium. (See Table 13-1.)

Equipment preparation

A special, sterilized salpingogram kit is provided by surgical supply or the referring gynecologist.

Examination

After the scout (survey) radiograph has been completed and checked, the patient is placed in the lithotomy* position at the foot-end of the table. The genitourinary region is cleansed by the nurse assistant. The doctor inserts a vaginal speculum and then introduces the special uterine cannula until the tip is engaged in the fallopian orifice. The legs are then extended and the patient is positioned for radiography.

Note: Some routine series call for fluoroscopy at this stage of progress if so, follow the equipment preparation procedures per the barium enema studies on pp. 410 and 411, prior to the examination.

---

*Lithotomy position has the patient on her back, the legs flexed on the thighs, the thighs flexed on the belly, and abducted.

ROUTINE RADIOGRAPHIC POSITION

Hysterosalpingography—posterior (A-P) view (Figs. 13-48 and 13-49)

Film size—10″ × 12″
Cassette
Lengthwise
Bucky
Collimate to cover

Technique

Factors	Screen film cassette (par)	Screen film cassette (par) High kVp—16:1 grid
mA	300	200
Time	0.3	0.1
mAs	90	20
Thickness in cm	20	20
kVp	68	120
Distance	40	40

Palpation point

Greater trochanter of the femur.

Procedure

The patient remains in the supine position with the median line of the body over the center line of the table. Center the film holder 2 inches above the greater trochanter.

Central ray

Direct the central ray perpendicular to the center of the film holder. Collimate to film holder.

Immobilization

Employ suspended expiration.

Right-left markers

Place the right marker on the right lateral center border of the film holder.

Examination

The injection of the contrast medium is performed by the doctor. After filling has been completed, the exposure is made.

Note: A 24-hour radiograph may be ordered to determine the presence of stasis.

Structures demonstrated

Posterior (A-P) view of the female pelvic region with the use of a catheter-injected contrast medium to demonstrate absence of patency of one or both uterine tubes, and other pathology associated with the ovaries, uterine tubes, and uterus.

Note: For oblique views of this region, follow routine procedures for R.P.O. and L.P.O. bicycle positions (see p. 452).

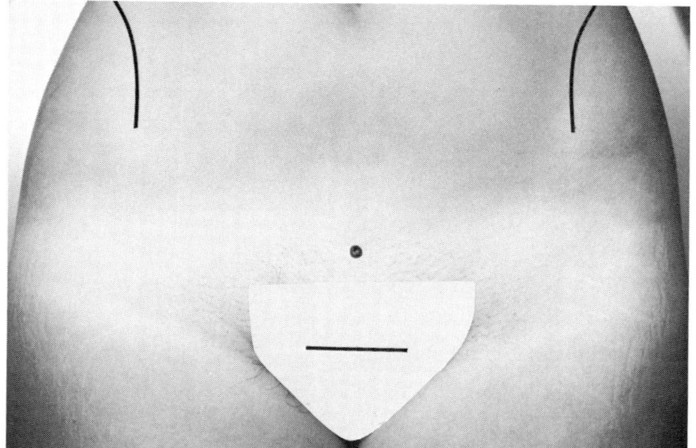

Fig. 13-48. Hysterosalpingogram—posterior (A-P) position.

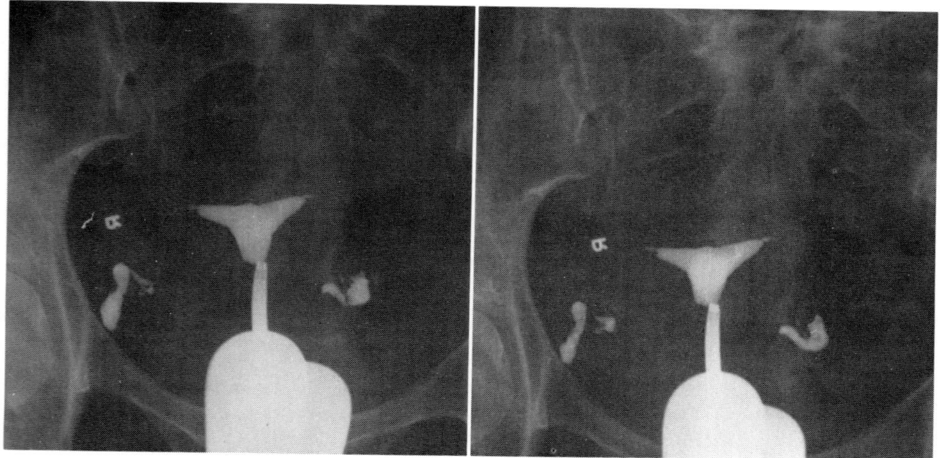

Fig. 13-49. Hysterosalpingogram—immediate posterior (A-P) and 3-minute posterior (A-P) views. (Courtesy Dr. E. I. L. Cilley, Dr. T. W. Crowell, Dr. R. E. Waud, and Dr. G. H. Hoffman.)

Fetography

A fetogram is a routine radiographic examination of the unborn fetus without the use of a contrast medium to determine the following:

1. Position of the fetus for possible placenta previa
2. Question of multiple pregnancy
3. Question of fetal age
4. Question of fetal pathology
5. Question of fetal death

ROUTINE RADIOGRAPHIC POSITIONS

Fetography—posterior (A-P) view (Figs. 13-50 and 13-51)

Film size—14″ × 17″
Cassette
Lengthwise

Bucky
Collimate to cover

Technique

Factors	Screen film cassette (par) Regular kVp—12:1 grid	Screen film cassette (par) High kVp—16:1 grid
mA	300	200
Time	0.3	0.2
mAs	90	40
Thickness in cm	28	28
kVp	80	120
Distance	40	40

Patient preparation

Remove all garments except shoes and socks. Provide a gown and instruct the patient to tie the open ends together in the back.

Palpation points

Crest of the ilium; symphysis pubis or greater trochanter.

Procedure

Place the patient in the supine position with the median line of the body over the center line of the table. Elevate the knees with a pillow or sponges to relieve strain on the spine. Center the film holder to the crest of the ilium.

Note: It is important that the inferior border of the film holder is aligned 2½ inches below the level of the symphysis pubis (or greater trochanter).

Central ray

Direct the central ray perpendicular to the center of the film holder. Collimate to film holder.

Immobilization

Use a compression band on large abdomens. Rapid, deep respiration prior to the exposure will reduce fetal movement. Employ suspended expiration.

Right-left markers

Place the right marker in the right lateral center border of the film holder.

Structures demonstrated

Posterior (A-P) view of the female abdomen and pelvis to demonstrate relationship, number, age, or pathology associated with the unborn fetus and placenta.

Note: A lateral view may be requested. However, most radiologists require the posterior (A-P) view only, to reduce radiation exposure to the fetus.

Pelvimetry, Colcher-Sussman method

Pelvimetry is a radiographic examination of the (unborn) fetus with the use of a pelvic measuring device (having a centimeter scale) to determine the size relationship of the fetal head with the pelvic outlet.

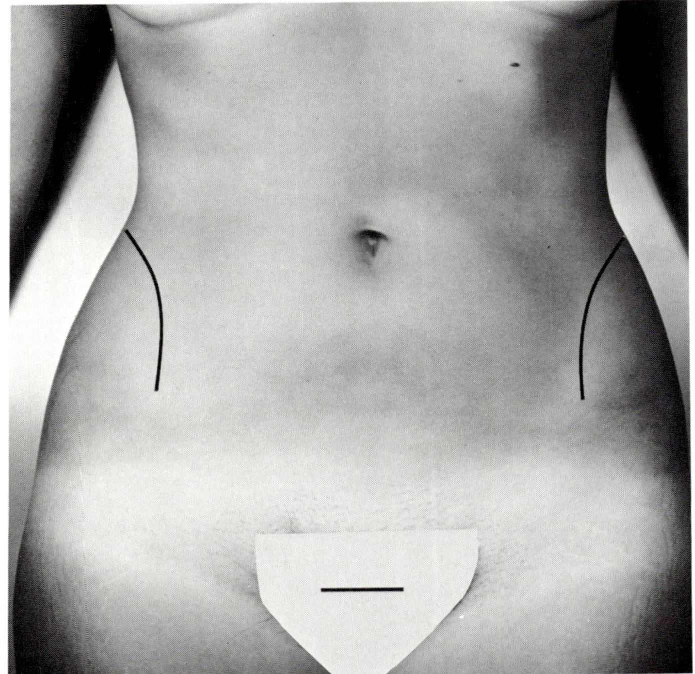

Fig. 13-50. Fetogram—posterior (A-P) position.

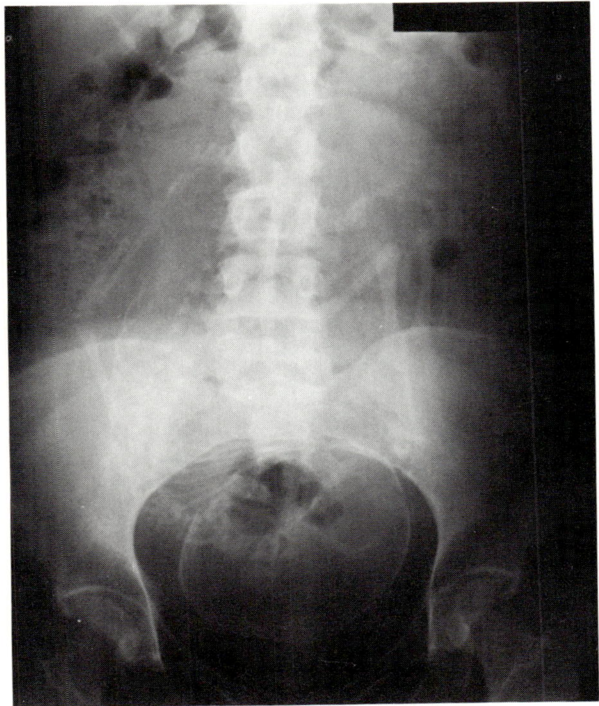

Fig. 13-51. Fetus—posterior (A-P) view. (Courtesy Dr. E. I. L. Cilley, Dr. T. W. Crowell, Dr. R. E. Waud, and Dr. G. H. Hoffman.)

ROUTINE RADIOGRAPHIC POSITIONS

Pelvimetry—Colcher-Sussman, posterior (A-P) view (Figs. 13-52 to 13-54)

Film size—14″ × 17″
Cassette
Lengthwise
Bucky
Collimate to cover

Technique

Factors	Screen film cassette (par) Regular kVp—12:1 grid	Screen film cassette (par) High kVp—16:1 grid
mA	300	200
Time	0.3	0.2
mAs	90	40
Thickness in cm	28	28
kVp	80	120
Distance	40	40

Patient preparation

Remove all garments except shoes and socks. Provide a gown and instruct the patient to tie the open ends together in the back.

Palpation points

Symphysis pubis; ischial tuberosities.

Procedure

Place the patient in the supine position with the median line of the body over the center line of the table. Flex the knees, placing the feet flat on the table. Separate the thighs and place the transverse scale of the pelvimeter against the buttocks at the level of the ischial tuberosities (10 cm below the upper border of the symphysis pubis). Secure the foot of the pelvimeter with a sandbag. Align the inferior border of the film holder 4 inches below the level of the transverse centimeter scale.

Central ray

Direct the central ray perpendicular to the center of the film holder. Collimate to film holder.

Immobilization

Use a compression band on large abdomens. Rapid, deep respiration prior to the exposure will reduce fetal movement. Employ suspended expiration.

Right-left markers

Place the right marker on the right lateral center border of the film holder.

Structures demonstrated

Posterior (A-P) view of the female pelvis to demonstrate size relationship of the fetal head with the maternal pelvic outlet.

E, Pelvic inlet

T, Pelvic outlet (ischial tuberosity)

F, Midpelvis

G, Top of symphysis pubis

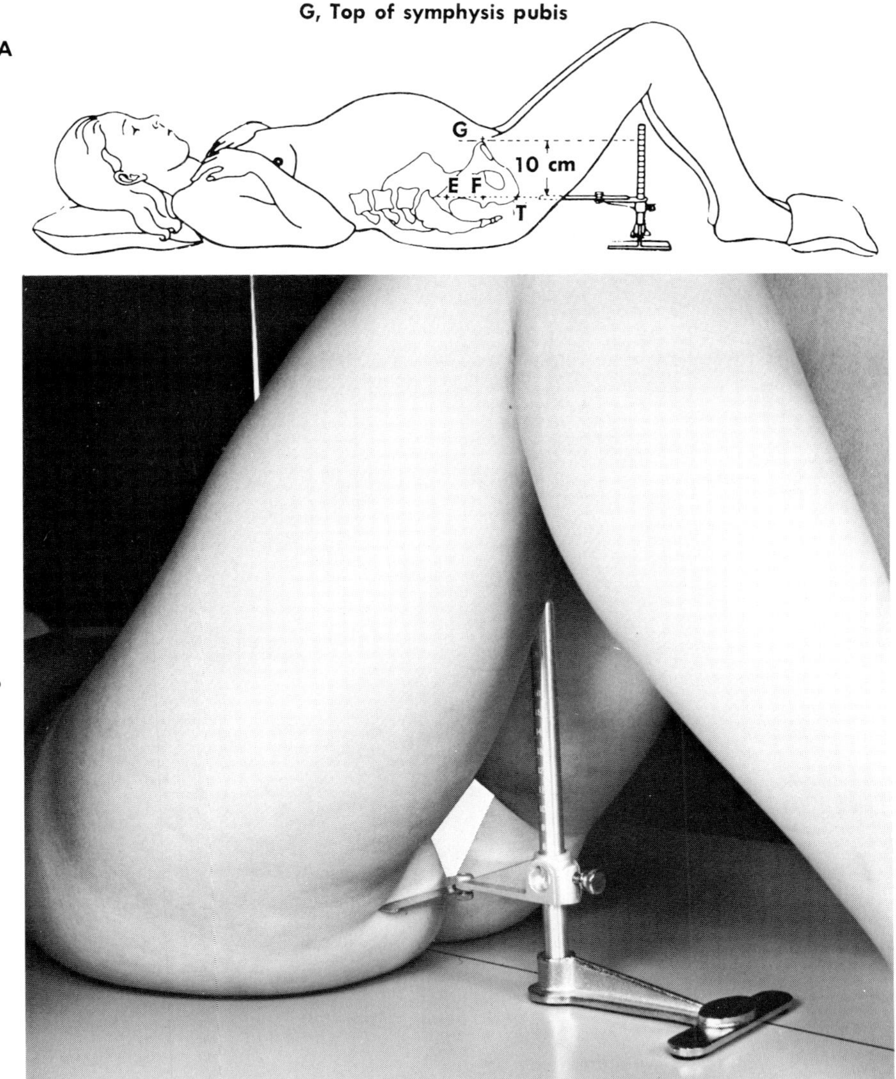

Fig. 13-52. Pelvimetry. A and B, Posterior (A-P) positions.

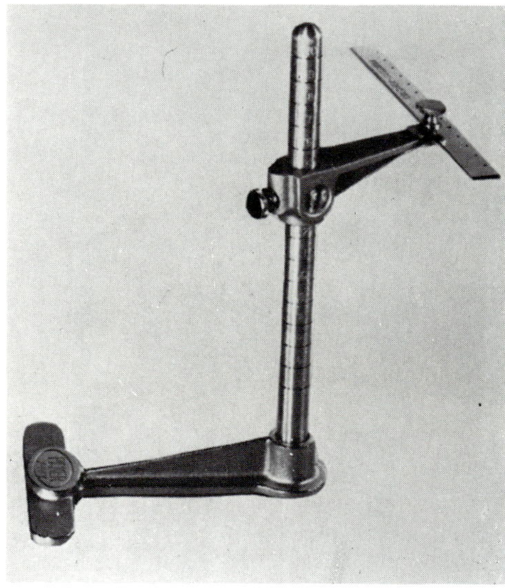

Fig. 13-53. Colcher-Sussman pelvimeter. (Courtesy Picker X-ray Corp.)

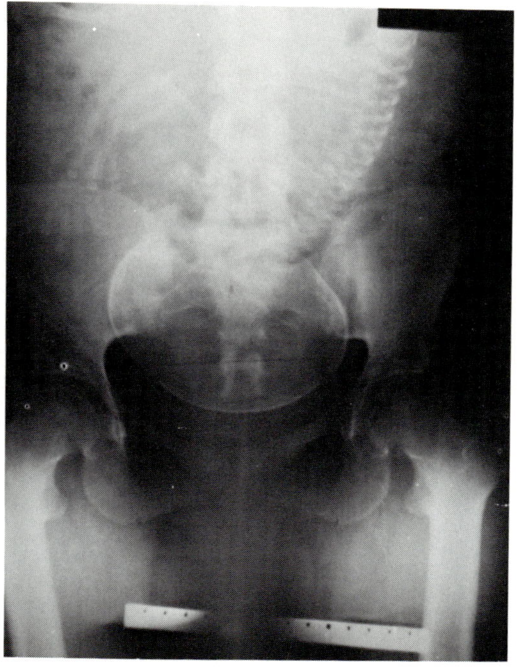

Fig. 13-54. Pelvimetry—posterior (A-P) view. (Courtesy Dr. E. I. L. Cilley, Dr. T. W. Crowell, Dr. R. E. Waud, and Dr. G. H. Hoffman.)

Pelvimetry—Colcher-Sussman, lateral view (Figs. 13-55 and 13-56)

Film size—14″ × 17″
Cassette
Lengthwise
Bucky
Collimate to cover

Technique

Factors	Screen film cassette (par) Regular kVp—12:1 grid	Screen film cassette (par) High kVp—16:1 grid
mA	300	200
Time	1	0.3
mAs	300	60
Thickness in cm	32	32
kVp	92	120
Distance	40	40

Patient preparation

Remove all garments except shoes and socks. Provide a gown and instruct the patient to tie the open ends together in the back.

Palpation points

Greater trochanter of the femur; posterior sacrum.

Procedure

Place the patient in a true left lateral position with the legs together, the knees flexed 90 degrees, and the hips flexed 45 degrees. Place the midaxillary line over the center line of the table. Adjust the height of the pelvimeter to insert the transverse centimeter scale between the gluteal folds. (The transverse centimeter scale should be parallel with the long axis of the femoral shaft. See Fig. 13-55.) Align the inferior border of the film holder 4 inches below the center level of the transverse centimeter scale.

Central ray

Direct the central ray perpendicular to the center of the film holder. Collimate to film holder.

Immobilization

Use a compression band. Rapid, deep respiration prior to the exposure will reduce fetal movement. Place sponges between the knees and between and beneath the ankles. Employ suspended expiration.

Right-left markers

Place the left marker on the anterior (patient) side, lateral center border of the film holder.

Structures demonstrated

Left lateral view of the female pelvis to demonstrate size relationship of the fetal head with the maternal pelvic outlet.

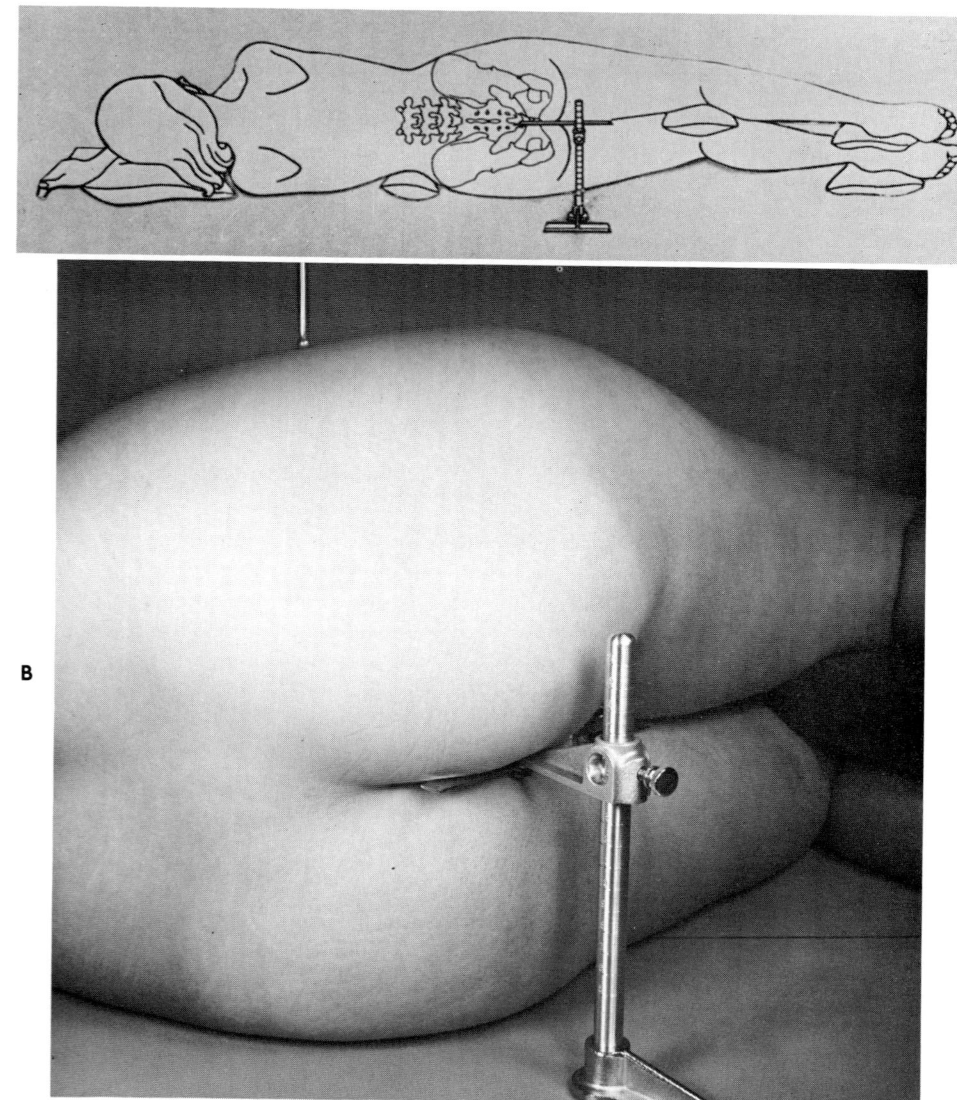

Fig. 13-55. Pelvimetry. **A** and **B,** Lateral positions.

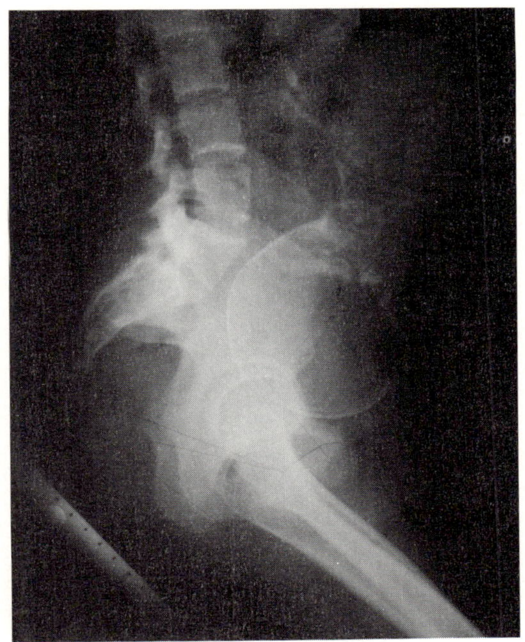

Fig. 13-56. Pelvimetry—lateral view. (Courtesy Dr. E. I. L. Cilley, Dr. T. W. Crowell, Dr. R. E. Waud, and Dr. G. H. Hoffman.)

MAMMOGRAPHY

Mammography is the routine soft tissue radiography of the breast to differentiate between benign and malignant neoplasms.

ROUTINE RADIOGRAPHIC POSITIONS

Mammography—axillary, posterior (A-P) view (Figs. 13-57 and 13-58)

Film size—10″ × 12″
No-screen film holder
Lengthwise
Tabletop
Extension cone

Technique

Factors	Screen film, no screen film holder
mA	200
Time	2.5
mAs	250
Thickness in cm	—
kVp	36
Distance	28–34

Patient preparation

Remove all garments down to the waist. Be certain that the breast region is free of any body powder. Tape a lead beebee to each breast just above the nipple for the purpose of indicating involuntary motion on the radiograph.

Palpation point

None.

Procedure

Place the patient in a supine position on the table. Place the film holder on the table in line with the sternomanubrial joint. Rotate the patient approximately 30 degrees towards the side being examined. Place the hand adjacent to the head, allowing the upper arm to rest on the table and to form a right angle, or greater, with the body.

Central ray

Direct the central ray perpendicular, tangent to the lateral rib cage, and to the center of the film holder.

Immobilization

Employ suspended expiration.

Right-left markers

Place the correct marker on the lateral center border of the film holder.

Structures demonstrated

Axillary projection of the lymph nodes.

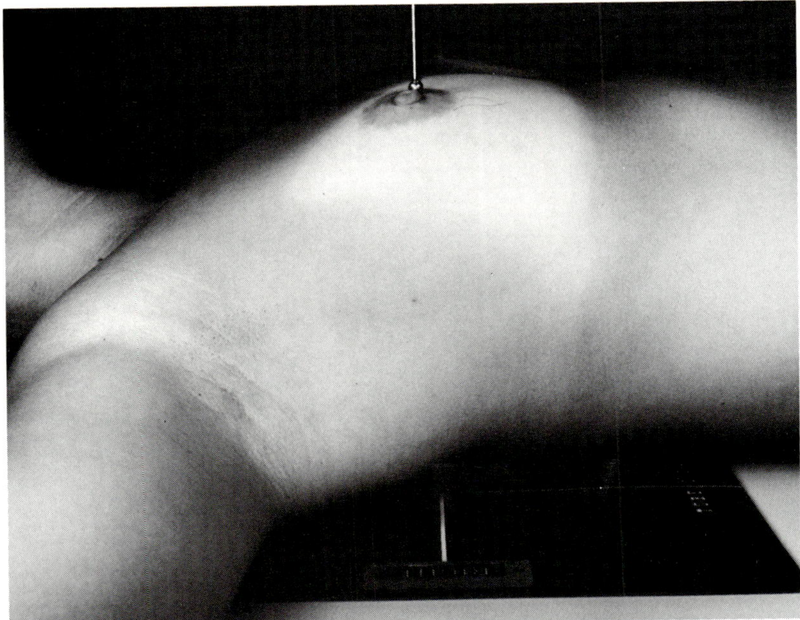

Fig. 13-57. Mammography—axillary, posterior (A-P) position.

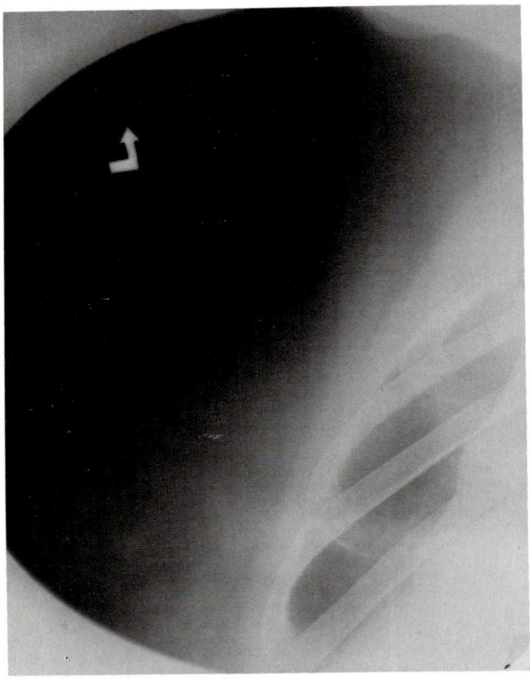

Fig. 13-58. Mammogram—axillary, posterior (A-P) view. (Courtesy Tucson Medical Center Hospital.)

Mammography—mediolateral view (Figs. 13-59 and 13-60)

Film size—8″ × 10″
No-screen film holder
Lengthwise
Tabletop
Extension cone

Technique

Factors	Screen film, no screen holder
mA	200
Time	2.5
mAs	250
Thickness in cm	—
kVp	36
Distance	28–34

Patient preparation

Remove all garments down to the waist. Be certain that the breast region is free of any body powder. Tape a lead beebee to each breast just above the nipple for the purpose of indicating involuntary motion on the radiograph.

Palpation point

None.

Procedure

Place the patient in the supine position on the table. Place the film holder on the table in line with the center of the breast. (It may be necessary to elevate the film holder on a sponge block for breast support.) Rotate the patient, toward the side being examined, into a semilateral position so that the breast and nipple are extended at their complete profile. Place the hand adjacent to the head, allowing the upper arm to rest on the table and to form a right angle with the body.

Central ray

Direct the central ray perpendicular through the center of the film holder.

Immobilization

Employ suspended expiration.

Right-left markers

Place the correct marker in an unobstructed lateral corner of the film holder.

Technical tips

In most cases it is necessary for the patient to retract the opposite breast to eliminate superimposition.

Structures demonstrated

Lateral profile of entire breast for soft tissue visualization.

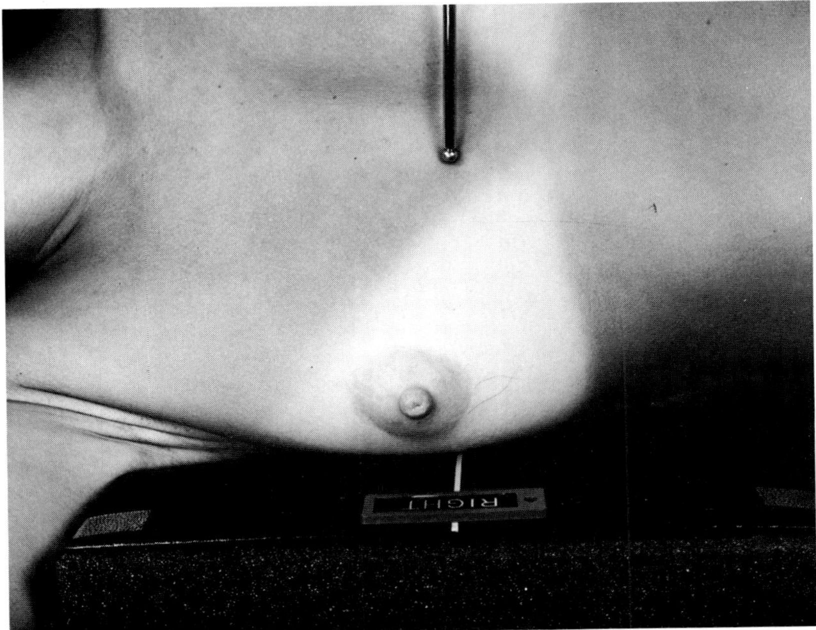

Fig. 13-59. Mammography—mediolateral position.

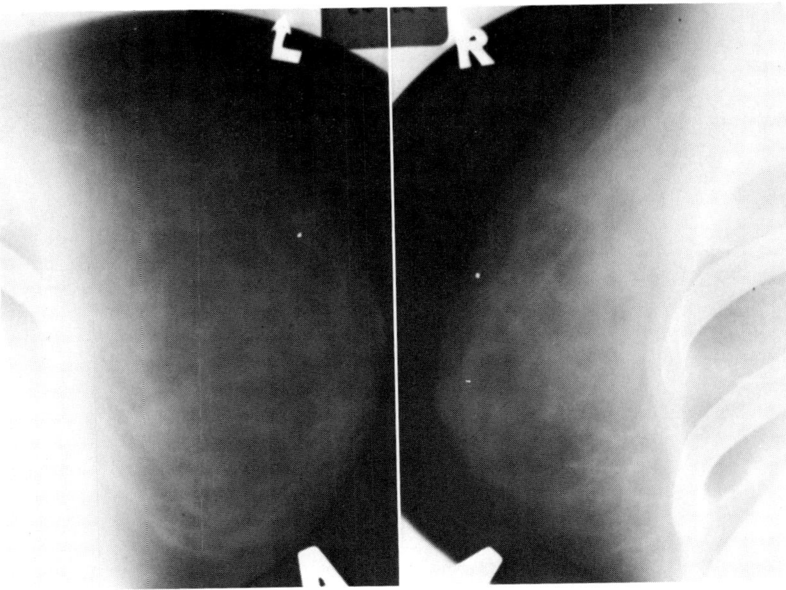

Fig. 13-60. Mammogram—mediolateral (bilateral) views. (Courtesy Tucson Medical Center Hospital.)

Mammography—craniocaudad view (Figs. 13-61 and 13-62)

Film size—8″ × 10″
No-screen film holder
Lengthwise
Tabletop
Extension cone

Technique

Factors	Screen film, no screen holder
mA	200
Time	2.5
mAs	250
Thickness in cm	—
kVp	36
Distance	28–34

Patient preparation

Remove all garments down to the waist. Be certain that the breast region is free of any body powder. Tape a lead beebee to each breast just above the nipple for the purpose of indicating involuntary motion on the radiograph.

Palpation point

None.

Procedure

Place the patient in an erect sitting position on an adjustable stool, and facing the end of the table. Adjust the height of the stool so that the lower border of the breast is at tabletop level. Place the film holder on the table beneath the breast with the edge firmly against the patient so that breast and nipple are extended at their complete profile. Tilt the head away from the side being examined.

Central ray

Direct the central ray perpendicular through the center of the breast to the film holder.

Immobilization

Instruct the patient to grasp the edge of the table. Employ suspended expiration.

Technical tips

Place a lead sheet under the film holder to help reduce backscatter and assist in patient protection.

Structures demonstrated

Craniocaudad profile of entire breast for soft tissue visualization.

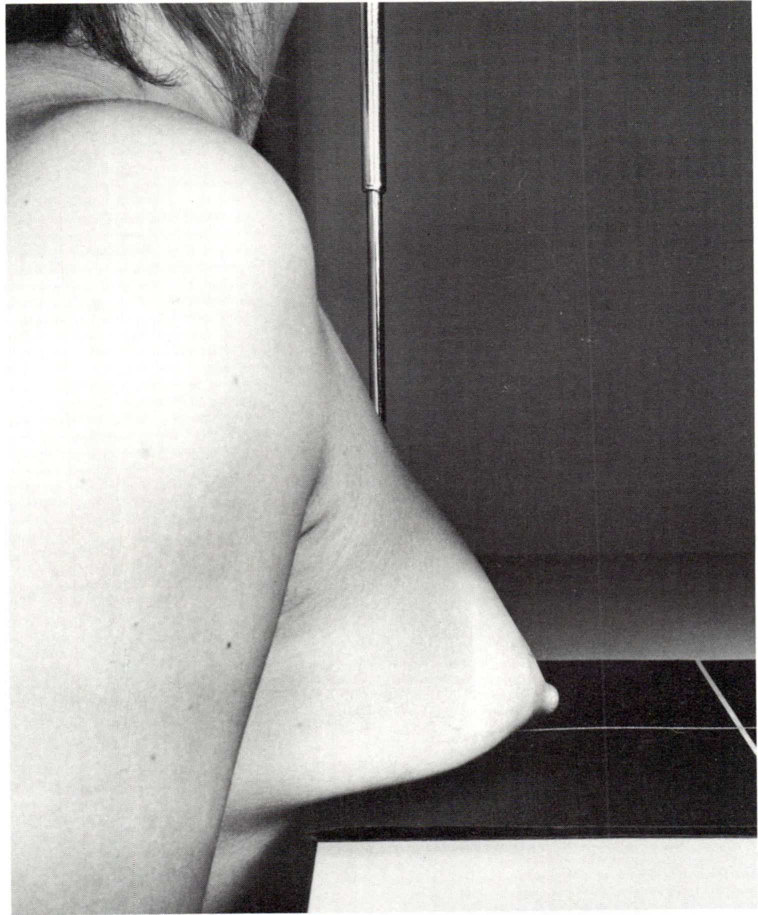

Fig. 13-61. Mammography—craniocaudad position.

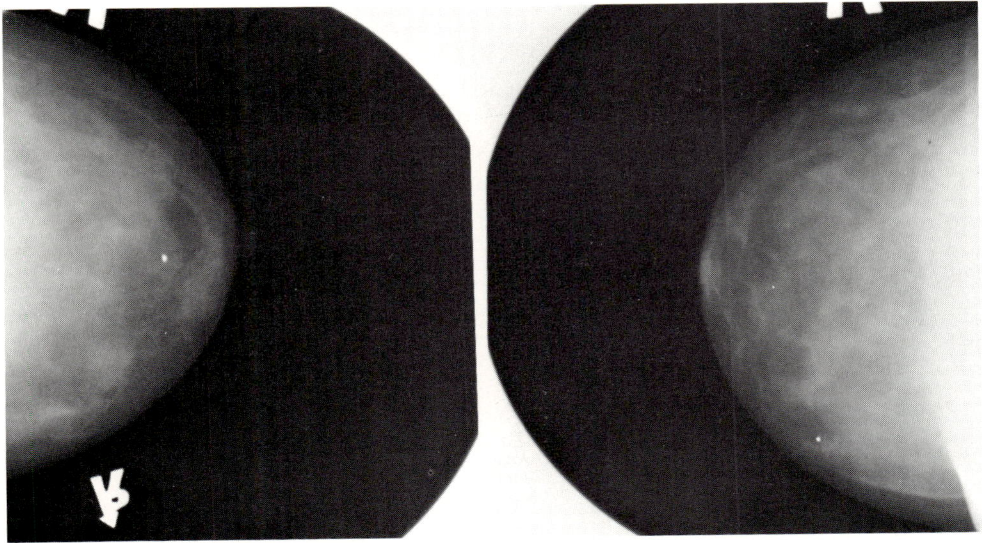

Fig. 13-62. Mammogram—craniocaudad views. (Courtesy Tucson Medical Center Hospital.)

BRONCHOGRAPHY

Bronchography is a nonfunctional fluoroscopic and radiographic examination of the lungs with the use of a directly injected contrast medium.

Patient preparation

When the patient is admitted, remove all garments down to the waist. Provide a gown for female patients and instruct the patient to tie the open ends together in the back.

Make routine anterior (P-A) and lateral radiographs of the lung fields.

Note: The patient may be admitted with nasal catheter preinserted and positioned by the referring physician.

Contrast media

1. Fill a sterile 20 cc syringe with Lipiodol, Dionosil, or other selected iodized oil that has been warmed to body temperature. (See Table 13-1.)
2. A sterilized bronchogram kit is provided by surgical supply or the referring physician.
3. The contrast medium may be injected by one of the following methods:
   a. Through the nasal pharynx by means of a nasal catheter (the most common method)
   b. Through the oral pharynx by means of a cannula
   c. Through the cricothyroid membrane by means of a needle

Equipment preparation

1. For fluoroscopy preparation, follow the same equipment preparation as for the esophageal examination, p. 398.
2. Provide a sterile 20 cc syringe with contrast medium.
3. Four to six loaded cassettes for spot films must be provided.

Examination

1. Position the patient erect, either sitting or standing, with his back against the fluoroscopy table.
2. Assist the radiologist with lead apron and lead gloves.
3. The assisting doctor or technologist will insert the contrast medium-filled syringe into the external opening of the nasal catheter and inject the iodized oil in small quantities.
4. The radiologist will fluoroscope the patient during this procedure (Step 3) while he is maneuvering (Churchill's maneuvers) the patient into different positions. The Trendelenburg position may also be used.
5. When one side has been filled satisfactorily, radiographs are then made with *essential speed.*
6. After satisfactory radiography of the region(s) being examined, the catheter is removed and the examination is concluded.

ROUTINE RADIOGRAPHIC POSITIONS

Bronchography—anterior (P-A) view (Figs. 13-63 and 13-64)

Film size—14″ × 17″
Cassette
Lengthwise
Erect film holder
Collimate to cover

Technique

Factors	Screen film cassette (par)
mA	300
Time	$0.0\overline{33}$
mAs	10
Thickness in cm	22
kVp	70
Distance	72

Palpation points

Acromion processes, lateral ribs.

Procedure

Place the patient in the erect position with the anterior surface of the chest against the film holder. Center the midline of the body over the center line of the film holder. Align the top of the film holder 3 inches above the acromion processes. Elevate the chin so that it rests on top of the film holder. Place the backs of the hands on the hips. Roll the shoulders anteriorly as far as possible.

Note: *Speed in obtaining this radiograph is essential.*

Central ray

Direct the central ray horizontal and perpendicular to the center of the film holder. Collimate to film holder.

Immobilization

A compression band may be used across the thoracic cage. Employ deep suspended inspiration.

Right-left markers

Place the *L* marker in the left superior corner of the film holder.

Structures demonstrated

Anterior (P-A) views of the lungs, heart, and the rib structures above the diaphragm. The bronchi and bronchioles are demonstrated with the injected contrast medium.

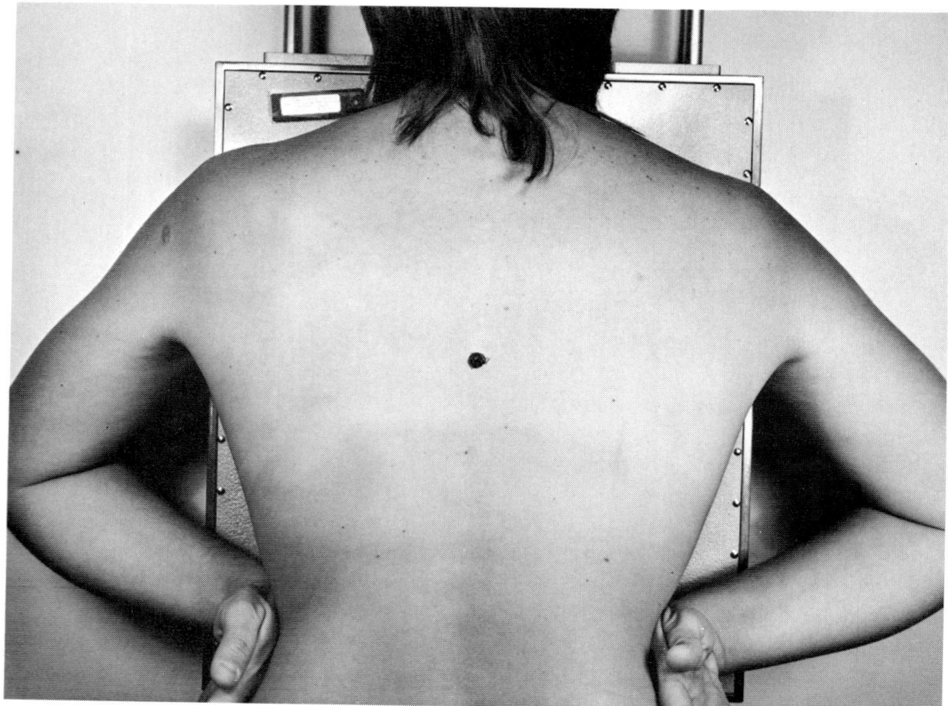

Fig. 13-63. Bronchography—anterior (P-A) position.

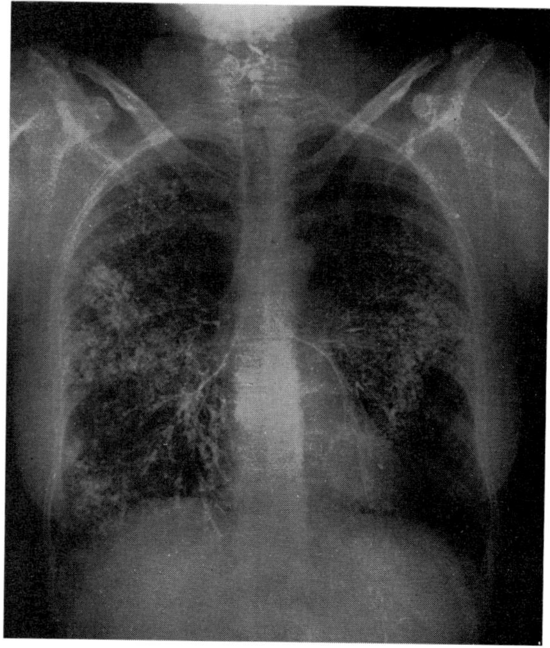

Fig. 13-64. Bronchogram—anterior (P-A) view. (Courtesy Dr. E. I. L. Cilley, Dr. T. W. Crowell, Dr. R. E. Waud, and Dr. G. H. Hoffman.)

Bronchography—lateral view (Figs. 13-65 and 13-66)

Film size—14″ × 17″
Cassette
Lengthwise
Erect film holder
Collimate to cover

Technique

Factors	Screen film cassette (par)
mA	300
Time	$0.\overline{066}$
mAs	20
Thickness in cm	30
kVp	78
Distance	72

Palpation points

Acromion processes; anterior and posterior ribs.

Procedure

Place the patient in the erect position with the lateral surface of the side of the chest being examined against the film holder. Center the midaxillary line of the body over the center line of the film holder. Align the top of the film holder 3 inches above the acromion processes. Cross the arms over the head and rest the forearms on top of the head. Rotate the body into a true lateral position.

Note: *Speed in obtaining this radiograph is essential.*

Central ray

Direct the central ray horizontal and perpendicular to the center of the film holder. Collimate to film holder.

Immobilization

A compression band may be used across the thoracic cage. Employ deep suspended inspiration.

Right-left markers

Place the correct marker in the left superior corner of the film holder.

Structures demonstrated

Lateral views of both lungs superimposed, heart and aorta, and the midthoracic spine. The bronchi and bronchioles are demonstrated with the injected contrast medium.

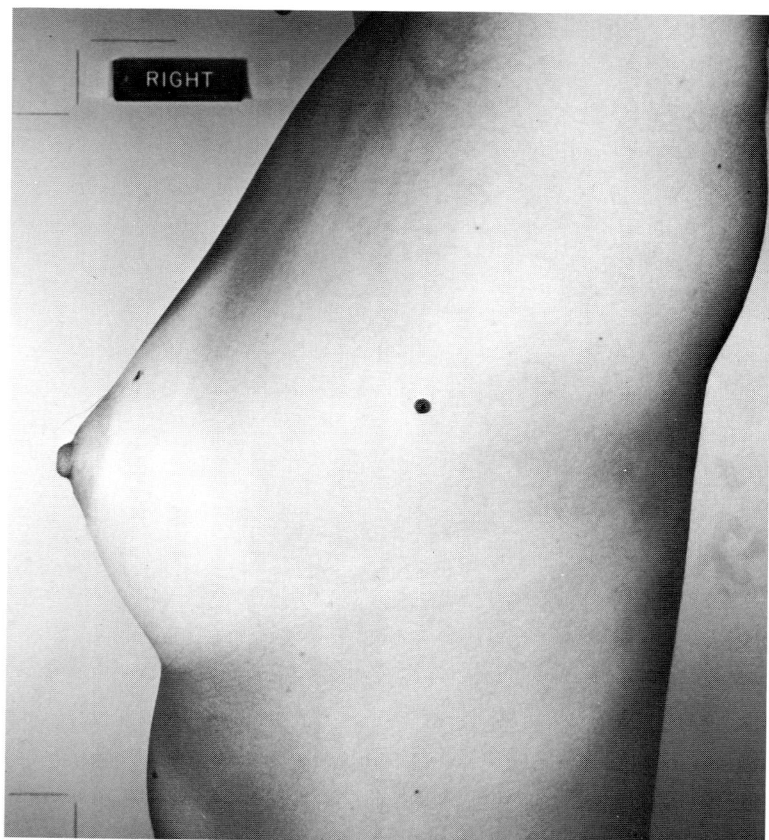

Fig. 13-65. Bronchography—lateral position.

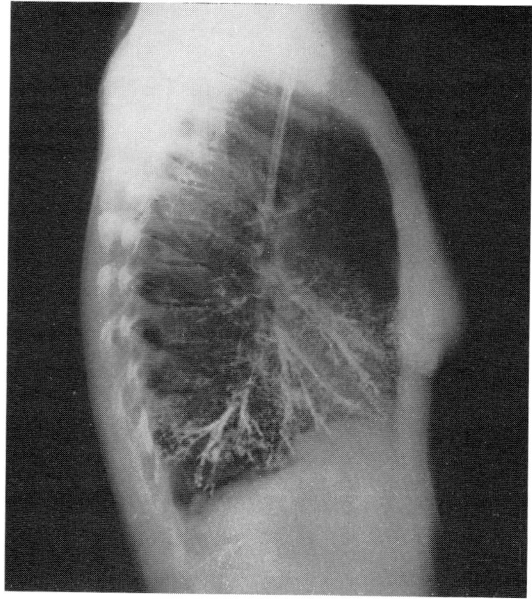

Fig. 13-66. Bronchogram—lateral view. (Courtesy Dr. E. I. L. Cilley, Dr. T. W. Crowell, Dr. R. E. Waud, and Dr. G. H. Hoffman.)

Bronchography—left-right anterior oblique (L.A.O.-R.A.O.) views (Figs. 13-67 and 13-68)

Film size—14″ × 17″
Cassette
Lengthwise
Erect film holder
Collimate to cover

Technique

Factors	Screen film cassette (par)
mA	300
Time	$0.0\overline{33}$
mAs	10
Thickness in cm	26
kVp	78
Distance	72

Palpation points

Acromion processes; lateral ribs; spinous processes.

Procedure

Place the patient in the erect position with the anterior surface of the chest against the film holder. Align the top of the film holder 3 inches above the acromion processes. Rotate the side of the chest being examined *away* from the film holder 35 degrees. Flex that elbow and place the patient's hand on top of the film holder. Flex the opposite elbow and place the hand on the hip. Align a point midway between the spinous processes and the erect lateral margin of the side being examined over the center line of the film holder.

Central ray

Direct the central ray horizontal and perpendicular to the center of the film holder. Collimate to film holder.

Immobilization

A compression band may be used across the thoracic cage. Employ deep, suspended inspiration.

Right-left markers

Place the correct marker in the left superior corner of the film holder.

Structures demonstrated

Left anterior oblique—Maximum view of the right lung field, the trachea, and left bronchial tree. The right bronchi and bronchioles are demonstrated with injected contrast medium.

Right anterior oblique—Maximum view of the left lung field, the trachea, the entire right bronchial tree, and left atrium and both ventricles of the heart. The left bronchi and bronchioles are demonstrated with injected contrast medium.

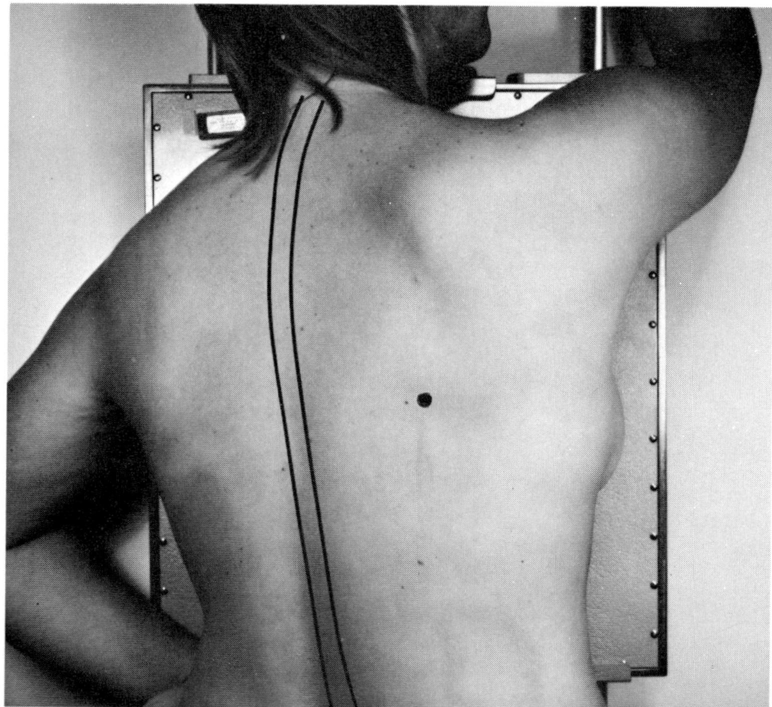

Fig. 13-67. Bronchography—left anterior oblique (L.A.O.) position.

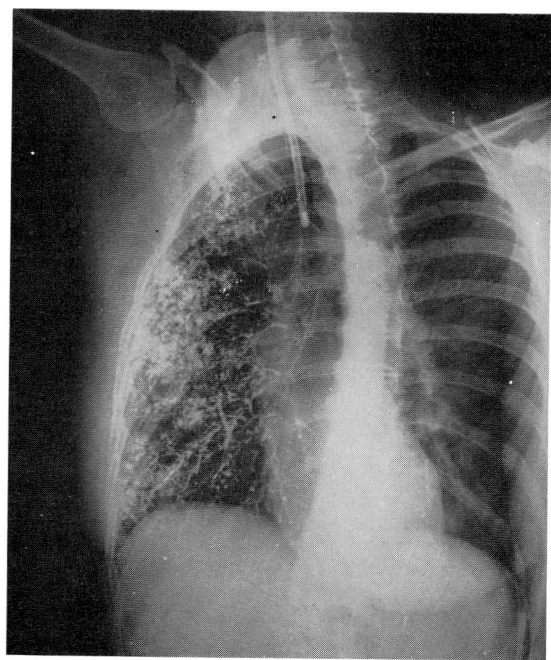

Fig. 13-68. Bronchogram—left anterior oblique (L.A.O.) view. (Courtesy Dr. E. I. L. Cilley, Dr. T. W. Crowell, Dr. R. E. Waud, and Dr. G. H. Hoffman.)

MYELOGRAPHY

Myelography is a nonfunctional fluoroscopic and radiographic examination of the spinal canal (cervical or lumbar injection sites) with the use of a directly injected contrast medium.

Patient preparation

The sterile preparation of the patient is conducted by the doctor or surgical scrub nurse after the patient has been delivered into the radiographic room.

Contrast media

One or more of the following three agents may be used, depending on the patient's situation and the type of examination:

1. Air or oxygen
2. A water-soluble medium
3. Pantopaque or another selected iodized oil-base contrast medium (See Table 13-1.)

The contrast medium may be furnished by surgical supply or the radiology department.

Equipment preparation

1. For fluoroscopy preparation, follow the same equipment preparation as for the colon examination, pp. 410 and 411.
2. Set the myelogram lock on the fluoroscopy tower.
3. A sterilized myelogram kit is provided by surgical supply.
4. Four to six loaded cassettes for spot films must be provided.

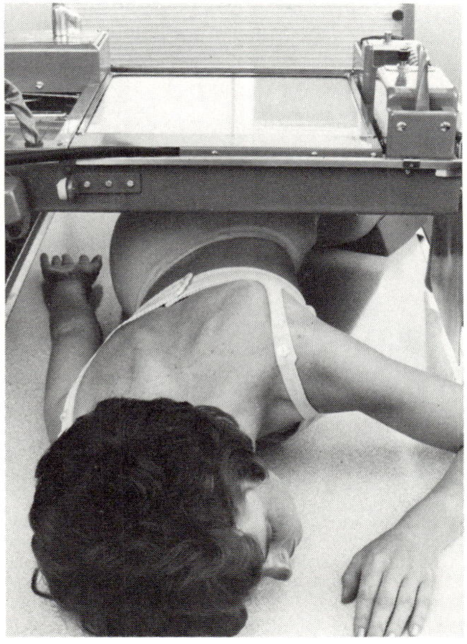

Fig. 13-69. Myelography—right anterior oblique (R.A.O.) position for fluoroscopic spot views.

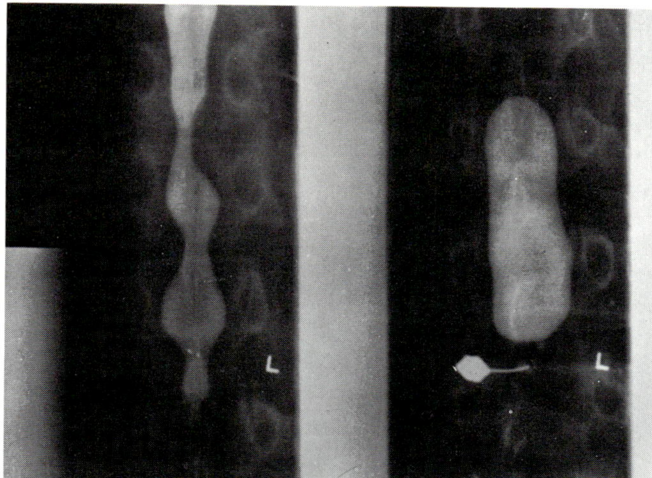

Fig. 13-70. Myelogram—fluoroscopic spot views. (Courtesy Dr. E. I. L. Cilley, Dr. T. W. Crowell, Dr. R. E. Waud, and Dr. G. H. Hoffman.)

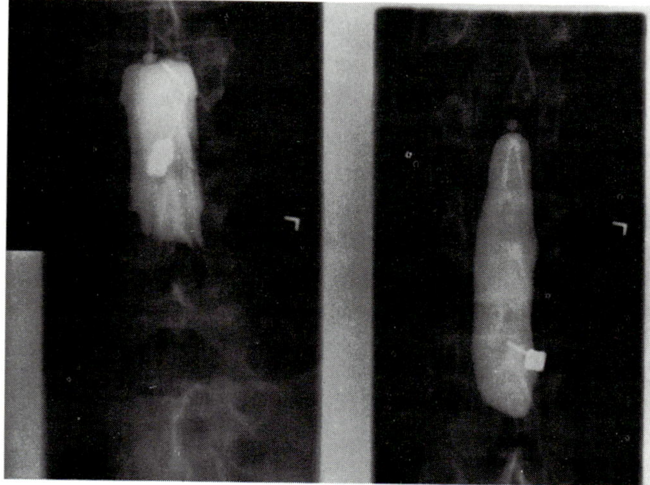

Fig. 13-71. Myelogram—fluoroscopic spot views. (Courtesy Dr. E. I. L. Cilley, Dr. T. W. Crowell, Dr. R. E. Waud, and Dr. G. H. Hoffman.)

Examination (Figs. 13-69 to 13-71)

1. The patient is placed in a lateral recumbent or a sitting position (depending on the region to be examined).
2. The doctor inserts a needle into a predetermined point in the spinal canal and collect spinal fluid for laboratory examination.
3. A similar quantity of the contrast medium is then injected.
4. After repeating this process, the patient is fluoroscoped in the lateral, anterior oblique, and prone positions with varying degrees of the Trendelenburg and semierect table positions.
5. Spot films are made periodically.
6. Upon completion of satisfactory spot films or radiographs, the doctor will aspirate as much of the contrast medium as possible, and the examination is concluded.

ANGIOGRAPHY

Percutaneous carotid arteriography

Percutaneous carotid arteriography (P.C.A.) is a special arteriographic examination of the carotid arteries in the neck and the intercranial circulation by injection of contrast media into the carotid arteries.

Patient preparation

1. The patient is admitted to the radiology department on a stretcher (wheeled gurney). Check the patient's records accurately for the following:
   a. Identification (patients with similar names)
   b. Complete blood work (laboratory report)
   c. Surgical permit
   d. Allergy report
2. Patient is placed on the radiographic table in a supine position with the occipital region resting on the A.P. film changer.
3. Make routine posterior (A-P) and lateral scout radiographs of the head and neck for technique and positioning.
4. The patient is then hyperextended by placing a pneumatic pillow under the shoulders for easy access to the carotid arteries.
5. The cervical region is sterilized and prepared.

Contrast media

Sterile 20 cc syringes are filled with 6 to 10 cc (per injection) of Hypaque 60%, Renografin 60%, or other suitable contrast medium (Table 13-1).

The contrast medium may be furnished by surgical supply or the radiology department.

Equipment preparation (Figs. 13-72 and 13-73)

1. Provide rapid film changer.
2. A sterilized arteriogram kit is usually provided by surgical supply.
3. Provide positioning accessories.
4. Provide lead aprons and gloves.
5. Select technique and energize controls.
6. The time factor is critical in this examination so all personnel must be alert.

Examination

1. The radiologist or neurosurgeon inserts the needle into the artery.
2. Technicians are alerted; a rapid injection is made for one of the following:
   a. For each position using manual or conventional exposure
   b. For posterior (A-P) and lateral positions when biplane rapid exposure is used
3. For manual exposure, three radiographs are necessary to demonstrate arterial, capillary, and venous phases in each position.
4. When one side has been demonstrated satisfactorily, the opposite side may be injected.
5. Following satisfactory studies of the region(s) being examined, the needle is removed and the examination concluded.

Note: Average circulation time from arterial through venous phase is approximately 4 seconds.

1. Manual exposure time should be less than .5 second.
2. Automatic exposure time should be less than .25 second.

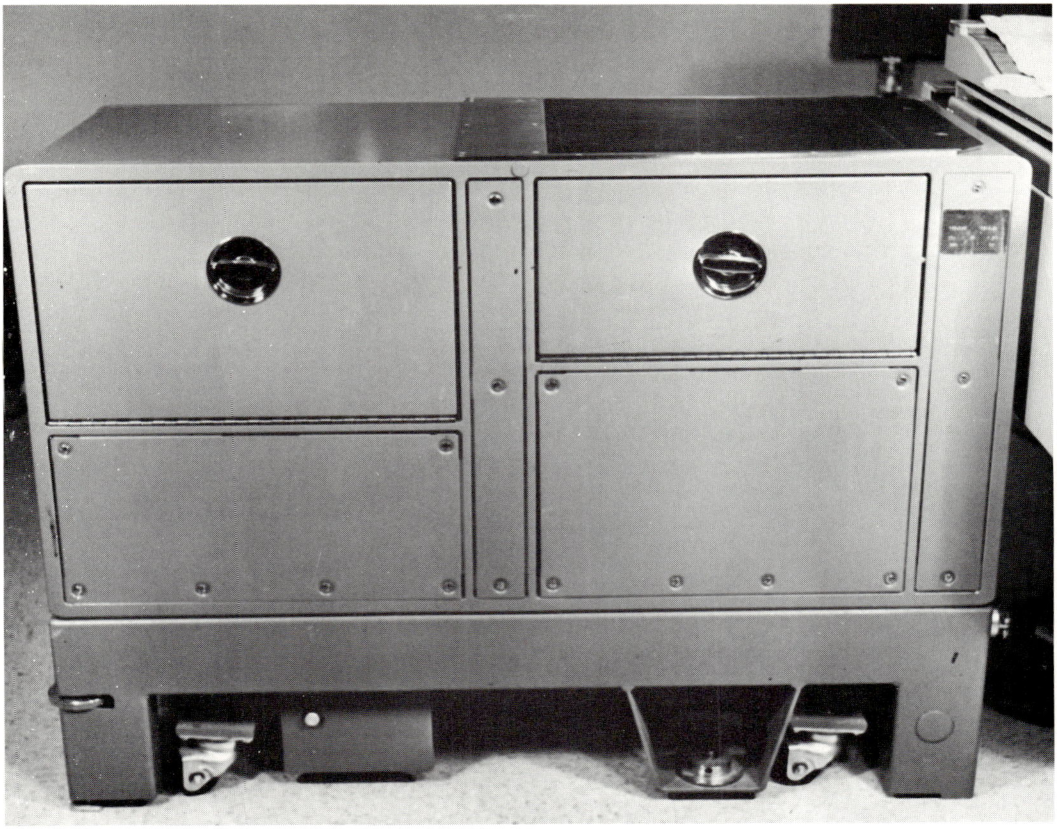

Fig. 13-72. Rapid (serial) film changer. (Courtesy St. Joseph's Hospital, Tucson.)

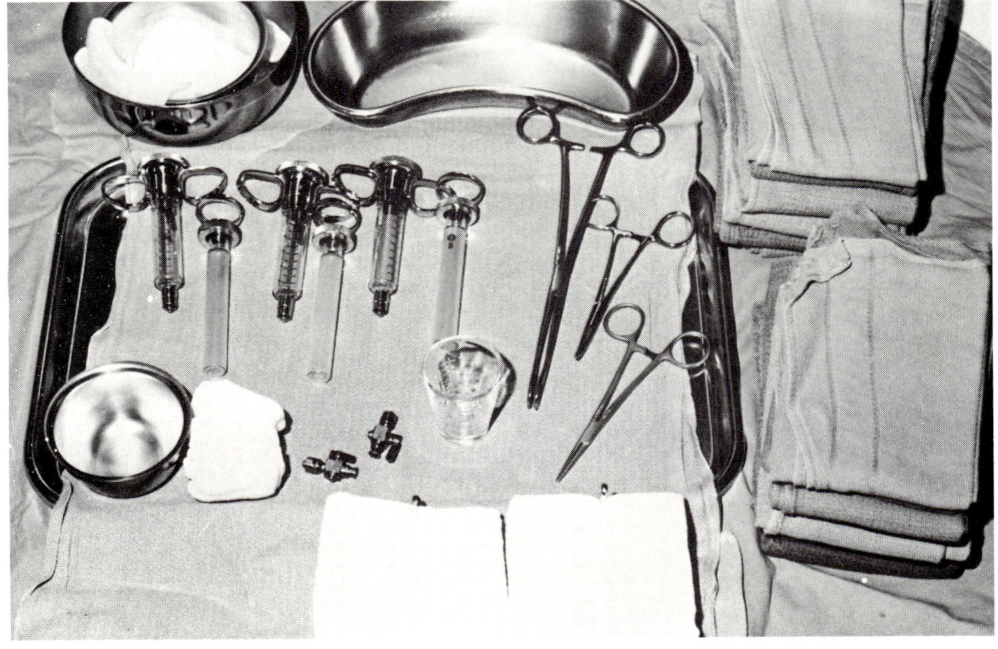

Fig. 13-73. Carotid arteriogram kit. (Courtesy Tucson Medical Center Hospital.)

ROUTINE RADIOGRAPHIC POSITIONS

Percutaneous carotid arteriography—posterior (A-P) view (Figs. 13-74 to 13-77)

Film size—10″ × 12″ (manual) *Film holder*
11″ × 14″ (on roll) *Autochanger*
Lengthwise
Collimate to cover
and/or skull diaphragm

Technique

Factors	Screen film cassette (par)
mA	300S
Time	.10
mAs	30
Thickness in cm	19
kVp	80
Distance	46

Palpation point

Vertex.

Procedure

Patient remains in the supine position with the vertex of the skull in line with the superior margin of the A.P. film changer. Both the midsagittal plane and the infraorbitomeatal line are perpendicular to the headrest.

Central ray

Direct the central ray caudad, 1 inch cranial to and parallel with a line extending from the supraorbital margin to the base of the occiput, to the film holder. Collimate to film holder.

Immobilization

Use tape or special head holder (Olympic type) across the frontal region.

Right-left markers

Place the *R* marker on the right lateral center border of the film holder or in an unobstructed corner of the film holder.

Structures demonstrated

Posterior (A-P) view of the intra- and extracranial circulation of the head and neck to demonstrate space-occupying lesions of the brain, intracranial aneurysms, A-V malformations, and extracranial vascular lesions of the carotid arteries.

Note: Variations of this view depend on the nature and location of the pathology in question.

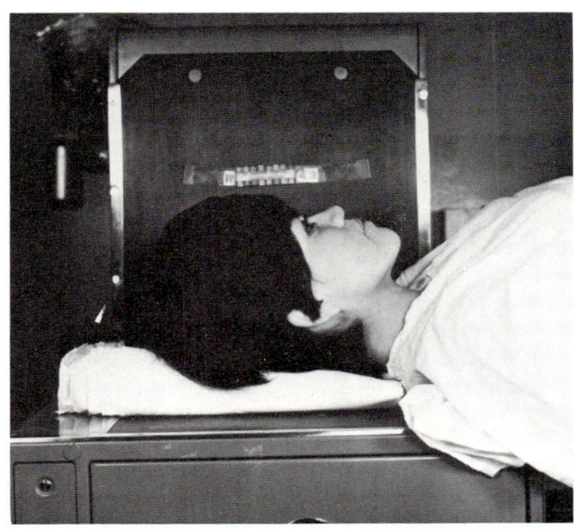

Fig. 13-74. Percutaneous carotid arteriography—posterior (A-P) position. (Courtesy St. Joseph's Hospital, Tucson.)

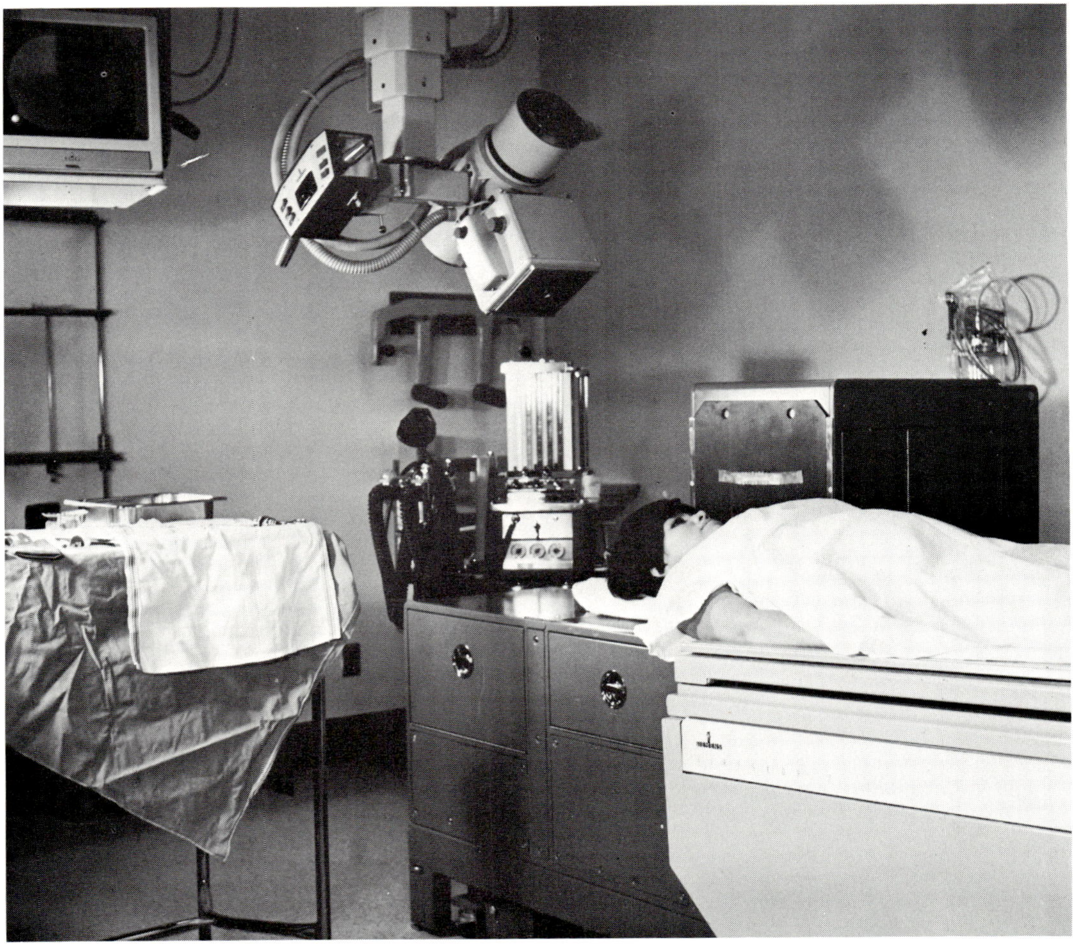

Fig. 13-75. Percutaneous carotid arteriography—posterior (A-P) axial position. (Courtesy St. Joseph's Hospital, Tucson.)

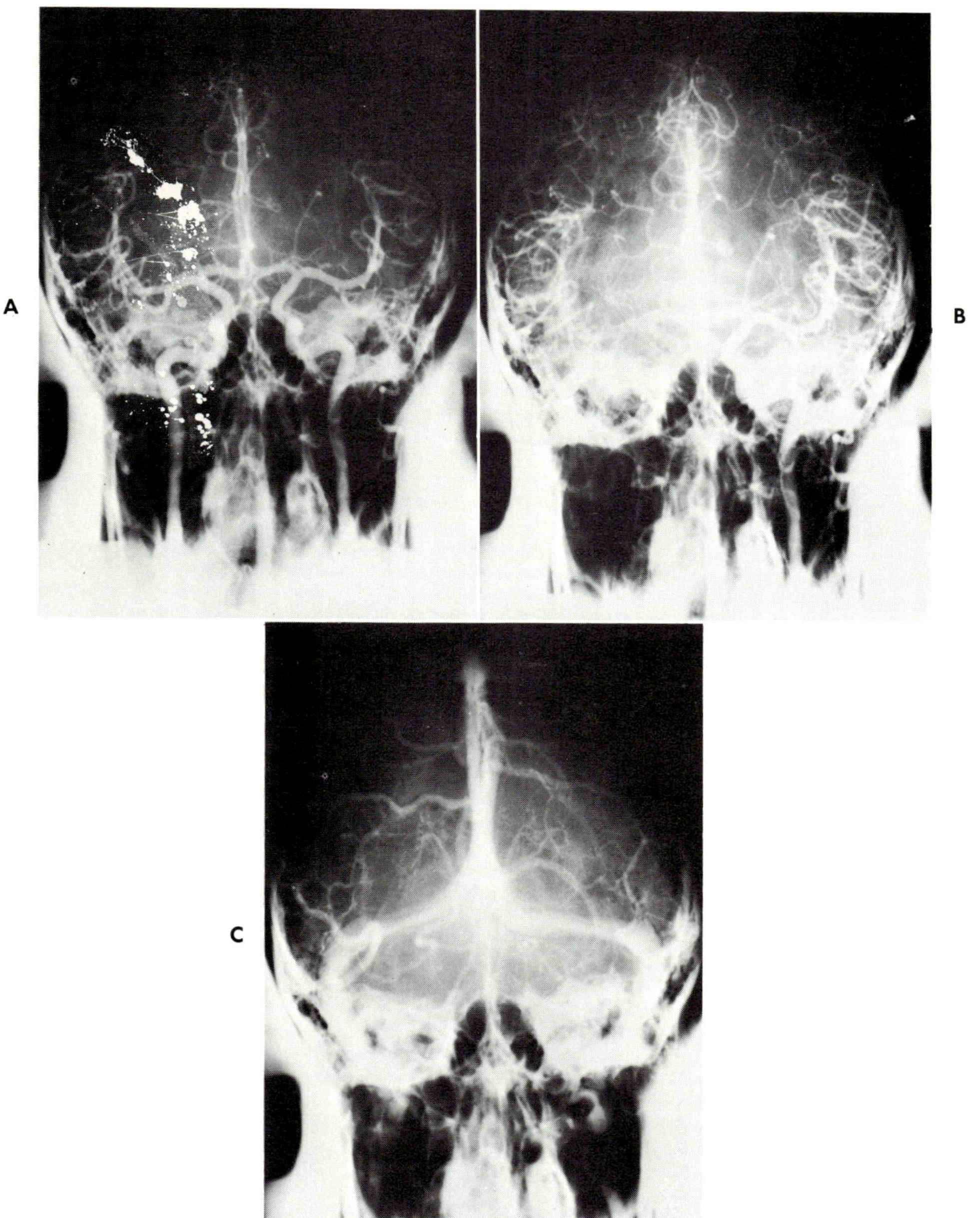

Fig. 13-76. Percutaneous carotid arteriograms—posterior (A-P) views. **A,** Arterial phase. **B,** Capillary phase. **C,** Venous phase. (Courtesy Tuscon Medical Center Hospital.)

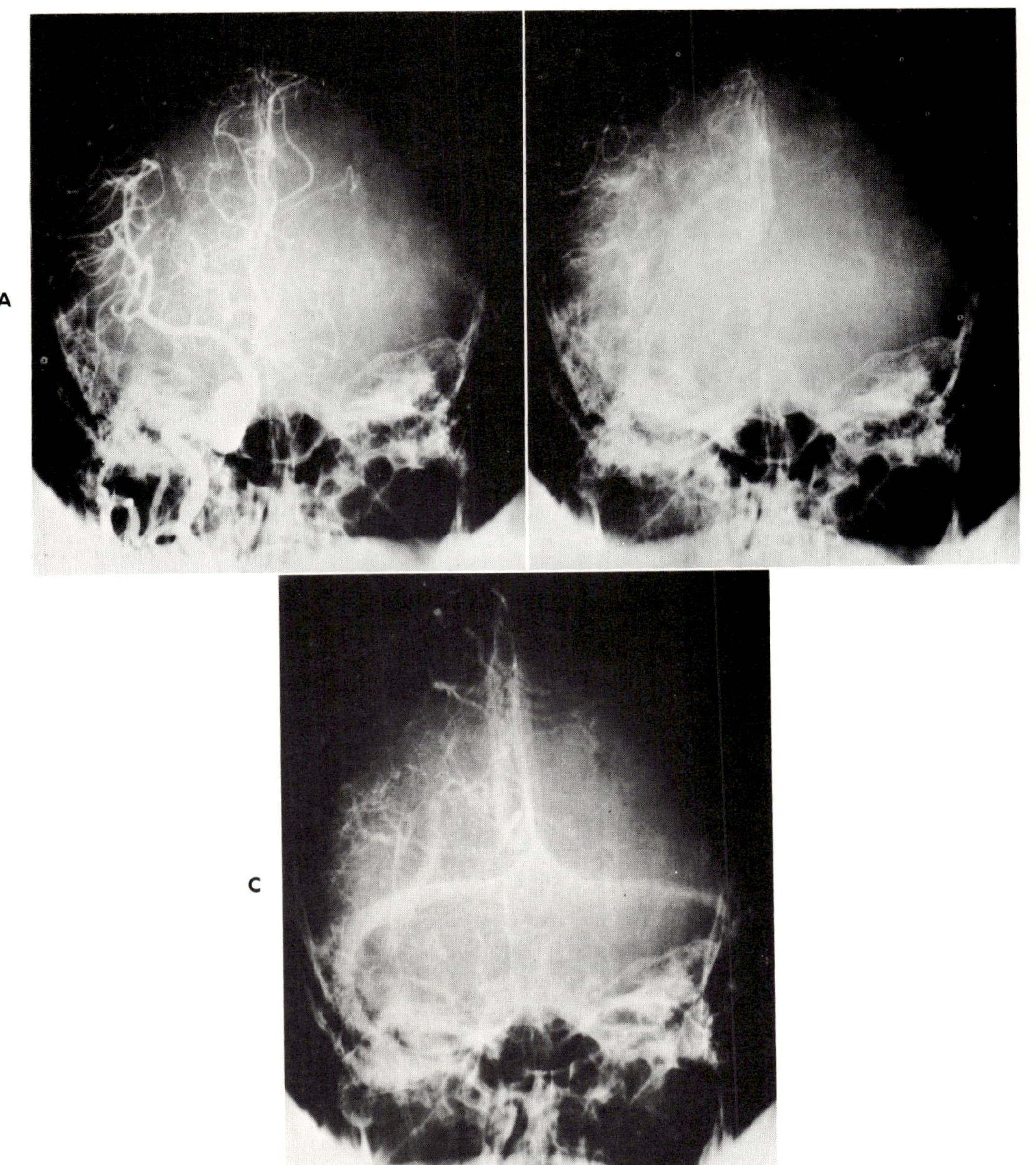

Fig. 13-77. Percutaneous carotid arteriograms—posterior (A-P) views. **A,** Arterial phase. **B,** Capillary phase. **C,** Venous phase. (Courtesy St. Joseph's Hospital, Tucson.)

Percutaneous carotid arteriography—lateral view (Figs. 13-78 to 13-80)

Film size—10″ × 12″ (manual) *Film holder*
11″ × 14″ (on roll) *Autochanger*
Lengthwise
Collimate to cover
and/or skull diaphragm

Technique

Factors	Screen film cassette (par)
mA	300S
Time	.10
mAs	30
Thickness in cm	16
kVp	74
Distance	46

Palpation point

Vertex.

Procedure

Place the patient in the supine position with the occipital region resting on an elevated (for example, sponge) support and centered to the midportion of the lateral film changer. Both the midsagittal plane and the infraorbitalmeatal line are perpendicular to the headrest.

Central ray

Direct the central ray horizontal and perpendicular through a point 2 inches superior and 1 inch anterior to the external auditory meatus to the film holder. Collimate to film holder.

Immobilization

Tape may be used around the cranium and fastened to the vertical changer.

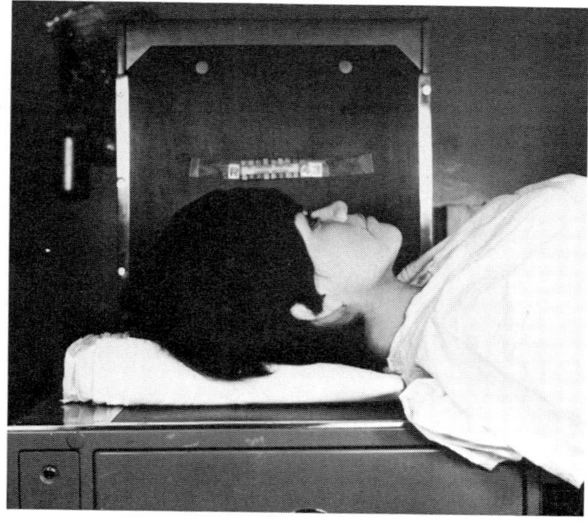

Fig. 13-78. Percutaneous carotid arteriography—lateral position. (Courtesy St. Joseph's Hospital, Tucson.)

Right-left markers

Place the correct marker on the anterior center border of the film holder.

Structures demonstrated

Lateral view of the intracranial circulation of the head to demonstrate space-occupying lesions of the brain, cranial aneurysms, and A-V malformations.

Percutaneous translumbar aortography

Percutaneous translumbar aortography (P.T.A.) is a special arteriographic examination of the abdominal aorta, pelvis, and lower circulatory system by direct injection into the aorta.

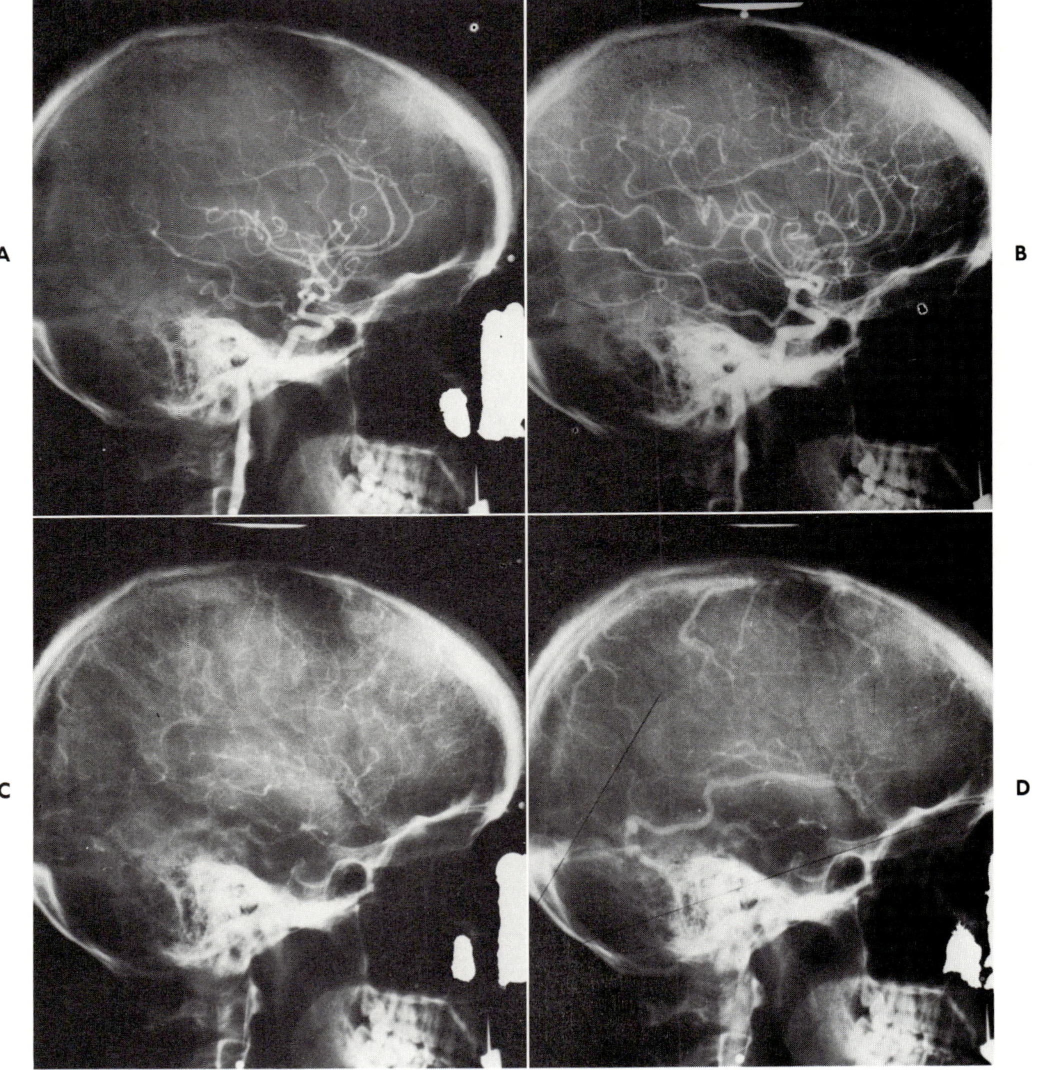

Fig. 13-79. Percutaneous carotid arteriogram—lateral views. **A** and **B**, Arterial phase. **C**, Capillary phase. **D**, Venous phase. (Courtesy Special Procedures Department, Southern Nevada Memorial Hospital, Las Vegas, Nevada.)

Patient preparation

1. The patient is admitted to the radiology department on a stretcher (wheeled gurney). Check the patient's records accurately for the following:
   a. Identification (patients with similar names)
   b. Complete blood work (laboratory report)
   c. Surgical permit
   d. Allergy report
2. The patient is placed on the cassette tunnel in a prone position.

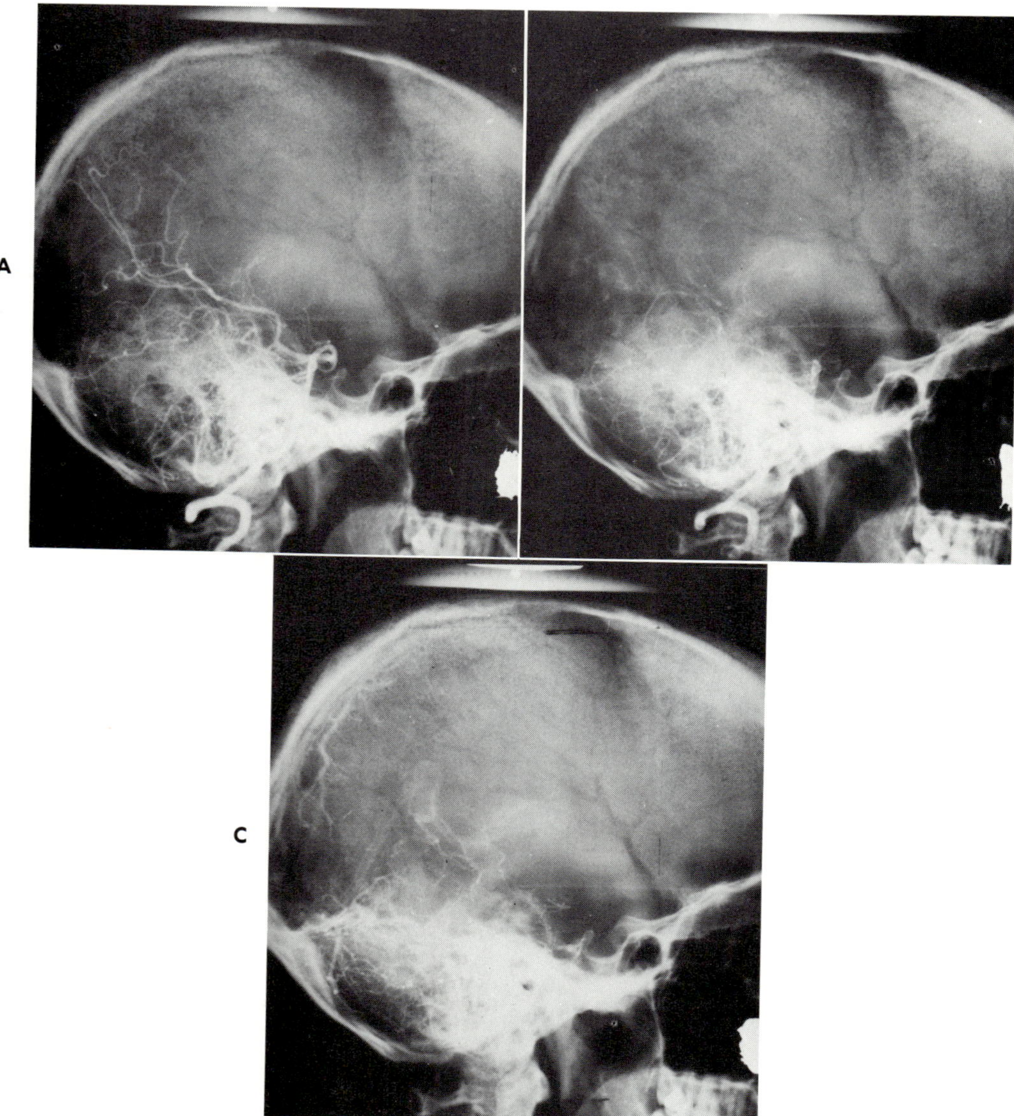

Fig. 13-80. Percutaneous arteriogram for posterior circulation—lateral views. **A,** Arterial phase. **B,** Capillary phase. **C,** Venous phase. (Courtesy Special Procedures Department, Southern Nevada Memorial Hospital, Las Vegas, Nevada.)

3. Make a routine anterior (P-A) scout film of the lower extremities.
4. The thoracolumbar region is sterilized and prepared.
5. An epidural block is usually performed by an anesthesiologist.

Contrast media

A sterile 50 cc syringe is filled with 30 to 50 cc of Hypaque 50%, Renografin 76%, or other suitable contrast medium (Table 13-1), and injected over a 5- to 10-second period.

The contrast medium may be furnished by surgical supply or the radiology department.

Equipment preparation (Fig. 13-81)

1. Provide rapid film changer and 14″ × 36″ cassette.
2. A sterilized arteriogram kit is provided by surgical supply.
3. Provide lead aprons and gloves.
4. Select technique and energize controls.
5. The time factor is important in this examination so all personnel must be alert.

Examination

1. The specialist inserts a large gauge needle into the aorta.
2. Technicians are alerted and an injection is made.
3. A series of selected radiographs are then taken of the abdomen, pelvis, and lower extremities.
4. After satisfactory studies of the region(s) being examined, the needle is removed and the examination concluded.

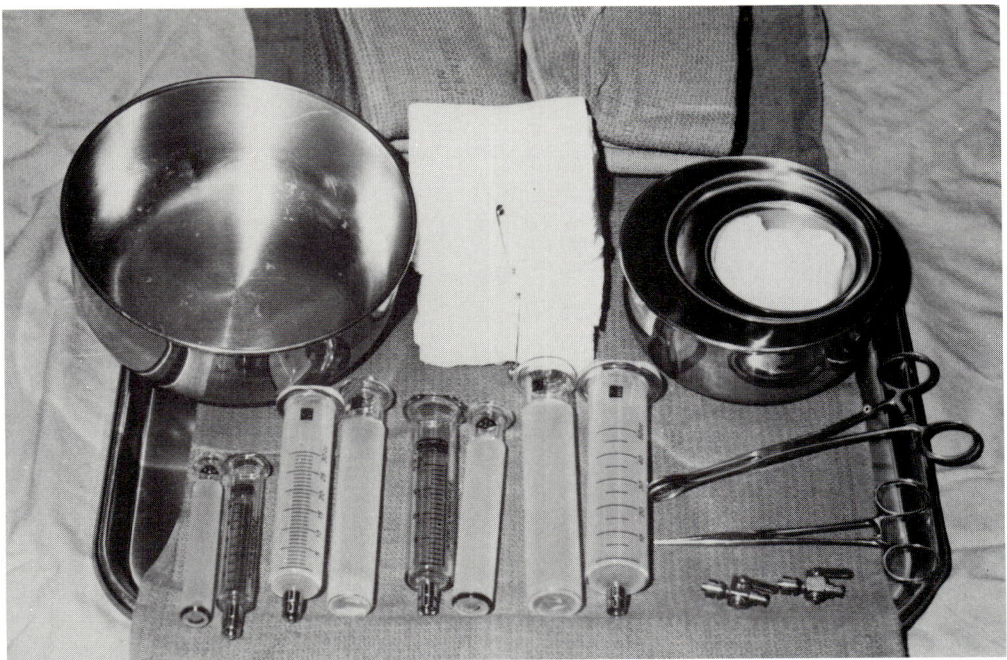

Fig. 13-81. Translumbar aortoarteriogram kit. (Courtesy Tucson Medical Center Hospital.)

ROUTINE RADIOGRAPHIC POSITION

Percutaneous translumbar aortography—anterior (P-A) view (Figs. 13-82 to 13-84)

Film size—14″ × 17″ and 14″ × 36″
Cassette
Lengthwise

Bucky
Collimate to cover

Technique

Factors	Screen film cassette (par)
mA	300
Time	.30
mAs	90
Thickness in cm	20
kVp	76
Distance	60

Palpation points

Crest of the ilium; apex of patella.

Procedure

Abdomen—Patient remains in the prone position with the median line of the body over the center line of the table. Center the 14″ × 17″ film holder to the crest of the ilium. Make exposure after bolus of 33 cc or more of contrast medium has been injected.

Lower extremities—Patient remains in the prone position with the legs centered over the cassette tunnel. Center the 14″ × 36″ film holder to cover from the distal pelvis to the popliteal trifurcation. Make exposure after slow injection of 30 to 50 cc of contrast medium.

Central ray

Direct the central ray perpendicular to the center of each film holder. Collimate to film holder.

Immobilization

Use tape across legs.

Right-left markers

Place the right marker on the right lateral center border of the film holder.

Structures demonstrated

Anterior (P-A) views of the abdomen, pelvis, and lower extremities to demonstrate aneurysms, plaques, and arteriosclerotic changes in the circulatory flow.

Note: The translumbar aortogram procedure can be used with a serial film changer for performing renal arteriographic examinations.

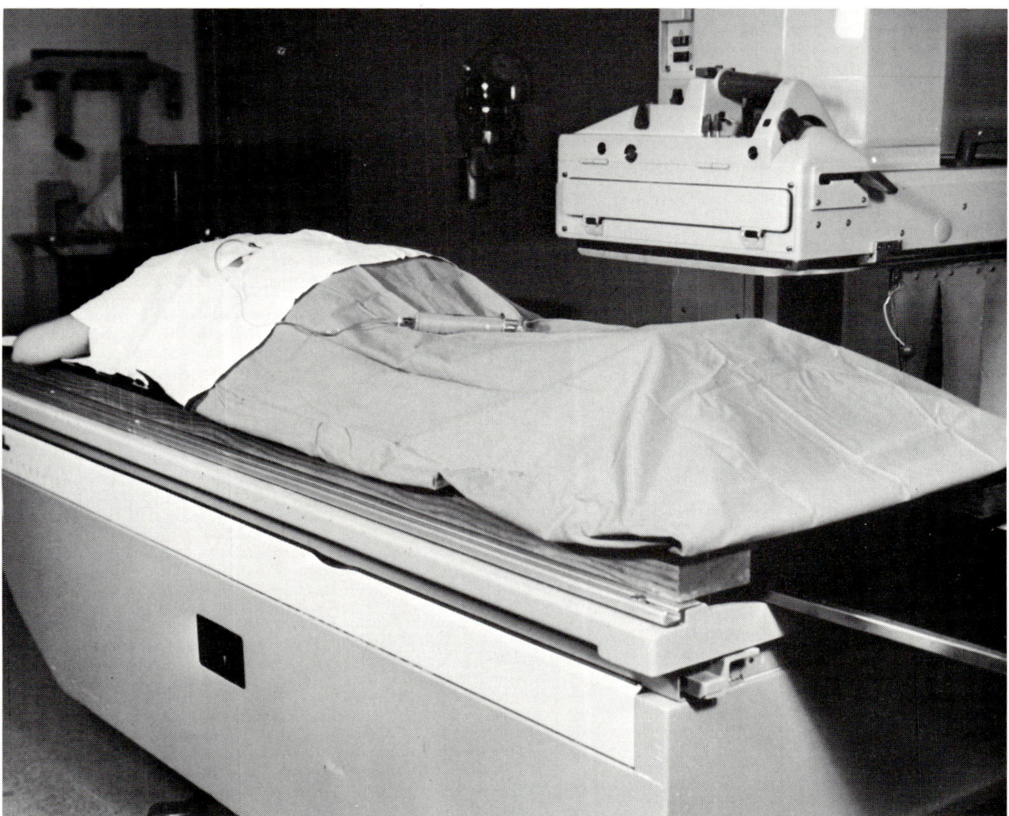

Fig. 13-82. Percutaneous translumbar aortography—anterior (P-A) position. (Courtesy St. Joseph's Hospital, Tucson.)

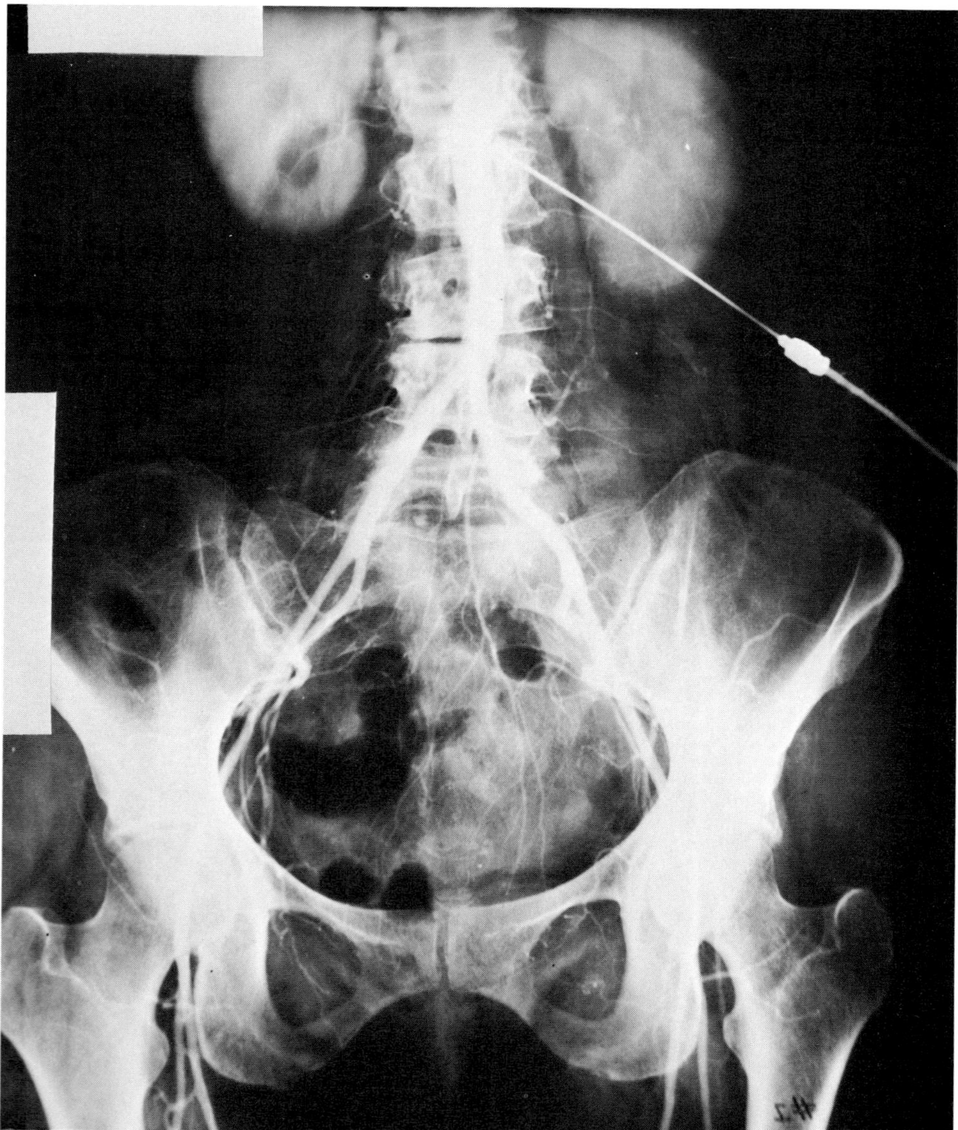

Fig. 13-83. Percutaneous translumbar aortogram—anterior (P-A) view. Early injection phase. (Courtesy St. Joseph's Hospital, Tucson.)

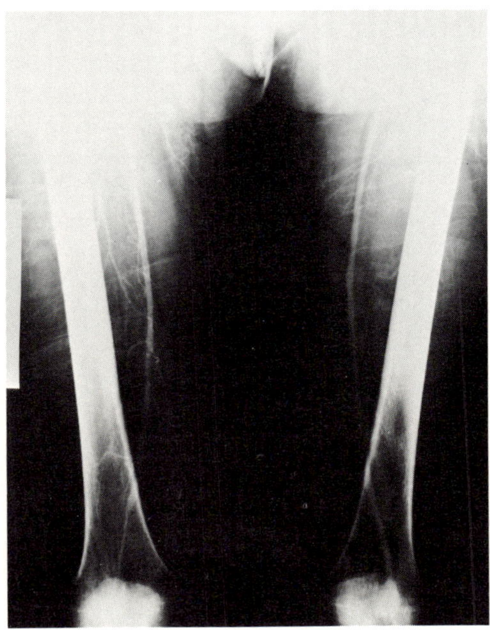

Fig. 13-84. Percutaneous translumbar aortogram—anterior (P-A) view. Late injection runoff. (Courtesy St. Joseph's Hospital, Tucson.)

Percutaneous transfemoral arteriography

Percutaneous transfemoral arteriography is a special retrograde arteriographic examination of the abdominal aorta and renal arteries by catheterization of the femoral artery.

Patient preparation

1. The patient is admitted to the radiology department on a stretcher (wheeled gurney). Check the patient's records accurately for the following:
   a. Identification (patients with similar names)
   b. Complete blood work (laboratory report)
   c. Surgical permit
   d. Allergy report
2. The posterior tibial and dorsalis pedis arterial pulses are checked and marked for emergency purposes.
3. The patient is placed on the radiographic table in a supine position.
4. The groin area is shaved and prepared for sterile draping.
5. A scout film of the abdomen is made to check for position, technique, and patient preparation. The groin area is then draped for the examination.
6. The artery is punctured and a guidewire is passed up the femoral artery into the abdominal aorta under fluoroscopy control.
7. The needle is removed and a selected catheter is passed over the wire into the abdominal aorta.
8. The wire is removed and a test injection of contrast medium is made to determine origin of arteries in question.

Contrast media

Use 30 to 50 cc of Hypaque 75%, Renografin 76%, or other suitable contrast medium (Table 13-1).

Equipment preparation (Figs. 13-85 and 13-86)

1. Provide rapid film changer.
2. Provide fluoroscopy equipment.
3. A sterilized arteriogram kit is usually provided by surgical supply.
4. Provide selected needles, guidewires, and catheters.
5. Provide pressure injector.
6. Provide lead aprons and gloves.
7. Select technique and energize controls.
8. The time factor is important in this examination so all personnel must be alert.

Examination

1. The specialist injects 30 to 50 cc of contrast medium.
2. Exposures are made; patient is then moved off changer and films are checked.
3. A decision may be made to take oblique views or to perform selective catheter studies.
4. Selective studies include the following:
   a. A guidewire is passed up the catheter.
   b. The catheter is removed and a special curved catheter passed over the wire.

   c. Under fluoroscopy, each renal artery can be selectively catheterized, and a coned down radiographic series of each kidney is performed.
5. Film sequence is as follows:
   a. 2 per second for 3 seconds
   b. 1 per second for 3 seconds
   c. 1 three-second and 1 five-second delayed
6. When satisfactory radiographs have been obtained, the catheter is removed, and the examination is concluded.

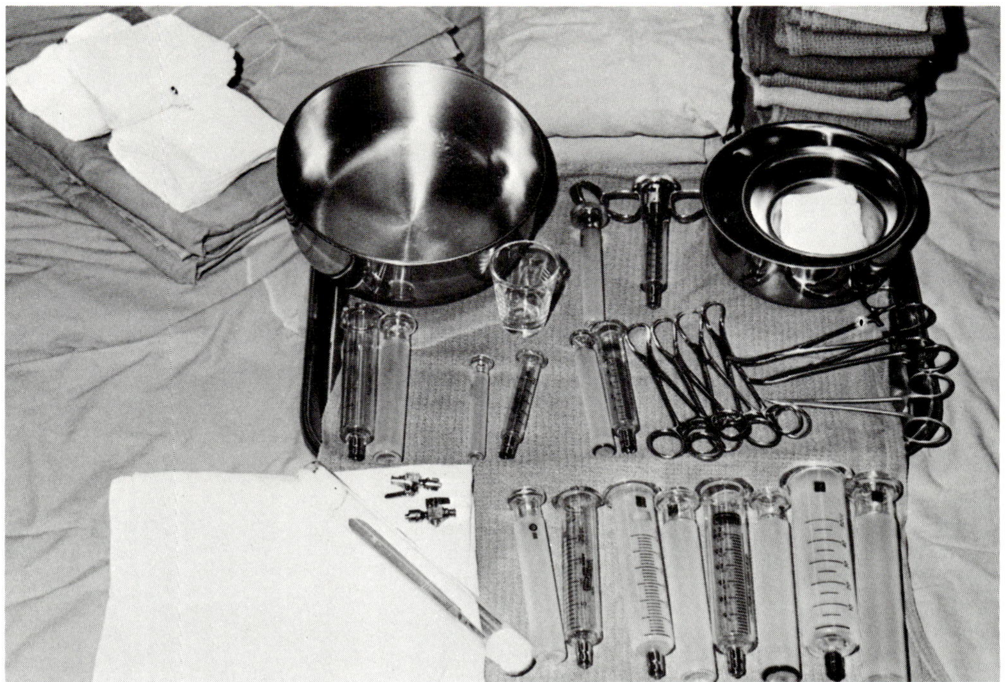

Fig. 13-85. Retrograde arteriogram kit. (Courtesy Tucson Medical Center Hospital.)

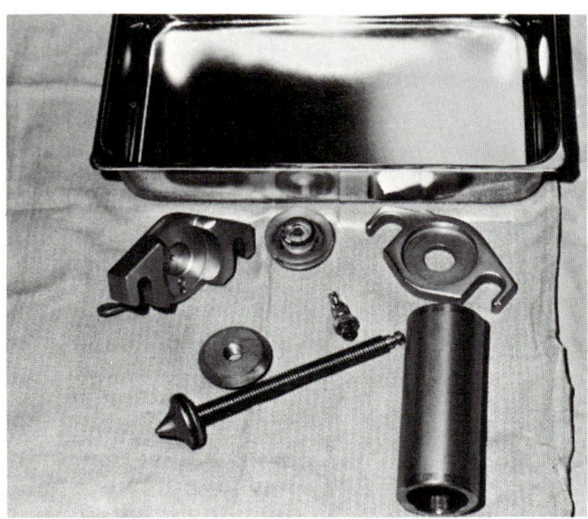

Fig. 13-86. Viamonte-Hobbs pressure injector syringe. (Courtesy Tucson Medical Center Hospital.)

RADIOGRAPHIC POSITION
Abdominal aorta and renal arteries—posterior (A-P) view (Figs. 13-87 to 13-95)

Film size—14″ × 14″ or 11″ × 14″ *Collimate to cover*
Serial changer
Lengthwise

Technique

Factors	Screen film-changer (par)
mA	640
Time	.10
mAs	64
Thickness in cm	20
kVp	70
Distance	40

Palpation points

Crest of the ilium; xiphoid process.

Procedure

From the supine position, center a point 1½ inches superior to the iliac crest over the film changer.

Central ray

Direct the central ray perpendicular to the center of the film changer. Collimate to film holder.

Immobilization

Suspended respiration.

Right-left markers

Place the right marker on the right lateral center border of the film holder.

Structures demonstrated

Posterior (A-P) views of the abdominal aorta and renal arteries to demonstrate renal vascular lesions, tumors, cysts, and other abnormalities.

Text continued on p. 506.

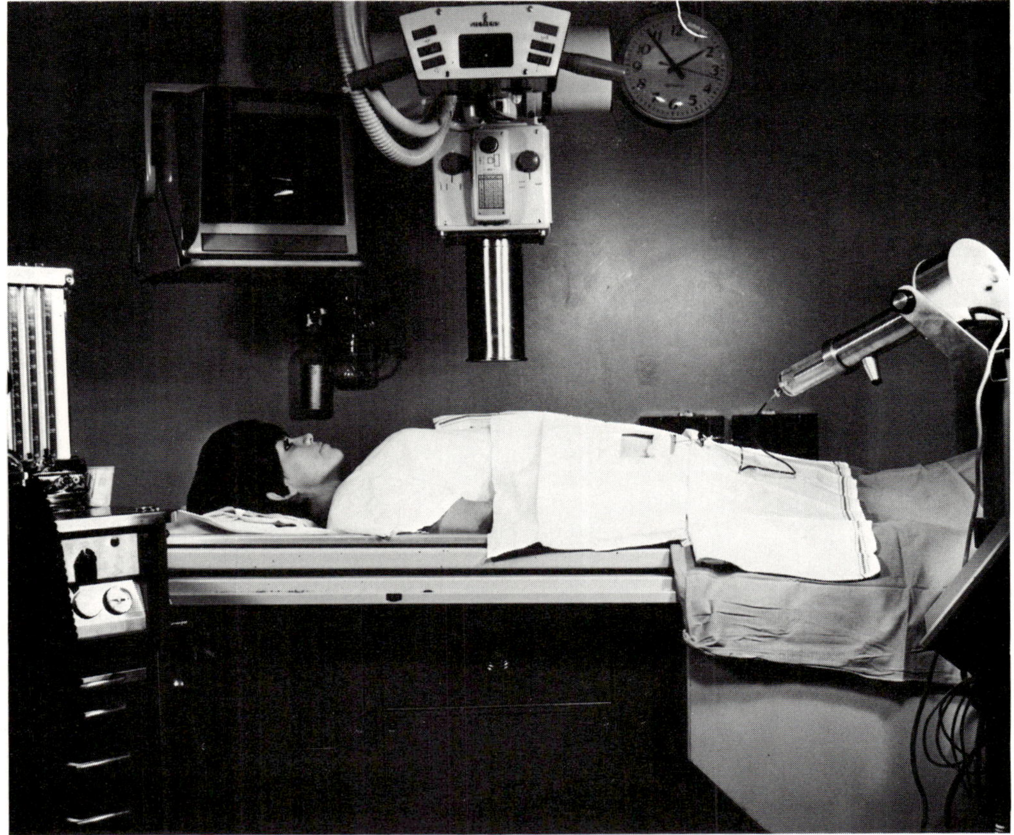

Fig. 13-87. Percutaneous transfemoral arteriography—posterior (A-P) position. (Courtesy St. Joseph's Hospital, Tucson.)

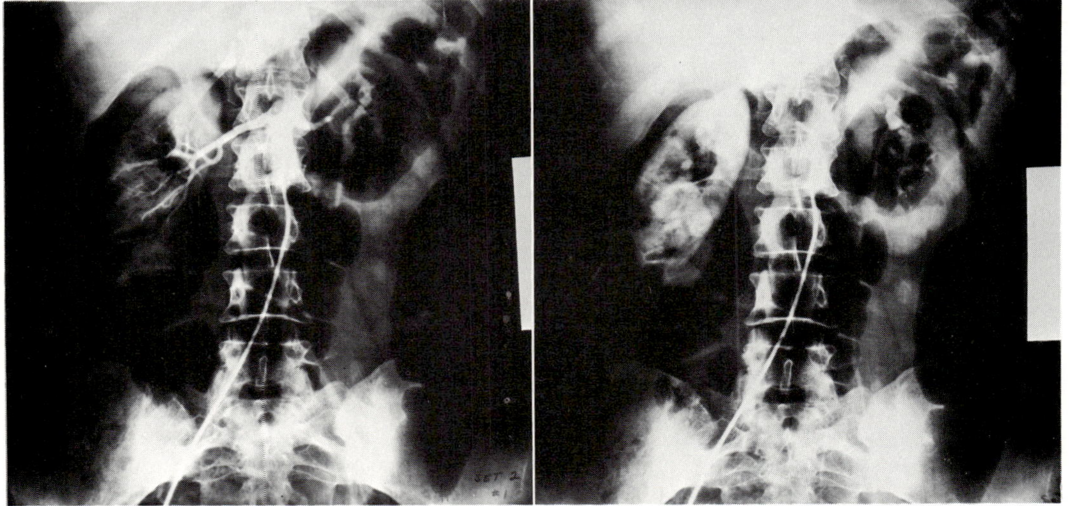

Fig. 13-88. Transfemoral selective renal artiogram—posterior (A-P) views. **A,** Early injection phase. **B,** Late injection phase. (Courtesy St. Joseph's Hospital, Tucson.)

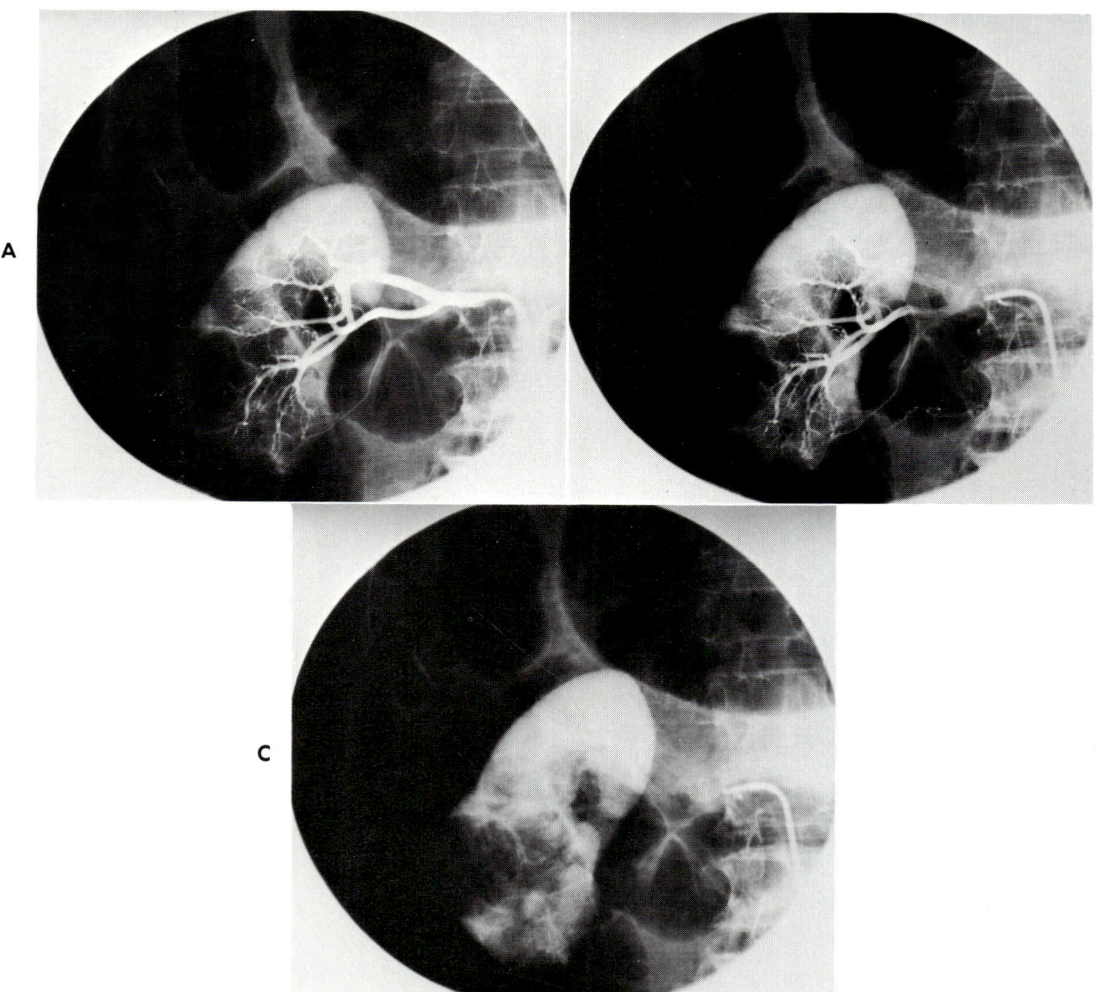

Fig. 13-89. Transfemoral selective renal arteriogram—posterior (A-P) views. **A,** Early injection phase. **B,** Postinjection phase. **C,** Late injection phase. (Courtesy St. Joseph's Hospital, Tucson.)

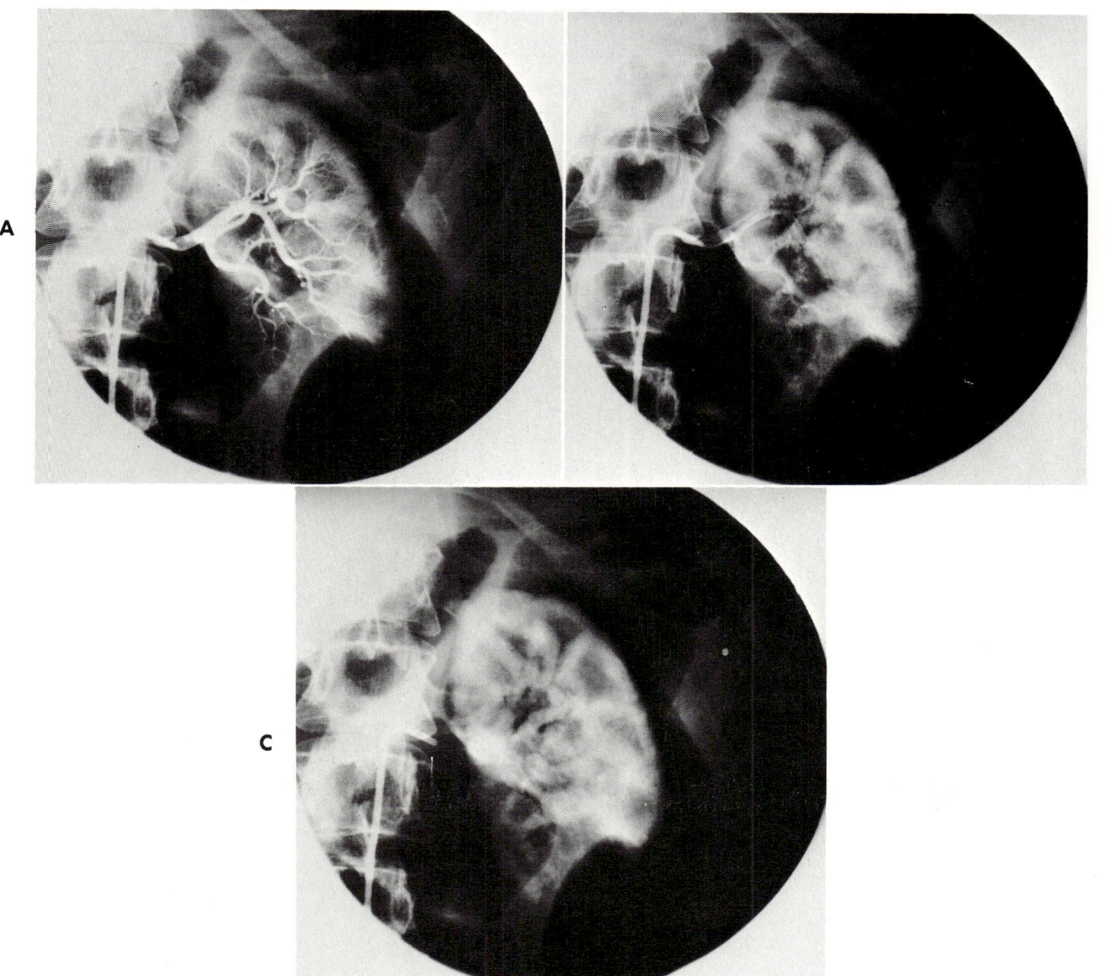

Fig. 13-90. Transfemoral selective renal arteriogram—posterior (A-P) views. **A,** Early injection phase. **B,** Postinjection phase. **C,** Late injection phase. (Courtesy St. Joseph's Hospital, Tucson.)

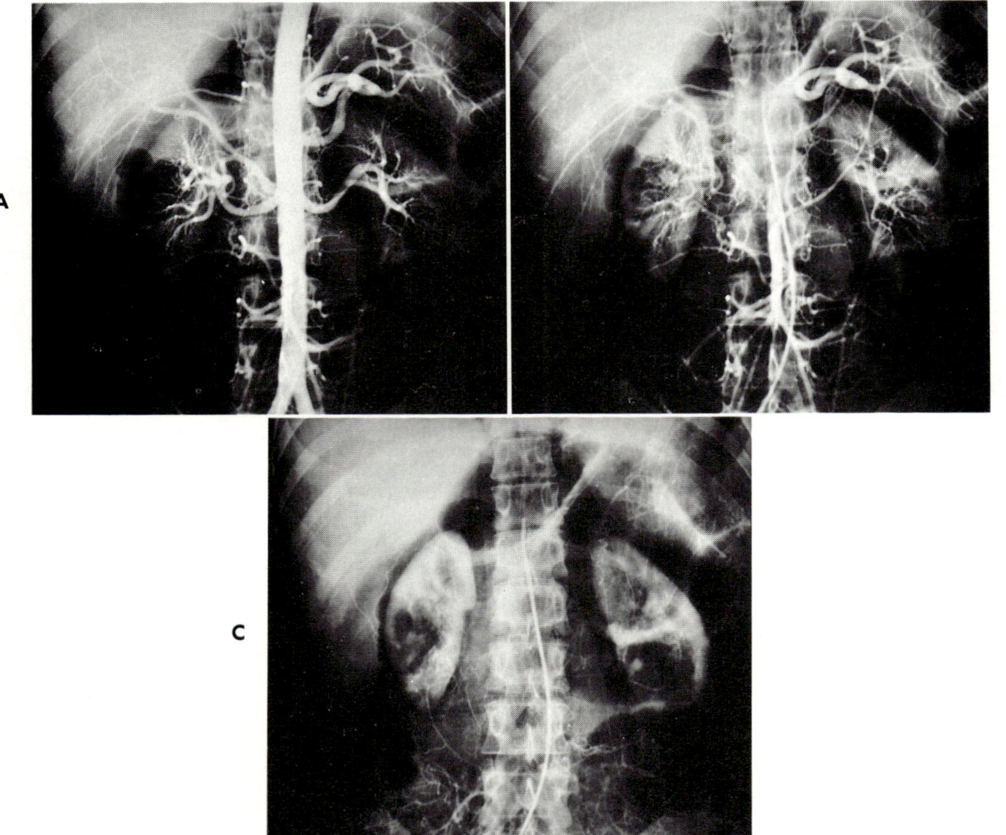

Fig. 13-91. Transfemoral catheter aortogram (flood study)—posterior (A-P) views. **A,** Early injection phase. **B,** Postinjection phase. **C,** Late injection phase. (Courtesy St. Joseph's Hospital, Tucson.)

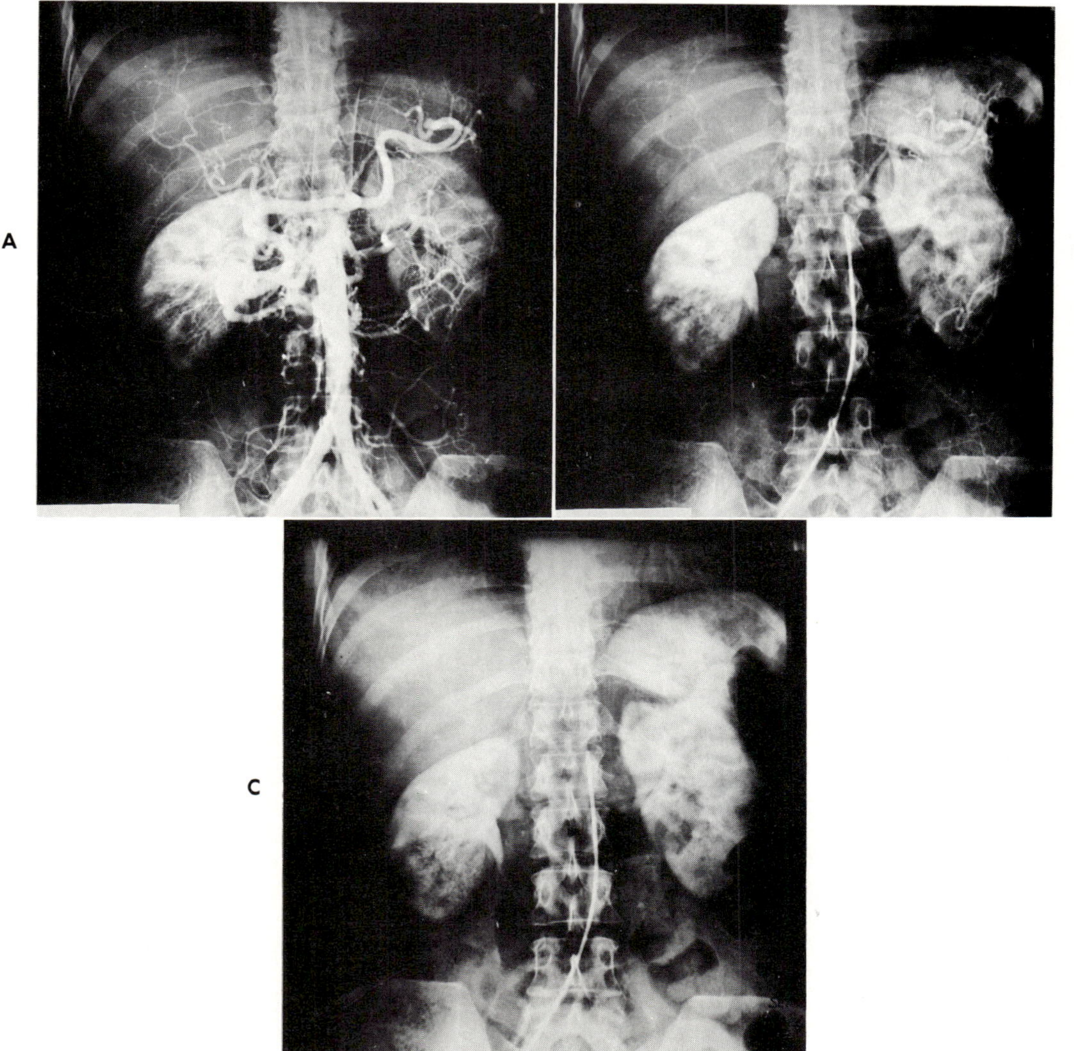

Fig. 13-92. Transfemoral catheter aortogram (flood study)—posterior (A-P) views. **A,** Early injection phase. **B,** Postinjection phase. **C,** Late injection phase. (Courtesy St. Joseph's Hospital, Tucson.)

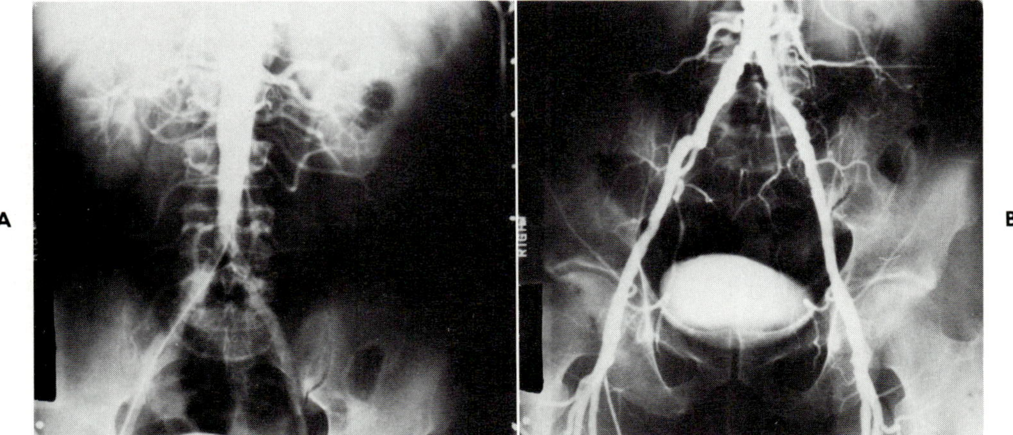

Fig. 13-93. Catheter aortography—posterior (A-P) views. **A,** Early injection phase. **B,** Abdominal runoff. (Courtesy Special Procedures Department, Southern Nevada Memorial Hospital, Las Vegas, Nevada.)

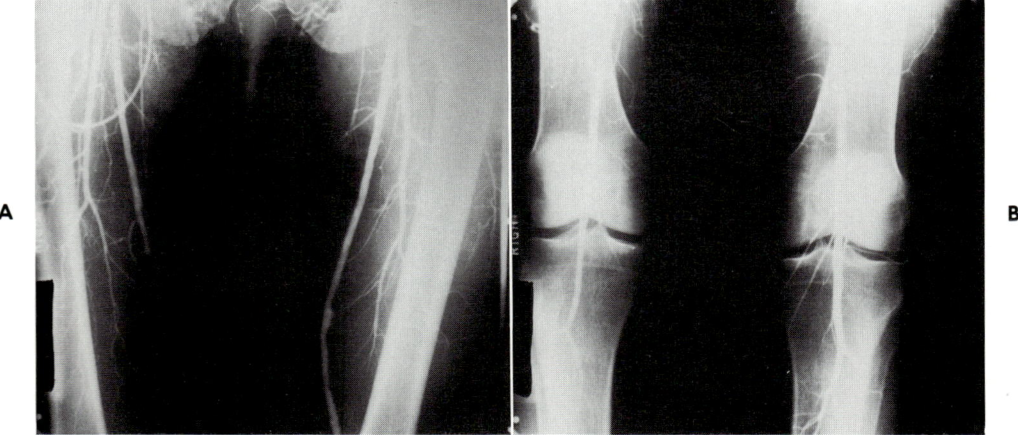

Fig. 13-94. Catheter aortography—posterior (A-P) views. **A** and **B,** Late injection runoff. (Courtesy Special Procedures Department, Southern Nevada Memorial Hospital, Las Vegas, Nevada.)

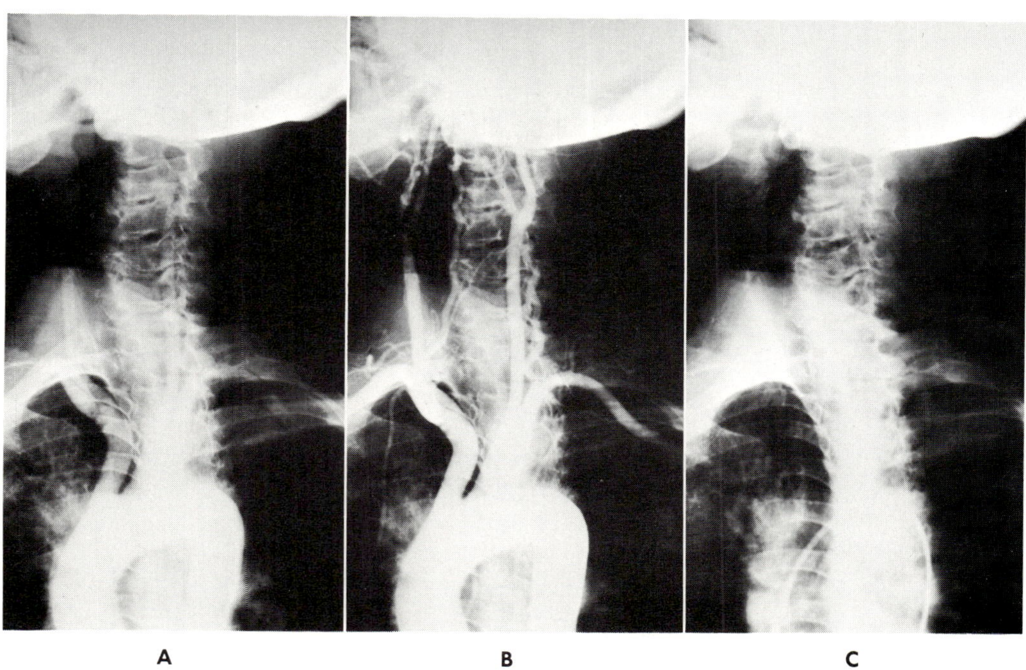

Fig. 13-95. Transfemoral aortic arch arteriogram—right oblique views. **A,** Early injection phase. **B,** Postinjection phase. **C,** Late injection phase. (Courtesy St. Joseph's Hospital, Tucson.)

PNEUMOENCEPHALOGRAPHY

Pneumoencephalography (Peg.) is a special radiographic examination of the ventricular system of the brain by the injection of a radiolucent medium (air, oxygen, or carbon dioxide) into the subarachnoid canal. The two puncture sites are (1) cisterna magna (cervical region) and (2) the lower lumbar (between third and fourth lumbar spinous processes).

Patient preparation (lumbar puncture)

1. The patient is admitted to the radiology department. Check the patient's record accurately for the following:
   a. Identification (patients with similar names)
   b. Complete blood work (laboratory report)
   c. Surgical permit
   d. Allergy report
2. The patient is strapped into the Peg. chair in an upright sitting position with the neck flexed and the frontal area resting against a vertical film changer.
3. The lumbar region is sterilized and prepared.

Contrast media

A selected quantity of air, oxygen, or carbon dioxide is determined and injected by the physician.

Equipment preparation

1. Provide autotomograph.
2. Provide a vertical film holder.
3. A sterilized pneumoencephalogram kit is usually provided by surgical supply.
4. Provide positioning accessories (sponges, compression bands, etc.).
5. Select technique and energize controls.

Examination

1. The physician introduces a large needle into the subarachnoid space, and a spinal tap is usually performed at this time.
2. Equal amounts of radiolucent contrast medium are injected after each aspiration of spinal fluid is made.
3. Routine exposures are then made to demonstrate the fourth ventricle, cerebral aqueduct, and the basal cisternae.
4. After additional fluid aspirations and contrast injections are completed, the needle is removed and exposures are made to demonstrate lateral and third ventricles.

Note: The radiographic series for this examination will vary in some departments. An example of one total series is as follows:

1. First injection—patient erect
   a. Translateral scout—CR horizontal
2. Second injection—patient erect
   a. Lateral autotomogram
   b. Frontal (P-A)—CR perpendicular
   c. Frontal (P-A)—CR caudad
   d. Frontal (P-A)—(reverse Towne)

3. Third injection and needle removed—patient supine—brow-up
   a. Translateral—CR horizontal
   b. Posterior (A-P)—CR perpendicular
   c. Occipital (A-P) Towne—CR 25 degrees caudad
4. Patient is then maneuvered through a complete forward somersault—patient supine—brow-up
   a. Translateral, hyperextension—CR horizontal
   b. Posterior (A-P)—CR perpendicular
   c. Occipital (A-P) Towne—CR 25 degrees caudad
5. Patient prone—brow-down
   a. Bilaterals—CR perpendicular
   b. Anterior (P-A)—CR perpendicular
   c. Anterior (P-A)—reverse Towne—CR 25 degrees cephalad

ROUTINE RADIOGRAPHIC POSITIONS

Pneumoencephalography—frontal (P-A) erect views (Figs. 13-96 and 13-97)

Film size—10″ × 12″
Cassette
Lengthwise

Bucky or grid
Collimate to cover

Technique

Factors	Screen film cassette (par)
mA	300S
Time	$0.0\overline{33}$
mAs	10
Thickness in cm	23
kVp	110
Distance	40

Palpation points

Frontal area; vertex; base of occiput.

Procedure

Position 1—Patient remains in the upright sitting position with the frontal area resting against the film changer. The midsagittal plane of the skull is perpendicular to the film holder. The canthomeatal line forms a 25-degree angle with the film holder.

CENTRAL RAY—Direct the central ray horizontal and perpendicular, in line with a point 4 cm cranial to the external auditory meatus to the center of the film holder. Collimate to film holder.

Position 2—Patient remains in position 1.

CENTRAL RAY—Direct the central ray slightly caudad (parallel with the glabellomeatal line), in line with a point 4 cm cranial to the external auditory meatus to the center of the film holder. Collimate to film holder.

Position 3—Patient remains in position 1.

CENTRAL RAY—Direct the central ray 5 degrees cephalad, in line with a point 4 cm cranial to the external auditory meatus to the center of the film holder. Collimate to film holder.

Immobilization

Compression band, suspended expiration.

Right-left markers

Place selected markers on lateral center border of the film holders.

Structures demonstrated

Positions 1 and 2—Frontal (P-A) view of fourth ventricle and vallecula.

Position 3—Frontal (P-A) view of the basal cisterns.

Note: All views are made for the purpose of demonstrating deep-seated lesion(s) of the brain, cerebral atrophy, and hydrocephalus.

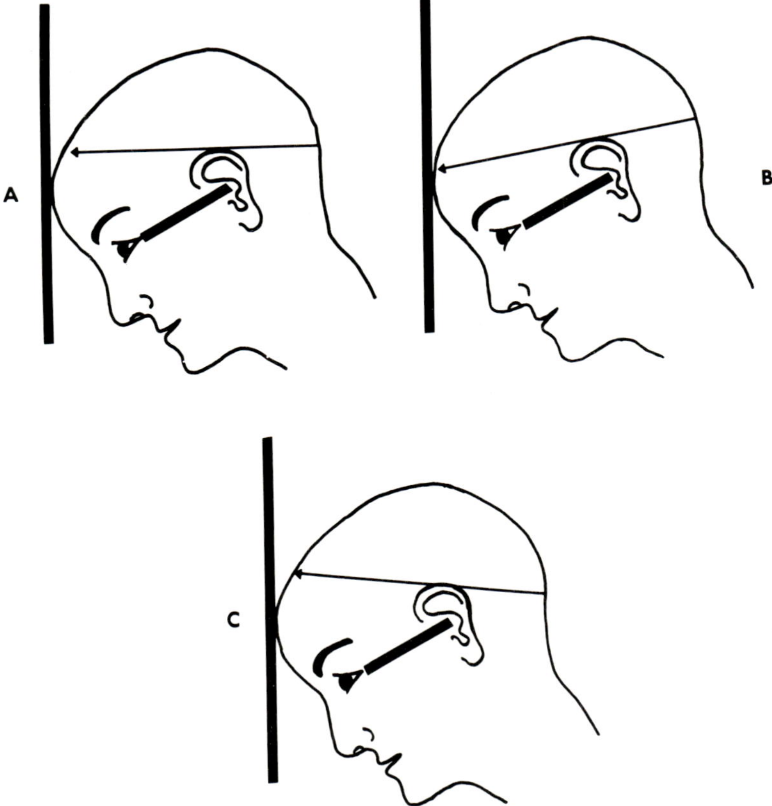

Fig. 13-96. Pneumoencephalography—frontal (P-A) erect positions. A, Central ray perpendicular. B, Central ray caudad. C, Central ray 5 degrees cephalad.

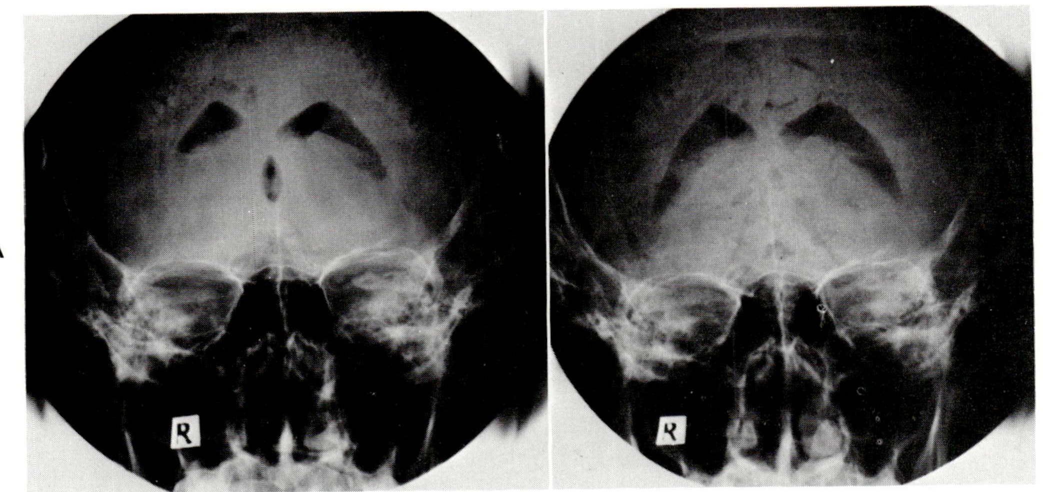

Fig. 13-97. Pneumoencephalogram. A, Anterior (P-A) erect view. B, Anterior (P-A) prone view. (Courtesy Tucson Medical Center Hospital.)

Pneumoencephalography—translateral, erect view (Figs. 13-98 and 13-99)

Film size—10″ × 12″
Cassette
Crosswise
Bucky or grid
Collimate to cover

Technique

Factors	Screen film cassette (par)
mA	300S
Time	.01$\bar{6}$
mAs	5
Thickness in cm	18
kVp	100
Distance	40

Palpation points

Vertex; base of occiput.

Procedure

Patient remains in the upright sitting position with the frontal area resting against the film changer or head support. Place a portable film changer, or attached film holder, against the side of the skull being examined and parallel with the midsagittal plane of the skull.

Central ray

Direct the central ray horizontal and perpendicular through a point 4 cm cranial to the external auditory meatus to the film holder. Collimate to film holder.

Immobilization

Employ suspended expiration.

Right-left markers

Place selected markers on the posterior center border of the film holder.

Structure demonstrated

Lateral view of the fourth ventricle.

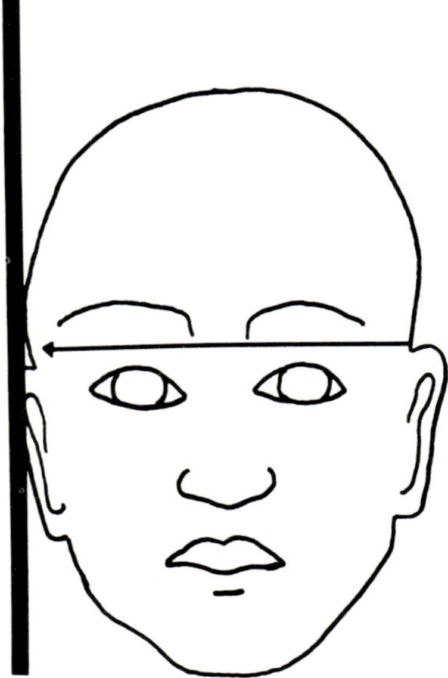

Fig. 13-98. Pneumoencephalography—translateral, erect position.

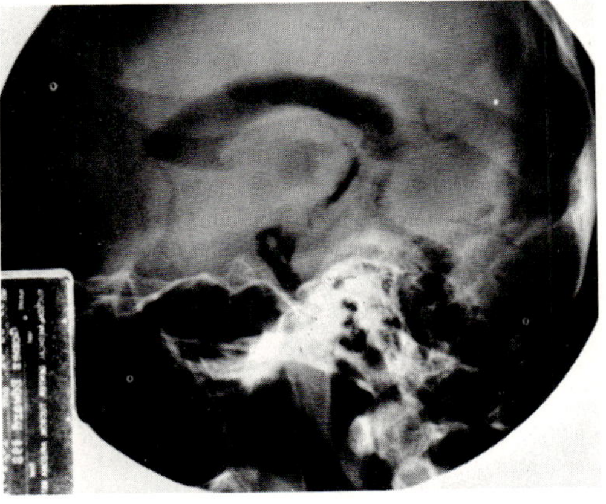

Fig. 13-99. Pneumoencephalogram—translateral, erect view. (Courtesy Tucson Medical Center Hospital.)

Pneumoencephalography—translateral, supine (brow-up) view (Fig. 13-100)

Film size—10″ × 12″
Cassette
Crosswise

Bucky or grid
Collimate to cover

Technique

Factors	Screen film cassette (par)
mA	300S
Time	$.01\bar{6}$
mAs	5
Thickness in cm	18
kVp	100
Distance	40

Palpation point

Vertex.

Procedure

Place the patient in the supine position with the head resting on a radiolucent sponge and with the median plane of the skull and body over the center line of the table. Flex the chin so that both the midsagittal plane and the canthomeatal line are perpendicular to the tabletop. Place a film holder against the side of the skull being examined and parallel with the midsagittal plane of the skull.

Central ray

Direct the central ray horizontal and perpendicular through a point 4 cm cranial to the external auditory meatus to the center of the film holder. Collimate to film holder.

Immobilization

Employ suspended expiration.

Right-left markers

Place the correct marker on the anterior center border of the film holder.

Structures demonstrated

Lateral view of the frontal and temporal horns (cornu) of the lateral ventricles.

Note: Posterior (A-P) and occipital (A-P) 25-degree Towne views may be positioned according to routine skull position (pp. 315 and 316).

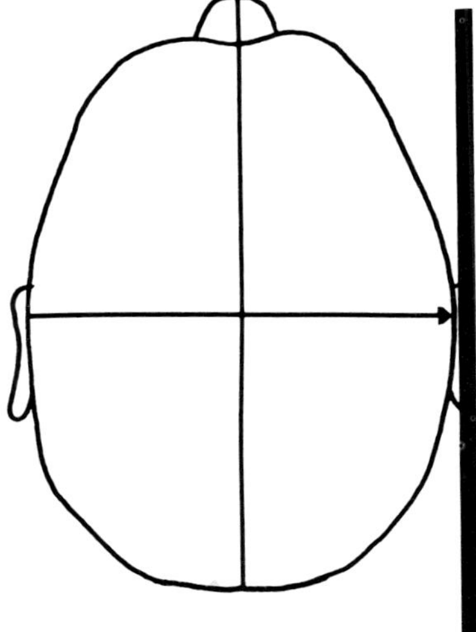

Fig. 13-100. Pneumoencephalography—translateral, supine (brow-up) position.

Pneumoencephalography—translateral, hyperextension view (Fig. 13-101)

Film size—10″ × 12″
Cassette
Crosswise
Bucky or grid
Collimate to cover

Technique

Factors	Screen film cassette (par)
mA	300S
Time	$.01\bar{6}$
mAs	5
Thickness in cm	18
kVp	100
Distance	40

Palpation points

Glabella; base of the occiput.

Procedure

From the supine position, hyperextend the patient's head over the end of the table with the vertex of the skull resting on a radiolucent sponge on top of a horizontal film changer or supporting table. The canthomeatal line is parallel with the surface of the head support. The midsagittal plane is perpendicular to the surface of the head support. Place a film holder against the side of the skull being examined and parallel with the midsagittal plane of the skull.

Central ray

Direct the central ray horizontal and perpendicular through a point ¾ inch anterior and ¾ inch cranial to the external auditory meatus to the center of the film holder. Collimate to film holder.

Immobilization

Employ suspended expiration.

Right-left markers

Place the correct marker on the anterior center border of the film holder.

Structures demonstrated

Lateral view of the third ventricle demonstrating the anteroinferior borders.

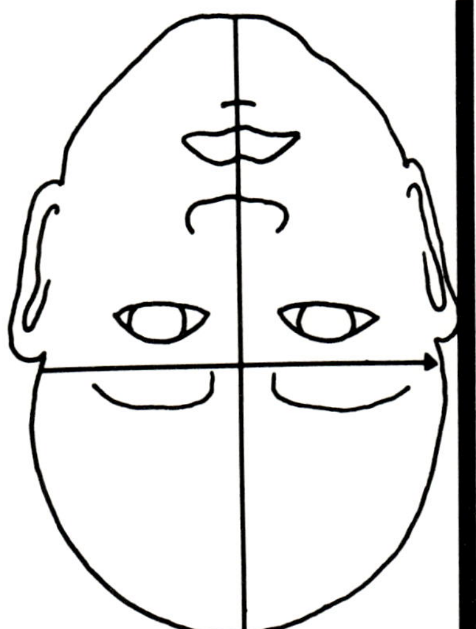

Fig. 13-101. Pneumoencephalography–translateral, hyperextension position.

Pneumoencephalography—posterior (A-P) and occipital (A-P) Towne views (Figs. 13-102 and 13-103)

Film size—10″ × 12″
Cassette
Lengthwise

Bucky
Collimate to cover

Technique

Factors	Screen film cassette (par)
mA	300S
Time	.0$\overline{66}$
mAs	10
Thickness in cm	23
kVp	110
Distance	40

Palpation point

Vertex.

Procedure

Place the patient in the supine position with the median line of the skull and body over the center line of the table. The midsagittal plane is perpendicular to the tabletop. Flex the chin so that the canthomeatal line is perpendicular to the tabletop.

Central ray

Position 1—Direct the central ray 25 degrees caudad in line with a point 2 cm cranial to the external auditory meatus to the center of the film holder. Collimate to film holder.

Position 2—Direct the central ray 10 degrees cephalad through the nasion to the center of the film holder. Collimate to film holder.

Immobilization

Compression band. Employ suspended expiration.

Right-left markers

Place the right marker on the right lateral center border of the film holder.

Structures demonstrated

Posterior (A-P) and occipital (A-P) Towne views to demonstrate the temporal horns and the bodies of the lateral ventricles.

Note: For additional prone views to demonstrate the lateral ventricles, refer to positioning instructions listed on p. 311.

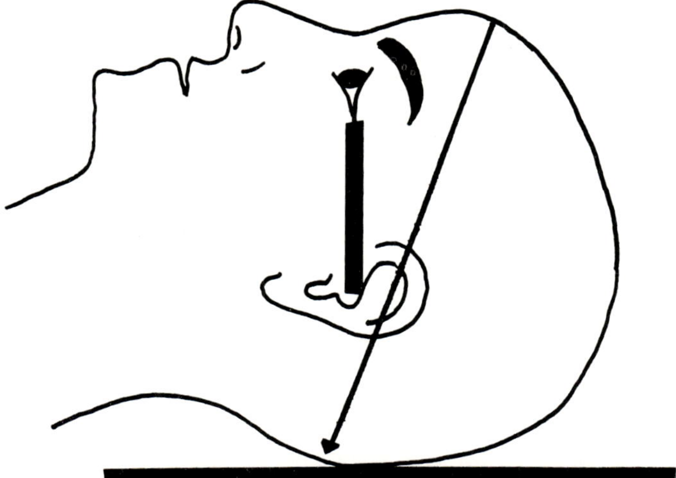

Fig. 13-102. Pneumoencephalography—occipital (A-P) Towne position.

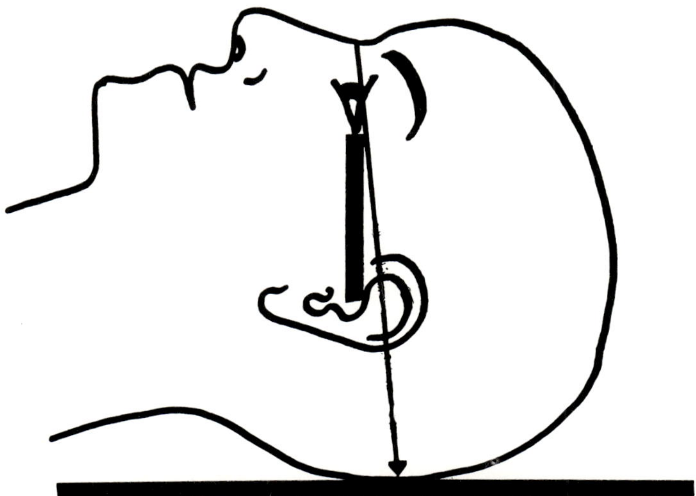

Fig. 13-103. Pneumoencephalography—posterior (A-P) position.

QUESTIONS

1. Name four advantages for using contrast media.
2. Name four different forms of contrast media.
3. Describe the radiographic procedure for the posteroanterior projection of the parotid gland.
4. Describe the equipment preparation for a routine fluoroscopy setup for gastrointestinal studies.
5. What precaution is necessary when making an R.A.O. stomach radiograph on a hypersthenic patient?
6. When can you determine that a small intestine study is completed?
7. List the basic equipment preparation necessary for a large intestine radiographic study.
8. What method may be employed to combat flaking or dehydration of the contrast medium in a double-contrast study of the intestine?
9. Define cholecystography.
10. Name five methods which may be employed to overcome gas shadows in the intestinal tract during an oral cholecystogram study.
11. Name five reasons why contrast medium may be absent in the gallbladder.
12. Explain the purpose for making a right lateral decubitus projection of the gallbladder during oral cholecystogram studies.
13. Define T-tube cholangiography.
14. Describe the radiographic procedure for the postoperative T-tube choledochogram.
15. Name three preparations that may be found in an emergency I.V. kit.
16. Explain the advantage of making a two-film radiographic K.U.B. series.
17. Explain the difference between functional and nonfunctional examinations of the urinary system.
18. Name four important structures that may be found in a routine retrograde pyelogram study.
19. Explain the purpose of the bicycle position in urethrography.
20. State five reasons for making a routine radiographic examination of the unborn fetus.
21. Describe the radiographic procedure for the anteroposterior Colcher-Sussman method of pelvimetry.
22. Describe the contrast media preparation for bronchography.
23. Name three routine radiographic positions for mammography.
24. Describe the radiographic procedures for the craniocaudad projection of the breast.
25. Define percutaneous carotid arteriography.
26. In carotid arteriography what is the average circulation time from arterial through venous phase?
27. Is it important to check the patient's allergy report when doing percutaneous translumbar aortography?
28. Give two reasons why it may be necessary to perform a percutaneous translumbar aortographic examination.
29. Locate the two injection sites that may be used in pneumoencephalography.
30. Name three contrast media which may be used in pneumoencephalography.

APPENDIX

MEANING OF GREEK LETTERS OFTEN USED

α **(alpha)** A positive particle consisting of two protons and two neutrons (the helium atom nucleus).

β **(beta)** A negative particle consisting of one electron.

γ **(gamma)** An electromagnetic wave from radioactive substance.

Δ **(delta)** To indicate the change, as in energy.

λ **(lambda)** Wavelength.

ν **(nu)** Frequency.

υ **(upsilon)** Velocity when less than that of light.

ϕ **(phi)** The work function of a given metal.

USEFUL CONSTANTS, LAWS, DEFINITIONS, AND FORMULAS

Planck's constant 6.62×10^{-27} erg-seconds; simply written as *h;* a mathematical value that represents the ratio of the energy of any quantum of radiation to its frequency.

c **(the speed of light)** 186,000 miles/second or 3×10^{10} cm/second.

Thermodynamics

Law I: When mechanical work is transformed into heat or heat into work, the amount of work is always equivalent to the quantity of heat (conservation of energy).

Law II: It is impossible by any continuous self-sustaining process for heat to be transferred from a colder to a hotter body.

Newton's laws

I. Law of inertia: A body at rest tends to remain at rest, while a body in motion tends to continue in motion in the same straight line unless acted upon by an outside force.

II. Law of momentum: When a force acts upon a body, it changes the momentum of that body. This change of momentum is proportional to the applied force and to the time it acts upon the body.

III. Law of reaction: Every action (force) is accompanied by an equal and opposite reaction (force).

IV. Law of gravitation: Every body in the universe attracts every other body with a force that is directly proportional to the product of the masses (weights) of the two bodies and inversely proportional to the square of the distance between their exact centers.

Density The ratio of the mass of a homogeneous portion of matter to its volume.

Mass-energy equivalence The mass of anything increases as its velocity increases, and if the velocity approaches that of light, the mass becomes infinitely large. Mass is constant only when there is no motion. The effect of velocity in mass is significant only when the velocity is near the speed of light. Einstein postulated that the energy of anything is equal to its mass times the square of the speed of light; this is written: $E = mc^2$, where E is the energy, m is the mass at rest, and c is the constant for the speed of light.

Melting point The temperature, under standard pressure, at which a solid substance begins to melt.

MPD The maximum permissible dose in rems to the most critical organs is $5(N - 18)$ where N is the age in years and is greater than 18; the MPD in rems to the skin of the whole body is $10(N - 18)$.

Quantum of radiant energy of frequency $W = h\nu$, where W is the quantum, h is Planck's constant, and ν is the frequency of the energy.

Specific heat The heat in calories required to raise the temperature of one gram of substance 1 degree centigrade.

Temperature of volatilization The temperature, under standard pressure, at which a substance begins to vaporize readily.

Thermal conductivity The quantity of heat that passes in unit time through a unit area of plate whose thickness is unity, when its opposite faces differ in temperature by one degree.

Z number The atomic number of any element.

Silver stain remover formula:

Water	750 ml
Thiourea	75 grams
Citric acid	75 grams
Water to make	1 liter

Temperature conversion formulas:

°C. = °F. − 32 × 5/9
°F. = °C. × 9/5 + 32
O°K. (Kelvin or absolute) = −273.18° C.

SEQUENCE OF THE ELEMENTS

Element	Symbol	Atomic number	Atomic weight*	Orbits with number of electrons contained K	L	M	N	O	P	Q
Hydrogen	H	1	1.008	1						
Helium	He	2	4.003	2						
Lithium	Li	3	6.940	2	1					
Beryllium	Be	4	9.013	2	2					
Boron	B	5	10.82	2	3					
Carbon	C	6	12.01	2	4					
Nitrogen	N	7	14.008	2	5					
Oxygen	O	8	16.000	2	6					
Fluorine	F	9	19.000	2	7					
Neon	Ne	10	20.183	2	8					
Sodium	Na	11	22.997	2	8	1				
Magnesium	Mg	12	24.32	2	8	2				
Aluminum	Al	13	26.98	2	8	3				
Silicon	Si	14	28.09	2	8	4				
Phosphorus	P	15	30.975	2	8	5				
Sulfur	S	16	32.006	2	8	6				
Chlorine	Cl	17	35.457	2	8	7				
Argon	A	18	39.994	2	8	8				
Potassium	K	19	39.100	2	8	8	1			
Calcium	Ca	20	40.08	2	8	8	2			
Scandium	Sc	21	44.96	2	8	9	2			
Titanium	Ti	22	47.90	2	8	10	2			
Vanadium	V	23	50.95	2	8	11	2			
Chromium	Cr	24	52.01	2	8	13	1			
Manganese	Mn	25	54.93	2	8	13	2			
Iron	Fe	26	55.85	2	8	14	2			
Cobalt	Co	27	58.94	2	8	15	2			
Nickel	Ni	28	58.69	2	8	16	2			
Copper	Cu	29	63.54	2	8	18	1			
Zinc	Zn	30	65.38	2	8	18	2			
Gallium	Ga	31	69.72	2	8	18	3			
Germanium	Ge	32	72.60	2	8	18	4			
Arsenic	As	33	74.91	2	8	18	5			
Selenium	Se	34	78.96	2	8	18	6			
Bromine	Br	35	79.916	2	8	18	7			
Krypton	Kr	36	83.80	2	8	18	8			
Rubidium	Rb	37	85.48	2	8	18	8	1		
Strontium	Sr	38	87.63	2	8	18	8	2		
Yttrium	Y	39	88.92	2	8	18	9	2		
Zirconium	Zr	40	91.22	2	8	18	10	2		
Niobium	Nb	41	92.91	2	8	18	12	1		
Molybdenum	Mo	42	95.95	2	8	18	13	1		
Technetium	Tc	43	99.000	2	8	18	14	1		
Ruthenium	Ru	44	101.7	2	8	18	15	1		
Rhodium	Rh	45	102.91	2	8	18	16	1		
Palladium	Pd	46	106.7	2	8	18	18	0		
Silver	Ag	47	107.880	2	8	18	18	1		
Cadmium	Cd	48	112.41	2	8	18	18	2		
Indium	In	49	114.76	2	8	18	18	3		
Tin	Sn	50	118.70	2	8	18	18	4		
Antimony	Sb	51	121.76	2	8	18	18	5		
Tellurium	Te	52	127.61	2	8	18	18	6		
Iodine	I	53	126.91	2	8	18	18	7		

*A number in parentheses indicates the mass number of the isotope of the longest known half-life.

SEQUENCE OF THE ELEMENTS—cont'd

Element	Symbol	Atomic number	Atomic weight*	K	L	M	N	O	P	Q
				Orbits with number of electrons contained						
Xenon	Xe	54	131.3	2	8	18	18	8		
Cesium	Cs	55	132.91	2	8	18	18	8	1	
Barium	Ba	56	137.36	2	8	18	18	8	2	
Lanthanum	La	57	138.92	2	8	18	18	9	2	
Cerium	Ce	58	140.13	2	8	18	20	8	2	
Praseodymium	Pr	59	140.92	2	8	18	21	8	2	
Neodymium	Nd	60	144.27	2	8	18	22	8	2	
Promethium	Pm	61	(145)	2	8	18	23	8	2	
Samarium	Sm	62	150.43	2	8	18	24	8	2	
Europium	Eu	63	152.0	2	8	18	25	8	2	
Gadolinium	Gd	64	156.9	2	8	18	25	9	2	
Terbium	Tb	65	159.2	2	8	18	27	8	2	
Dysprosium	Dy	66	162.46	2	8	18	28	8	2	
Holmium	Ho	67	164.94	2	8	18	29	8	2	
Erbium	Er	68	167.2	2	8	18	30	8	2	
Thulium	Tm	69	169.4	2	8	18	31	8	2	
Ytterbium	Yb	70	173.04	2	8	18	32	8	2	
Lutetium	Lu	71	174.99	2	8	18	32	9	2	
Hafnium	Hf	72	178.6	2	8	18	32	10	2	
Tantalum	Ta	73	180.88	2	8	18	32	11	2	
Tungsten	W	74	183.92	2	8	18	32	12	2	
Rhenium	Re	75	186.31	2	8	18	32	13	2	
Osmium	Os	76	190.2	2	8	18	32	14	2	
Iridium	Ir	77	193.1	2	8	18	32	15	2	
Platinum	Pt	78	195.23	2	8	18	32	17	1	
Gold	Au	79	197.2	2	8	18	32	18	1	
Mercury	Hg	80	200.61	2	8	18	32	18	2	
Thallium	Tl	81	204.39	2	8	18	32	18	3	
Lead	Pb	82	207.21	2	8	18	32	18	4	
Bismuth	Bi	83	209.00	2	8	18	32	18	5	
Polonium	Po	84	(210)	2	8	18	32	18	6	
Astatine	At	85	(210)	2	8	18	32	18	7	
Radon	Rn	86	(222)	2	8	18	32	18	8	
Francium	Fr	87	(223)	2	8	18	32	18	8	1
Radium	Ra	88	(226)	2	8	18	32	18	8	2
Actinium	Ac	89	(227)	2	8	18	32	18	9	2
Thorium	Th	90	(232)	2	8	18	32	18	10	2
Protactinium	Pa	91	(231)	2	8	18	32	20	9	2
Uranium	U	92	(238)	2	8	18	32	21	9	2
Neptunium	Np	93	(237)	2	8	18	32	22	9	2
Plutonium	Pu	94	(242)	2	8	18	32	23	9	2
Americium	Am	95	(243)	2	8	18	32	24	9	2
Curium	Cm	96	(247)	2	8	18	32	25	9	2
Berkelium	Bk	97	(249)							
Californium	Cf	98	(251)							
Einsteinium	Es	99	(254)							
Fermium	Fm	100	(253)							
Mendelevium	Md	101	(256)							
Nobelium	No	102	(254)							
Lawrencium	Lw	103								

COMPARISON OF TUNGSTEN WITH SOME OTHER ELEMENTS AS A TARGET

Symbol	Z	Density Gm/cm³	Melting point °C.	Temp. of volatilization at 0° C.	Thermal conductivity	Specific heat	Efficiency of anode at 100 kVp
Co	27	8.9	1480			0.09	0.378%
Ni	28	8.9	1450		0.14	0.10	0.392%
Cu	29	8.92	1084		0.92	0.09	0.406%
Mo	42	10.2	2620		0.346	0.07	0.588%
Ag	47	10.5	960.5		0.992	0.05	0.658%
W	**74**	**19.3**	**3370**	**1800**	**0.35**	**0.03**	**1.036%**
Os	76	22.5	2700	2300	0.17	0.03	1.064%
Ir	77	22.4	2350	1400	0.17	0.03	1.078%
Pt	78	21.5	1750	1200	0.17	0.03	1.092%
Pb	82	11.34	327.43		0.082	0.03	1.148%

USEFUL ELECTRICAL SYMBOLS*

Number	American standard number	Description	Symbol
1	1.	Adjustable	↗
2	6.	Battery	
3	6.3	Battery, multicell	
4	7.1	Circuit breaker	
5	12.	Coil, operating	
6	14.1	Connector, female contact	
7	14.2	Connector, male contact	
8	14.4	Connectors, separable	
9	15.1.2	Contact, fixed, for switch	
10	15.3.2	Contact, open	
11	15.4	Contact, open, with time closing	TC
12	15.5	Contact, closed, with time opening	TO
13	16.2	Contactor, electrically operated with series blowout coil (magnetic contactor)	
14	27.	Fuse	
15	28.	Ground	

*Adapted from American standard graphical symbols for electrical diagrams, American Standards Association, Inc., New York. Courtesy Institute of Radio Engineers, Inc., New York.

USEFUL ELECTRICAL SYMBOLS—cont'd

Number	American standard number	Description	Symbol
16	31.1	Inductor, winding	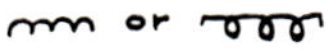
17	31.2	Inductor, winding, with magnetic core	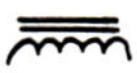
18	31.5	Inductor, adjustable	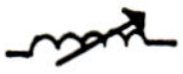
19	43.5	Crossed wires, not connected	
20	43.6.2	Crossed wires, connected	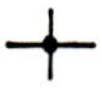
21	50.1	Resistor	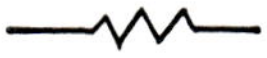
22	50.4	Resistor, variable	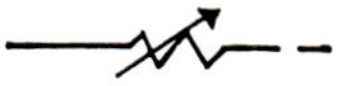
23	56.1	Switch, single throw	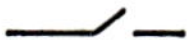
24	56.2	Switch, double throw	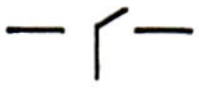
25	56.2.1	Switch, double throw, two-pole	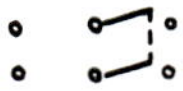
26	63.	Transformer	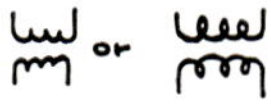
27	63.2	Transformer, magnetic core	
28	63.7.1	Autotransformer, adjustable	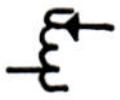
29	64.1.1	Emitting electrode, directly heated	
30	64.3.1	Anode or plate	
31	64.3.2	Target or x-ray anode	
32	64.6.1	Glass envelope	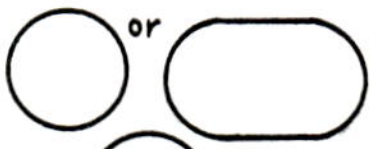
33	64.11.6.1	Single unit vacuum tube	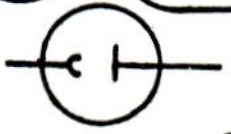
34	64.11.12.1	X-ray tube with filamentary cathode and focusing cup	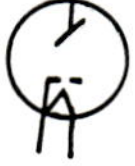
35	37.	Meter instrument symbols†	
		Ammeter	A
		Galvanometer	G
		Milliammeter	MA
		Voltmeter	V
		Prereading voltmeter	PV

†The symbols for these instruments are included in the circle located where the meter would be located.

GLOSSARY

ANATOMY, PHYSIOLOGY, AND RELATED TERMS

A

ab- A prefix indicating off or away from.

abdomen (ab-do'men) The large inferior cavity of the trunk bounded superiorly by the diaphragm, anteriorly by the ribs and abdominal muscles, bilaterally by the ribs and abdominal muscles, and posteriorly by the vertebral column, psoas, and quadratus lumborum muscles.

aberration (ab-er-a'shun) Deviation from the usual course.

acetabulum (as-e-tab'u-lum) The fossa or depression in the lateral and anterior surface of the pelvis for the articulation of the head of the femur.

acoustic (ah-koos'tik) Pertaining to sound or to the sense of hearing.

acromion (ah-kro'me-on) Process of the scapula, part of the shoulder girdle.

adipose (ad'e-pos) Fatty tissue; obese.

aerated (a'er-at-ed) Filled with air.

afferent (af'er-ent) Leading toward the center.

alveolar (al-ve'o-lar) Pertaining to an alveolus. The alveolar process is the process from which the teeth erupt.

ambulatory (am'bu-la-to-re) Able to walk.

ampulla (am-pul'ah) A dilatation of a canal or duct.

anastomosis (a-nas'to-mo"sis) A communication between two vessels.

anatomy (ah-nat'o-me) The science of the structure of organs or of organic bodies.

anion (an'i-on) An ion carrying a negative charge.

ankylosis (ang-kil-o'sis) Stiffness of a joint resulting from either traumatic or intentional union of the joint surfaces.

antecubital space (an-te-ku'be-tal) The space in the bend of the elbow on the volar surface of the forearm.

antrum (an'trum) A cavity or chamber; one of the paranasal sinuses in the maxillae. It is also called the maxillary sinus.

anus (a'nus) The terminus and outlet of the digestive tract.

aorta (a-or'tah) The very large artery arising from the left ventricle of the heart. All the lesser arteries, except the coronary arteries, arise from it.

apex (a'peks) The top or summit of any organ; also the pointed end.

apophyseal joint (ap-o-fiz'e-al) The true intervertebral joint between the articular processes.

arachnoid (ah-rak'noid) The delicate membrane of the brain and spinal cord between the dura and pia maters; weblike.

areolar (ah-re'o-lar) Containing minute interspaces.

artery (ar'ter-e) A vessel that conveys blood from the heart.

arthritic (ar-thrit'ik) Pertaining to or affected with arthritis.

arthritis (ar-thri'tis) Inflammation of a joint.

arthroclasia (ar-thro-kla'ze-ah) The breaking down of an ankylosis to secure free movement of the joint.

arthrodesis (ar-throd'e-sis) The surgical fixation of a joint.

articulate (ar-tik'u-lat) To unite so as to form a joint.

articulation (ar-tik-u-la'shun) Usually indicates motion between two or more bones; any naturally occurring union between two or more bones. The types of articulations are synarthroses—immovable; schindyleses—grooved; gomphoses—sockets; suturae—sutures; diarthroses—movable; arthrodia—gliding; ginglymus—hinge; enarthroses—ball-and-socket; and amphiarthroses—mixed or combinations.

atlas (at'las) The first cervical vertebra.

atrium (a'tre-um) The auricle of the heart; a vessel that receives venous blood.

atypical (a-tip'e-kal) Not conformable to type.

auditory meatus (aw'de-to-re) The opening of the ear.

auricle (aw're-kl) The pinna or flap of the ear; also one of the upper chambers of the heart that receives the blood from the circulatory system.

axilla (ak-sil'ah) The armpit.

axis (ak'sis) The second cervical vertebra.

B

biliary (bil'e-a-re) Pertaining to the bile or its production.

binary fission (bi'na-re) Division into two equal parts.

brachial (bra'ke-al) Brachium; belonging to the arm.

bronchiole (brong'ke-ol) One of the finer subdivisions of the branched bronchial tree.

bronchus (brong'kus) An air tube; one of the divisions of the trachea.

C

calcaneus (kal-ka'ne-us) The heel bone, largest bone of the tarsus.

calcareous (kal-ka're-us) Pertaining to or containing calcium or lime.

calcigerous (kal-sij'er-us) Producing or carrying calcium salts.

calvarium (kal-va're-um) The cranium.

calyx (ka'liks) One of the cuplike divisions of the pelvis of the kidney.

canaliculus (kan-al-ik'u-lus) Any one of a system of minute channels connected with each haversian canal.

cancellous bone (kan'sel-us) Bone having a reticular, spongy, or latticelike structure.

carpus (kar'pus) The bones of the wrist.

cartilage (kar'ti-lij) Connective tissue containing no vascular network.

cation (kat'i-on) An ion carrying a positive charge.

cerebellum (ser-e-bel'um) That division of the brain behind the cerebrum and above the pons and fourth ventricle concerned with coordination of movements.

cerebrum (ser'e-brum) The main portion of the brain.

choana (ko'a-nah) Funnel; opening of the posterior nares into the pharynx.

chromosome (kro'mo-som) One of several small, dark-staining bodies that appear in the nucleus of a cell especially during mitosis.

chyle (kil) The milk-white fluid absorbed by the lacteals during digestion; lymph containing absorbed fat.

chyme (kīm) Food having undergone gastric digestion only.

coccyx (kok'siks) The caudal and vestigial terminus of the spinal column.

colon (ko'lon) The large part of the intestine, beginning with the cecum and terminating at the end of the sigmoid flexure.

compact bone Bone having very dense structure; true bone.

condyle (kon'dil) Rounded eminence of bone, usually articular.

congenital (kon-gen'i-tal) Existing at or before birth.

coracoid (kor'ah-koid) Shaped like a crow's beak; a process of the scapula.

coronoid (kor'o-noid) Crown-shaped; processes found on the mandible and ulna.

cortex (kor'teks) The outer layer of an organ as distinguished from its inner substance.

cribriform plate (krib're-form) The sievelike upper plate of the ethmoid.

crista galli (kris'tah gal'le) A ridge on the ethmoid bone to which the falx cerebri is attached.

cuboid (ku'boid) The lateral bone of the tarsus between the calcaneus and fourth and fifth metatarsals.

cuneiform (ku-ne'e-form) Wedge-shaped; bones of the tarsus.

D

dactyl (dak'til) A digit, either finger or toe.

deglutition (deg-loo-tish'un) The act of swallowing, consumated in three steps: the larynx is elevated; the pharyngeal space is briefly closed while the food bolus is shot back over the tongue; the pharyngeal space then opens to receive the bolus, which is rapidly forced into the upper one third of the esophagus where peristaltic action begins. True peristalsis does not begin in the esophagus. The first step in deglutition is voluntary; the next two steps are involuntary. The entire elapsed time when no respiration occurs is from 5 to 6 seconds.

dermis (der'mis) The corium or true skin.

diaphragm (di'ah-fram) The wall that separates the thorax from the abdomen. It is muscular at the circumference and tendinous in the center.

diaphysis (di-af'is-is) The shaft of a long bone.

diastole (di-as'to-le) The heart at rest; the period of dilation of one of the heart chambers.

digestion (di-jest'yun) The process of converting food into materials for absorption and assimilation.

digit (dij'it) A finger or toe.

diverticulum (di-ver-tik'u-lum) A small pouch or blind sac arising from a main structure.

duodenum (du-o-de'num) The first part of the small intestine between the pylorus and jejunum.

dura mater (du'rah ma'ter) Durable or hard mother. The fibrous outer membrane covering of the brain and spinal cord.

E

efferent (ef'er-ent) Carrying away from.

endocrine gland (en'do-krin) A gland that secretes a substance or substances directly into the bloodstream. The gland has no common ducts.

endosteum (en-dos'te-um) The vascular membranous layer of connective tissue lining the medullary cavity of bones.

epicondyle (ep-e-kon'dil) An eminence upon a bone above its condyle. It is usually roughened for attachment with muscles or tendons.

epidermis (ep-e-der'mis) The outer and nonvascular layer of the skin. It is protective and comprised of four layers. From inside out the layers are stratum germinativum, stratum granulosum, stratum lucidum, and stratum corneum.

epigastrium (ep-e-gas'tre-um) Upper and midparts of the abdomen relating to the position of the stomach.

epiphyseal line (ep-e-fiz'e-al) The line of junction

between the epiphysis and the body of the bone; often confusing in the determination of hairline fractures in this region.

epiphysis (e-pif'is-is) A process of bone that is attached for a time to the body of the bone by cartilage, but that later completely ossifies to the body of the bone. The growth in length of the long bones occurs at this cartilaginous joint before maturity of the individual is reached.

epipteric bone (e-pip-ter'ik) A wormian (supernumerary) bone in the region of the pterion.

esophagus (e-sof'ah-gus) That portion of the digestive tract between the pharynx and the stomach.

eversion (e-ver'zhun) Of the foot, turning the foot outwardly or laterally.

F

facet (fas'et) A small plane surface.

femur (fe'mur) The largest bone of the body, the thigh bone.

fetus (fe'tus) The unborn offspring of any viviparous animal; in man, the term applies after the second month.

foramen (fo-ra'men) Perforation or opening (usually in a bone) through which nerves or blood vessels pass.

fossa (fos'ah) A pit or depression.

G

glabella (glah-bel'ah) A point midway between the supraorbital ridges.

gland An organ that secretes or excretes a substance that may be beneficial or detrimental to life.

glottis (glot'is) Upper opening of the larynx; the epiglottis is the fibrocartilaginous structure that aids in the prevention of solids and liquids from entering the larynx and trachea. The glottis is situated upon the upper border of the larynx and is leaf shaped.

H

haversian system (ha-ver'shan) From the English anatomist, Havers; system of small canals in the bones.

hiatus (hi-a'tus) Normal perforation through the diaphragm.

hilum (hi'lum) Point of entrance and exit, into and from the lung and kidney, of the nerves and blood vessels.

hydrolysis (hi-drol'is-is) The decomposition of water.

hyoid (hi-oid') The bone between the root of the tongue and the larynx. The hyoid supports the tongue and gives attachment to its muscles. The hyoid is U shaped.

hypochondrium (hi-po-kon'dre-um) The region below either costal arch.

hypogastrium (hi-po-gas'tre-um) The lower region of the abdomen, located anteriorly in the median area.

hypophysis (hi-pof'is-is) The pituitary gland located in the sella turcica under the hypothalamus.

I

ileum (il'e-um) The third part of the small intestine between the jejunum and cecum.

ilium (il'e-um) The proximal part of the pelvic bone, one of the bones of the pelvis.

incisura angularis (in-si-su'rah ang-gu-lar'is) The notch formed in the lesser curvature of the stomach at the angle of the junction of the body and the pyloric third. Peristaltic waves on the lesser curvature become quite pronounced as they pass through the incisura.

inguinal (ing'gwi-nal) Pertaining to the thigh or inguinal region.

inion (in'e-on) The external occipital protuberance.

ischium (is'ke-um) The inferior and posterior part of the pelvic bone.

J

jejunum (je-joo'num) The second part of the small intestine beginning at the terminal end of the duodenum and terminating at the junction with the ileum.

L

labium (la'be-um) A lip.

lacrimal (lak're-mal) One of the bones of the facial section of the skull. Pertaining to tears.

lambdoid (lam'doid) A suture between the occiput, parietal, and temporal bones; similar in shape to the Greek letter lambda.

larynx (lar'inks) The voice box. The cartilaginous portion of the air passages extending from the base of the tongue to the trachea.

lobe (lob) A division of the lungs, liver, and brain.

lumen (lu'men) The cavity or hollow space in an organ or tube.

lymph (limf) The clear fluid of the lymphatic system.

M

malar (ma'lar) The malar bone, same as the zygoma.

mammary gland (mam'er-e) One of the two or more large compound glands, characteristic of the Mammalia, which, in the female, secrete milk for the nourishment of the young.

mandible (man'di-bl) The bone of the lower jaw.

manubrium (mah-nu'bre-um) The first part of the sternum; a handle.

mastoid (mas'toid) Part of the temporal bone; shaped like a breast.

maxilla (mak-sil'ah) The bone of the upper jaw.

mediastinum (me"de-as-ti'num) Midspace of the thoracic cavity, containing the following viscera: bronchi, ascending aorta, aortic arch, upper part of the descending aorta, inferior vena cava, esophagus, thoracic duct, lymphatic duct, and azygos veins.

medulla (me-dul'ah) The central part of a gland or organ.
medullary canal (med'u-lar-e). The central canal of the shaft of any long bone; carries the nutritive and nervous supplies; the marrow.
meninges (me-nin'jez) The membranes of the brain and spinal cord.
metabolism (me-tab'o-lizm) Life processes; the chemical changes associated with the assimilation of energy materials into cell protoplasm and the elimination of the waste products of cellular activity. A combination of the processes of anabolism and catabolism.
metacarpus (met-ah-kar'pus) The bones of the hand.
metaphysis (me-taf'i-sis) The line of junction of the epiphysis with the diaphysis of a long bone; the epiphyseal line.
metatarsus (met-ah-tar'sus) The bones of the foot.
mitral valve (mi'tral) The left atrioventricular valve of the heart, shaped like a miter.
multipara (mul-tip'ah-rah) A woman who has given birth to two or more children.

N

naris (na'ris) The nostril.
nasal (na'zal) The bone of the nose; also pertaining to the nose.
navicular (na-vik'u-lar) A bone of the tarsus; boat shaped.
neural (nu'ral) Pertaining to the nerves.
node (nod) A knob or protuberance.
nucha (nu'kah) The nape of the neck.

O

obese (o-bes') Extremely fat, corpulent.
occiput (ok'si-put) A bone of the cranial section of the skull; forms the posterior portion and base of the skull.
occlusion (ok-klu'shun) Complete meeting or meshing of the teeth of the upper and lower jaws.
occult (ok-kult') Hidden or concealed.
odontoid process (o-don'toid) Process of the second vertebral body, which extends superiorly through the bony ring of the atlas.
olecranon process (o-lek'rah-non) The large bony process located proximally on the ulna.
organ (or'gan) Any part of the body having a definite function to perform.
orifice (or'i-fis) An opening or aperture.
os Bone; mouth.
osseous (os'e-us) Bony.
ossification (os"i-fi-ka'shun) Bone formation, growth.

P

palatine (pal'ah-tin) One of the bones of the facial section of the skull; also a process of the maxilla.
palmar (pah'mar) Palm surface of the hand.
patella (pah-tel'ah) Kneecap; largest sesamoid bone in the body; the only sesamoid necessary for normal function.
pelvic straits (pel'vik strates)
 inferior The plane of the pelvic outlet. The anteroposterior diameter extends from the tip of the coccyx to the subpubic ligament and is 9.5 cm. The transverse diameter extends between the ischial tuberosities and is 11 cm.
 superior The plane of the pelvic inlet. The anteroposterior, or conjugate, diameter extends from the superior border of the first sacral vertebra to a point ⅜ inch inferior to the superior border of the symphysis pubis and is 11 cm. The transverse diameter at the widest point is 13.5 cm.
pericardium (per-i-kar'de-um) The closed membranous sac enveloping the heart.
perineum (per-i-ne'um) The area of the body bounded anteriorly by the pubic arch, posteriorly by the coccyx, and bilaterally by the ischial tuberosities.
periosteum (per-e-os'te-um) The fibrous membrane covering bone surfaces except at points of tendinous and ligamentous attachment and articular surfaces.
peritoneum (per"i-to-ne'um) The serous membrane lining the abdomen and surrounding the viscera.
phalanx (fa'lanks) One of the bones of the fingers or toes.
pharynx (far'inks) The throat. The musculomembranous pouch situated posteriorly to the nose, mouth, and larynx.
phrenic (fren'ik) Pertaining to the diaphragm.
pia mater (pi'ah ma'ter) The innermost membrane of the meninges containing the blood supply; tender mother.
plantar (plan'tar) The sole surface of the foot.
pleura (ploor'ah) The serous membrane surrounding the lungs.
pubis (pu'bis) One of the pelvic bones.
pyknic (pik'nik) Having a short, thick, stocky build.
pylorus (pi-lo'rus) The muscular and circular opening of the stomach into the duodenum.

Q

quadrate (kwod'rat) Four-sided.

R

radius (ra'de-us) The lateral bone of the forearm.
ramus (ra'mus) A branch; slender process of bone projecting from the main part.
ruga (roo'gah) A fold of the mucosa in the stomach, visible radiographically after barium ingestion.

S

sacrum (sa'krum) A curved triangular bone comprised of five united segments situated between the fifth lumbar vertebra above and the coccyx below and the pelves on each side; forms the posterior boundary of the pelvis.
scapula (skap'u-lah) The large, flat, triangular bone forming the back of the shoulder.

sella turcica (sel'ah tur'si-kah) The saddle-shaped fossa in the sphenoid in which the pituitary gland is situated.

semilunar (sem-e-lu'nar) Half-moon shaped.

septum (sep'tum) A partition or division wall.

sesamoid (ses'ah-moid) A small bone shaped like a grain; auxiliary bones found at articular surfaces, especially in the manus or pedis. The patella is the largest of these.

sigmoid (sig'moid) S shaped.

sinus (si'nus) A normal cavity in a bone or organ; pathologically in tissues and normally containing pus.

sphenoid (sfe'noid) Wedge shaped; one of the bones of the cranial section of the skull.

sphincter (sfingk'ter) A muscle that closes an orifice.

splenic (splen'ik) Pertaining to the spleen.

squamous (skwa'mus) Flat, or scale shaped.

sternum (ster'num) The breast bone. There are three parts: manubrium—handle or first part; body or gladiolus—midportion; xiphoid (xyphoid) process—distal portion.

sthenic (sthen'ik) Active, strong.

styloid (sti'loid) Pointed like a stylus.

subarachnoid space (sub-ah-rak'noid) The space beneath the arachnoid membrane, which is filled with cerebrospinal fluid.

sulcus (sul'kus) A groove or narrow depression.

sustentaculum tali (sus-ten-tak'u-lum ta'li) A process of the calcaneus that supports the talus.

suture line (su'tur) A line of joining or closure.

symphysis (sim'fi-sis) A line of junction of two bones.

synovia (si-no've-ah) The clear fluid secreted within the synovial membrane.

synovial (si-no've-al) Pertaining to the synovia.

T

talus (ta'lus) The second largest bone of the tarsus; the major weight-supporting bone of the body.

tarsus (tahr'sus) The bones of the ankle.

thoracic (tho-ras'ik) Pertaining to or situated in the chest or thorax.

thyroid (thi'roid) One of the endocrine glands situated anterior to the trachea.

tissue (tis'u) A group of cells of similar origin, structure, and function.

tonus (to'nus) The state of mild contraction exhibited by all healthy muscles.

torsion (tor'shun) Twisting.

trabecula (trah-bek'u-lah) A small beam or line visible radiographically in bones. Any one of the fibrous bands extending from the capsule into the interior of an organ.

trachea (tra'ke-ah) The windpipe.

tragus (tra'gus) The small prominence of cartilage projecting over the meatus of the external ear.

trochlea (trok'le-ah) Grooved convexity at the distal end of the humerus for articulation of the sigmoid of the olecranon process of the ulna.

tubercle (tu'ber-kl) A small bony projection; a small nodule.

tuberosity (tu-ber-os'i-te) A large bony projection.

tuft (tuft) The terminal end of the terminal phalanx.

U

ulna (ul'nah) The medial bone of the forearm.

umbilicus (um-bi-li'kus, umbil'i-cus) The navel; the round, depressed cicatrix in the median line of the abdomen; the former site of attachment of the umbilical cord.

ureter (u-re'ter) The tube that conveys the urine from the kidney to the bladder.

urethra (u-re'thrah) Canal through which the urine is eliminated from the bladder.

uterus (u'ter-us) The pear-shaped, muscular organ of the female reproductive system in which the fetus develops.

V

vagina (vah-ji'nah) Sheath; passageway from the cervix (neck) of the uterus to the vulva.

vascular (vas'ku-lar) Containing numerous blood vessels.

vein (van) A blood vessel carrying blood from the tissues to the heart.

vena cava (ve'nah ca'vah) A very large hollow vein.

ventricle (ven'tre-k'l A small cavity or pouch.

vertebra (ver'te-brah) Any one of the bones that compose the spinal column.

vertebra prominens (prom'i-nens) The seventh cervical vertebra.

vertex (ver'teks) The crown of the head; a summit or top.

vestigial (ves-tij'e-al) Rudimentary; a trace remaining.

villus (vil'us) Vascular, fingerlike projection of the mucosa.

viscera (vis'er-ah) Plural of viscus.

viscus (vis'kus) (pl. **viscera**) Any organ that is enclosed within one of the three great cavities.

void (void) To cast out as waste matter, as in voiding urine.

vulva (vul'vah) The external female genitalia, comprised of the labia majora and minora.

W

wormian bones (wer'me-an) Small supernumerary bones in the skull sutures; those found in the region of the pterion are called epipteric bones.

X

xiphoid (zīf'oid) Sword shaped; the distal portion of the sternum.

Z

zygoma (zi-go'mah) One of the bones of the facial section of the skull.

PATHOLOGIC, SURGICAL, AND RELATED TERMS

A

abrasion (ah-bra'zhun) Excoriation of the cutaneous or mucous surface by mechanical means.

abscess (ab'ses) A localized collection of pus surrounded by a wall of lymph; an inflammatory exudate.

acromegaly (ak-ro-meg'a-le) A disease of the pituitary gland in adults that produces overgrowth of bone, especially in the jaws and hands.

adenoma (ad-e-no'mah) A tumor of glandlike structure.

amputation (am'pu-ta"shun) The condition that follows the removal (usually surgical) of part or all of an appendage.

aneurysm (an'u-rizm) A circumscribed dilation of the walls of an artery.

aphagia (ah-fa'je-ah) Loss of the power of swallowing.

aphasia (ah-fa'ze-ah) Defect or loss of the power of expression by speech, writing, or signs, or of comprehending spoken or written language, due to injury or disease of the brain centers.

apnea (ap-ne'ah) A partial privation or suspension of breath.

ataxia (ah-tak'se-ah) Failure or irregularity of muscular coordination.

atelectasis (at-e-lek'tah-sis) Imperfect expansion or collapse of the air vesicles of the lungs

atony (at'o-ne) The lack of normal tone or strength.

atresia (ah-tre'ze-ah) The absence or closure of a normal opening.

atrophy (at'ro-fe) Diminution in size of a tissue, organ, or part due to degeneration or decrease in cell size.

autopsy (aw'top-se) The postmortem examination of a body.

B

benign (be-nin') Not endangering health or life.

bezoar (be'zor) A concretion of various compositions, sometimes found in the stomach or intestines. There are four types: (1) trichobezoar—hair; (2) phytobezoar—fruit and vegetable fibers and skins; (3) trichophytobezoar—combination of 1 and 2; and (4) concretions of shellac.

biopsy (bi'op-se) The removal and examination of tissue from the living body for diagnostic purposes.

bronchiectasis (brong-ke-ek'tah-sis) Dilatation of the walls of the bronchi.

bursitis (bur-si'tis) Inflammation of a bursa. The inflammation may be the result of a foreign substance.

C

Ca Abbreviation for cancer and for calcium.

calculus (kal'ku-lus) A stonelike concretion found in the body.

cancer (kan'ser) Any type of malignant growth.

caries (ka're-ez) Decay of bone or teeth.

cholecystitis (ko"le-sis-ti'tis) Inflammation of the gallbladder.

cholelithiasis (ko"le-le-thi'ah-sis) The presence of, or a condition associated with, calculi in the gallbladder or bile duct.

cicatrix (sik-a'triks) A scar; connective tissue that replaces a localized loss of substance.

coarctation (ko-ark-ta'shun) A straightening or pressing together; a condition of stricture or contracture.

contusion (kon-tu'zhun) a bruise; an injury attended with more or less disorganization of the subcutaneous tissue and effusion of blood beneath the skin, but without breaking of the skin.

crepitus, bony (krep'i-tus) The crackling sound produced by the rubbing together of fragments of fractured bone.

cyanosis (si-ah-no'sis) Bluish discoloration of the skin resulting from insufficient quantity of oxygen in the blood.

cyst, dermoid (sist) A pouch or sac of developmental origin, consisting of a fibrous wall lined with stratified epithelium and containing hair follicles, sweat glands, and sebaceous glands.

D

desquamation (des-kwah-ma'shun) The shedding of epithelial elements, chiefly of the skin, in scales or sheets.

DU Abbreviation for duodenal ulcer.

dyspnea (disp-ne'ah) Difficult breathing.

E

ecchymosis (ek-e-mo'sis) An extravasation of blood; also a discoloration of the skin caused by the extravasation of blood.

edema (e-de'mah) Infiltration of serum in a part.

effusion (ef-u'zhun) A pouring out.

embolism (em'bo-lizm) Clot formation causing a stoppage of the flow of blood in a blood vessel.

emphysema (em-fi-se'mah) Air or gas in a normally airless tissue or an excess of air in normally aerated tissues.

empyema (em-pi-e'mah) Pus in a cavity.

etiology (e"te-ol'o-je) The study or the theory of causation of any disease; the sum of knowledge regarding causes.

exacerbation (eg-sas-er-ba'shun) An increase in the severity of any symptoms or disease.

exudate (eks'u-dat) A collection of material that has filtered through the walls of vessels into the surrounding tissues.

F

fibrosis (fi-bro'sis) Development of fibrous tissue.

fistula (fis'tu-lah) A narrow canal or tube left by incomplete healing of a wound, incision, or abscess.

H

hiatus hernia The protrusion of any structure through the esophageal hiatus of the diaphragm.

hypermotility (hi'per-mo-til'i-te) Excessive motility.

hypersthenic (hi-per-sthen'ik) Marked by exalted strength or tonicity.

hypertrophy (hi-per'tro-fe) Excessive growth or overgrowth.

hyposthenic (hi-po-sthen'ik) Not well developed; feeble, weak.

I

ileus (il'e-us) An obstruction of the intestine producing severe colic.

induration (in-du-ra'shun) Hardening of a tissue or part.

infarct (in'farkt) A wedge-shaped area of either hemorrhage or necrosis into an organ caused by loss of blood supply or obstruction of a terminal vessel.

intussusception (in"tus-sus-sep'shun) The invagination or indigitation of a portion of the intestine into an adjacent portion.

J

jaundice (jawn'dis) Yellow discoloration of the skin, mucous membranes, and excretions as a result of bile pigments in the blood.

K

keloid (ke'loid) A new growth or tumor of the skin, consisting of whitish ridges, nodules, and plates of dense tissue.

kyphosis (ki-fo'sis) The condition called humpback; convexity turned dorsally.

L

laceration (las-er-a'shun) A tear.

lordosis (lor-do'sis) Curvature of the spine with the convexity forward.

luxation (luks-a'shun) The displacement of any part, especially of a bone.

-lysis (li'sis) A suffix meaning gradual decline of a fever; splitting or destruction of a substance or cell.

M

malignant (mah-lig'nant) Virulent; compromising or threatening life.

mastectomy (mas-tek'to-me) Excision of the breast.

radical mastectomy A surgical procedure in which all of the related lymph glands, nodes, and ducts are removed in addition to the mammary gland.

simple mastectomy A surgical procedure in which only the mammary gland is removed.

metastasis (me-tas'tah-sis) The translocation of disease from its primary site to a second site via the blood or lymph. From the Greek word meaning "to transpose."

moribund (mor'e-bund) In a dying state.

N

necropsy (nek'rop-se) A postmortem examination.

necrosis (ne-kro'sis) The death of a portion of tissue.

neoplasm (ne'o-plazm) Any new and abnormal growth, such as a tumor.

O

osteolith (os'te-o-lith) Petrified bone.

osteomyelitis (os"te-o-mi-e-li'tis) Inflammation or infection of bone marrow.

osteoporosis (os"te-o-po-ro'sis) Abnormal porosity or rarefaction of bone by the enlargement of its canals or the formation of abnormal spaces.

P

pan All, whole, or completely; usually joined with a second element, sometimes by a hyphen.

panhysterectomy (pan"his-ter-ek'to-me) Complete extirpation of the uterus and cervix.

paracentesis (par"ah-sen-te'sis) The puncture of the wall of a cavity of the body.

paralysis (pah-ral'is-is) Loss or impairment of motor function in a part due to lesion of the neural or muscular mechanism.

path An abbreviation for the pathology.

pathology (pah-thol'o-je) The branch of medical science dealing with the modifications of functions and changes in structure caused by disease.

phleboliths (fleb'o-liths) Small rounded calcium deposits in the walls of veins.

phytobezoar (fi"to-be'zor) A gastric concretion composed of vegetable matter such as skins, seeds, and fibers of fruits and vegetables.

pneumoperitoneum (nu"mo-per-i-to-ne'um) The presence of air or gas in the peritoneal cavity.

pneumothorax (nu-mo-tho'raks) The presence of air or gas in the pleural cavity.

P-O Abbreviation for postoperative.

polyp (pol'ip) A smooth, pedunculated growth from a mucous surface, as of the nose, bladder, rectum, etc. Polyps are the result of hypertrophy of the mucous membrane, or are true tumors.

prosthesis (pros'the-sis) Replacement of a missing part by an artificial substitute.

pyogenic (pi-o-jen'ik) Producing pus.

R

rigor mortis (ri'gor mor'tis) The muscular rigidity that occurs after death.

S

Schmorl's nodule (schmorlz) A nodule seen in roentgenograms of the spine, due to prolapse of a nucleus pulposus into an adjoining vertebra.

sclerosis (skle-ro'sis) Hardening.
scoliosis (sko-le-o'sis) Morbid lateral curvature of the spine.
sepsis (sep'sis) Poisoning caused by the products of a putrefactive process.
sequela (se-kwe'lah) Any lesion or affection after or caused by an attack of disease.
sequestrum (se-kwes'trum) A detached or dead piece of bone within a cavity, abscess, or wound.
spina bifida occulta (spi'nah bif'i-da o-kul'ta) A congenital cleft in the neural arch that is hidden or that has no visible protrusion of the spinal membranes.
spondylolisthesis (spon"di-lo-lis-the'sis) Forward displacement of one vertebra over another, especially pertaining to a separation of the fifth lumbar vertebra from and a slipping forward on the first sacral vertebra.
stasis (sta'sis) A standing still or stoppage of movement or flow.
stenosis (ste-no'sis) The narrowing or constriction of a passage.
sterile (ster'il) Not fertile; infertile; barren; not producing young. Aseptic; not producing microorganisms; free from microorganisms.
subluxation (sub-luk-sa'shun) Incomplete luxation; sprain.
suppuration (sup-u-ra'shun) Pus formation.
syndrome (sin'drom) A typical set of conditions that characterize a deficiency or disease.

T

tenaculum (te-nak'u-lum) A hooklike instrument for seizing and holding parts.
tetanus (tet'ah-nus) Sustained contraction of a muscle.
tetany (tet'ah-ne) A syndrome manifested by sharp flexion of the wrist and ankle joints, cramps, muscle twitchings, and convulsions.
thoracentesis (tho"rah-sen-te'sis) Surgical puncture or tapping of the chest wall.
thoracoplasty (tho-ra'ko-plas-te) A plastic operation on the thorax.
thrombus (throm'bus) A clot of blood formed within the heart or vessels.
trauma (traw'mah) A wound or injury.

W

wound (woond) A rupture of the continuity of an inner or outer surface of the body.

PHYSICS, ELECTRICITY, AND RELATED TERMS

A

Å Abbreviation for angstrom unit.
a.c. Abbreviation for alternating current.
actinic (ak-tin'ik) A type of radiation that is capable of producing a chemical change.
alpha particle (al'fa) A positively charged particle, consisting of two protons and two neutrons, which is ejected at high speed in certain radioactive disintegrations.
alternating current (**a.c.**) Electric current that flows for a given length of time in one direction and immediately flows in the opposite direction for the same length of time. It usually consists of 60 complete cycles per second.
ampere (am'per) The unit of intensity of an electric current, being the current produced by 1 volt acting through a resistance of 1 ohm.
angstrom unit (awng'strem) One one-hundred millionth of a centimeter; the unit of measure of wavelengths.
anode (an'od) The positive part of the x-ray tube in the secondary circuit, made of tungsten imbedded in a copper bar; also called the target.
atom (at'om) The ultimate particle of an element; one of the divisions of a molecule that is the smallest quantity of a substance that can exist free or uncombined.
atomic number (ah-tom'ik) The total number of protons in the nucleus of an atom.
atomic weight The sum of the protons plus the neutrons in the nucleus of an atom.
attenuation (a-ten'u-a"shun) The decrease in dose rate of radiation in passing through a material.
autotransformer A transformer with a single wrapping or winding of wire, with both ends of the wire attached to the primary alternating current.

B

background radiation In a given area, the sum total of radioactivity from cosmic rays, natural radioactive materials, and whatever may have been introduced into the area.
backscatter A term used to describe the rays that are generated when the x rays capable of penetrating the object strike the surface upon which the film holder lies.
barn The unit of cross section of a nuclear reaction; 10^{-24} sq. cm. The term describes the target area or cross section in a nuclear reaction.
beta particle (ba'tah) An electron.

C

cathode (kath'od) The negative part of the x-ray tube from which the electrons are emitted.
characteristic fluorescent rays (floo"o-res'ent) Rays that are generated in an absorbing material (fluoresce from) as a result of primary x-ray photon bombardment.
characteristic x rays X rays of definite wavelengths, characteristic of a pure substance and emitted by it under proper excitation.
Compton effect A change in the wavelength of scattered rays and emission of recoil electrons in deep radiation.
coulomb (koo'lom) The unit of quantity in current

electricity. The quantity afforded by 1 ampere of current in 1 second flowing against 1 ohm of resistance with a force of 1 volt.

D

d.c. Abbreviation for direct current.

E

eddy current (ed'e) An induced electric current circulating wholly within a mass of metal. Such currents are converted into heat, and thus cause serious waste.

electricity (e-lek-tris'i-te) One of the forces of nature developed by chemism, magnetism, or friction; also said to be electrons in motion.

electrolyte (e-lek'tro-lit) A substance capable of conducting an electric current and being decomposed by it.

electromagnetic wave A wave produced by the oscillation of an electric charge.

electron (e-lek'tron) The ultimate particle of negative electricity.

electron volt An energy unit; the amount of energy acquired when a particle having a charge equal to the fundamental or electronic unit falls through a potential difference of 1 volt.

energy (en'er-je) The capacity for doing work. There are two kinds of energy: kinetic, the power of a body in motion; and latent or potential, the power possessed by a body at rest. Radiant energy is a form of kinetic energy that is emitted by all bodies in proportion to their temperature and is propagated by undulations in the luminiferous ether.

erg A unit of work. The work done in moving a body 1 cm against a force of 1 dyne.

F

fission (fish'un) The act of splitting.

fluorescence (floo"o-res'ens) The ability of a chemical (calcium tungstate) to give off light in the presence of an active source.

frequency (fre'kwen-se) In harmonic motions, the number of vibrations or cycles in a unit of time.

fusion (fu'zhun) The union or blending of things as if melted together.

G

gamma ray (gam'a) A type of ray (similar to an x ray but of shorter wavelength) emitted by certain radioactive substances.

H

half-value layer The thickness of a standard material (pure metal, etc.) required to reduce the intensity of a beam of x rays (when passing through the absorber at right angles to its longitudinal axis) to exactly one-half of its original value.

heel effect Rays from the cathode end of the x-ray tube have a slightly visible tendency to make a more dense image than those from the anode end.

heterogeneous (het-er-o-je'ne-us) Composed of different substances.

heterogeneous radiation Beam of x rays consisting of many x rays of different wavelengths.

hysteresis (his-ter-e'sis) A lagging or retardation of the effect. The magnetization of a piece of iron or steel due to a magnetic field that is made to vary through a cycle of values; lags behind the field.

I

intensification factor The quantity of intensification, expressed numerically as light energy, of the applied source of energy when it passes through the screen emulsion. To find the factor of intensification of an unknown screen: expose a plain film in cardboard with the regular factors; expose an identical film in the cassette containing the unknown screens and using the same factors and object. When the radiographs are dry, place them on an illuminator and check the overall density, or light transmission, with a light meter or densitometer. Give a value of 1.0 to the quantity of light transmitted through the plain film radiograph that was exposed in the cardboard holder.

ion (i'on) An atom or group of atoms carrying an electric charge, formed by the dissociation of a dissolved molecule by the action of a solvent.

ionization (i-on-i-za'shun) Electrolytic dissociation; the production of ions. An atom is said to be ionized when an electron is either gained or lost.

isobar (i'so-bar) One of two or more chemical elements that have identical atomic weights but different atomic numbers.

isotope (i'so-top) Of a collection of atoms of a given element (having the same number of protons), those atoms possessing a different number of neutrons are the different isotopes of the element.

M

molecule (mol'e-kul) The smallest quantity into which a subtsance can be divided and retain its characteristic properties.

MPD Abbreviation for the maxmum permissible dose.

N

neutron (nu'tron) An atomic particle having the same weight as a proton of the same atom but having no electric charge.

nucleus (nu'kle-us) The essential part or positive particle (atomic) of any atom carrying a positive charge. It may consist of a single proton, or protons and neutrons.

O

ohm (om) The unit of electric resistance.

P

phosphorescence (fos-fo-res′ens) The ability of a chemical (zinc sulfate) to continue to give off light after the activating source has ceased.

photon (fo′ton) A quantum of gamma radiation or light; also used in reference to x ray.

physics (fiz′iks) The science of matter and forces.

positron (pos′i-tron) An atomic particle having the same mass as an electron, but having a positive electric charge.

proton (pro′ton) The nuclear positive corpuscle of electricity.

Q

quantum (kwon′tum) An elemental unit of energy according to the quantum theory. Its value is $h\nu$, where h is Planck's constant (6.62×10^{-27}), and ν is the frequency of the vibrations or waves with which the energy is associated.

R

R Abbreviation for roentgen unit.

rad The unit of absorbed x-ray dose; its quantity is 100 ergs per gram.

radiation (ra-de-a′shun) The act of radiating or diverging from a central point, such as light rays radiate from a source of light.

radioactive fallout (ra″de-o-ak′tiv) The dust and other debris rendered radioactive by nuclear fission or neutron bombardment that settles out of the atmosphere while the material is still highly active.

Rem The abbreviation for roentgen-equivalent-man.

remnant radiation (rem′nant) That ionizing radiation that produces the radiographic image.

Rep The abbreviation for roentgen-equivalent-physical.

roentgen unit The unit of measure of x ray; the amount of conductivity of 1 ml of atmospheric air (at saturation) at 0° C. and 760 mm of mercury pressure, exclusive of the wall effect of the chamber.

roentgen-meter A device that incorporates the principle of a gold-leaf galvanometer to measure a given amount of radiation, or R. Radiation causes ionization. Ionization causes an increase in conductivity or electric charges in air.

S

scattered radiation Secondary rays. They may be of the same wavelength, or longer, than the primary. They may be characteristic fluorescent rays.

secondary rays The rays that are generated in the patient as the x rays pass through the patient.

substance (sub′stans) A solid body; a material object as distinguished from something visionary or shadowy. Any particular kind of matter, whether element, compound, or mixture; any chemical material of which bodies are composed; some authorities restrict a substance to elements and compounds.

T

thermionic emission (ther-me-on′ik e-mish′un) Release of electrons from the cathode filament by heat.

Thoraeus filter (tho′re-us) A filter used for x-ray therapy. Composition: tin, copper, and aluminum. This kind of filter is used primarily in deep therapy.

transformer (trans-for′mer) An electrical device for increasing or decreasing the incoming voltage.

filament transformer The filament transformer is immersed in oil (in the generator), and is a step-down type transformer to supply the x-ray tube filament with a current of no more than 5 amperes at not more than 15 volts. In older valve-rectified equipment, there are separate filament transformers for the valve tube filaments.

V

velocity (ve-los′i-te) The ratio of displacement to the time required for this displacement. Time rate of motion in a given direction and sense. Average velocity equals the total distance passed over, divided by the whole time taken.

volt The unit of electric pressure or electromotive force; the force necessary to cause 1 ampere of current to flow against 1 ohm of resistance.

W

watt The unit of electric power, the result of multiplying volts times amperes.

wavelength The distance between the peaks or troughs of any two adjacent and like waves.

X

x ray The rays discovered by Dr. Roentgen on Nov. 8, 1895. The roentgen (R) is the unit of measurement. The quantity of roentgen radiation (x rays) which, when the secondary electrons are fully utilized, and the wall effect of the chamber is avoided, produces in 1 ml of atmospheric air at 0° C. and 760 mm of mercury pressure such a degree of conductivity that one electrostatic unit is measured at saturation point. (Actually, it amounts to the degree of ionization produced in 1 ml of air by exposing the chamber to x rays.)

x rays One form of energy released from an x-ray tube as a result of the sudden deceleration of electrons.

PROCESSING, TECHNIQUE, AND RELATED TERMS

A

acid (as′id) A compound of an electronegative element with one or more atoms of hydrogen that can be replaced by electropositive atoms when a salt is formed.

acid stop bath A 28% solution of acetic acid used between the developer and fixer to stop development in manual processing.

alkali (al'kah-li) Opposite of acid; strongly electropositive.

artifact (ar'te-fakt) Foreign or artificial marks on radiographs caused by improper processing or faulty equipment.

C

catalyst (kat'ah-list) A substance that alters the velocity of a chemical reaction without undergoing any apparent physical or chemical change itself and without becoming a part of the product formed.

D

developer (de-vel'op-er) The solution in which the films are developed. It brings out the latent image.

E

emulsion (e-mul'shun) A liquid, usually water, containing an insoluble substance in suspension; it may be used in a dehydrated form.

F

film emulsion A dehydrated emulsion of the silver salts of three of the halogens—bromine, chlorine, and iodine—on a suitable base. The base is comprised of either cellulose acetate or one of the newer synthetics, each of which is *safe,* that is, it generates no poisonous gases when burned.

fixer The solution, incorrectly called hypo, in which the manifest image is fixed and hardened.

G

graininess (gran'i-nes) A mottling of the radiographic image.

L

latent image (la'tent) The invisible image in the x-ray film emulsion of the radiographed object caused by the remnant rays.

M

manifest image (man'i-fest) Visible image in the film emulsion after the reducing action of the developer.

maximum tissue differentiation The ultimate in diagnostic quality of any radiograph, present only when each of the controlling factors is present in its utmost degree. The two major factors are definition (sharpness) and visibility of detail.

N

no-screen film Any x-ray film with a different and faster speed emulsion than the emulsion of plain film. It was used in cardboard holders for radiographing thin parts (less than 13 cm) where great detail and contrast are desired. It is generally neither available nor used in modern practice.

P

pH A shortened term introduced by Sörenson to avoid confusion; refers to a total dissociation of ions always totaling 14. As the hydrogen ions increase, the hydroxyl ions decrease in reverse ratio. pH is based on the hydrogen ion concentration. A pH of 7.0 is neutral, the ions of both hydrogen and hydroxyl radicals being even. Any value above 7.0 is alkaline or base, and any value below 7.0 is acidic.

plain film The type film commonly used in cassettes having intensifying screens.

Q

Q.S. Quantity sufficient to fill to volume.

R

radiographic quality The characteristic summation of the various factors that combine to produce a radiograph.

replenisher (re-plen'ish-er) Solutions for replenishing, strengthening, and prolonging the life of the developer and fixer. There is a specific replenisher for each of the two solutions.

S

sandbags Bags of sand (or rice) of various sizes and shapes used for immobilization of the part to be x-rayed.

screen speed A term used to describe the speed of intensification of the applied energy as it passes through the screen emulsion.

sp.gr. Abbreviation for specific gravity; the weight of a substance judged in comparison with that of a specific standard, usually distilled water at 20° C. and 760 mm of mercury pressure.

RADIOGRAPHY AND RADIOGRAPHIC RELATED TERMS

A

abduct (ab-dukt') To move away from the midline of the body, or outwardly.

acanthion (ah-kan'the-on) A point at the base of the anterior nasal spine.

ad A prefix indicating toward the midline.

adduct (ah-dukt') To move toward the midline of the body, or inwardly.

amniography (am"ni-og'rah-fe) The process of making a radiograph after the replacement of some of the amniotic fluid surrounding the fetus with a contrast medium.

amphi- (am'fe) A prefix indicating a bilateral condition; double.

anesthesia (an-es-the'ze-ah) Loss of feeling or sensation.

anesthesiologist (an-es-the-ze-ol'-jist) A specialist in anesthesia.

anesthetic (an-es-thet'ik) Without the sense of pain or touch.

anesthetist (an-es'the-tist) An expert in administering anesthetics.

angio- (an'je-o) A prefix pertaining to a vessel, usually a blood vessel.

angiocardiography (an"je-o-kar-de-og'rah-fe) A radiographic study of the heart and great vessels after being made radiopaque by injection of suitable contrast media.

angiogram (an'je-o-gram) A radiograph of blood vessels.

angle board A device used in certain radiographic procedures enabling the technologist to place the patient's head in particular angles.

ante- A prefix indicating previous or in front of.

anterior (an-te're-or) Nearest the head or front.

anti- A prefix indicating opposition to or against.

antiseptic (an-te-sep'tik) A substance that will inhibit the growth and development of microorganisms without necessarily destroying them.

A-P Abbreviation for anteroposterior position or projection.

arteriography (ar"te-re-og'rah-fe) The radiographic examination and study of the arteries by injection of a radiopaque solution.

arthro- A prefix indicating relationship with a joint.

asterion (as-te're-on) The point of junction on the superior surface of the skull of the lambdoidal, parietomastoid, and occipitomastoid sutures.

B

barium sulfate (ba're-um sul'fat) A radiopaque compound used in gastrointestinal studies.

B.E. Abbreviation for barium enema.

bi- A prefix indicating two, twofold, or twice.

bilateral (bi-lat'er-al) Pertaining to or affecting both sides of the body.

bio- A prefix indicating life or its processes.

bolus (bo'lus) a rounded mass. The term used for the food mass in the act of deglutition and digestion.

broncho- A prefix indicating association with the trachea.

bronchography (brong-kog'rah-fe) The radiographic examination and study of the bronchial tree after injection of suitable radiopaque material.

bursa (bur'sah) A small sac interposed between parts that move upon one another.

C

c̄ The symbol indicating with.

callus (kal'us) A new growth of incomplete osseous tissue surrounding the ends of a fractured bone that is in the process of healing.

cannula (kan'u-lah) A tube for insertion into the body, its lumen being usually occupied by a trocar during the act of insertion.

canthus (kan'thus) The angle, either temporal (outer) or nasal (inner), formed by the junction of the eyelids.

cardboard holder A lightproof holder made of cardboard used for holding certain types of x-ray film. The back side has in it a thin sheet of lead that prevents backscatter. It is used to produce high contrast and detail in extremity radiographs.

cardio- (kar'de-o) A prefix pertaining to the heart.

cassette (kah-set') A device for holding x-ray films during exposure. Cassettes are made in several sizes. The tube side is composed of radiolucent substance, and the back side contains a thin lead sheet. The back is hinged and fits into the tube side, sealing out all light. Two intensifying screens are mounted inside, one on each side, between which the film is sandwiched.

catheter (kath'e-ter) A tubular surgical instrument for withdrawing fluids from a cavity of the body.

catheterization (kath"e-ter-i-za'shun) The employment or passage of a catheter.

caudad (kaw'dad) Toward the tail or cauda; in man, downward.

caudal (kaw'dal) Referring to a position near the tail end of the long axis of the body.

cephalad (sef'ah-lad) Toward the head.

cephalic (se-fal'ik) Pertaining to the head.

cholangiogram, operative (ko-lan'je-o-gram) Radiography of the gallbladder and associated ducts during surgery.

chole- (ko'le) A combining form denoting relationship to the bile.

cholecystography (ko"le-sis-tog'rah-fe) Radiography of the gallbladder after opacification.

circumduction (ser-kum-duk'shun) The movement of a limb in such a manner that its distal part describes a circle, the proximal end being fixed.

circumflex (ser'kum-fleks) Winding around.

collimate (kall-i-mate) To control the size of the x-ray beam through the use of lead shutters mounted inside a mechanical device which is attached to the diaphragm opening on the tube housing.

cone A funnel-shaped attachment on the x-ray tube shielding aperture. Used to control the scattering of x rays in the air and to limit the x rays in any given area. Generally replaced on modern equipment with a collimator.

contrast (kon'trast) Defined radiographically, the visible difference between adjacent densities resulting from subject and film characteristics. Generally, contrast is the property of a photographic material that determines the magnitude of the density difference resulting from a given exposure difference.

coronal plane (ko-ro'nal) A vertical plane extending

from left to right and separating anterior from posterior.

costal (kos'tal) Pertaining to the ribs.

costophrenic angle (kos'to-fren'ik) The angle formed by the lateral junction of the ribs with the diaphragm.

cysto- (sis'to) A prefix pertaining to the urinary bladder. Abbreviation for bladder examination.

D

decubitus (de-ku'be-tus) Recumbent or horizontal position.

definition Distinctness with which images of anatomic structures are recorded; detail, sharpness.

density, radiographic The degree of gradation of blackness in a radiograph; the amount of film blackening.

dermo- (der'mo) A prefix pertaining to the skin or integument.

detail The quantity of visibility of the fine structures and marginal sharpness that is demonstrated radiographically.

di- A prefix indicating twice or double.

discography (disk-og'rah-fe) The roentgen examination, by use of contrast media, of the intervertebral discs.

distal (dis'tal) Farthest from the body or origin; opposite to proximal.

distortion (dis-tor'shun) The perversion of shape in a radiographic image.

dorsal (dor'sal) Posterior or rear.

E

ec-, ecto- Prefixes indicating outside or away from.

-ectomy (ek'to-me) A suffix indicating removal of or excision.

em-, en- Prefixes indicating inside of or within.

emesis (em'e-sis) Vomitus; the act of vomiting.

emetic (e-met'ik) Having the power to cause vomiting.

encephalography (en-sef-ah-log'rah-fe) Radiographic examination of the head after a given quantity of spinal fluid has been withdrawn and replaced by an equal quantity of radiopaque or radiolucent contrast media.

epi- A prefix indicating the position upon or above.

erythema (er-e-the'mah) A redness of the skin after exposure to certain irritants. It is due to congestion of the capillaries.

erythema dose The minimum quantity of x or gamma radiation that will produce the appearance of erythema to a particular part of the integument. The quantity of the dose will vary from part to part on the same individual and among different individuals.

E.S.D. The abbreviation for the radiographic examination of the esophagus, stomach, and duodenum.

eversion (e-ver'zhun) Of the foot, turning outwardly or laterally.

excrete (eks-kret') To eliminate by means of a duct, tube, tract, or into a common opening.

excretion pyelography or urography (eks-kre'shun) The radiographic examination of the urinary system after intravenous injection of the radiopaque solution. The solution is eliminated by normal processes.

exhale (eks'hal) To breathe out.

exostosis (ek-sos-to'sis) An abnormal bony or osseous outgrowth from a bone surface.

expiration (eks-pira'shun) Expelling air from the lungs.

extension (eks-ten'shun) Straightening out; stretching.

external rotation (eks-ter'nal) Of the humerus; to rotate the hand laterally with the palm forward in the true anteroposterior (posterior) position.

F

filter Usually a 1- or 2-mm-thick sheet of aluminum (Al), placed in the tube housing aperture. It is used to filter out the softer rays and reduce the amount of radiation to the patient's skin.

flexion (flek'shun) The act of bending or contracting.

fluoroscopy (floo-or-os'ko-pe) The process of examining the tissues by means of a fluorescent screen.

focal spot Commonly called the spot, meaning the area on the anode from which the x rays radiate.

fog A general or local deposit of silver or silver compound, formed as the result of exposure to extraneous radiation or by chemical action; it is in addition to the legitimate image. Defined radiographically, fog is undesirable cloudiness of a radiographic image.

fracture (frak'tur) A breaking; a break in continuity of the margin of a bone.

fracture types:

- **bumper** In pedestrians, approximately 2 inches distal to the knee.
- **buttonhole** Caused by a flying object knocking an actual hole in a bone.
- **Colles'** Of the radius, from ½ to 1 inch above the distal end, with posterior and lateral displacement of the hand.
- **comminuted** The bone broken into more than two pieces at one site.
- **compound** Puncture of the skin at the fracture site.
- **compression** Occurring in the vertebrae, smashing part or all of the bone to a lesser thickness.
- **contrecoup** Away from the point of trauma, generally opposite, as on the opposite side of the skull from the point of trauma.
- **dentate** The fracture presents a serrated surface.
- **double** Two fractures at two locations, one each, in any one bone.
- **greenstick** In young persons, one side of the bone remains whole, but the other side is fractured.
- **impacted** Usually at one end of a long bone, the

end being driven into the adjacent end or surface of another bone.

incomplete Similar to greenstick fracture, also a hairline not extending through the entire bone.

oblique At an angle other than horizontal or vertical.

Pott's In the fibula approximately 3 inches above the distal end, with splitting of the internal malleolus.

reverse Pott's In the tibia, approximately 3 inches above the distal end, with splitting of the external malleolus.

simple A noncomplicated fracture.

Smith's Same as Colles' fracture except about 5 cm above the distal end of the radius.

spiral One complete fracture in a spiral shape around the shaft of the bone.

spontaneous Occurring spontaneously, as in bones having pathology.

ununited In which there has been no union.

fundus (fun'dus) Base; often located at the top of the organ.

G

gastro- A prefix pertaining to the gastric region, especially the stomach.

G.B. Abbreviation for gallbladder.

G.I. Abbreviation for gastrointestinal.

glenoid (gle'noid) Having the shape of a shallow cavity.

gluteal (gloo'te-al) The region of the buttocks.

-graphy A suffix pertaining to a graphic record.

grid A stationary arrangement of thin lead strips. Grids may be an integral part of the Potter-Bucky diaphragm, in which they move across the table; they may be used as stationary devices between the tube and film holder in situations where a Bucky could not be employed.

H

haustra (haws'trah) Sacculations of the colon.

hema-, hemo- Prefixes pertaining to the blood.

hepat- A prefix pertaining to the liver.

hernia (her'ne-ah) A protrusion of a part of an organ through an opening.

htt, HTT Abbreviations for high-tension transformer.

hyper- (hi'per) A prefix pertaining to an excess.

hypo- A prefix pertaining to deficient or beneath.

hypothenar (hi-poth'e-nar) The ridge on the palm of the hand along the bases of the fingers and the ulnar margin.

I

ileo- (il'e-o) A prefix pertaining to the ileum.

ilio- (il'e-o) A prefix pertaining to the ilium.

inferior (in-fe're-or) Lower or below.

inhale (in-hal') To breathe in.

inherent filter The filtering effect built into modern, shockproof x-ray tube shieldings. The quantity of filtration must be equivalent to a minimum of 0.5 mm of aluminum.

inspiration (in-spi-ra'shun) The drawing in of the breath.

insufflation (in-suf-fla'shun) The blowing of air into a cavity.

intensifying screen A dehydrated emulsion of certain chemicals (phosphors) that fluoresce in the presence of x rays. The emulsion is coated upon a suitable base.

intermediate The term applied to tissues that are between radiopaque and radiolucent in regard to x-ray penetration.

internal rotation (in-ter'nal) Of the humerus; to rotate the hand medially with the palm facing laterally.

inversion (in-ver'zhun) Of the foot, turning of the foot inwardly or medially.

-itis A suffix pertaining to inflammation or irritation of some specific tissue, gland, or organ.

I.V.P. Abbreviation for intravenous pyelography, the injection of a radiopaque solution into one of the antecubital veins. The opacifying medium enters the kidneys via normal circulation, and the calyces, pelves, uterers, and bladder of the urinary system are visualized.

K

kilovolt (kV) (kil'o-volt) 1,000 volts.

K.U.B. Abbreviation for radiography of the kidneys, ureters, and bladder.

kV Abbreviation for kilovolt or kilovoltage.

kVp Abbreviation for kilovolts peak or kilovoltage; the peak kilovoltage used in making any x ray exposure.

L

L Abbreviation for left or left side.

L.A.O. Abbreviation for left anterior oblique.

lateral Outside surface, that is, outside of the leg; away from the midsagittal plane.

latitude (lat'i-tud) The range in exposure factors that will produce a diagnostic radiographic image; the extent of variation between maximum and minimum density in a radiograph consistent with the diagnostic quality of the radiograph. Radiographic latitude increases with *long-scale* contrast.

L.P.O. Abbreviation for left posterior oblique.

M

mA Abbreviation for milliampere or milliamperage.

magnification (mag'ni-fi-ka"shun) The symmetrical enlargement of the image on the radiograph.

malingerer (mah-ling'ger-er) One who feigns illness.

mAs, MAS Abbreviation for milliampere-seconds. The result of multiplying milliamperes by the time in seconds.

meatus (me-a'tus) An opening or passage.

medial (me'de-al) Middle or medial, side as opposite to lateral, that is, inside of leg; toward the midsagittal plane.

micturate (mik'tu-rat) To urinate.

midaxillary line (mid-ak'sil-ar-e) An imaginary line drawn or extending from the axilla to the crest of the ilium.

milliampere (mA) (mil"e-am-per') 1/1,000 part of an ampere.

myelo- (mi'el-o) A prefix indicating relationship with the spinal cord or bone marrow.

myelogram (mi'el-o-gram) A radiograph of the spinal cord or a part of it after opacification.

myo- A prefix pertaining to muscle.

N

nasion (na'ze-on) The median point of the nasofrontal suture.

nephro- (nef'ro) The prefix pertaining to the kidney.

neuro- (nu'ro) A prefix pertaining to the nerves.

O

object-film distance (ofd, OFD) Distance in centimeters between the object or skin and the cassette or film.

oblique (ob-lik', ob-lek') Angular view of a surface or object, not a true anteroposterior (posterior) or lateral position, toward the midsagittal plane.

occlusal plane (ok-klu'sal) The plane of the masticating surfaces of the molar and bicsupid teeth of the upper and lower jaws when the jaws are closed.

odonto- (o-don'to) A prefix pertaining to a tooth, or meaning like a tooth.

ofd, OFD (sfd, SFD) Abbreviation for object-film distance (skin-film distance).

O.G.C. Abbreviation for oral Graham-Cole.

oral Graham-Cole A method of administration of gallbladder contrast medium.

orthodiagraphy (or"tho-di-ag'rah-fe) The radiographic examination and study of the internal organs to record and measure the size and location; also of foreign bodies.

-osis (o-sis) A suffix indicating condition caused by, or presence of.

osteo- (os'te-o) A prefix pertaining to a bone.

osteogenesis (os"te-o-jen'e-sis) The development of bony tissue.

-ostomy (os'to-me) A suffix pertaining to the surgical removal of a diseased tissue.

oto- A prefix denoting relationship to the ear.

P

P-A Abbreviation for posteroanterior (anterior) position or projection.

palliate (pal'e-at) To reduce the severity of; to relieve.

palliative therapy (pal'e-a-tiv) To afford relief, but not to cure.

para- A prefix pertaining to a place beyond.

patent (pa'tent) Open or exposed.

P.E., PE, pe Abbreviation for photographic effect.

peak kilovoltage The peak kilovoltage used in making any x-ray exposure.

pelvimetry (pel-vim'e-tre) A method of measurement of the size of the bony pelvis.

peri- A prefix meaning surrounding or around.

peristalsis (per-e-stal'sis) The peculiar wavelike contractions of tubular structures as in the digestive tract.

photographic effect (P.E., PE, pe) The ability of a source of energy to cause a latent image formation in the film emulsion in the shape or image of the object through which or from which the energy rays pass to the film.

pkV Abbreviation for peak kilovoltage.

placentography (plas-en-tog'rah-fe) Radiologic visualization of the placenta after the injection of a contrast medium.

planigram (pla'ne-gram) A roentgenogram of a selected layer of the body made by planigraphy.

post- A prefix meaning behind or following.

posterior (pos-te're-or) Nearest the back or rear.

pre- A prefix meaning in front of or preceding.

primipara (pri-mip'ah-rah) A woman who has given birth to her first child.

proc-, procto- Prefixes pertaining to the rectum.

pronate (pro'nat) Lying prone or face down.

pronation (pro-na'shun) The act of being in the prone position; of the hand, with the palm down.

prone (pron) Lying with the anterior or ventral surface of the face down.

proximal (prok'si-mal) Nearest the body or origin.

ptosis (to'sis) Dropping, prolapse, or abnormal depression.

pyelography (pi-el-og'rah-fe) The radiographic examination of the renal pelves, ureters, and bladder after opacifying same with a suitable radiopaque solution.

pyo- A prefix pertaining to pus.

R

R Abbreviation for right or right side, and for roentgen.

radiograph (ra'de-o-graf) A permanent photographic record of the structures through which a beam of ionizing radiation has passed.

radiographer (ra"de-og'rah-fer) A person who is skilled in the art of producing radiographs.

radiography (ra"de-og'rah-fe) The science and art of producing radiographs and skiagraphs.

radiologist (ra-de-ol'o-jist) A physician who has had specialized training in the use of radiant energy for treatment and diagnosis; this includes x rays, radium, etc.

radiology (ra-de-ol'o-je) The science of radiant energy.

radiolucent (ra-de-o-lu'sent) Permitting the passage of radiant energy or waves.

radiopaque (ra-de-o-pak') Not permitting the passage of radiant energy or waves.

R.A.O. Abbreviation for right anterior oblique.

Reid's base line A line from the infraorbital ridge to the external auditory meatus and the middle line of the occiput.

renal (re'nal) Pertaining to the kidney.

retro- A prefix indicating back or backward.

retrograde pyelography (ret'ro-grad) Radiography of the renal calyces, pelves, ureters, and bladder after opacification has been accomplished by injection via the urethra.

retrograde urography (u-rog'rah-fe) Radiography of the urinary bladder after injection of opacifying material via the urethra.

roentgenologist (rent-gen-ol'o-jist) A physician who has had specialized training in the use of x rays.

R.P.O. Abbreviation meaning right posterior oblique.

S

s̄ The symbol indicating without.

sagittal plane (saj'i-tal) A vertical plane extending from anterior to posterior and separating right from left.

sfd, SFD (ofd, OFD) see ofd.

solarization (so'ler-i-za"shun) A process of transferring the manifest image from a radiograph as either a negative or a positive image to another film by employing either sun or artificial light. A reversal of gradation sequence in the image (usually very dense) obtained on the normal development of films, plates, and papers after giving a very intense or long-continued exposure. A greater exposure than this appears to restore the original sequence of gradation, and a still greater one has been stated to bring about a second reversal.

sub- A prefix meaning beneath.

super- A prefix meaning above.

superior (su-pe're-or) Proximal, upper border or surface.

supination (su-pi-na'shun) In relation to the hand, the palm turned upward.

supine (su'pin') Lying with the face or ventral surface upward.

supra- A prefix meaning above.

T

target (focal)—film distance (tfd, TFD) The distance in inches between the x-ray tube anode and the film.

target (focal)—skin distance (tsd, TSD) The distance in inches between the x ray tube anode and the skin of the patient. It is used more frequently in x-ray therapy than in radiography.

teleroentgenography (tel"e-rent-gen-og'rah-fe) Radiography at a long target-film distance, usually 6 feet, and of the chest, to avoid magnification.

thenar (the'nar) The fleshy prominence of the palm of the hand corresponding to the thumb base.

therapeutic dose (ther-ah-pu'tik) a curative dose.

tomography (to-mog'rah-fe) A special technique to show in detail images of structures lying in a predetermined plane of tissue, while blurring or eliminating detail in images of structures in other planes.

transverse (trans-vers') At right angles to the longitudinal axis of the body.

Trendelenburg position (tren-del'en-berg) A recumbent position of the patient on the table; the patient is usually supine, with the pelvis above the head.

tube target The target of the anode, usually made of tungsten imbedded in a copper block. This is the part of the x-ray tube bombarded by the electron beams to produce x rays.

U

U.G.I. The abbreviation for an upper gastrointestinal study.

V

ventral (ven'tral) Anterior or front.

ventriculography (ven-trik-u-log'rah-fe) The radiographic examination of the brain ventricles after replacement of a specific quantity of spinal fluid with air or gas.

volar (vo'lar) The palm surface of the forearm.

vt, VT Abbreviations for valve tube.

X

xeroradiography (ze-ro-ra"de-og'rah-fe) From the Greek word xeros meaning "dry"; physical, rather than chemical, production of a permanent radiograph; production of radiographs without the use of water and other solutions.

xrt, XRT Abbreviations for x-ray tube.

INDEX

*Indicates term in glossary.

S

T